Understanding Nursing Care

Understanding Nursing Care

EDITED BY

Anne M. Chilman

Director of Nurse Education,
North Lothian College of Nursing and Midwifery,
Edinburgh

Margaret Thomas

Principal Officer,
Committee for Clinical Nursing Studies,
Edinburgh

SECOND EDITION

CHURCHILL LIVINGSTONE
EDINBURGH LONDON MELBOURNE AND NEW YORK 1981

CHURCHILL LIVINGSTONE
Medical Division of Longman Group Limited

Distributed in the United States of America by
Churchill Livingstone Inc., 19 West 44th Street, New
York, N.Y. 10036, and by associated companies,
branches and representatives throughout the world.

First edition 1978
Second edition 1981
  Reprinted 1982

ISBN 0 443 02563 0 (Cased)
ISBN 0 443 02160 0 (Limp)

British Library Cataloguing in Publication Data
Understanding nursing care. 2nd ed.
  1. Pathology
  I. Chilman, Anne M.
  II. Thomas, Margaret, *1924–*
  616'.0024613   RT65

Printed in Hong Kong by
Wilture Enterprises (International) Ltd

Preface to the Second Edition

The second edition of *Understanding Nursing Care* provides a welcome opportunity for updating the text and for considering the requests made by readers for additional material. The purpose of the book remains as stated in the preface to the first edition — to help nurses to understand why certain treatments and nursing care are required and to foster a perceptive, sympathetic and empathetic approach to the patient and his relatives.

Some sections have had to be rewritten because of changes in methods of investigation and treatment which influence the nurse's contribution to patient care. Certain drawings have been altered and more up-to-date photographs have been included where it was considered helpful to do so. The chapters on the urogenital system and mental disorder in particular have benefited from an increase in their illustrative content.

Tumours of the nervous system and some other common causes of distress such as Parkinson's disease are now discussed, and the anatomy and physiology necessary to understand the alterations in function characteristic of these disorders have been included. Particular attention has been paid to the nursing management of patients with joint disorders, those undergoing breast surgery and those with skin disturbances.

Nursing requires many skills, a great number of which are common to the care of people in differently designated wards and hospitals and in the community. These skills constitute what is usually known as 'general nursing care'. Some cross references pointedly indicate this aspect of constancy in nursing, and in other places it should be apparent on reflection. Always it is understood, however, that 'general nursing care' means the special tailoring of a general principle to meet an individual's need.

1981

Anne M. Chilman
Margaret Thomas

Preface to the First Edition

The contributors to *Understanding Nursing Care* believe that the panoramic view of nursing which a broadly based primary programme encourages should be supplemented by a guide with a similar breadth of view. The purpose of the book is to help nurses to understand more fully why certain treatments and nursing care are required and to foster a perceptive, sympathetic and empathetic approach to the patient and his relatives. No attempt has been made to replace specialized texts; they will still be necessary for those needing detailed knowledge of particular subjects.

It has been assumed that the reader has some knowledge of biological sciences, and Section A explains the relationship of common disorders of biological systems to nursing care. Section B contains descriptions of needs and resources that are of particular relevance to different age groups. Some titles for further reading appear at the end of each chapter, and suggestions for either written assignments or topics for discussion have been made for chapters in Section A. Terms printed in *italics* are included in the glossary at the end of the book.

Two words—'patient' and 'reassurance'—appear repeatedly in any nursing textbook, and this is no exception. 'Patient' is a word which nurses and doctors find convenient to use, as a kind of shorthand, for an individual who is deemed to need their help. But each patient is essentially a person with experiences and needs that distinguish him from all other members of the human race. We have tried to emphasize throughout the book the nurse's responsibility to respect her 'patient's' individuality, even when performing the most routine of hospital procedures.

The second word, 'reassurance', is used here to mean restoration of courage or confidence. Possible approaches have been indicated in some chapters, but there are no words which are appropriate for all people and from all nurses, and words alone may not convey the right message. This important professional responsibility demands skills which come more easily to some nurses than others. Observation of experienced staff—from many disciplines—and perception of the various strategies used should enable the student to add to her own repertoire of supporting and encouraging tactics.

Patients are not the only people who have needs a nurse should meet and expectations she should learn to fulfil. Nursing and other health staff colleagues, relatives and friends of patients and men and women engaged in official and voluntary services all deserve willing help and a friendly response.

We have had much help and encouragement in preparing this book and are grateful to many medical practitioners and other experts who have given generously of their time and advice. Our thanks are due, too, to Miss Moira Alexander, Mrs Anne Davies, Miss M. Rea Johnston and Miss Kathleen Wright for their contributions. There would, however, have been no book without the great assistance we received from the publishers, and we wish, in particular, to thank Miss Mary Emmerson and Mrs Ellen Green for their invariable support, professional advice and, most of all, for their patience with us. We thank them, too, for recruiting Mr Douglas Kirk to illustrate the book; his work has given us great pleasure and we are confident that his unique contribution will add to its usefulness. Finally, we wish to acknowledge the help of the staff of the Medical Photography Department of the Western General Hospital, Edinburgh.

1977

Anne M. Chilman
Margaret Thomas

Contributors

Noelle I. Cairns R.F.N., R.G.N., S.C.M., R.N.T.
Tutor, North Lothian College of Nursing and Midwifery

Mary Clements R.G.N., R.S.C.N., S.C.M.
Nursing Officer, Western General Hospital, Edinburgh

Elizabeth Cumming R.G.N., R.C.T.
Clinical Teacher, North Lothian College of Nursing and Midwifery

Celia J. Dodds R.G.N., R.C.T., R.N.T.
Tutor, North Lothian College of Nursing and Midwifery

Isobel M. Gibson R.G.N., S.C.M., R.C.T.
Clinical Teacher, North Lothian College of Nursing and Midwifery

Christina E. Gillies R.G.N., R.C.T., R.N.T., D.N.(London)
Tutor, North Lothian College of Nursing and Midwifery

Mary K. Gillon B.A., R.G.N., R.M.N., R.N.T.
Senior Tutor, North Lothian College of Nursing and Midwifery

Margaret C. Grubb R.G.N., R.C.T.
Clinical Teacher, North Lothian College of Nursing and Midwifery

Jane Innes R.G.N., S.C.M., R.N.T.
Assistant Director of Nurse Education, North Lothian College of Nursing and Midwifery

George J. McKenzie B.A., R.G.N., R.M.N., R.N.T.
Lecturer in Nursing Studies, Dundee College of Technology

Patricia I. Peattie B.Sc., R.S.C.N., R.G.N., R.N.T.
Senior Lecturer in Clinical Nursing Education, Queen Margaret College, Edinburgh

Stephen J. Rigby R.G.N., R.M.N., R.C.T., R.N.T.
Tutor, North Lothian College of Nursing and Midwifery

Sister Eleanor E. Rodgers R.G.N., R.N.M.D., R.N.T., D.N.(London)
St Joseph's Hospital, Rosewell, Midlothian

Phyllis J. Runciman B.Sc., M.Phil., R.G.N., S.C.M., H.V.
Research Associate — Health Visitor, Nursing Research Unit, University of Edinburgh

Christine M. Slater R.G.N., R.N.T.
Tutor, North Lothian College of Nursing and Midwifery

Jean M. N. Smith R.G.N., R.C.T., D.N.(London)
Ward Sister, Beechmount Hospital, Edinburgh

Norah J. Stephen R.G.N., R.S.C.N., S.C.M., M.T.D.
Divisional Nursing Officer (Midwifery), North Lothian District

Williamina W. Thomson B.Sc., R.G.N., S.C.M., O.N.C., R.N.T., Dip.Admin.
Nursing Officer (Education), Scottish Home and Health Department

James Wiley B.A., R.M.N., R.G.N., R.N.T.
Senior Tutor, North Lothian College of Nursing and Midwifery

Contents

Section A

Physical and Mental Disorders

1. The Nature of Infection

This chapter is a selection of those aspects of infection which are most relevant to nurses. The subject is not as mysterious as it may appear, nor is it a daunting task to discover the principles of nursing which have been derived from the science of medical microbiology. For those who wish to pursue the subject further after reading this chapter, a reading list is given at the end which offers a wider perspective for increasing understanding.

INFECTION

Babies are normally born free of micro-organisms. However, they quickly acquire a population of various types, which they retain for the rest of their lives and to which others may be added. It might be expected, then, that infection would be extremely common, caused by either one's own micro-organisms or those from someone else. Indeed, everyone at some time or another has an infection, such as German measles or the common cold, although in most cases it is fortunately mild. Serious infections do occur, but they are surprisingly uncommon. The reason we do not all die from infections is the ability of the human body to protect itself. This ability is known as **resistance**. Some of its many aspects will be discussed in this chapter.

All micro-organisms have a point of origin. This is known as the **source of infection**. In order to infect others they must spread in one of several well-known ways. Further, they must invade the body of another person, again in one of a number of ways. Of course, they must not be overcome by this person's resistance. The newly infected person is known as the **host**, and now acts also as a source. Knowledge about sources, methods of spread and ways of invasion of the host is gained from scientific study of the biological characteristics and the natural history of micro-organisms. Tried and tested ways of prevention and treatment of infection are based on this study.

In the community the nurse is especially involved with the protection of individuals through immunization. In hospital, she is very much concerned with prevention of spread between patients, a process known as cross-infection. She is the guardian of her patients and must ensure, through her awareness and the intelligent application of knowledge, that no patient is exposed unnecessarily to infection from either her own actions or the behaviour of others. The community nurse is in the unique position of being able to educate the public about the dangers of infection and the ways to prevent it, particularly through elementary hygiene.

The meticulous application of sound principles is largely a matter for the conscience of the individual. Nurses must therefore embody a positive attitude towards preventing infection in their philosophy of nursing. Further, knowledge never stands still and the problems that have to be solved vary with the times. The profile of infection has altered considerably over a relatively short period. Old enemies such as tuberculosis and diphtheria are under control, as can be seen from the figures given in Table 1.1 of cases occurring in Great Britain since 1951. But new problems are always appearing, such as increasing numbers of wound, urinary and respiratory tract infections with Gram-negative bacilli. These are currently causing concern, as is the increasing resistance of many bacteria to antibiotics. And there is evidence that the old enemies spoken of are not dead but merely sleeping, waiting for the unguarded moment.

Table 1.1
The changing incidence of infectious diseases

Disease	Cases by year notified in Great Britain			
	1951	1961	1971	1976
(thousands)				
Pulmonary tuberculosis	50·3	22·2	10·5	9·0
Whooping cough	192·3	26·9	18·5	4·3
Measles	628·6	776·4	150·6	67·9
(numbers)				
Diphtheria	826	51	17	2
Poliomyelitis	2925	904	8	15

THE NATURE OF MICRO-ORGANISMS

Micro-organisms, as the name proclaims, are microscopic living things. Although widely dispersed in nature, fortunately only a small fraction of the total number of species causes disease in humans. Included among those that do are bacteria, viruses and fungi.

Bacteria

These are unicellular organisms. That is, they are each composed of one cell only. They vary in size, but are larger than viruses and can be seen through the ordinary light microscope. Reproduction occurs by simple binary fission. This means that each cell divides to form two, both of which divide in turn. Rates of reproduction vary considerably, one factor influencing the rate being the suitability of the environment. Even under optimum conditions different species vary considerably, for instance *Escherichia coli* divides about every 20 minutes, while *Mycobacterium tuberculosis* may take several days to reproduce itself.

In order to multiply, bacteria require a favourable environment. In fact, measures to kill bacteria or prevent growth depend on rendering their surroundings as unfavourable as possible. Broadly speaking, pathogenic bacteria survive best in the sort of environment that the human body provides. This includes a temperature of around 37°C, moisture, a supply of food and slight alkalinity. Some bacteria are absolutely dependent on a supply of oxygen (obligatory aerobes). Others can survive but not thrive in its absence (facultative anaerobes). Still others (obligatory anaerobes) require oxygen to be absent. Clearly, then, an anaerobic bacillus such as *Clostridium tetani* will be more likely to cause infection if it enters the body in a deep wound, say, a puncture wound contaminated with dirt or soil.

Bacteria require moisture; most types will be killed by drying. The gonococcus, which causes a form of sexually transmitted disease, is especially sensitive to lack of moisture. Stories of having 'caught it from a lavatory seat', while not impossible, are regarded with some scepticism since the bacteria are unlikely to survive there for long. On the other hand, certain bacilli have the ability to change into a form which is extremely resistant to adverse conditions. This resistant form is known as a **spore** (Fig. 1.1) Shown on the diagram as clear areas, the spores, which house the materials necessary for reproduction, shed the rest of the bacterial cell. When conditions become favourable, the organism can return to its original form and begin to reproduce again. Two of the most important bacilli to have this ability are *Cl. tetani* and *Cl. welchii*, which cause tetanus and gas gangrene respectively.

Much of the effect of bacterial infection on the body is caused by products of the bacteria. These harmful substances are called **toxins**; when released they circulate in the bloodstream. In a severe infection they cause serious symptoms, collectively referred to as toxaemia. There are two types of toxins: endotoxins, released only when the bacterial cell dies and disintegrates, and exotoxins, released continually by the bacteria. Endotoxins are not likely to cause damage unless present in large quantities, when local tissue destruction may occur. A small number of bacteria, including *Cl. tetani*, *Cl. welchii* and diphtheria bacillus produce exotoxins. These travel in the bloodstream to

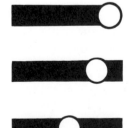

Figure 1.1
Bacilli showing sites of spore formation

distant parts and exert their effects there. Thus, the characteristic muscle spasm of tetanus is due to the effect of the exotoxin on the nervous system.

Enzymes play a large part in the life processes of bacteria, as in other living things. Some bacteria produce enzymes which can influence the course of an infection. *Staphylococcus aureus*, for example, produces an enzyme called coagulase. This protects the bacteria by creating a fibrin barrier around them. Another enzyme produced by *Staph. aureus* is penicillinase, which destroys penicillin thus rendering the bacteria resistant to it. *Streptococcus pyogenes* produces streptokinase, which helps it to spread through tissues.

Classification of bacteria

The importance of classification lies in the need to be able to identify bacteria so that the most effective methods can be used to prevent spread and to treat infections.

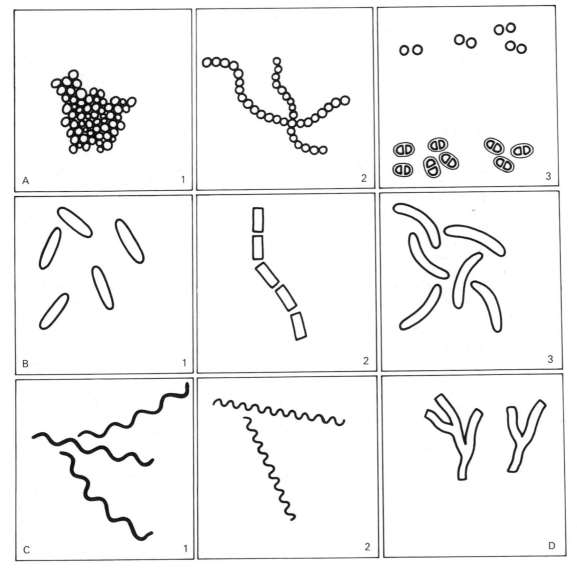

Figure 1.2
Classification of bacteria by shape
A. Cocci (spherical bacteria)
   1. Staphylococci
   2. Streptococci
   3. Diplococci
B. 1, 2 and 3 Bacilli
C. 1 and 2 Spirochaetes
D. Actinomyces

Shape is the most elementary method of classification. Figure 1.2 shows the various shapes of bacteria.

Cocci are spherical bacteria. The various types are (1) staphylococci, which are found arranged in clusters; (2) streptococci, which grow in chains; and (3) diplococci, which grow in pairs and may be encapsulated.

Bacilli are bacteria which are rod-shaped, or nearly rod-shaped. Some of these are capable of producing spores.

Corkscrew-shaped or spiral bacteria are known as **spirochaetes**. In different spirochaetes, the coils of the spiral may be either tight or loose.

Actinomyces are branching micro-organisms, sometimes regarded as fungi, although they have some characteristics in common with bacteria.

Another simple method of classifying bacteria, which divides them into only two categories, is Gram-staining. This technique involves a number of steps, but briefly it means that a prepared slide of bacteria is stained with a violet dye, washed, then stained with a red dye and washed again. Some bacteria will retain the violet dye and are referred to as Gram-positive. Others lose it but retain the red dye and are called Gram-negative.

Microbiologists use other more sophisticated methods which identify bacteria according to their characteristics. These include the appearance of colonies when grown on nutrient media, biochemical activities such as carbohydrate fermentation, and phage-typing (see p. 8). Some common bacteria, how they spread and the infections they cause are listed in Table 1.2.

Table 1.2
Some common bacteria

Bacteria	Reservoir	Spread	Infections caused
		Gram-positive cocci	
Staphylococcus aureus	Noses; perinei; infected lesions	Autoinfection; directly by contact; indirectly by hands, dust, other articles	Boils, styes, wound infections, osteomyelitis, pneumonia septicaemia, food poisoning
Streptococcus pyogenes (haemolytic streptococcus)	Noses and throats of healthy carriers; infected lesions	Airborne in droplets; dust; contact with contaminated articles	Tonsillitis, otitis media, impetigo, scarlet fever, wound infections, associated with acute nephritis, rheumatic fever
Streptococcus viridans	Commensal in mouth.	Enters bloodstream after dental extraction	Dental abscess; subacute bacterial endocarditis where heart valves have been previously damaged
Streptococcus pneumoniae (pneumococcus)	Commensal in upper respiratory tract	Airborne in droplets; endogenous infection	Pneumonia, otitis media, meningitis, conjunctivitis
		Gram-negative cocci	
Neisseria gonorrhoeae (gonococcus)	Infected genitourinary tract	Direct contact in sexual intercourse	Gonorrhoea
Neisseria meningitidis (meningococcus)	Commensal in nasopharynx	Endogenous infection; airborne from carrier or infected person	Meningococcal meningitis, septicaemia

Table 1.2
Some common bateria (*continued*)

Bacteria	Reservoir	Spread	Infections caused
		Gram-positive bacilli	
Bacillus anthracis	Cattle; sheep; animal hides	Direct contact	Anthrax
Clostridium tetani	Faeces of humans and animals; soil and dust	Direct contact of wounds with soil or dust	Tetanus
Clostridium perfringens (*Ci. welchii*)	Animal faeces; soil and dust	Direct contact; ingestion	Gas gangrene, food poisoning
Mycobacterium tuberculosis	Infected cattle; respiratory tract of infected person	Airborne by droplets or contaminated dust; infected milk	Tuberculosis
		Gram-negative bacilli	
Haemorphilus influenzae	Commensal of upper respiratory tract	Endogenous opportunist infection	Chronic bronchitis, pneumonia, meningitis in children
Bordetella pertussis	Nasopharynx of infected child	Droplet spread	Whooping cough
Salmonella typhi (and *paratyphi* A & B)	Faeces of infected persons and carriers	Contaminated food, water or milk	Typhoid, paratyphoid A or B
Salmonella typhimurium (and many others)	Faeces of infected persons, infected cattle, pigs, poultry, mice	Contaminated food including meat products, poultry, milk and duck eggs	Food poisoning
Shigella sonnei	Faeces of infected humans	Direct or indirect contamination of food or feeding bottles; hand-to-mouth routes	Bacillary dysentery.
Escherichia coli	Commensal in large intestine	Endogenous infection; direct or indirect spread	Wound infections, urinary tract infections, peritonitis, septicaemia, infant gastroenteritis.
Proteus mirabilis Proteus vulgaris	Commensal in large intestine; soil	Endogenous infection; hands, dust or other articles	Wound and burn infections, urinary tract infections, septicaemia (resistant to many antibiotics)
Pseudomonas pyocyanea	Human intestines; soil, water; survives in disinfectant bottles, respirators and humidifiers	Endogenous infections; direct or indirect spread	Wound and burn infections; urinary tract infections; septicaemia (also resistant to many antibiotics)
Spirochaetes			
Borrelia vincenti	Commensal in mouth	Endogenous infection; direct contact	Vincent's angina

Table 1.2
Some common bacteria *(continued)*

Treponema pallidum	Infected genital tract	Direct contact in sexual intercourse; intrauterine infection of fetus	Syphilis
Leptospira icterohaemor- rhagiae	Infected rats.	Contact with water contaminated by rat's urine, e.g. sewers	Weil's disease (haemolytic jaundice)

Viruses

Viruses are so much smaller than bacteria that a special type of microscope, the electron microscope, must be used in order to see them. Many infections, including the common cold, influenza and a large number of what are called 'communicable diseases', are caused by viruses. There is, too, a growing body of evidence which suggests that viruses play a part in causing some types of cancer and leukaemia.

Viruses differ from bacteria in the way they reproduce. Reproduction can only take place inside a living cell, which the virus has invaded. Bacteria are, of course, living cells and can be invaded by certain viruses called bacteriophages. Indeed, bacteria can be labelled according to the viruses which are capable of invading them. Another method of identification of different strains of bacteria has, consequently, evolved.

Bacteria are to a greater or lesser degree sensitive to antibiotics, while viruses are very little affected by them. There are only a few antiviral drugs at present, but others are being developed. Viruses themselves cause cells to produce a substance called interferon. This passes to neighbouring cells, providing a temporary resistance and probably limiting the course of the infection. Interferon has not yet been used therapeutically to any significant extent although its potential as an anti-cancer agent is currently being evaluated.

Viruses consist of either *DNA* or *RNA* inside a protein covering. When a cell is invaded, its nucleic acids are diverted from normal activities to make the nucleic acid and protein of the virus. These are assembled into new viruses, which are released to invade new cells (Fig. 1.3).

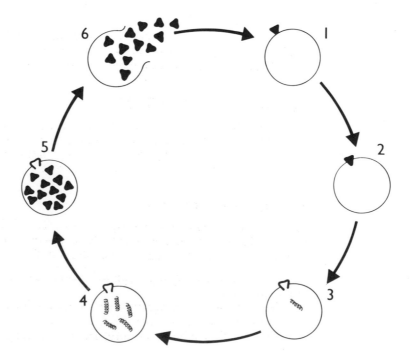

Figure 1.3
Replication of viruses

Within the body, viruses spread in various ways. A wart is an example of local spread from cell to cell. More extensive spread may occur in the respiratory tract, for instance in influenza. Spread by lymphatics and bloodstream (viraemia) causes symptoms of a generalized infection. Viruses often attack particular target organs, for example the spinal cord in poliomyelitis with resultant paralysis. Great advances have been made in the study of viruses. The effort being put into this research reflects a growing awareness of the importance of viruses as infecting agents. Many respiratory infections such as bronchitis and bronchopneumonia, as well as many cases of diarrhoeal infection, are known to be caused in this way.

Fungi

From the nurse's point of view, fungal infections are less important than those caused by bacteria or viruses. The common fungal infections are of the hair, skin and mucous membranes. Occasionally some infections are of a serious and generalized nature.

Actinomycosis

Actinomyces israeli is an anaerobic branching organism. In pus it gives the appearance of gold-coloured granules. It can cause an infection of the jaw, often after injury. Infections of lungs and abdominal organs may also occur.

Moniliasis

Candida albicans, the causative micro-organism, is a *commensal* of the mouth, and often of the skin. The predisposing conditions which must exist before this infection occurs include:

1. Antibiotic therapy which suppresses normal flora.
2. Corticosteroid therapy given over a long period.
3. Diabetes mellitus.
4. General debility such as is found in subnutrition.

The common sites of moniliasis are the mouth (thrush), the vagina (vulvovaginitis) and skin folds.

Ringworm

Fungi causing ringworm are known as dermatophytes. They infect tissue which is keratinized, that is, hair, nails and skin. Animals such as cats, dogs, cattle and horses may act as sources, though the infection can be spread from person to person.

Athlete's foot (*Tinea pedis*)

This is a fungus infection of the skin, commonly spread during communal bathing. It is a particularly difficult infection to cure, and so measures are necessary to prevent spread, for instance in a household, by using separate bath towels and sponges.

SPREAD OF INFECTION

As already stated, the control of infection depends on an understanding of the ways in which spread occurs (Fig. 1.4). All pathogenic micro-organisms have a source. They must have a way of leaving that source, a way of travelling to a new host and a way of entering his body. The new host then becomes a source as well.

Sources of infection

Most infections originate with people who are either suffering from the infection or are carriers. Carriers are persons who harbour and disseminate micro-organisms without themselves showing any signs of the infection. Four categories are described:

1. Those who are incubating an infection and in whom features of the illness have not yet appeared.
2. Those who are recovering from the infection (convalescent carriers).
3. Permanent carriers (as distinct from types 1 and 2, who are temporary carriers).
4. Those with a subclinical, and therefore unrecognised infection.

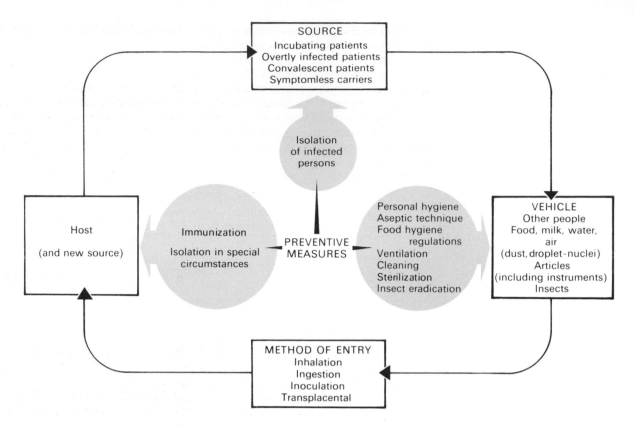

Figure 1.4
Methods of spread of infection
and some preventive measures

Animals provide another, though less common, source of infection. Hens, mice and ducks may be sources of Salmonella, cattle of tuberculosis and brucellosis, dogs of rabies and parrots and budgerigars of psittacosis.

The route of exit

The way in which micro-organisms leave the body of an infected person depends on the part of the body which is the seat of the infection. Skin infections leave directly from the lesions. In respiratory infections micro-organisms leave in discharges from that tract, that is, in droplets (see below) and in sputum. Bacteria from infected wounds leave in pus, from urinary tract infections in urine. Micro-organisms causing a number of infections leave in faeces—food poisoning, dysentery, enteric fevers, poliomyelitis and infectious hepatitis. The virus of serum hepatitis leaves in blood or blood products.

Modes of spread

Infection is spread from one person to another either directly or indirectly. Direct spread is relatively uncommon and requires direct contact of the appropriate nature, say, kissing in the case of herpes simplex and sexual intercourse in gonorrhoea or syphilis. Spread by indirect means accounts for most cases of transmission of infection. This includes indirect contact, that is, another person such as a nurse acting as an intermediary. Also included in indirect methods of spread are the following:

Fomites
These are any articles which have been used by or in contact with an infected person. If these are shared or passed on to another person without being disinfected, they may act as vehicles for transfer of pathogenic micro-organisms.

Food and drink
These can be instrumental in the spread of faecal-borne diseases, if they have been contaminated by some person engaged in food preparation or cooking. Some

infections originating in animals, such as tuberculosis, brucellosis and Salmonella food poisoning, are also transmitted in this way.

Air

Micro-organisms are being constantly discharged into the air from individuals' respiratory tracts. Coughing and sneezing are responsible for the spread of more micro-organisms than talking. They are expelled into the air in minute water droplets of varying size. The smallest dry up, remain suspended for long periods and may be inhaled. Larger droplets fall to the floor and dry up, leaving the dust contaminated. The dust can then be dispersed during cleaning. Airborne infections include tuberculosis, pneumonia, influenza, measles, the common cold and diphtheria.

Dust

As well as being contaminated in the way described, dust acquires micro-organisms from clothing, bed clothes, skin, hair and faecal matter.

Soil

Soil is a reservoir for micro-organisms deposited in it from animal faeces, including *Cl. tetani* and *Cl. welchii*.

Portals of entry

Infection may enter the body by inhalation, ingestion or through abrasions in skin or mucous membrane. Each of these portals of entry possesses protective mechanisms which help to prevent infection or to contain it locally if it occurs.

The fetus can acquire infections from which the mother is suffering. They enter the bloodstream of the fetus by means of the placenta. Examples are rubella and congenital syphilis.

RESISTANCE TO INFECTION

Resistance means the body's ability to defend itself against infection. It depends on a number of factors, some non-specific and others specific to a particular micro-organism. There are three principal lines of defence: outer defences, mainly mechanical barriers; inflammatory responses; and immunity.

Outer defences

Skin provides a mechanical barrier to most micro-organisms but bacteria are found in hair follicles where they may set up infections. The resident population of skin bacteria prevents other pathogenic ones from living on it by competing with them for food.

Mucous membrane lines all body passages which open on to the surface. The mucus produced is a trap for micro-organisms. In the respiratory tract, cilia move this mucus to the outside. In the stomach, strong hydrochloric acid is produced, lethal to many bacteria. The outward flow of urine protects the urinary tract, while the acidity of the adult vagina renders it unsuitable for bacterial growth. Eyes are protected by the flow of tears, which contain an antibacterial substance called lysozyme.

Despite these defences, pathogenic micro-organisms do gain access to the tissues. Then the second line of defence comes into action.

Inflammatory responses

Although most often associated with infection, inflammation is the body's response to any form of injury. The result of this process is that large numbers of phagocytic cells, i.e., polymorphonuclear leucocytes, and antibacterial substances are concentrated at the site of the infection or injury. First a dilatation of small blood vessels occurs in the affected area. The flow of blood is slowed down, and the area becomes hot and red. Capillary walls become more permeable, and an exudate composed of fluid and polymorphonuclear leucocytes leaves the bloodstream. This results in swelling, which in turn causes pain by pressure on nerve endings. The exudate provides several defence mechanisms. The fluid helps to dilute toxins. Fibrinogen becomes converted to fibrin, creating a barrier to the local spread of the micro-organisms. Antibodies may also be present. The polymorphonuclear leucocytes destroy bacteria by ingesting them.

Immunity

When the body is invaded by pathogenic micro-organisms, it reacts by producing either antibodies or immune cells. **Antibodies** are protein substances—gamma globulins, fractions of one of the plasma proteins. **Immune cells** are lymphocytes with antibodies attached. The production of antibodies is known as the humoral response, that of immune cells the cellular response. In both cases, the protection provided is effective only against the specific micro-organism provoking the response, which is referred to as the **antigen**.

Antigens are recognized by the body as 'not-self' and thus they must be rejected. About 7 days after invasion by the antigen, antibodies appear in the bloodstream. At the site of local infections they leave the bloodstream through capillary walls. The way in which antibodies work depends on the nature of the antigen. If it is a bacterial toxin, it is neutralized. If the bacterial capsule is the antigenic substance, it is removed, exposing the bacteria to phagocytosis. Where the bacterial cell wall is the antigen, the bacteria are caused to clump together facilitating phagocytosis. Immune cells carry a chemical which attracts phagocytes to the antigen.

When this process has occurred in response to a particular antigen, the individual is said to have developed immunity to it. A second exposure to the micro-organism results in rapid production of specific antibodies and an abortive or very mild attack of the disease.

Thus one way of developing immunity is to have the infection. The immunity produced in this way is usually long-lasting and may even be life-long. Subclinical infections produce a similar immunity. Because the process of disease is a natural one, immunity gained in this way is said to have been acquired naturally. And since the individual's own body has been active in producing the antibodies, the immunity is called **active immunity**. Active immunity may also be acquired artificially. This is what happens when we are vaccinated. A harmless form of the antigen is introduced into the body to provoke the immune response. These antigens may be toxoids, that is toxins treated with formalin, or vaccines made up of micro-organisms that have been either killed or weakened (attenuated).

Sometimes an individual may acquire antibodies from another source. In this case, the individual's body has not been active in the antibody production and the immunity is thus known as **passive immunity**. It is usually very short-lived because such donated antibodies are themselves foreign, and are consequently destroyed by the body. Like active immunity, passive immunity can be acquired naturally or artificially. Passive immunity is acquired naturally by the fetus, which is supplied with the antibodies possessed by the mother and is thus, at birth, temporarily immune to the same infections to which the mother is immune. When a person requires immediate protection from infection for a short period, antibodies (in the form of gamma globulin) are injected — an example of artificially acquired, passive immunity. The types of acquired immunity are summarized in Table 1.3.

Table 1.3
Acquired immunity

Acquired by	Nature	Duration
Infection	Natural active immunity	Long-lasting
Vaccination	Artificial active immunity	Long-lasting
Transplacental transfer	Natural passive immunity	Short-lasting
Injection of gamma globulin	Artificial passive immunity	Short-lasting

Other factors

Other factors influence the body's ability to resist infection.

Age. The very young and the very old are more susceptible to infections than other age groups.

Hormones. Patients having corticosteroid therapy are more prone to infection, as are diabetics. In women, the protective acidity of the vagina is maintained by normal levels of oestrogen.

Malnutrition. Although often quoted as a reason for increased susceptibility to infection, there is no direct evidence to substantiate this. However, subnutrition is often found in conjunction with other factors which do predispose to spread of infection, such as overcrowding.

HOSPITAL-ACQUIRED INFECTION

Hospitals provide unparalleled opportunities for infection to occur. A large number of people are brought together, each with his own population of micro-organisms. The pathogenic micro-organisms which are commonly found in hospitals are both virulent and resistant to many antibiotics, and are therefore extremely dangerous. In addition, patients in hospitals are usually more susceptible to infection. They include the very young and the very old, those whose defences have been weakened by illness, or whose skin is been breached by surgery. Some treatments increase the hazard — radiotherapy, cytotoxic agents and immuno-suppressive therapy all interfere with white cell production and the immune response, while antibiotics destroy the body's normal protective bacteria.

Broadly speaking, hospital-acquired infections fall into three categories:

Wound infections.
Chest infections.
Urinary tract infections.

But this list is not exclusive. Other types of infection also occur, including gastrointestinal infections and serum or viral type B hepatitis (a particular hazard to hospital staff).

Wound infections

Surgical wounds are normally uncontaminated and heal without infection. Some, such as incisions for abscesses, should be regarded as infected or potentially so. As such they are sources of infection for others and require special precautions to be taken. Most clean wounds which become infected, do so in the ward. Burns become infected in the same way, and the risk is even greater because of the loss of the mechanical barrier — skin and the presence of an admirable nutrient medium, the exudate. The micro-organisms involved in wound and burn infections include staphylococcus, streptococcus, proteus, pseudomonas and, less frequently, *E. coli*. Sources are almost always other humans, though autoinfection can occur. An obvious source is another infected wound, dispersing bacteria on to bedding, or dust, which may be picked up on hands or uniforms and transported to a new host. Pyogenic infections among staff, such as boils, styes or hand infections, are also ready sources. The one source not readily recognizable is the nasal carrier. Sixty per cent of persons who work in hospital carry staphylococci in their noses, thus presenting a potential hazard. A significant number also carry the haemolytic streptococcus in their noses and throats.

Chest infections

Chest infections acquired in hospital are frequently preventable. They may be the result of lack of attention to detail in carrying out nursing procedures. Patients may have difficulty in breathing either because of their illness or from postoperative pain. The inadequate lung ventilation which results, leads to a retention of secretions that provide an admirable breeding ground for bacteria. Patients who are especially prone to chest infections include the following:

Postoperative patients
Operations on the thorax or upper abdomen carry a particular risk of infection because pain prevents deep breathing. Reduced mobility, for any reason, also increases the danger.

Unconscious patients
Loss of the cough reflex and incorrect positioning of the patient in bed increase the risk of infection.

Patients on ventilators
These patients must be protected by the removal of bronchial secretions by suction. If a tracheostomy has been performed, natural defences in the upper respiratory tract are by-passed. It is worth noting that *Pseudomonas pyocyanea* can survive happily in water and may colonize humidifiers and respirators.

Very ill patients
The lowered resistance, the weakness which prevents proper lung ventilation and some specific features of severe illness, such as pulmonary oedema, all predispose to chest infection. Micro-organisms responsible for chest infections include:
   Pneumoccoci. These are found in the throats of many healthy people. They can cause pneumonia following virus infections or following the inhalation of saliva or vomitus.
   Staphylococcus aureus. The widespread distribution of this micro-organism in hospitals makes it likely to cause chest infections in any of the circumstances discussed above.
   Klebsiella pneumoniae. This sometimes causes pneumonia secondary to other infections.
   Spread of pathogens causing chest infections is by airborne means, though opportunist infection by the patient's own commensals may occur.

Urinary tract infections
Urine is normally sterile, but bacteria gaining access to it can grow successfully. These include *E. coli, Strept. faecalis, Bacillus proteus* and pseudomonas. Infection by blood or lymphatic spread can occur, but in most cases it is due to ascending infection. Many cases are caused by the patient's own intestinal bacteria, particularly in a woman since she has a short urethra, the orifice of which is in close proximity to the anus. It is also more likely to occur in patients confined to bed because the bottom sheet may act as a vehicle for transfer of bacteria; in addition there may be stasis of urine. The passage of any instrument such as a catheter or cystoscope into the bladder can introduce bacteria. The longer a catheter is left in the bladder, the greater the possibility of infection. It is also believed that clamping of catheters is more likely to lead to infection than free drainage. Any form of contamination of the catheter, the drainage tubing interior, the collecting bags, or of irrigation equipment also constitutes a hazard.

PREVENTION OF HOSPITAL-ACQUIRED INFECTION

Since micro-organisms cannot be eliminated completely from the hospital environment, prevention of infection must depend on governing the behaviour of workers and manipulating the environment. In this way, sources of infection can be controlled, the channels of spread blocked and susceptible persons protected.

Wound infections
In preventing wound infections, the overall aim is to prevent contamination with pathogenic bacteria. Contamination can occur during dressing procedures, so a technique which prevents this is necessary. Most hospitals have evolved their own methods; they vary in detail, but all are based on the principles of asepsis. Control of nasal carriers among the staff is essential, and provision must be made for their detection and treatment. There is considerable advantage in having a dressing-room separate from the ward. It is easier to clean thoroughly, and will not house the same concentrations of bacteria as a ward. Protection of clean wounds from infected ones may require isolation of patients with septic lesions.

Principles of aseptic technique are most often applied when carrying out a surgical dressing, but they are of equal importance in any procedure which is likely to permit the entry of micro-organisms into the tissues, including catheterization, bladder irrigation, venesection, intravenous infusion, lumbar puncture and marrow puncture. The risk of introducing infection during any invasive technique cannot be over-emphasised. The most important principles of asepsis are:

1. Nurses with infected lesions of skin or throat should not participate.

2. Packs from central sterile supply departments or from commercial suppliers should be checked for damage and expiry dates.

3. Equipment must be collected in advance, as any interruption to the smooth flow of the procedure may create a hazard, for instance, by causing a wound to be exposed unnecessarily.

4. Prescribed methods of cleaning dressing trolleys and dressingrooms must be followed. These may vary from hospital to hospital.

5. Controversy exists regarding the wearing of masks; however, hair must be covered and clean gowns worn.

6. Hands must be washed at the beginning of the procedure and at any time during it when an unsterile article is touched.

7. Different types of packs require different methods of opening. The correct method that will avoid contaminating the contents should be ascertained.

8. Soiled dressings must be removed carefully from the wound, to prevent scattering of micro-organisms into the air. In most units the outer covering is removed by an assistant and the inner covering by the dresser, using forceps which are then discarded.

9. Used dressings should be put straight into a paper or plastic bag provided for the purpose and later incinerated.

10. Neither the wound nor any sterile material may be touched by hand.

11. Opportunity for infection is minimized by:

No unnecessary talking.
No unnecessary movement.
Minimum exposure of wounds.
Minimum disturbance of clothing and linen.

Chest infections

The prevention of chest infections depends to a large extent on the exercise of good basic nursing principles for ill, postoperative and unconscious patients. Consideration must be given to the patient's position in bed, changes of position, physiotherapy, and the use of suction to keep the respiratory passages clear. Details of this aspect of nursing care will be found in Chapter 6.

A patient suffering from a chest infection is an obvious source of infection for others and may need to be nursed in a single room. Collection of sputum requires special precautions. Disposable cartons with lids should be used and changed frequently. They should be handled carefully, collected into waterproof sacks and incinerated. Paper tissues should be used in place of handkerchiefs and disposed of in a similar manner. Hands should be thoroughly washed after handling sputum containers, not only to protect other patients, but also to protect the nurse herself.

Urinary tract infections

One of the most important ways of preventing urinary tract infections is to avoid passing catheters if at all possible. When such a procedure is necessary, it should be carried out strictly in accordance with the principles of asepsis. Indwelling catheters present a greater risk of infection than those removed immediately after insertion. At the same time it must be recognized that each time a catheter is passed, another opportunity for infection is created. Some authorities recommend weekly changing of indwelling catheters. Others believe that they may safely be left in place longer, if drainage bags capable of being emptied without disconnecting the catheter are used. If the system remains closed in this way, less opportunity for the entrance of micro-organisms is provided.

Obstruction to the flow of urine should be avoided, since urine which remains in the bladder will act as a culture medium for bacteria. Tubing must, therefore, be kept free of kinks and other interference which would occlude the lumen. At no time should spigots be used, as this will mean not only interfering with the closed drainage system, but also the possibility of introducing micro-organisms. If it becomes necessary to interrupt the flow of urine temporarily, a gate-clip should be used. Changes of drainage bags, when this becomes necessary, should be carried out with due attention to asepsis. In particular, care must be taken not to contaminate the catheter lumen at this time.

Backward flow of urine into the bladder is undesirable, and is prevented by maintaining the position of the drainage tubing and bag below the level of the bladder.

Cleansing of the urethral meatus, and perineal toilet for women is necessary several times a day. Thorough cleansing of the perineum for women after defaecation is especially important, not only for those with catheters, but also those who are confined to bed. Frequent changing of bottom sheets on the bed will also help prevent the transfer of micro-organisms from anus to urethra.

Environmental control

Control of the environment and of activities of staff, with the object of reducing infection in hospital, is best carried out by a Control of Infection Committee headed by a bacteriologist and including a nurse. Rules can be laid down governing all practices which might constitute an infection hazard. Policies regarding the use of antiseptics and antibiotics can also be drawn up. Among its tasks should be the education of all grades of staff in preventive measures.

Several aspects of environmental control merit further discussion.

Cleaning

Dust is a reservoir of bacteria, so cleaning must ensure its removal not its redistribution. Domestic workers must be educated in the importance of their role in infection control and in the safest methods of cleaning. To prevent dust dispersal, floor cleaning must be carried out by vacuum cleaners fitted with filters. Mops, if not cleaned properly, can be dangerous breeding grounds for bacteria and can actually increase the number of bacteria on floors. Mops should be thoroughly washed in hot water, steeped in a strong solution of phenol disinfectant such as Sudol 1 per cent and then rinsed and dried.

Dishes should only be washed in a dishwashing machine. The importance of very hot water cannot be overemphasized. Dish cloths and drying cloths should be prohibited.

Dirty linen

Careful handling of soiled linen is necessary to prevent the dissemination of bacteria into the air. On removal from a bed, linen must be put straight into a container before being carried out. Careful and quiet making of beds is necessary for the same reason. A colour-coding system for laundry bags is necessary, so that infected or contaminated linen is clearly recognizable by the laundry staff. Proper steps to protect laundry workers and to disinfect the linen can then be taken.

Bedpans and urinals

Problems can be avoided if disposable types are used. These, however, create the difficulty of finding space for storage. Stainless steel bedpans and glass urinals are adequately treated in normal circumstances by automatic washers. Where disinfection of bedpan contents is considered necessary, for example in typhoid, it is customary to fill the bedpan with a phenol disinfectant (Sudol 1 per cent) and leave it for at least an hour. It can then be cleaned in the bedpan washer. Some authorities, however, question the value of this practice.

Waste disposal

Certain types of used materials are an infection risk and their disposal must be carefully controlled. These include used dressings, infusion sets, syringes and needles. Dressings must be put into a waterproof paper sack of distinctive colour, sealed and incinerated. Sharp objects such as glass ampoules, scalpel blades and needles must be placed in a rigid cardboard box before disposal to avoid accidental injury to handlers and the risk of serum hepatitis.

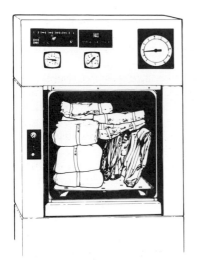

Figure 1.5
A fully automatic high vacuum autoclave

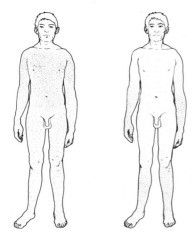

Figure 1.6
Distribution of the rash—chickenpox and smallpox (see Table 1.4)

Sterilization

Much hospital equipment needs to be sterile, that is, free from all living micro-organisms. A good deal of this equipment is supplied commercially and is disposable, for instance syringes, needles, infusion sets, catheters and dressings. These items are generally sterilized by gamma radiation. Equipment which is reused is sterilized locally in hospital central sterile supply departments. This category includes surgical instruments, glassware, surgical gowns and towels.

Boiling as a means of sterilization is not effective and is seldom used in hospitals. Most materials requiring sterilization are suitable for treatment by either steam under pressure or dry heat.

The autoclave (Fig. 1.5) is used to sterilize by steam under pressure. It employs the same principle as the pressure cooker—the greater the pressure steam is subjected to, the higher the temperature that can be achieved. Articles must be held at a predetermined temperature for a given time; the higher the temperature, the shorter the time, thus:

Temperature	Holding time
121 °C	15 min
126 °C	10 min
135 °C	3 min

Dry heat is only suitable for sterilizing materials which will not burn, such as all-glass syringes, metal instruments, powders and oils. A variety of methods is employed ranging from a Bunsen burner flame, used in laboratories to sterilize platinum wire loops, to hot air ovens and infrared heated conveyer ovens.

Whatever the method of sterilization, the articles must be thoroughly cleaned first, as bacteria protected by dirt or blood are likely to survive.

Disinfectants are extremely unreliable as a means of killing bacteria. They are therefore not normally used for articles which must be sterile. Disinfectants are also unsafe for the storage of sterile instruments and, as a rule, should only be used where no other treatment is suitable.

INFECTION IN THE COMMUNITY

Infectious or communicable diseases are no longer the threat to life that they once were. This is mainly due to the institution of immunization programmes against many of these diseases, particularly the more serious ones such as diphtheria and poliomyelitis. To some extent, the advent of antibiotics and the improvement in living standards have also contributed to this change.

The number of infections that come under the category of communicable disease is considerable and cannot be discussed at any great length in this chapter. Emphasis has been placed on those diseases which occur most commonly and those which by their nature are serious hazards. Although it is customary to discuss sexually transmitted diseases separately, they are communicable diseases and, as such, have been included here. A list of the main communicable diseases and their distinguishing features is given in Table 1.4.

Sexually transmitted diseases

Gonorrhoea
The increasing incidence of gonorrhoea in many countries is giving rise to concern (Fig. 1.7). The causative micro-organism is the *Neisseria gonorrhoeae* (gonococcus), most often transmitted during sexual intercourse. A form of non-sexual contact is the infection of a newborn baby by its mother, causing ophthalmia neonatorum. On rare occasions indirect spread may occur, for example by using communal towels. Among the reasons suggested for the increasing incidence of gonorrhoea are:

1. Decreasing use of the sheath as a means of contraception (a sheath is a useful mechanical barrier to infection).
2. Ease of availability of the contraceptive pill.
3. Increasing promiscuity among young women (who provide an often undetected reservoir of infection).

Table 1.4
Summary of communicable diseases

Disease and cause	Spread	Incubation period	Rash	Other features	Treatment	Other remarks
Measles Measles virus	Droplet (Affects mainly young children).	8–11 days.	Rapidly spreading, blotchy rash about fourth day. Coalescent macular spots. Fades in few days, followed by desquamation.	Catarrhal symptoms during 3- or 4-day prodromal period, i.e., sneezing, coughing, watery eyes and nose. Photophobia. Koplik's spots. Temperature rises to 40°C by about 4 days. Falls when rash fades.	No specific treatment. Nurse in warm, well-ventilated room. Shade from bright light. Encourage fluids. Isolate until rash disappears.	Complications may include: stomatitis, laryngitis, bronchitis, otitis media, corneal ulceration, convulsions, encephalitis. Routine vaccination available. Gamma globulin given to protect very young or ill children who are contacts. Notifiable.
Rubella Rubella virus	Droplet.	About 17 days.	Appears on first day. Small pink spots which coalesce. Fades in about 48 hours.	Sudden onset, sneezing, coughing, watery eyes and sore throat. Temperature rises to about 38°C. Falls when rash fades. Often a very mild disease.	No specific treatment. None usually required.	Complications are rare. Rubella is known to be liable to cause congenital defects in the offspring if contracted by pregnant women in first 3 months of pregnancy. In this situation, passive immunity with gamma globulin may be tried but is not very successful. Active immunization is available for girls of about 13.
Chickenpox Varicella virus	Direct contact or droplet.	14–21 days.	Mainly confined to the trunk (Fig. 1.6). Rash appears on first day. Progresses through papular, vesicular and pustular stages. Successive crops permit spots at all stages to be seen together. Crusting precedes healing.	Symptoms in children may be very mild, in adults more severe. Headache, malaise, sore throat, fever. In adults, this virus causes shingles.	No specific treatment. Isolation at home until rash heals. Itching and irritation is treated with calamine lotion; antibiotics only for secondary bacterial infection.	Probably advantageous for children to have chickenpox, since the resulting immunity is life-long. Secondary bacterial infection with haemolytic streptococci or with staphylococci may occur. Other complications are rare.
Mumps Mumps virus	Droplet, direct contact, food contaminated by saliva from infected person.	14–21 days.		Tender swelling of salivary glands, headache, difficulty in chewing. Temperature may reach 39°C.	No specific treatment. Rest in bed, with soft diet and plenty of fluids. Analgesics and frequent mouth washes. Observation for complications.	Complications include orchitis, oophoritis and pancreatitis.
Smallpox Variola virus	Droplet. Contact with discharges from skin lesions or respiratory discharges of infected person. Indirect contact with articles contaminated by above.	About 12 days.	Rash appears on third day and is distributed mainly on face, scalp and limbs (Fig. 1.6). Progresses through papular, vesicular and pustular stages, taking about 24 hours. Pustules dry to scabs in 8 or 9 days. These leave pock marks.	Prodromal symptoms are malaise, shivering, headache, backache, sore throat. Ulcers of upper respiratory mucosa may occur. Temperature rises again in pustular stage of rash and toxaemia is common. Pneumonia is common.	There is no specific treatment. Good nursing care by staff recently vaccinated. Isolation in infectious diseases unit is essential. Antibiotics may be given to prevent secondary bacterial infection. Correction of water and electrolyte balance may be necessary. Care of skin and mouth is essential.	Complications include heart failure, secondary bacteria infection of respiratory tract leading to bronchopneumonia, delirium, convulsions, corneal ulcers. Routine vaccination has recently been discontinued. A notifiable disease.

	Spread	Incubation	Rash	Clinical features	Treatment	Complications
Infectious Mononucleosis (Glandular Fever) Probably caused by a virus.	Affects many young people. Spread occurs probably as the result of exchange of saliva such as occurs in kissing or sharing drinking utensils.	5–10 days	Some cases present with a macular rash.	A variety of types occurs. Fever may be accompanied by a sore throat, by malaise, anorexia, headache and rash, or by enlargement of superficial lymph glands and the spleen. In some instances jaundice appears.	No specific treatment. Rest in bed is advisable during the febrile period. A soft diet may be helpful and adequate hydration is essential. In very severe cases corticosteroids may be used. Antibiotics are only useful in secondary bacterial infection.	Recovery always occurs, though the illness can persist for weeks or months. Complications are rare, the most serious being accidental injury to an enlarged spleen.
Diphtheria *Corynebacterium diphtheriae*	Droplet from infected persons or carriers.	2–5 days.		Usually begins with malaise, headache and sore throat. Infection is local and general symptoms are due to exotoxins. Grey membrane forms across pharynx and may cause respiratory obstruction. Tachycardia with fall in blood pressure occurs due to effect of toxin on myocardium. Effects on nervous system may show as swallowing difficulties and disturbance of visual accommodation. Only a slight elevation of temperature occurs	Immediate antitoxin, intravenously in severe or moderate cases intramuscularly in mild. A trial dose may be used to detect sensitivity to horse serum. Patients and carriers should be isolated until 3 consecutive negative swabs are taken. The bacillus, but not the toxin, is sensitive to penicillin, which is given intramuscularly for 5–7 days. Respiratory obstruction due to membrane requires immediate tracheostomy	Active immunization, begun in 1942, has reduced the incidence dramatically. This should be carried out for all young children. Complications are involvement of the myocardium, nervous system, respiratory obstruction and pneumonia. Notifiable.
Scarlet fever Haemolytic streptococcus	Droplet. Occasionally by contaminated milk or ice cream.	2–4 days.	The rash appears in 24–36 hours. The face is flushed with pale area round the mouth. The erythema, which spreads over the body, has dark red points. Fades in about 3 days. After first week, skin peels.	Sudden onset. Temperature rises, throat becomes sore. There may be vomiting. Tonsils are red and swollen, covered with 'exudate'. The tongue, furred in beginning, peels, leaving strawberry appearance. Condition improves when rash fades. In some children, disease is very mild.	Penicillin is effective against the streptococcus. Most cases can be cared for at home. Rest, with plenty of fluids and analgesia, is generally all the care required.	Complications are less common nowadays. These include otitis media and skin infections. Acute glomerulonephritis and rheumatic fever are due to sensitivity to the streptococcus. Notifiable.
Whooping cough *Bordetella pertussis*	Droplet. Direct contact.	7–14 days.		Onset is gradual. Two steps occur 1. Catarrhal stage with cough, vomiting, slight elevation of temperature and possible convulsions. This lasts about 10 days. 2. The second stage is characterized by paroxysms of coughing, each series of coughs followed by inspiratory 'whoop'. The child is usually better after 4–6 weeks.	No specific treatment. Antibiotics to control secondary infection is necessary. Mild disease in children best cared for at home. Light sedation may be helpful. In severe illness, admission to hospital may be necessary in case of pneumonia.	Complications such as hernia, rectal prolapse and sub-conjunctival haemorrhage are due to increased intra-abdominal or intrathoracic pressure. Laryngitis, bronchitis and bronchopneumonia may occur. Active immunization is given to children as part of triple vaccine. Notifiable.

Table 1.4
Summary of communicable diseases (*continued*)

Disease and cause	Spread	Incubation period	Rash	Other features	Treatment	Other remarks
Bacillary dysentery *Shigella sonnei* *Shigella flexneri*	Food contaminated by carriers or cases.	3–7 days (may be less).		Sudden onset with abdominal pain, diarrhoea. Vomiting not common. The temperature may be elevated. In about a third of patients blood and mucus appear in stools.	Antibiotics are usually better reserved for seriously ill patients. Most people recover in a few days. Adequate hydration is important, and in young infants and those very ill, intravenous correction of electrolyte balance may be necessary.	Control of spread includes notification. Prevention of spread depends on strict hygiene, especially after defaecation. Only the very ill need be admitted to hospital, where isolation techniques should be practised. Children with dysentery should be kept from school.
Typhoid *Salmonella typhi*	Water, milk and food which have been contaminated by cases or carriers. Occurs in U.K. usually only if imported.	7–21 days	Scattered rose pink spots appear about seventh day and last for 3 or 4 days.	Insidious onset, with anorexia, headache, malaise, gastrointestinal upset. Temperature rises over a week to about 40°C (step-ladder phenomenon). Remains high for a week then falls during third and fourth week. The pulse is slow. Spleen is enlarged. Haemorrhage or perforation of the intestine is a danger.	Chloramphenicol is effective, as may be Ampicillin. Corticosteroids, e.g. prednisone, may be used. Admission to infectious diseases unit is essential. Nursing is mainly basic care, with particular attention paid to fluid balance and oral hygiene. Measures to prevent spread are essential.	A carrier state develops in about 5% of cases, 2% being chronic. Measures to prevent spread by carriers are essential, notification is obligatory. It enables investigation into the source and institution of measures to control spread of the disease. Prophylactic vaccine is given to those entering areas where typhoid is endemic.

4. Lack of parental control.
5. Falling moral standards.

Gonorrhoea has a short incubation period of 3 to 6 days. In men, a purulent urethral discharge is the main feature, but if left untreated, more serious complications will develop including urethral stricture, arthritis and sterility. In women an ascending infection of the reproductive tract occurs which can involve the ovaries and the Fallopian tubes. Treatment with penicillin is still effective, although the gonococcus is becoming increasingly resistant, necessitating the use of broad spectrum antibiotics. Education and contact tracing is an important part of the control of this infection.

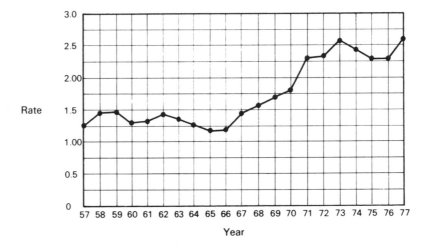

Figure 1.7
New cases of gonorrhoea occurring in Scotland (1957–77.) rate per 1000 population

Syphilis
Syphilis is caused by the *Treponema pallidum*. The incidence is less than that of gonorrhoea but it is a much more serious disease. There is an increasing incidence of syphilis on a world-wide basis, although in Great Britain the number of new cases each year remains fairly constant. Spread is again mainly by sexual intercourse; however, the spirochaete can enter through an abrasion in the skin and may infect a nurse or doctor caring for infected persons. Fortunately this is a very rare occurrence, but it nevertheless dictates extreme caution.

Congenital syphilis occurs in babies born of infected mothers who have been untreated. Screening by means of blood tests is now carried out to detect such women and give them early treatment. The incubation period of syphilis varies from 10 days to 3 months, after which the primary sore or chancre, appears at the site of infection, which may be the penis, labia or lips. In the secondary stage, skin manifestations such as an erythematous rash, condylomata and snail-track ulcers of the buccal mucosa appear. The third stage may occur from 2 to 20 years later and be manifested in lesions anywhere, but particularly in the cardiovascular and central nervous systems. Treatment over a period of 12 days by penicillin is still effective, though other drugs may be necessary.

Nursing care
Nursing the patient with a sexually transmitted disease requires a very special type of person. Much of the contact with these patients is in out-patient departments, which are usually open in the evenings. The extent to which patients will be willing to come forward for treatment depends very much on the reception they meet in these treatment centres. Nurses should be very careful not to let their own personal feelings affect their attitudes to their patients. No moral judgments must be made or expressed. Further, all confidences must be respected and information divulged only for the purpose of treatment. This applies especially to employers, relatives and also to the patient's husband or wife, though usually the spouse will be in the same course of investigation or treatment.

The nurse must be particularly careful not to risk becoming accidentally infected herself. She must avoid contact with any discharges, observe scrupulous hygiene of her hands and wear gloves when attending patients if she has any cuts or abrasions. She should also be careful when handling syringes, needles and specimens. Nurses may be asked for advice by members of the public. They therefore must have an understanding of the subject and a knowledge of the facilities available for treatment.

Contact tracing is an important part of controlling sexually transmitted disease. This is usually carried out by trained personnel, including social workers and health visitors who have had specific preparation for this work. A social worker should be employed in clinics where these diseases are treated, since they are often only one aspect of a social problem which may include marital difficulties and separation.

Controlling infection in the community

Broadly speaking, control consists of dealing with two aspects: the prevention of importation of diseases from abroad, and the prevention of spread of those diseases endemic to a country.

Imported infections

Travellers going abroad

The speed of modern travel means that a person may go abroad, acquire an infection and return home before the incubation period is over. The most effective way of dealing with this is to ensure that travellers are vaccinated against diseases endemic in those regions they propose to visit. International health regulations provide for requirements to be made for travellers to such areas to be in possession of a valid international certificate of vaccination against appropriate infections.

At the time of writing, one of the most significant achievements of the World Health Organisation has been announced — that the world is now completely free of smallpox. Consequently, regulations regarding vaccination of travellers against smallpox are now being revised. At present there are only four countries — Chad, Cambodia, Djibouti and Madagascar — which still officially require international certificates of vaccination against smallpox.

Three groups of people in the United Kingdom regarded in some way at risk to smallpox are:

1. those working in research laboratories
2. those engaged in the manufacture of vaccines against the disease
3. those who are likely to be working in a hospital in which suspected or confirmed sufferers from smallpox will be treated.

The current recommendation is for vaccination to be provided for these categories.

For other communicable diseases which travellers are likely to encounter precautions are also necessary. Yellow fever still exists, and advice should be sought regarding any vaccination requirements. Visitors to central Africa, central and south America, Asia and parts of the Middle-East are recommened to take precautions regarding malaria. Vaccination against typhoid, paratyphoid and poliomyelitis is also advised for travellers to areas other than Canada, the United States, Australia, New Zealand and northern Europe.

Much responsibility rests with port and airport medical officers to ensure that no person with a serious infection is allowed to land undetected in the country. They will have advance information available regarding any outbreaks or epidemics of infections in areas from which ships or planes are arriving, and so will be on the alert. Captains of ships and planes are required to make a declaration of the health of passengers and crew on arrival, and nobody may land until the medical officer is satisfied.

Immigrants

As well as the infections discussed above, immigrants may be suffering from other infections, particularly tuberculosis. This may be detected by screening on arrival, and treatment is provided.

Imported food
Medical officers at disembarkation points are responsible for inspecting and taking samples of all food imported into the country. Many people in Britain will recall the 1964 outbreak of typhoid in Aberdeen, where more than 300 people were infected by one can of corned beef containing *Salmonella typhi*. This sort of outbreak is rare but it shows what could happen if vigilance were relaxed.

Imported livestock
Importation of live animals is rarely a cause of infection in Great Britain. Hides, wool and bone meal are frequently infected with *Bacillus anthracis*. This is a risk for handlers, though infections are surprisingly uncommon. Parrots and budgerigars can bring with them psittacosis and dogs can carry rabies. The increasing illegal importation into Great Britain of pets such as dogs has caused considerable anxiety because of the danger of rabies being introduced into the country.

Endemic infections
Prevention of these can be considered under the following headings: immunization; notification; source and contact tracing; food hygiene; health education.

Immunization
As already pointed out, immunization has been greatly responsible for the decline of communicable disease in the U.K. and many other countries. Infant immunization for diphtheria, whooping cough, tetanus and poliomyelitis is routine. To this may be added BCG vaccination for tuberculosis. A typical schedule is given in Chapter 18.

Notification
This is required by law for certain specified infections. There are a number of reasons for its importance. By means of notification, the effectiveness of immunization, medical policies and services can be assessed. Also, the relationship of infections to factors such as occupation and social grouping can be judged and the geographical distribution of cases seen. Notification is made to the area's chief medical officer by the doctor who diagnoses the condition. Included in the list of notifiable diseases are:

Acute poliomyelitis	Malaria
Anthrax	Measles
Cholera	Ophthalmia neonatorum
Diphtheria	Puerperal fever
Dysentery	Rubella
Enteric fever	Scarlet fever
Erysipelas	Smallpox
Infective jaundice	Tuberculosis
	Whooping cough

Source and contact tracing
Until the source of an infection is identified, spread can still occur. Contact tracing is especially important in food poisoning and in serious infections such as typhoid or smallpox, since it identifies further possible sources of the infection. In tuberculosis, known contacts must be screened by X-ray. Contacts of persons who develop poliomyelitis must be immunized, and a booster immunization is given to diphtheria contacts, who must also be screened to detect whether they are carriers of the micro-organisms.

Food hygiene
Infections spread by food are mainly preventable and common sense hygiene is all that is required. Water-borne diseases are virtually unknown in most Western countries due to the reliability of water supplies and the efficiency of methods of sewage disposal. Most food-borne infections are the result of contamination by either a carrier or an infected person during the cooking or the preparation of food. Contamination at source also occurs; for example duck eggs may be infected with Salmonella, as may be

poultry. Carriers and those with infected skin lesions must not be permitted to work in any food trade. Simple hygiene measures which will prevent food poisoning include:

Preparing food under clean conditions.
Frequent handwashing, especially after defaecation.
Eating cooked food immediately, or storing it under refrigerated conditions.
Avoiding precooking meat for heating later.
Thorough cooking of food and, if frozen, thorough defrosting before cooking.

Health education
Awareness is increasing of the importance of health education as a means of preventing many forms of illness, including communicable diseases. Its purpose is to convince people of the need for measures to promote health and to persuade them to change their style of living if it is likely to lead to ill health. Health education is carried out by many workers, including local authority health education officers, health visitors, general practitioners, teachers and social workers. Much teaching is also carried out informally by nurses in contact with their patients. A wide variety of methods is used in health education, each designed to meet a particular situation. A back-up service of posters, films and tape recordings is often provided by resource centres. Most of us are familiar with mass media techniques that use radio and television extensively for informing the public on topics such as immunization and sexually transmitted disease. Where a special need exists, say, to encourage immunization in a particular area, a concentrated campaign using a number of techniques may be mounted.

PRINCIPLES OF NURSING IN COMMUNICABLE DISEASE

Many of the minor communicable diseases do not require admission to hospital, and such has been the decline in serious infections that fever hospitals, once busy, have now been converted to other types of work, leaving perhaps one or two wards to be used for the original purpose.

The basic principles of nursing care are the same for these diseases as for all forms of illness. However, they have a special importance in serious infections where, apart from treatment with antibiotics, the patient's progress depends to a large extent on good nursing.

Rest
This is an important part of the treatment of any illness. In serious infections the need for rest is even greater because, as a result of the disease, the respiratory rate, pulse rate and temperature are increased. In order to prevent further strain on the heart, rest is essential. A quiet, non-stimulating atmosphere is necessary because of the heightened irritability which often accompanies fevers. It is necessary to encourage sleep by all means at the nurse's disposal, avoiding the use of drugs if possible.

Hygiene
High temperatures are accompanied by profuse sweating, which leads to much discomfort. The daily bed-bath is therefore of considerable importance. A wash at intervals during the day is also helpful. While an increased temperature is the body's way of combating the infecting micro-organisms, a temperature of over 40°C can be harmful to its own cells. Tepid sponging and other temperature-reducing treatments must therefore be employed to prevent body temperature from exceeding this level. Clothing should be light and loose, cotton being more comfortable than other materials. It will be necessary to change bed linen frequently.

Oral hygiene
Sweating, increased respiratory rates and high temperature cause water to be lost from the body, and the mouth will become dry and uncomfortable. Since the patient is unlikely to be eating much, salivation will also be diminished. Some infections may be accompanied by lesions in the mouth or lips. Frequent and careful oral hygiene is therefore necessary, and a mouth wash should be available at all times.

Fluid balance

The loss of water by seriously ill patients (noted above) is greatly increased if vomiting or diarrhoea are features of the disease, and these features may also cause severe electrolyte deficiency. At least 3 litres of fluids should be taken daily, and in cases of severe loss, replacement by intravenous means may be necessary with additives such as potassium chloride to correct the electrolyte imbalance. Oral fluids should include glucose drinks and fruit juices, which provide vitamin C and potassium.

Diet

Various proprietary protein supplements are available to be added to milk; these should be given when the patient is disinclined to eat. Once the patient's temperature has begun to fall and his appetite returns, a light diet, attractively presented, can be given, supplemented as described.

Skin care

The essentials of skin care are fully discussed in Chapter 14. It is worth remembering that cleanliness and change of position are two of the most important principles. Itching, such as occurs in chickenpox, leads to scratching and consequent secondary infection. To minimize irritation soothing lotions should be freely used. Anal tenderness will accompany diarrhoeal diseases, and a suitable barrier cream should be provided.

Observation and records

Pulse, temperature and respiratory rates must be recorded at intervals as requested by the doctor. This may be hourly or less frequently. In serious infections, blood pressure readings may be needed, and daily urine testing may be required. A fluid balance record is a useful guide in preventing dehydration. In diarrhoeal diseases, a record should be kept of the frequency and nature of stools.

Prevention of spread

The protection of other patients and of the staff is an important part of nursing infected patients. All staff should be recently vaccinated against any serious infection that is being nursed. These patients also require isolation in an infectious diseases unit. Ideally, this should be carried out in a single room, the door of which is kept closed. Rooms specially designed for this purpose may have vestibules as air-locks, so that air from the room which may be carrying micro-organisms does not enter the rest of the ward. Air must not be recycled by air conditioning systems, but should be expelled to the outside.

All persons entering the room should wear protective gowns, and masks are necessary when the micro-organism is spread by air. For infections spread by the faecal route, urine or blood, gowns need only be worn when in actual contact with the patient, his bed or excreta. Gloves should also be worn for highly infectious and serious infections such as diphtheria, as well as when removing sanitary utensils containing infected faeces or urine. Hands should be washed immediately before and after removing gowns and masks. Gowns should be hung on hooks inside the room or in the vestibule, spaced in such a way that they do not touch each other.

Cleaning of the rooms should be carried out in the usual way, but separate utensils must be kept stored in a cupboard in each room. Terminal cleaning must include washing floors and walls with hot water and soap, and fumigation may be necessary. Linen should be disposed of as indicated on page 16, in appropriately identified plastic bags. The advice of the central sterile supply superintendent should be sought when it is necessary to use any equipment from that department, as, even though expensive, it may be desirable to use disposable equipment. Disposable items must also be collected in colour-coded plastic bags in the room, put into another bag when being removed and incinerated.

Disposal of excreta can be a problem in the enteric fevers. Separate bedpans and urinals are essential. The conventional method of disinfection is described on page 16.

Prevention of spread of infection depends ultimately on knowing the methods by which micro-organisms are transmitted and adjusting behaviour accordingly. If the rules that are laid down are observed, then prevention of spread is a simple matter and can be accomplished even in the most unsatisfactory conditions.

SUGGESTED ASSIGNMENTS

1. Imagine that you have been invited to talk to a young wives group at your local church. Outline how you would explain to them the purpose and advantages of infant immunization.

2. Read the prescribed procedure for carrying out a simple surgical dressing in your own hospital. Demonstrate how it complies with the principles set out on page 15 for practising aseptic technique. (A simple method is to label each stage of the procedure with code letters or numbers representing the appropriate principle or principles.)

3. The protection of hospital staff from infection is very important. How are staff in your hospital protected in regard to:

Collection and transport to the laboratories of specimens of sputum, blood and pus?

Arrangements for disposal of used intravenous infusion sets, hypodermic syringes and needles and scalpel blades?

Removal of used linen from wards?

4. Nurses play a vital part in the prevention of infection in hospital wards and in the community. Could their preparation for this responsibility be improved? If *yes*, how?

FURTHER READING

Catterall R D 1979 Venereology and genitourinary medicine, 2nd edn. Hodder & Stoughton, London.
Gibson G L (ed) 1974 Infection in hospital. A code of practice, 2nd edn. Churchill Livingstone, Edinburgh
Hare R, Cooke E Mary 1979 Bacteriology and immunity for nurses, 5th edn. Churchill Livingstone, Edinburgh
Maurer I M 1978 Hospital hygiene, 2nd edn. Arnold, London
Parker M J 1978 Microbiology for nurses, 5th edn. Bailliere Tindall, London
Parry W H 1979 Communicable diseases, 3rd edn. Hodder & Stoughton, London
Schofield C B S 1979 Sexually transmitted diseases, 3rd edn. Churchill Livingstone, Edinburgh

2. The Locomotor System

In health a person must be able to stand upright, sit, walk, run, jump and perform the many complex movements necessary in everyday life. To do this it is vital that the bones, joints, voluntary muscles, sensory and motor nerves are all healthy and in perfect working order. Distortions and malfunctioning of any part of these systems will cause a proportionate reduction in locomotor efficiency.

Orthopaedic conditions, their prevention, treatment and nursing, is a speciality in its own right, and there are many excellent textbooks on the subject from which a detailed knowledge of such disorders can be gained. The purpose of this chapter is to provide some basic information about the working of the locomotor system which can be applied in general nursing care and some guidelines to the treatment of a limited number of orthopaedic conditions which the nurse may meet in a general hospital.

ANATOMY AND PHYSIOLOGY

Maintenance of body shape and the protection of vital organs are two of the functions of the skeleton. A third function is that it forms a system of levers and joints so that the action of voluntary muscles, stimulated by motor nerve fibres, will cause movement of a part of the body.

How joints and muscles work

A joint is any place in the body where two or more bones touch (or articulate). Some joints are fixed, such as the joints between the bones of the adult skull. These sutures, as they are called ossify early in childhood and, of course, movement is not possible at such joints.

A second type of articulation is the slightly movable joint; here the union between the bones is formed by cartilage. Examples of such joints can be seen at the symphysis pubis of the pelvis, or the union between the bodies of the vertebrae. Cartilaginous joints allow very slight movement to occur between the bones; for example, the movement between any two vertebral bodies is very limited and in some cases non-existent, though the composite range of movement of the whole spinal column is fairly wide.

It is the third type of joint, however, which is of major importance in locomotion, namely the freely movable joint.

Characteristics of a freely movable joint

The articulating surfaces are smooth and complementary to each other — as in the shoulder, hip and knee joints on the skeleton. These surfaces are made even smoother by a covering of tough resilient cartilage which also acts to some extent as a shock-absorber. The bones which form a joint are held together by bands of fibrous tissue called ligaments. All freely movable joints are enclosed in a sleeve of this fibrous tissue. This is called the joint capsule, or capsular ligament, because it encapsulates the joint and holds the bones in place without unduly restricting movement (Fig. 2.1).

Some freely movable joints have additional ligaments situated within the capsule (intracapsular ligaments) and others which lie outside the capsule (extracapsular ligaments). These ligaments lend extra stability to the joint and prevent undesirable movement. Intracapsular ligaments hold the bones together without limitation of movement. An example of this is the hip joint, where a ligament passes from the small notch on the head of femur to the roughened depression which can be seen clearly in the base of the cup-like acetabulum of the innominate bone of the pelvis. This effectively tethers the ball-like head of the femur to the socket-shaped acetabulum.

Though freedom of movement is essential, excessive movement or movement in undesirable directions must be prevented. For instance it would be difficult to walk if the knee joint allowed lateral movement, so that at every step the leg bowed or went into a knock-kneed position. This is where the extracapsular ligaments come into play. Strong bands of fibrous tissue called collateral ligaments on the medial and lateral aspect of the knee prevent this undesirable movement. The patellar ligament (though technically a tendon) performs a similar function anteriorly.

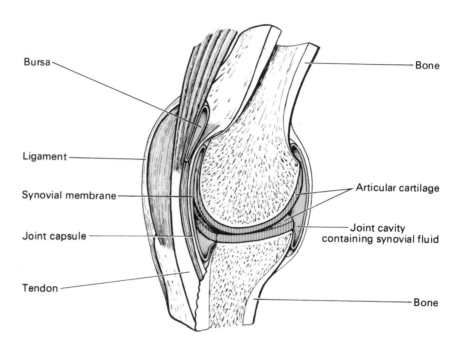

Figure 2.1
A freely movable joint

Sometimes, in addition to the stability conferred on a joint by the shape of the articulating surfaces and the supportive ligaments, joints are further stabilized by structures within the capsule. These are commonly wedges or pads of cartilage which deepen a socket or build up an area deficient in bone. Examples of these intracapsular structures are found in the shoulder and hip joint where the glenoid and acetabular labra deepen the respective sockets. Similarly in the knee joint, the half-moon shaped (semilunar) cartilages known as menisci build up the medial and lateral aspects of the table-like head of the tibia, thus increasing the stability of the joint.

All joints, mechanical or biological, require lubrication to cut down friction and wear and to permit free action. In mechanical joints lubricants such as oil, grease, silicone or graphite have to be regularly maintained and replaced, as motorists know to their cost. Freely movable joints are lubricated by a clear, viscid fluid called synovial fluid. It is secreted by a specialized tissue, the synovial membrane, which lines and covers all non-articular surfaces within a joint capsule. In health the secretion of synovial fluid by this tissue is sufficient to provide a small lubricant cushion between joint surfaces. As with other secretory membranes, like the pleura for example, irritation — mechanical, chemical or bacteriological —will stimulate an increase in production of the exudate. Thus, as pleural effusion is associated with pleurisy, so joint effusion may be associated with infection or injury.

Bursae

Some joints, due to the type of load they are required to bear, are subject to excessive friction or pressure, for instance the knee in the kneeling position. In such cases small, fluid-filled sacs or bursae of synovial tissue act as cushions to buffer the joint from a jarring shock.

The action of muscles of locomotion

The groups of muscles which produce movement act synchronously — when the flexor muscles in the upper arm contract to bend the elbow, the extensor muscles relax to permit the action. The jerky movements of the child suffering from cerebral palsy are due to malfunctioning of the neural control, the system that allows this synchronous action to occur.

Terminology

Muscle contraction
Increased stimulation by motor nerve fibres causes muscle fibres either:

> 1. To shorten the muscle, the tension remaining the same (isotonic contraction), or
> 2. To increase the tension, the length of the muscle remaining the same (isometric contraction).

Muscle relaxation
Decreased stimulation by the motor nerve results in either lengthening of the muscle or decrease in the tone.

Muscle tone
In health all muscle fibres are held in a state midway between contraction and relaxation and are ready for instant action to produce a smooth movement. This state is referred to as muscle tone (Fig. 2.2).

Maximum muscle contraction potential does not occur during activity in normal body states.

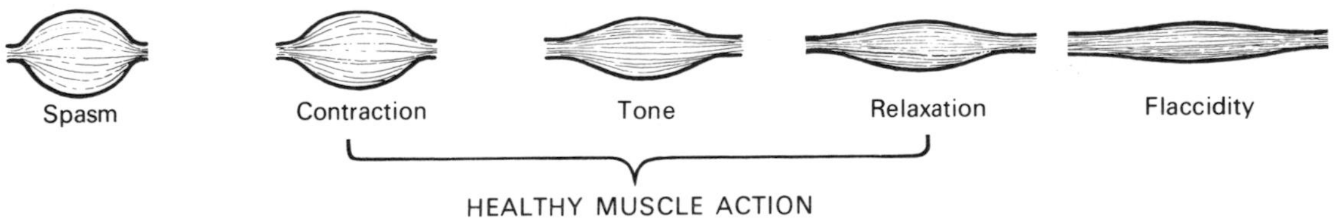

Spasm   Contraction   Tone   Relaxation   Flaccidity

HEALTHY MUSCLE ACTION

Figure 2.2
Muscle action

Abnormal muscle action

Muscle spasm
Excessive muscle contraction is referred to as muscle spasm. In this state the affected muscles are rigid and stone-like in quality. Muscle spasm can also occur in conditions other than orthopaedic disorders. The board-like abdomen of the patient with a perforated peptic ulcer or the painful and disabling leg cramp sometimes experienced by swimmers are other examples of muscle spasm.

Sudden dramatic muscle contraction, say, when a mother lifts a very heavy object to free her trapped child, can be sufficiently violent to fracture bones or to tear muscle tendons from their bony attachments. One reason patients undergoing electro-convulsive therapy in psychiatric hospitals are given relaxant drugs as part of their anaesthetic is to prevent the violent muscle contractions which would otherwise be produced by the passage of the electric current through the body.

Muscle spasm is always acutely painful. It immobilizes the affected joint and can spread to adjacent muscles causing further pain and immobility.

Flaccidity
Just as muscles do not normally fully contract, similarly muscles do not normally fully relax. When a muscle cannot contract due to a disorder of its nerve supply, the muscle is said to be flaccid or paralysed. When a patient is unable to contract any of the muscle groups around a joint, that joint is said to be flail. Such a situation can arise in patients suffering from poliomyelitis. In this case the joint must be protected, because without support the limb will fall into abnormal positions causing stretching of ligaments and tendons.

Simple measures to relieve muscle spasm
Muscle spasm caused by inflammatory or other painful lesions can often be relieved by the application of local heat.

Local heat
Local heat applications all aim to increase the circulation to the affected muscle thus raising the temperature locally. The nurse should realize that there is always the danger that skin may be burnt in the process and take care to prevent this. The following are some methods of applying local heat:

1. A carefully protected hot water bottle or electric heat pad.
2. Hot baths — total immersion or immersion of the affected part only.
3. Wax baths — similar to item 2 but the heat is retained for longer by the wax and only the affected part is immersed.
4. Poultices — preparations such as Kaolin contain a counter-irritant, thus the action is two-fold; these need frequent reapplication.
5. Hot fomentations ⎫
6. Warm wool   ⎬   largely superseded by other methods.
7. Counter-irritants ⎭
8. Infrared rays from a special lamp — superficial heat.
9. Ultrasonic massage: very high frequency sound waves penetrate tissue to the required depth and increase blood flow to the affected part.

Correcting posture
It is useful to remember that the patient having bed rest and skin traction may complain of acute lumbar or groin pain due to abnormal positioning of the pelvis. By gently altering the patient's position in bed so that the anterior iliac spines are level and the hips abducted, the muscle spasm can often be relieved. The importance of correct posture in bed or in a chair is discussed later in this chapter.

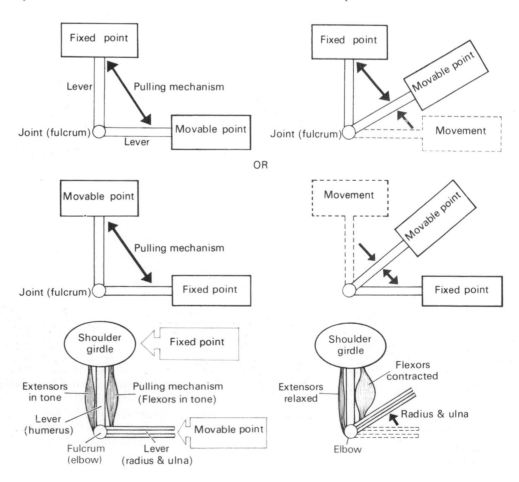

Figure 2.3
Movement

Types of Lever Action (Figs. 2.4 A–C)

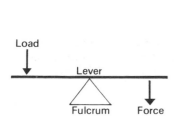

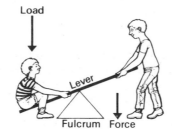

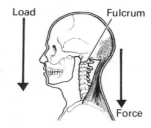

Figure 2.4A

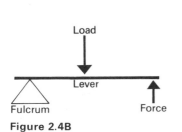

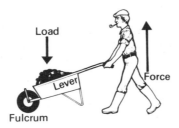

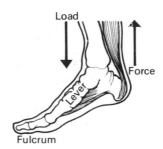

Figure 2.4B

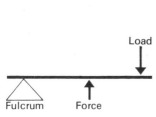

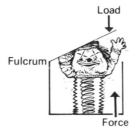

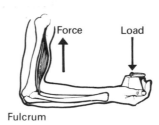

Figure 2.4C

Joint Movements (Figs. 2.5 A–H)

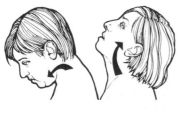

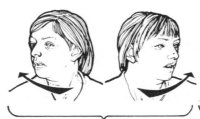

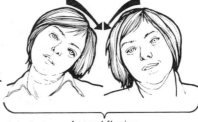

Flexion   Extension   Rotation   Lateral flexion

Figure 2.5A
Head and neck movements

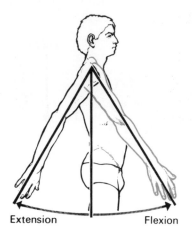
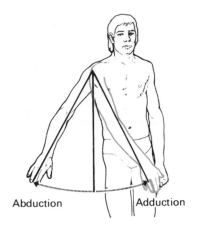

Extension   Flexion

Abduction   Adduction

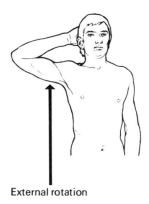
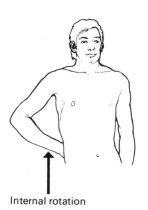

External rotation

Internal rotation

Figure 2.5B
Shoulder movements

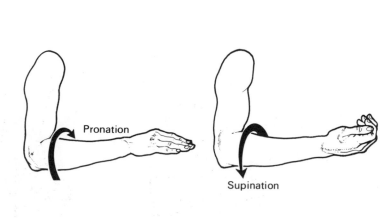

Flexion

Pronation

Supination

Extension

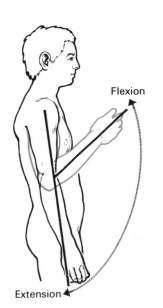
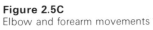

Figure 2.5C
Elbow and forearm movements

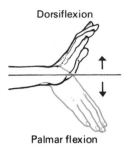

Dorsiflexion

Palmar flexion

Ulnar deviation   Radial deviation

Figure 2.5D
Wrist movements

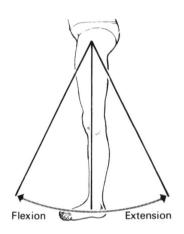

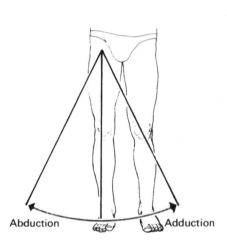

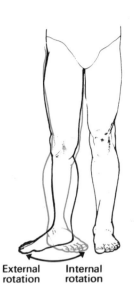

Flexion   Extension

Abduction   Adduction

External rotation   Internal rotation

Figure 2.5E
Hip movements

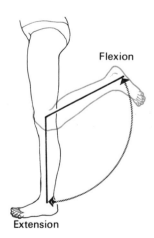

Flexion

Extension

Figure 2.5F
Knee movements

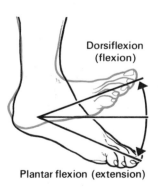

Dorsiflexion (flexion)

Plantar flexion (extension)

Figure 2.5G
Ankle movements

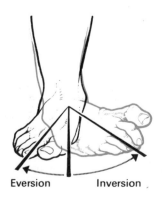

Eversion   Inversion

Figure 2.5H
Forefoot movements

Movement

A muscle or group of muscles producing movement must obviously be attached on either side of the joint so that when the muscle length is decreased the effect is to pull the two bones into a position where the angle between them is decreased. (At the same time the opposing set of muscles relaxes.) The muscle passes from a fixed point, across a joint to its attachment on the other bone(s), and when it contracts movement is produced (Fig. 2.3). The pulling force (or muscle) causes movement of the lever (bone) at the fulcrum (joint). The lever and fulcrum principle has been used in man's engineering feats for thousands of years: it enables great weights to be moved by minimum force.

Positions of rest

Excessive muscle contraction can be caused solely by abnormal joint position. It is, therefore, important that the nurse should know the position of rest for each of the major joints. In this position no undue tension is put on the muscles or strain on the ligaments of the joint. By gently moving a joint into the correct position, muscle spasm can often be relieved or minimized. It is also important when the patient has a flail limb. As the muscles are unable to support the limb it will tend to flop into abnormal positions which will strain the joint and can cause deformity. The nurse must ensure that when she is working with such a patient she holds the limb in a normal position at all times, and that when she leaves the patient the limb is gently but firmly supported by pillows and pads so that the desired position will be maintained.

Positions of rest for important joints (Figs. 2.6A–I)

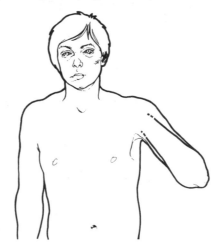

Figure 2.6A
Position of rest—shoulder
60 degrees abduction
30 degrees forward flexion
45 degrees rotation

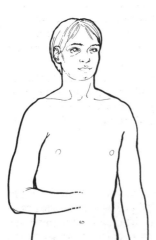

Figure 2.6B
Position of rest—elbow
90 degrees flexion
Forearm midway between
pronation and supination

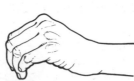

Figure 2.6C
Position of rest—wrist
30 degrees dorsiflexion
Slight ulnar deviation

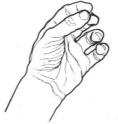

Figure 2.6D
Position of rest—thumb
45 degrees abduction
Thumb opposed to fingers

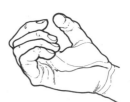

Figure 2.6E
Position of rest—fingers
Lightly curled

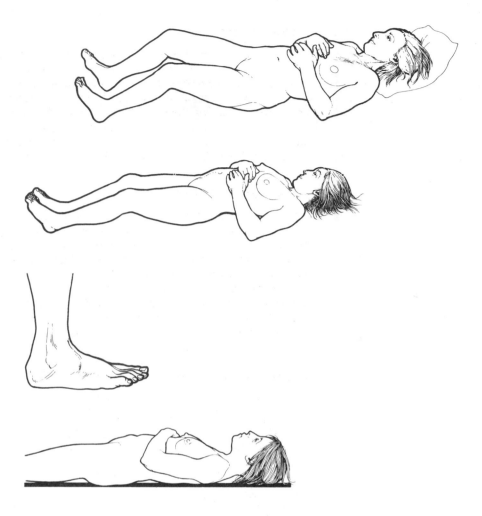

Figure 2.6F
Position of rest—hip
5–15 degrees abduction
30 degrees forward flexion
No rotation (toes point to ceiling)

Figure 2.6G
Position of rest—knee
5–15 degrees flexion
Patella points to ceiling

Figure 2.6H
Position of rest—ankle
Neutral—90 degree angle
(No inversion or eversion)

Figure 2.6I
Position of rest—spinal column
Shoulders level; pelvis level; no rotation
Support lumbar and cervical curves

LOCOMOTOR EFFICIENCY

The information in the preceding section gives guidance about the positions of rest and positions of function for the major joints in the body. The importance of knowledge in this area cannot be overemphasized. The nurse who uses this information to observe the patient, in bed or in a chair, to ensure that all joints are maintained in the best possible (optimum) position not only contributes to therapy, but does much to ensure the patient's comfort and sense of well-being.

The ability to ensure correct body alignment and joint position is a skill which the nurse may undervalue. There are some who may regard the ability to position supports and pillows as trivial. This is not the case, as is evident when one compares the efforts of the junior trainee with the deft movements of the experienced nurse, and the evident comfort of the patient after such expert attentions.

POSTURE AND BODY MECHANICS

In order to maintain the upright position with minimum effort, it is vital that weight transmission and balance are efficient. If the head, thorax and pelvis are thought of as loads which have to be carried by the legs, it is obvious that if the weights are piled in a straight column and balanced on straight legs, the amount of muscular effort needed to maintain this position will be minimal. The load is further stabilized when the feet are apart, as this gives a broader base for weight transmission (Fig. 2.7). The same is true of sitting positions. Strange as it may seem the slouching position is more tiring as it causes strain and muscle tension (Fig. 2.8).

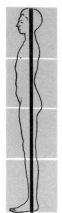
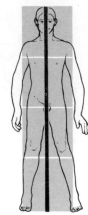
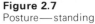
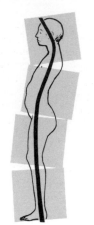
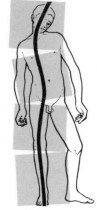

STABLE COLUMN
Body alignment allows gravitational pull
to pass straight down weight-bearing line

UNSTABLE COLUMN
Poor alignment causes fatigue due
to muscle and ligamentous strain

Figure 2.7
Posture—standing

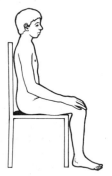
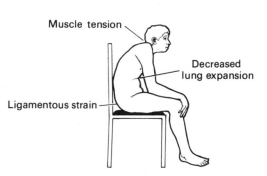

Muscle tension

Decreased
lung expansion

Ligamentous strain

Figure 2.8
Posture—sitting

Posture during normal activity

Good postural habits are vital to nurses since, by minimizing the amount of muscular effort needed for work, they help the nurse not only to complete the task with less fatigue, but also to avoid the possibility of joint strain. The major points of good posture are:

1. Head held high.
2. Chin tucked in.
3. Shoulders level.
4. Lower abdomen flat.
5. Curves of the spine maintained without exaggeration.
6. Pelvis level.
7. Knees relaxed.
8. Feet pointing straight ahead.

Good posture and body alignment must, however, be maintained not only when standing and sitting but during activity. The following summary may help the student to learn postural habits which will utilize efficiently the body's system of levers and joints.

1. When carrying or lifting, the load should be held close to the body. This simplifies weight transmission and thus minimizes effort.
2. When carrying a load, the elbows should be flexed and held close to the side of the body. This utilizes the stronger muscles of the upper arm, rather than demanding a combined effort from arm and shoulder muscles.
3. When lifting, the load should be faced, thus avoiding rotary strains of the spine.
4. Shoulders and pelvis should be held on the same plane and never twisted.

5. A broader base of support increases stability. By placing one foot in front of the other, the base of support is increased towards the object to be lifted.

6. To lift objects from a lower work level, the knees should be bent and the spine kept straight. This allows the load to be carried by the stronger thigh and buttock muscles rather than the weaker spinal muscles.

7. Stand close to the object to be moved. This helps to maintain the body's centre of gravity over the base of support and so increases stability.

8. When strenuous effort is required, prepare for it by 'fixing' the pelvis, that is contract the abdominal and gluteal muscles. Wherever possible, brace the flexed knee(s) against a solid object such as a chair or a bed frame.

9. The flexor muscles of the arm are usually stronger than the extensors, so always lift or turn objects towards oneself.

10. Whenever possible, turn or slide the object to be moved. Extra effort is needed to lift a load against the force of gravity.

11. Always use smooth, continuous movements as opposed to jerky, stop-start manoeuvres. Less effort is required to keep an object moving than to start the movement.

12. Try to move a patient on a level surface. Unless contraindicated, lower the back-rest before moving a patient towards the head of the bed.

13. A lifting or turning sheet is often helpful as it reduces the amount of contact surface and therefore friction. When using a lifting sheet, it is helpful if the patient is able to flex knees, hips and neck.

14. Never attempt to lift a heavy load without help. To do so is to put both your own and the patient's safety at risk.

Posture in bed or in chair

It is just as important for the patient to maintain good posture and body alignment in bed or when sitting in a chair. A sagging mattress can cause flexion contractures of the hip in an amazingly short time. Improperly placed pillows at head and neck can lead to round shoulders and decreased chest expansion. Knees permanently flexed will cause shortening of the hamstring tendons and therefore knee flexion contractures. These deformities do not take long to develop so the vigilant nurse must be aware of the hazards and take steps to prevent them. This means constant intelligent observation of the patient in bed. Untrained observation is of little use to the nurse. Knowledge of normal body function must be applied to each observation. Only by constant awareness of potential malfunctioning or dangers can the warning signs be detected soon enough.

Observation and maintenance of the best possible position for the patient is, of course, not only applicable to orthopaedic care. The nurse's knowledge of physiology and body mechanics must be interrelated. It should be obvious that a patient having oxygen therapy who is allowed to slip from the upright sitting position into a slumped position is no longer able to gain the full benefit of the therapy.

Complications of enforced inactivity

Problems associated with inactivity and bed rest are many and varied, and it is perhaps appropriate at this point to summarize the major problems which the observant nurse can prevent or minimize.

Muscle atrophy

Inactivity results in muscle atrophy. The muscle becomes smaller and its circulation diminishes, resulting in decreased endurance and rapid fatigue. The individual becomes less active and further atrophy occurs. A dramatic example of this can be seen in the patient who has had a plaster cast removed after several weeks of immobilization; the same process of atrophy will occur in the bed-fast patient after only a few days.

Joint contractures

Joints which are held immobile will soon become stiff. This may result from shortening of muscle tendons, capsular ligaments or the muscles themselves. In terms of the patient's well-being, the consequences may mean longer convalescence, discomfort or pain during rehabilitation, and possibly a persistent deformity. It is, therefore, an important nursing responsibility to prevent joint contractures, whenever possible, by good positioning and regular exercise.

Drop foot deformity

The nurse should note that if the foot is not supported, tendons of the calf muscles tend to shorten while the muscles of the anterior portion of the leg lengthen. Even a mild degree of drop foot can cause many weeks of painful rehabilitation. If severe, it will mean that the patient cannot put the heel to the gound when attempting to stand. Maintenance of the foot in a functional position at all times should be ensured, and special appliances should be used to maintain this position if the bed rest is prolonged.

Hypostatic pneumonia

A slouched or horizontal position in bed; lack of mobility; tight bandages around the chest and upper abdomen all cause a decrease in chest expansion. Severe pain and the administration of analgesics which depress the respiratory centre in the medulla can contribute to lung congestion. Inactivity lowers the basal metabolic rate, therefore CO_2 production is less, resulting in a further reduction in respiratory stimulus. The horizontal position allows pooling of secretions in the bronchial tree and if dehydration occurs, these secretions become tenacious and difficult to expectorate. This bronchial stasis provides an ideal medium for the growth of pathogenic organisms. Thus the stage is set for the development of hypostatic pneumonia and chest infections.

Pressure necrosis

The effect of prolonged pressure on vulnerable areas of tissue is well known and is fully discussed on page 446.

Disuse osteoporosis

The exact mechanism of calcium deposition and bone formation is not known. It is known that inactivity and lack of weight-bearing results in loss of calcium from the skeletal system. To minimize this loss, patients on prolonged bed rest, unless contraindicated, have the head of the bed raised for several hours per day, as this produces weight-bearing stress.

Renal calculi

The calcium lost from the skeletal system is excreted by the kidneys. Research has shown that increased calcium excretion begins as early as the third or fourth day of bed rest and reaches a peak by the fourth or fifth week. This increased calcium excretion may lead to the formation of kidney stones. Other precipitating factors are stasis of urine, decreased urinary output, urinary tract infection and an alkaline urine which is associated with decreased muscular activity. Raising the head of the bed will aid gravitational drainage and this, plus a high fluid intake, helps to minimize the problem.

Bladder and bowel problems

The patient confined to bed in the supine position has particular difficulty with elimination. Lack of privacy and attempting to use a bedpan or urinal in an unnatural position make it difficult for the patient to relax the perineal and sphincter muscles.

The nurse must recognize that the patient who asks for frequent bedpans but passes only small amounts of urine, or the older patient who is frequently incontinent, may be suffering from retention of urine with overflow (p.308).

Constipation and faecal impaction are also common problems with the immobilized patient. Neither lying supine nor sitting with the knees extended will promote the normal reflexes necessary for defaecation. The patient with faecal impaction may pass frequent small amounts of liquid faecal material which can be misinterpreted as diarrhoea.

Thrombosis
The problems of phlebothrombosis and thrombophlebitis associated with bed rest are fully discussed on page 254. Pulmonary embolism as a result of thrombosis formation can also occur (p. 255).

Fat embolus
When a large bone is fractured, fat globules from the bone marrow may enter the circulation and give rise to symptoms 24 to 48 hours after the fracture. The first sign may be a sudden or progressive pyrexia followed by restlessness, chest pain and dyspnoea. Tachycardia and cerebral symptoms develop and, if a large quantity of fat has been released into the circulation, the prognosis is poor. Other signs which the nurse must report urgently are urinary incontinence or the appearance of a petechial rash especially over the chest, neck and shoulders.

Postural hypotension
Patients who have been confined to bed for long periods may experience vertigo on assuming the upright position. Sometimes fainting will occur. This is known as postural hypotension and is due to sudden pooling of blood in the abdominal viscera and legs. Before ambulation, therefore, the nurse should prepare the patient gradually by raising the head of the bed for short periods or allowing him to sit up if permitted. The application of support bandages or stockings may also help to minimize the pooling of blood in the peripheral circulation and to prevent oedema of the dependent extremities.

Body position as part of therapy

There are many occasions in which the nurse's knowledge of optimum joint position plays a vital part in treatment. Perhaps a few instances would start the learner thinking about the relationship between anatomy, types of therapy, the aims of the treatment, and the constraints imposed upon such treatment. For example, a patient may be suffering from osteoarthritis of the left hip. If you look at the effect that the pain caused by this disease has had upon the patient's posture you will usually see that the hip is held in an unnatural position. It is often flexed, so that the patient has difficulty in placing the foot flat on the floor. Pain and muscle spasm often cause external rotation and adduction of the hip joint so that the knee-cap (patella) points away from the opposite leg instead of straight ahead. Flexion and external rotation of the hip will also cause tilting of the pelvis and alteration of the spinal curve in the lumbar region. This vicious circle of stiffness, due to distortion of joint surfaces, pain, spasm and shortening of ligaments and tendons, places the patient in a very unhappy situation. Attention paid to pillows which will support the joints in their most comfortable position will do much for the patient's comfort. If the admission is for surgical correction, for example, by arthroplasty, the pre-operative period will be one in which the nurse strives to achieve a position of comfort for the patient. Position of function is not possible at this stage, therefore the joints must be supported in the position the patient prefers and prevented from falling into a strained position. If the hip is flexed and externally rotated it should be supported in this position. Unsupported the weight of the leg will cause pulling on the shortened ligaments and will cause further pain and resultant spasm. Whether the patient is up or in bed, dorsal or in a lateral position, the observant nurse should ensure that all joints are supported in the best possible position.

   In the early stages after surgery to relieve the condition, there is a danger of dislocation of the joint. The patient is, therefore, nursed with the hip supported in its most stable position, that of slight internal rotation, and this position must be maintained at all times and during all nursing procedures.

TRAUMA AND THE PROCESS OF REPAIR

The repair process for soft tissues and bone is fundamental to any consideration of the remote complications of injury or surgery. Tissues vary in their capacity for true repair. In connective tissue such as bone, repair is almost perfect. A year after a fracture it may be impossible to identify the site of the injury. Other tissues, however, are so highly specialized that it is impossible for them to regenerate — for instance the nerve cells of the brain. Notable exceptions to this rule are the cells of the liver and kidney, which are capable of dramatic proliferation, though the structure may be disorganised.

The process of repair for all tissues is basically the same but is influenced by the degree of specialization of the cells, the vascularity of the part, the presence or absence of infection and the degree of tissue destruction. There are, of course, a number of other factors involved, many of which are as yet ill-understood and the subject of much experimental work.

Methods of repair

It is convenient to discuss tissue repair under two headings:

1. Healing by primary union.
2. Healing by granulation tissue.

Healing by primary union

This occurs in clean, incised wounds, such as a stitched, surgical incision, where there is little or no loss of tissue and the cut edges of the wound are in close opposition.

The space between the cut surfaces fills with plasma, which forms a sticky medium into which two types of cells grow: (1) fibroblasts and (2) vascular endothelial cells. This occurs very rapidly (within the first 24 hours or so). At the same time small blood vessels of the injured part enter a phase of great activity. The endothelial lining of the capillaries proliferates and these capillary buds join up with neighbouring buds to form a branching network. The buds quickly multiply and a lumen is established which communicates with the parent vessel. In the same way the lymphatic endothelial cells divide rapidly to establish a primitive lymphatic system.

The narrow gap on the skin surface is bridged by epithelial cells which grow in from the wound edges. Hair follicles and sweat glands (specialized cells) are not reproduced. Healing is complete and the resultant scar tissue gradually shrinks.

Healing by granulation tissue

Where there has been loss of tissue or infection the fibroblasts are unable to 'sew' the wound surfaces together and repair starts at the base of the wound.

The wound defect is filled by a blood clot, plasma and inflammatory exudate. As in healing by primary union fibroblasts and vascular endothelial cells proliferate, but in addition wandering, scavenger cells play an important part in the process. The resulting granulation tissue is highly vascular and easily damaged. It is, therefore, very vulnerable to careless dressing technique or inappropriate dressings.

The scavenger cells at first are mainly polymorphonuclear leucocytes. They ingest bacteria and debris and keep the surface of the wound free from serious infection. A granulating surface has remarkable powers to resist serious bacterial infection, but if there are foreign bodies or dead tissue in the wound, suppuration occurs and the process of healing will not take place.

When the wound is 'clean' (though not necessarily bacteriologically sterile) epithelial cells begin to grow in from the wound edges to cover the granulation tissue. As healing proceeds the granulation tissue contracts (collagen formation) and becomes less vascular. Parts of the wound may fail to heal because of avascularity or the presence of a foreign body. Persistent infection will also delay healing. Ulcer formation is associated with the former and the development of a sinus with the latter.

Factors which influence repair

Nutrition

When suffering from a major injury, malnutrition or starvation, the body is in negative nitrogen balance (Ch. 4) and wound repair is slow. Thus, unless contraindicated due to another disease condition, a high protein diet is indicated following trauma or surgery. The part played by vitamins in tissue development and repair should not be ignored, and vitamins C and D may be prescribed as a nutritional supplement.

Hormonal control
Endocrine glands influence repair either by systemic effects on metabolism or by direct action on the affected tissue. Cortisone, for example, inhibits vascular changes and discourages collagen formation, therefore patients having cortisone therapy may show evidence of slow healing.

Local vascularity
Tissues which have a good blood supply heal well. If vascularity is normally poor or has become so because of disease, healing is slow. Wounds of face or scalp, therefore, heal quickly while those on ankle or shin are notoriously slow.

Lymphatic drainage
Obstruction to the lymphatic drainage will cause oedema which delays healing.

Mechanical factors
Excessive movement tears young granulation tissue. In soft tissue, this tends to produce a dense thickened scar. In bony tissue, movement at a fracture site may convert osteoid tissue into fibrous tissue, and a pseudarthrosis or false joint may be formed.

Anchorage to subjacent structures
Where layers of tissue are firmly bound to other tissue, healing is slow. Wounds over the 'shin', for instance, heal badly.

Repair of specific tissues

Bone
Despite the specialized nature of the tissue, bone heals well. It is worth remembering that bone is not merely a rigid skeleton but is constantly changing in response to the physical or chemical demands of the body. An area of bone constantly subjected to extra stress will, over time, develop a buttress system to strengthen the area. The repair of bone consists of two processes:

1. The formation of osteoid tissue.
2. The deposition of calcium and phosphorus (ossification).

Granulation tissue forms in the haematoma which surrounds the broken bone ends. Very quickly the fibrous tissue so formed differentiates into fibrocartilage. Almost simultaneously, specialized cells called osteoblasts proliferate and a loosely woven osteoid tissue called callus forms a sleeve round the fractured bone ends. This tissue unites and helps to stabilize the fracture, but it is not strong enough to permit weight-bearing or prevent movement without additional splintage. Gradually more calcium and phosphorus salts are laid down in the tissue so that true bone is reformed. Restructuring and remodelling occur; eventually the bone is restored to its former shape.

Muscle
Voluntary muscle may regenerate to a very limited extent depending on the type of injury. When involuntary muscle is damaged, repair is by fibrous tissue replacement.

Tendons
Collagen fibres heal very well provided that the gap is not too great. Divided tendons are therefore sutured to facilitate repair. Tendon sheaths repair by fibrous tissue and if there is extensive destruction of the sheath adhesions tend to form.

Serous membrane
These tissues heal by fibrous tissue formation. The surface endothelium *may* cover the fibrous scar to restore the smooth membrane. Sometimes two or more adjacent surfaces are involved, and the fibrous tissues coalesce and become adherent. This is particularly likely if infection is present.

Articular cartilage
Repair is poor due to the relative avascularity of this tissue. The repair is usually by formation of fibrous tissue rather than articular cartilage.

Central nervous system
The brain and spinal cord have no power of regeneration.

Peripheral nerves
The repair process is complex and occurs after an extended period of time. If a peripheral nerve has been divided by an injury the nerve sheath must be sutured for regeneration to occur.

Skin
Small defects are quickly covered by epithelium, but the scar is thinner than normal skin and often unstable.

Fat
If fat cells have been destroyed they do not usually regenerate.

Solid organs
Specialized cells have little capacity for true healing. Repair is affected by connective tissue replacement.

DISORDERS OF THE LOCOMOTOR SYSTEM

As in other systems of the body, the locomotor system can become disordered by injury, disease or congenital malformation. In broad terms and excluding the neurological manifestations that affect locomotion, the system will be unable to function efficiently if its structure is altered. For example, if a long bone is fractured the muscles cannot pull upon it as a lever, therefore movement is impossible. Similarly if the smooth surface of a joint is destroyed due to osteoarthritis movement is reduced. Pain and resultant muscle spasm lead to further limitation of function.

Inflammatory responses give rise to swelling and exudate, which again result in loss of movement. In a less direct way the same effect is produced by congenital deformities or deformity as a result of trauma. Distortion of the shape of, say, the femur can lead to alteration of the lines of weight transmission, muscle spasm, extra wear and tear on joints, arthritis, pain and limitation of movement.

The purposes of orthopaedic treatment

The aims of orthopaedic treatment are:

1. To restore or maintain function.
2. To increase movement.
3. To prevent deformity.
4. To restore stability.
5. To correct deformity, if present.
6. To relieve pain.
7. To aid diagnosis.
8. To excise dead or infected tissue.
9. To develop powers of adaptation or compensation if loss of function or disability is inevitable.

Multidisciplinary management
Care of the person suffering from an orthopaedic condition requires the involvement of a team of people with a wide range of skills (Fig. 2.9). If an operation is necessary it is only one step in a carefully planned campaign from conservative management right through to the patient's independence and rehabilitation. At all times, the nurse must encourage and give explanations to the orthopaedic patient, whose road to recovery may be prolonged, painful and sometimes discouraging.

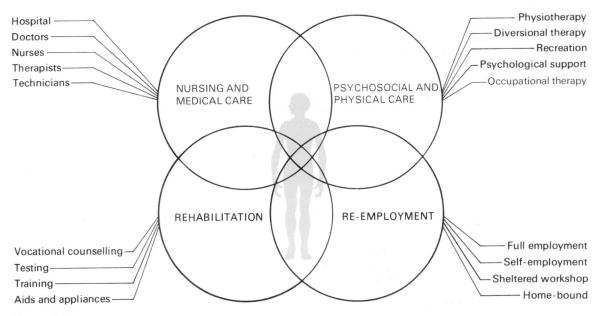

Hospital
Doctors
Nurses
Therapists
Technicians

NURSING AND MEDICAL CARE

PSYCHOSOCIAL AND PHYSICAL CARE

Physiotherapy
Diversional therapy
Recreation
Psychological support
Occupational therapy

REHABILITATION

RE-EMPLOYMENT

Vocational counselling
Testing
Training
Aids and appliances

Full employment
Self-employment
Sheltered workshop
Home-bound

Figure 2.9
The orthopaedic team

Orthopaedic treatment can be categorized as either conservative or operative, though often a combination of the two is required.

Conservative treatment

Active exercises

Normal joint function requires good muscle control. Specific exercises aimed at one muscle or group of muscles will be required if:

1. The muscles are weak and deformity is liable to occur due to the pull of the antagonist group of muscles. This can be caused by (a) nerve or muscle tissue damage; (b) brain or spinal cord lesions; (c) tendon injuries.
2. The joint has limited mobility following injury.

Passive movements

The therapist gently moves the joint through its full range of normal movement. Often this is combined with active exercise, when it is known as assisted movement. The manipulation is always gentle, never forced and can be used for the following reasons:

1. To prevent stiffening of the joints in a paralysed limb (hemiplegia following a cerebrovascular accident).
2. To correct deformity (club foot).
3. To restore joint movement (following immobilization).
4. To relieve muscle spasm (leg cramp).

Active exercise is encouraged whenever possible. It is only when the patient is unable to contract his muscles that passive movements would be carried out by the nurse or therapist in an attempt to maintain joint mobility. N.B. the term 'passive exercise' is a misnomer, as 'exercise' is always *active*.

Splinting

Sometimes it is necessary that certain joints or a limb should be held immobile in a prescribed position, using various appliances and materials. Splinting is used to:

1. Relieve pain.
2. Diminish muscle spasm.
3. Prevent undesirable movements.
4. Immobilize fractures in alignment until healed.
5. Maintain stable joint position after dislocation until the capsule is healed.

Operative treatment

Aseptic precautions

The outcome of most orthopaedic operations depends upon bone healing, and bones will not heal in the presence of infection. Infections of bone can lead to life-long crippling deformity or disablement. Prevention of infection, important in all surgery, is of paramount importance in orthopaedics. Every nurse should know that the prevention of wound infection depends to a large extent upon the following:

1. Careful and meticulous preoperative skin preparation.
2. Scrupulous surgical techniques in the operating theatre.
3. Care and attention to keep dressings efficient and intact.
4. Careful wound dressing technique.
5. Rigorous separation of patients with clean wounds from any whose wounds have become infected.

In addition, however, the nurse must remember the less obvious links in the chain of transmission of infection. Bandages which are unwound instead of being cut let loose a cloud of airborne micro-organisms. Unclean scissors used indiscriminately are another well-known hazard. It is the nurse's ability to predict potential sources of contamination which does much to avoid the disastrous results of wound infection in orthopaedics.

Orthopaedic operations can be classified under the following headings.

Operations on bones

1. Division of the bone (osteotomy) to alter its shape or correct deformity.
2. Internal fixation — metal plates, screws or special nails used to immobilize divided bone after fracture or osteotomy.
3. Bone graft. A piece of bone or bone chips used to support or encourage healing after fractures (especially if non-union occurs), osteotomy or removal of a bone tumour.
4. Removal of pieces of bone: for histological examination (biopsy) or because excess bone is pressing on adjacent structures and causing pain.
5. Operations for bone infections. It may be necessary to remove dead pieces of bone (sequestrectomy) which act as foreign bodies and delay healing, or to drain abscesses.

Operations on joints

1. Division of capsule or fascia to correct deformity (capsulotomy or fasciotomy).
2. Excision of synovial membrane for investigative reasons (biopsy) or therapeutic reasons (synovectomy).
3. Excision of joint surfaces to create a false joint and permit movement (pseudarthrosis).
4. Fixation of a badly damaged or painful joint (arthrodesis).
5. Refashioning of a joint by insertion of a prosthesis (arthroplasty).
6. Stabilization of a flail joint or one where there is recurrent dislocation.

Operation on muscles and tendons

1. Suturing where structures have been divided.
2. Division of a tendon to correct deformities (tenotomy).
3. Tendon transplant to restore function to a joint.

Operations on peripheral nerves

1. Suturing of a nerve sheath when a nerve has been divided.
2. Dissection to free a nerve from pressure due to ganglia, fascia, bone or tumour.
3. Division of nerve supply to overactive muscles.

Operations to repair skin defects and deficient blood supply

Amputation
This may be necessary when a limb or part of a limb has become a useless encumbrance because of one of the following:

1. Death of tissue.
2. Gross and intractable sepsis.
3. Gross deformity.

Diseases affecting joints

The multidisciplinary nature of care and therapy required by people with disorders of the locomotor system is perhaps best illustrated in the management of patients with joint disorders. It is not possible here to describe and discuss all the diseases which may affect joints but as rheumatoid arthritis is one of the major crippling diseases, perhaps this condition could be used to illustrate some important points of nursing management of patients with joint disorders in general.

Throughout this section the reader will be referred back to general points which have been discussed more fully elsewhere.

The physician initiates the plan of treatment which involves the nurse, physiotherapist, occupational therapist and medical social worker in a team effort. All have an important job to do as they make their own specialist contribution but the nurse has a major role to play, as she contributes to every aspect of treatment.

Rheumatoid arthritis

Rheumatoid arthritis is a chronic form of polyarthritis characterized in the majority of patients by exacerbations and remissions. The cause is still unknown but research suggests that disorders of the immune system play an important part in the development and perpetuation of the joint inflammation as well as the extra-articular manifestations such as skin nodules. What initiates and maintains the disease process is not clear. What has been established is that rheumatoid arthritis is an inflammatory disease unlike osteoarthritis which also affects synovial joints but in which inflammation does not play a major role. In this section some important facets of the nursing care of adult patients with rheumatoid arthritis will be described. Most of the text reflects experience gained from nursing such patients in a specialized hospital unit but much of what is suggested would, with appropriate modification, be equally applicable to the care of patients at home.

The first thing that the nurse must appreciate is that the patient is suffering from a chronic disease and is worried and often very bitter. Questions spoken and unspoken fill the air. Will I become a helpless cripple? Am I going to lead a normal life again? What did the doctor mean? The nurse plays an important role in listening to the patient and identifying the hidden fears and misconceptions he may have. This requires a great deal of time, patience and understanding coupled with factual knowledge about the disease process and the prospects for individual patients. The nurse must inspire in the person confidence and belief that even if cure is not possible, the treatment will lead to improvement in his condition.

A regime of medical treatment will be prescribed and nurses must ensure that the total programme is tailored to suit the individual needs of the patient. The role of the nurse in this blending of treatment and care to form an integrated pattern cannot be overemphasized. In any situation where cure is not possible, good and skilful nursing is of supreme importance. Although it is the doctor who prescribes the appropriate therapeutic regime for each individual patient, it is the nurse who organizes the therapy, diet, environment, rest and other aspects of the patient's day so that the needs of the individual are met. The processes of assessment, planning, teaching, explanation, reassurance and encouragement all play an important part in the building up of the patient's confidence to face the future.

For convenience the usual treatment can be described in three stages and at each one the nurse's attention to detail and knowledge of the person plays a major part. The three stages of management of a patient suffering from early active rheumatoid arthritis are:

1. Rest phase.
2. Remobilization.
3. Rehabilitative phase.

Patients with less active disease, for example the elderly and severely crippled, have a modified regime of treatment. The nursing care required may be classified under the following headings:

1. General care and comfort of the patient.
2. Alleviation of pain.
3. Prevention of deformity (in a specialist unit nurses would also participate in the correction of deformity).
4. Careful observation.
5. Support, teaching and encouragement of the patient and the maintenance of his morale.
6. Rehabilitation of the patient.
7. In a specialist unit nurses would also be involved in the maintenance of improvement and the provision of continuing support.

Phase 1 — Rest

General care
A bright, well-ventilated room with a good outlook is essential. The bed must have a firm mattress and fracture boards may be used to ensure this. A back rest with the necessary number of pillows is used to keep the patient in an upright position. The minimum number of pillows required for comfort should be allowed. This position is maintained for most of the day except for rest and treatment periods. The limbs must be correctly positioned (see pp. 34–35). A large cage with a padded foot board should be placed over the legs and feet. This should be anchored in position by straps if possible. (Fig. 2.10). The bedclothes should be light and a soft blanket next to the patient is warm and comforting. The patient's own clothing should be light and easy to put on.

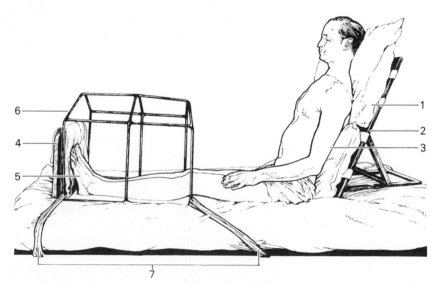

Figure 2.10
1. As few pillows as necessary for comfort
2. Back rest
3. Upright position
4. Padded footboard
5. Foot and ankle in position of function
6. Bed cage
7. Anchoring straps

The nurse must always remember that in the acute phase of the disease the joints are swollen, inflamed and painful. Movement will inevitably cause an increase in pain and muscle spasm, therefore the patient must be lifted and turned very carefully to avoid jarring of the joints. As this person is completely bedfast special care must be exercised when assisting with elimination. Great care must be taken to ensure that bed pans are positioned accurately and comfortably and that they are removed as soon as the patient wishes this. The limbs should be placed as close to the position of function as possible (see pp. 34–35). Skintight plaster of Paris splints are used to ensure this. (Fig. 2.11 A and B) During this phase, of rest and immobilization, the patient is totally dependent upon the nurse, therefore he will require assistance with most of the activities of daily living. Daily bed bathing, oral hygiene and hair care are all necessary but special attention must be paid to pressure areas (see p. 446). The patient is unable to move about the bed and often perspires excessively due to active disease or as a result of the administration of salicylates. The patient with subcutaneous nodules requires particularly good skin care as the area over the nodules is very prone to breakdown. (Fig. 2.12) Nodules are frequently found at the elbows but may occur over any bony prominence and they may become ulcerated following a minor knock or merely pressure. If skin breakdown does occur it often becomes infected and difficult to heal. The use of aids such as foam pads, air-rings, sheepskins or polystyrene bead bags can be of great assistance in the plan for skin care.

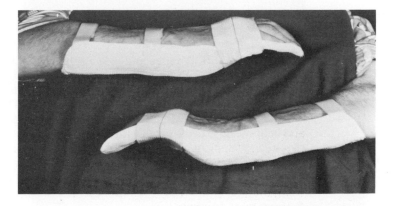

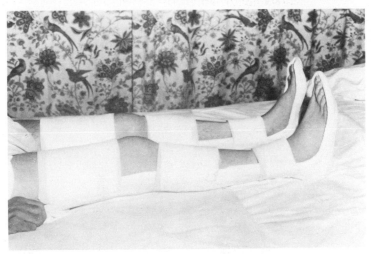

Figure 2.11A & B
Skin tight POP splints (Courtesy of Dr T. M. Chalmers, Consultant Rheumatologist, Northern General Hospital, Edinburgh)

A well-balanced diet is given. If the patient is underweight extra milk and protein are added. Often however the patient is obese and it is most important to restrict carbohydrate to reduce weight. This is necessary if weight-bearing joints are involved. An adequate fluid intake will help to prevent urinary tract infections and constipation (see p. 38). Assistance with feeding must be given in an unhurried fashion. The nurse should always sit by the bedside and give her full attention to the patient at mealtimes.

Alleviation of pain
1. Rest splints are used for the relief of pain.
2. Special procedures such as the aspiration of effusions and local injections into the joints are carried out by the doctor.
3. Many drugs have been used to alleviate the pain characteristic of rheumatoid arthritis and one of the most useful is acetylsalicylic acid (Aspirin). No pharmacological agent has yet been found to cure the condition and nurses must have a

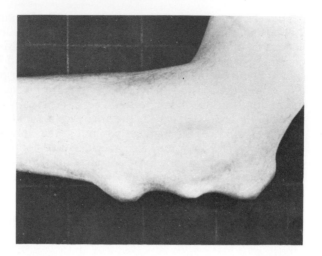

Figure 2.12
Subcutaneous nodules
(Courtesy of Dr T. M. Chalmers)

wide knowledge of the uses and side effects of the drugs prescribed so that they can detect and report any undesirable signs at the earliest possible moment. Accurate timing of drug administration is important. This means a departure from the traditional medicine round of three times a day. The drugs must be given with or immediately after a meal to reduce irritation of the gastric mucosa, the early morning and bedtime dose being given with a glass of milk or a small snack. If extra analgesia is required to supplement the antirheumatic medication it is best given between the usual medicine times and at bedtime. A mild sedative is often required in the initial stages but it is undesirable to use strong hypnotics or drugs of addiction.

Prevention of deformity
Good posture and position in bed are essential at all times (see p. 37). Skintight unpadded rest splints designed to hold the affected joint in the position of function without muscle strain, should be used to prevent further flexion deformities of the knees or wrists and to prevent ulnar deviation of the fingers (Fig. 2.13).

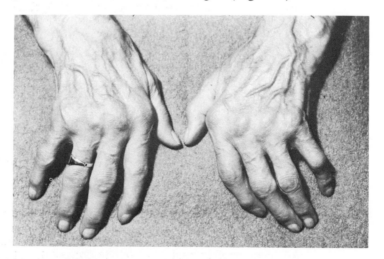

Figure 2.13
Ulnar deviation of the fingers
(Courtesy of Dr T. H. Chalmers)

Observation
As rheumatoid arthritis is an inflammatory disease temperature, pulse and respiration rate are normally recorded twice per day or four hourly if the patient is febrile. The nurse must note and report the duration of early morning stiffness, any increase in pain, tenderness or involvement of other joints. (Fig. 2.14)

Any signs of the plaster being too tight (see p. 55) such as colour changes, swelling or pain, should be reported immediately; if the plaster is too tight it will need to be removed at once. Pressure or rubbing of the plaster on bony prominences or rubbing at the edges of the plaster must be avoided lest abrasion of the skin occurs (see p. 57). The nurse must be able to report on the effectiveness of the prescribed drugs or any

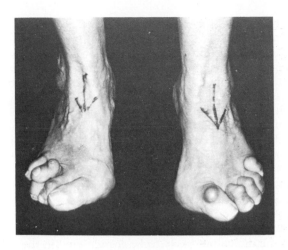

Figure 2.14
Deformities and stiffness of the feet (Courtesy of Dr T. M. Chalmers)

untoward effect which they may produce. Urine testing is important. Albuminuria may be present if there is renal involvement. Certain drugs, for example gold or D-penicillamine, may also produce protein in the urine. Glycosuria may develop in patients receiving high doses of steroids. The nurse must always be on the alert for any of the other possible complications that can arise due to immobilization and bed rest (see pp. 37–39).

Maintenance of morale
During this period of rest and immobilization the patient requires support and encouragement and her mind must be kept occupied. In addition to listening, talking and conversation between nurse and patient simple measures such as changing the position of the bed so that there is a view from the window will help. Full use can be made of television, books from the library and other diversions which all help to pass the time. Some patients who are ambulant may be of the greatest assistance simply by sitting and chatting with the bedfast patients. Visitors can also be of help and they too need support and advice from nursing staff. At this stage anxiety about the family and about the home may dominate the patient's outlook. The nurse may seek the help of the medical social worker to relieve the patient's worries.

The duration of phase 1 is usually about three weeks and towards the end of this period rest splints will be removed for short intervals during the day but are firmly and carefully secured at night.

Phase 2 — Remobilization
After the period of immobilization the physiotherapist starts a programme of graduated, non weight-bearing exercises beginning with general exercises designed to regain muscle tone and progressing to exercises designed to build muscle strength and joint mobility. Some patients may be over enthusiastic and may therefore have to be carefully supervised as too much exercise can cause a recurrence of joint inflammation.

It is the physiotherapist who will regulate the progression from day to day. Some increase in pain and stiffness is usual following unaccustomed exercise but if it is confined to the muscles it is not a contraindication to further treatment. Once again reassurance, support and encouragement from the nurse is essential. The patient is still very dependent at this stage but is now able to be taken in a chair to the bath and toilet. Less assistance will be required with feeding each day and the person must be encouraged towards greater independence. He is now able to sit out of bed and weight-bearing is permitted when adequate muscle strength has been developed. Each day activities are slowly increased, and when the physician is satisfied that disease activity has been controlled, the last phase of the treatment begins.

Phase 3 — Rehabilitation
At this stage patients are up for much of the day. They dress in their own clothes, wear shoes and go to the day room for meals and recreation. Physiotherapy is still carried out in the ward but in addition the patient now attends the physiotherapy department

for further treatment and training in the performance of essential activities such as climbing stairs and rising from a chair. A simple series of exercises, free and against resistance, must be learned by the patient. These will need to be performed daily at home to maintain movement, joint stability and to prevent contractures. The occupational therapist is also concerned in the rehabilitation programme. The patient is assessed in the activities of daily living by nursing staff. Where there are problems with personal and domestic activities, special retraining may be necessary. The occupational therapist's contribution to this aspect of rehabilitation is when the patient needs to use special aids and equipment such as modified cutlery or tools. Modification of the home may also be required, for example rails to help rising from the lavatory or bath or to negotiate stairs.

Both physiotherapist and occupational therapist have an important role in the final assessment of the functional level obtained, and translating this in terms of capacity for employment or work in the home. They collaborate with the nurse and medical social worker who will by now have a thorough knowledge of the patient's social background and the difficulties likely to be encountered in the process of resettlement. When the patient has reached the maximum degree of improvement the nurse as part of the team must help prepare him to face the future. By the time of discharge from the ward careful instructions should have been given about exercise and the wearing of splints at night, the limits of physical activity, the continuation of regular doses of anti-inflammatory drugs and the importance of returning to the follow-up clinic so that the physician can adjust the regime of treatment as required. Hospital admission as well as establishing reasonable control over the manifestations of the disease provides an opportunity for educating the patient to take a realistic view of the limitations within which he or she may have to live.

Joint injuries

In order to function efficiently the articular surfaces of a joint must be smooth, held in the correct position and able to slide one upon the other. Congenital abnormalities may be responsible for joint disorders, but the commonest cause is trauma.

Strains
If a joint is forced beyond its normal position but there is no tissue damage, the joint has been strained. The sufferer will complain of pain when he attempts specific actions, but there will be no evidence of swelling, deformity or loss of function. Local heat may give comfort by relieving muscle spasm and mild analgesics help the patient to persist with gentle exercise of the part.

Sprains
When a joint is forced into an abnormal position and some fibres of muscle, tendon or ligament are torn, the body response is pain, local swelling, limitation of movement and often local bruising. But there is no deformity or loss of function. This injury is referred to as a sprain. X-ray investigation will rule out the possibility of fracture. Though any joint can, technically, be sprained the commonest site is the ankle joint. Treatment is usually the application of a support bandage with the joint in the position of rest. The amount of exercise allowed during the process of healing depends upon the severity of the sprain.

Torn ligaments
This term is used when the traumatic force has been severe enough to tear ligaments or dislodge them from their bony attachments. Such an injury is much more serious as the joint is now unstable. If the ligament has been wrenched from its bony attachment and has taken with it a flake of bone, immobilization of the joint may allow bone healing to occur, thus reattaching the ligament. If, on the other hand, the ligament has been divided at some point along its length and that ligament is a vital factor in the affected joint's stability, surgery may be necessary so that the ligament can be sutured. Common sites for this injury are the knee and ankle joint. Treatment involves splintage in the rest position, then remobilization of the joint when sound healing has occurred.

Subluxation and dislocation

When the ligaments which support the joint are torn or cut the joint is unstable. In consequence the bones are able to slip from their normal position of close alignment of articular surfaces into an abnormal position. When the articular surfaces are completely out of alignment the term dislocation is used. If the disarticulation is only partial, the term subluxation is used.

The degree of damage to the ligaments is an important consideration in this type of trauma, whether due to surgery or accidental injury. The young man who sustains a dislocated hip in a road traffic accident may require similar nursing care in the early stages to the elderly lady who has undergone surgery to replace the head of the femur by a prosthesis. The accident may, and the operation certainly will, have divided the ligament which tethers the femoral head to the acetabulum. In either event the joint is potentially unstable, that is, liable to dislocate.

Most often the head of the bone is forced out through the capsule like a button through a button-hole. When the bone is relocated, healing of the capsule by fibrous tissue can occur and the joint is once more stable. Sometimes, however, the damage to the supporting ligaments is extensive and spontaneous repair is impossible. The joint never regains its stability and the patient has recurrent dislocations which occur during the performance of simple, everyday movements. The commonest site for this unusual injury is the shoulder joint and the sufferer may find that as he tries to put on his coat the joint slips out of position. In this situation surgical repair of the joint supports will be required.

When a joint is dislocated the features are pain, deformity and loss of function. Obvious swelling and bruising vary with the affected part. The treatment is to realign the articular surfaces as soon as possible (before oedema of the injured tissue makes this more difficult) and to support the limb in its most stable position. The stable positions of joints such as the fingers, thumb, wrist, elbow, ankle and knee are often similar to their positions of rest. Sometimes, however, due to the shape of the bones involved, exaggeration of certain planes of movement will make the joint less likely to dislocate.

When healing has occurred, either spontaneously or following surgical repair, intensive physiotherapy will be required to mobilize the joint fully so that the former range of movement is restored.

Complications of joint injuries

Synovial effusions

Response to injury causes increased secretion of synovial fluid. This can be felt as a fluctuant swelling around the joint. A common site is the knee, especially when the injury has torn part of the meniscus from its attachment. If effusion persists, it may require aspiration.

Haemarthrosis

In severe joint injuries, particularly where a fracture line involves the joint, bleeding may occur. This usually requires aspiration.

Damage to adjacent nerves

This is particularly liable to happen in shoulder injuries where damage to the circumflex nerve leads to paralysis of the deltoid muscle.

Osteoarthritis

This can be a late complication when a fracture has disrupted the smooth articular surface.

Fractures

A fracture is an interruption in the continuity of a bone. Fractures can be caused by direct violence, indirect violence, muscular effort and pathological defects of bone (Fig. 2.15A–D).

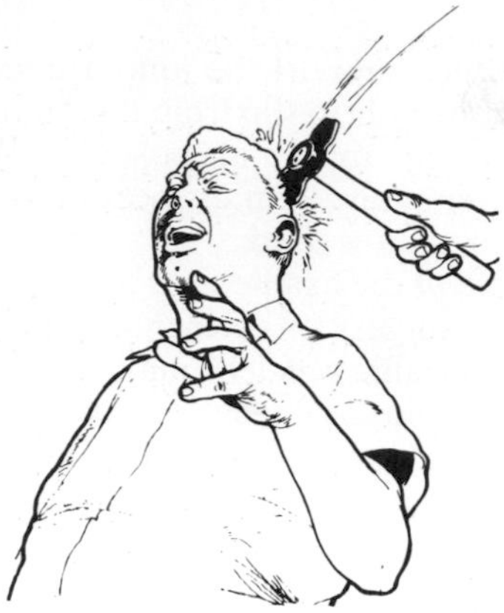

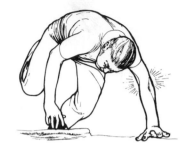

Figure 2.15A
Causes of fractures—direct violence

Figure 2.15B
Causes of fractures—indirect violence

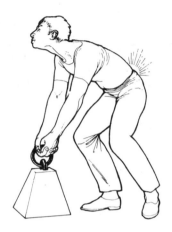

Figure 2.15C
Causes of fractures—indirect violence: muscular effort

Figure 2.15D
Causes of fractures—pathological defect of bone

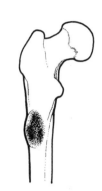

Types

Fractures can be closed (simple fractures) or open (compound fractures — where a wound allows the fractured bone to communicate with the air). The anatomical variations of fractures which can occur are: oblique, transverse, comminuted, greenstick and impacted, and complicated (Fig. 2.16). Fractures are considered complicated when they involve damage to some other tissue or structure, such as muscle or nerve. Both open and closed fractures can be complicated.

Fractures may be described as 'closed' (where the skin over the fracture site remains intact) or 'open' (where a wound over the fracture site allows communication between the bone and the air. This is sometimes referred to as a compound fracture). Fractures may also be described as simple or complicated. A simple fracture as the name implies is a break in the continuity of a bone which does not involve any other structure. A

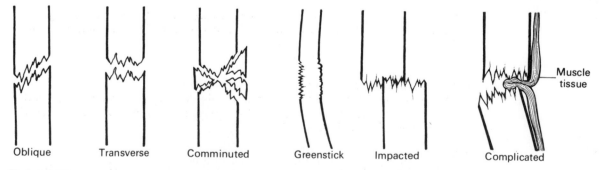

Figure 2.16
Types of fracture

complicated fracture, however, involves injury to other adjacent structures thus a compound fracture is always complicated as by definition it involves injury to the muscle and surrounding tissue while a closed fracture may be simple or complicated. Other words are attached to fractures and some of these are anatomical descriptions of the line of the fracture. The words transverse and spiral are self explanatory as are 'hairline' or 'crack' fractures.

Other descriptive terms refer to the *way* in which the bone has broken rather than site and line of the fracture. For example, the injury which causes some fractures may be such that the bone ends are driven into each other. This is described as impacted or compressed fracture. Another example of this type of description would be the so-called 'greenstick fracture' seen in young children. The bone being less brittle in children tends to bend and crack like a green stick rather than snap like a dry twig.

A further example of the words used to describe the way in which a bone breaks is the term comminuted which refers to a fracture which appears splintered on X-ray or visual inspection.

Lastly, words may be used to describe the exact site of the fracture. Sometimes they are anatomical terms such as a pertrochanteric or an intertrochanteric fracture of the femur, or a supracondylar fracture of the humerus. On other occasions a special fracture may bear the name of the doctor who first described it such as the 'Pott's fracture' of the ankle or the 'Colles' fracture' of the wrist. These doctors' names are only used to describe a particular fracture or specific injury to the ankle and wrist respectively.

Signs and symptoms of a fracture
1. Loss of function.
2. Deformity.
3. Shortening of the affected limb.
4. Abnormal mobility.
5. Local tenderness.
6. Swelling and bruising.

Complications of fractures
1. Early: injury to blood vessels, joints, nerves, viscera.
2. Late: infection, mal-union, non-union.

Sequelae of fractures
Shock (first 24 hours).
Fat emboli (first 48 hours). (p.39).
Pulmonary infarction (2 to 3 weeks after injury). (p. 255).
Hypostatic pneumonia ⎫
Pressure necrosis (p. 446) ⎬ (any time during bed rest).
Renal calculi (p. 302) ⎭

Principles of treatment of fractures

Figure 2.17 illustrates what happens when a fracture deformity occurs. There are three basic principles to be observed in the treatment of this type of injury:

1. Reduction of the fracture. The surgeon, by the application of traction and gentle manipulation, counteracts the muscle force and restores normal alignment to the bone.
2. Immobilization until healing occurs.
3. Restoration of full physical function.

Methods of immobilizing a fracture
Some form of fixation or splintage is required to hold the bone ends in alignment until healing occurs. This may be achieved by internal fixation involving surgical intervention or external splinting.

Internal fixation
Various devices have been invented to hold a fracture securely. These are commonly made of special metal that does not cause an inflammatory response in the body. Figure 2.18 shows some of the more common types of internal fixation.

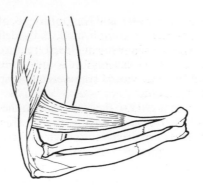
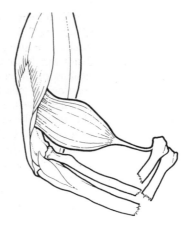

Figure 2.17
Fracture deformity

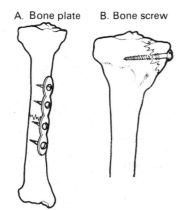

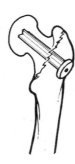
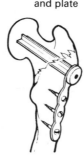
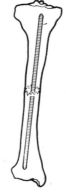

A. Bone plate B. Bone screw C. Tri-flange nail D. Tri-flange nail and plate E. Intramedullary bone nail

Figure 2.18
Common types of internal fixation

External splinting

There are many splints which can be applied to immobilize a fracture, but the commonest is plaster of Paris. Therefore special attention is given here to the care of patients wearing plaster casts.

Care of patients in plaster

The diagnosis, reduction and immobilization of fractures is the province of the medical practitioner. The decision about whether to use internal fixation by screws, pins, plates or nails is his, and he will perform the necessary operation. Similarly, if external splintage of the fracture is the chosen method of immobilization, the doctor will be closely involved with its application. Diagnosis, reduction and immobilization all take place in a matter of a few hours or, at most, a day or two. The period of immobilization necessary to allow healing to occur extends for many weeks (6 to 8 weeks for an upper limb; 3 months and longer for a major weight-bearing bone). It is this period of healing which is the prime concern of the nurse.

The commonest method of immobilization is the application of a plaster of Paris cast to the affected part. These casts are often extensive and may encase the whole lower limb (above knee plaster) the limb and torso (hip spica, which can be single- or double-legged), the torso alone (plaster jacket), the torso and shoulder (shoulder spica) or the torso and head (Minerva jacket). Preserving the efficiency of the cast and at the same time keeping the patient clean and comfortable can tax the ingenuity of the most skilful nurse. No single 'best' method can be defined — nurses working in orthopaedic centres are continually devising better ways of solving recurrent problems. What follows is merely an outline of some points which may help the inexperienced nurse who finds herself working for a short period in an orthopaedic unit.

The first thing to remember is that, although we shall be talking in terms of the plaster's efficiency and well-being, it is really the patient inside the cast who is our prime concern. Every complaint of pain or discomfort made by the patient must have prompt attention. It may be that the discomfort is only fleeting and insignificant, but on the other hand it could be a warning of imminent danger. A patient in a newly applied cast may complain of all manner of sensations at first — sharp pain, dull ache, throbbing sensation, sensations of heat, cold, itch or swelling. These impressions may be merely the brain trying to identify just exactly what the leg is feeling at the time. However, amongst all these sensations there may be one which is significant; therefore all must be heeded, lest the one important complaint be missed. If pressure is present under a plaster the patient will only experience discomfort for a few hours. After this time the part becomes numb, and although the patient says he is now comfortable, the pressure persists and the damage continues. Warning signs are **numbness and tingling**, a **burning sensation** or **persistent pain** over one part of the plaster. Remember it is not only the bony eminences which are vulnerable now. Any part of a plaster may have a ridge or dent in its inner surface that can cause pressure.

Observation of the circulation

The need for close observation of the circulation to the extremity when a plaster has been newly applied cannot be overstressed. It may be difficult for the inexperienced nurse to comprehend the speed with which the situation can deteriorate from impaired circulation to permanent damage. A paralysis of such severity that the patient may never regain the use of his hand or foot can occur within 24 hours. Inspecting the fingers or toes after application of a plaster is as important as checking the pulse after surgery. They should be warm and of good colour. Nurses should be familiar with the blanching test (capillary flush). The nails of the fingers or toes are each compressed in turn. When the pressure is released, blood should rush back into the nail bed, that is the nail should turn from white to pink **at once**. If the return of colour to the nail is sluggish, then the circulation is for some reason impaired. This state must be reported immediately. Inspection and the blanching test should be carried out $\frac{1}{2}$ to 1 hourly for 24 hours and should be observed regularly for several days. If there is any sign of circulatory impairment, the observations must be done every 10 to 15 minutes.

Cardinal signs of circulatory impairment
These are:
> Coldness.
> Blueness or pallor.
> Oedema.
> Loss of movement or stiffness.
> Numbness or pain.
> Sluggish return of blood after blanching test.

If several of these signs are present together, the situation is urgent and the doctor must take steps to relieve the pressure immediately.

Care of the cast

Plaster of Paris bandages are made by impregnating an open weave material with anhydrous gypsum, which we call plaster of Paris (calcium sulphate from which the water of crystallization has been removed). Plaster casts are made by wetting the bandages and applying them smoothly and evenly to the area to be encased. Great care is taken to mould the plaster to the contours of the patient so that pressure is avoided. The addition of water to anhydrous gypsum allows a chemical reaction to occur which reconverts the plaster of Paris to the rock-like gypsum. Setting occurs quite rapidly, but the full potential strength of the cast is not achieved until all the excess water has been removed by evaporation. At this stage, when the plaster is set but not yet dry, it is very susceptible to damage by cracking or denting.

Supporting the wet cast
Care of the cast begins before the patient returns from the plaster room. It begins with the preparation of the bed. A firm mattress and fracture boards are vital. Pillows to

support the cast will also be needed. Mattress and pillows will need waterproof protection to prevent dampness and mustiness caused by the wet plaster. For a plaster jacket, three pillows laid across the bed should be sufficient. For a hip spica, one pillow at waist level and two pillows laid lengthwise to support the leg are required. If both legs are encased in plaster, two or more pillows will be needed for the second leg. A pillow for head and shoulders will be needed for the patient who has not had an anaesthetic.

The nurse should never lay a damp plaster cast directly on to a mattress. If she does, the cast will become flattened over bony prominences such as the sacrum or the heel and damage to the underlying tissue will be unavoidable. It is essential that the pillows are positioned to support the contours of the plaster. Any sharp break in pillow alignment and support might cause the plaster to sag and crack at some strategic point. This is particularly likely to happen at the leg and body junction of the hip spica but may also occur at the knee.

When lifting the patient on to the bed, care must be taken to support the cast with the palms of the hand and not the fingers. Fingers can make indentations in a recently set plaster.

Drying the cast
Natural evaporation of moisture by exposing the cast to the air is preferred by many surgeons, as this gives the cast a chance to develop its full potential strength. Accelerated drying using heat lamps or a heat cradle is not usually recommended but is sometimes used in out-patient work. Though slow drying by exposure to the air is desirable for the cast, from the patient's point of view it is a lengthy, tedious and uncomfortable time. There is not a great deal that can be done about his enforced lack of mobility at this stage, but the nurse should give him reassurance and company as well as access to any diversion or entertainment the ward can provide.

The physical discomfort may be due to unaccustomed immobility, and ease can sometimes be gained by helping or encouraging the patient to move the parts of the body that are not encased in plaster into different positions. Much discomfort is caused by the fact that the patient has a large, wet, cold object in bed with him — namely the plaster. During application, due to the chemical reaction which is taking place, heat is generated and the plaster feels nice and warm. The patient may even feel that it is too hot and sometimes needs reassurance that he is not being burnt. Very soon, however, as the water evaporates, the plaster becomes profoundly cold. As water evaporates from the plaster heat is lost from the whole body. It should not be surprising, therefore, that the patient soon feels cold and shivery. Even with a relatively small cast such as an above the knee plaster, both legs will feel the chill badly. Make sure that all areas of the body not encased in plaster are warmly wrapped up. Use of small blankets next to the skin and a warm sock will not only help to prevent draughts but will stop the patient placing his 'good leg' on a sodden area of bed linen.

Turning the patient
The patient with an extensive cast in position must be turned from dorsal to prone position to allow drying of the back of the plaster and care of the pressure areas. Timing of the first turn requires professional judgment. During this first turn, more help will be needed than with subsequent turns, as the plaster must be fully supported to prevent cracking. Turning should always be done on the leg which is **not** encased or, in the case of a double hip spica, over the side which has **not** been operated on. Pillows to support the entire length of the cast must be positioned in readiness so that lifting the patient once he is turned is avoided. Lifting at this stage is uncomfortable for the patient, endangers the soft cast and places an unnecessary strain on the nurses' backs.

As soon as the turn is completed, the nurses should check the patient's position to see that the toes are not pressing against the mattress. Note should also be made of the body position. Too many pillows at head and shoulders will cause the cast to dig into the chest. If the pillow under the lumbar curve is not positioned correctly, the plaster edge may cut into the soft tissue of the buttocks.

When the cast has hardened regular turning can be managed by two or even one nurse. The patient soon becomes skilled at helping, and some manage to turn themselves without assistance. Pillows are no longer necessary for plaster protection but are used for the comfort of the patient. Support at the upper edge of a body plaster lifts the pressure from the patient's chest and makes breathing easier. Pillow support at buttock level prevents the plaster cutting into soft tissues. Lumbar support prevents pressure which would otherwise occur in this area if the patient was left with only the top and bottom of the plaster supported. Similarly with leg plasters, the heel must be supported clear of the bed, but the wearer of the plaster will be more comfortable if the plaster is supported along its length. If allowed to hang with only the foot supported, the top edge will cut into the front of the thigh. A pillow between the legs is also useful as it prevents the sound leg banging against the plaster.

Placing the patient on a bedpan

The plaster will be carefully trimmed and bound to allow the patient to use a bedpan or urinal and to leave access for perineal and anal toilet. To prevent soiling or wetting of the plaster, however, the nurse must develop some skill in the positioning of sanitary utensils. The following points will help to prevent accidents.

1. Elevate the head of the bed or place extra pillows under the shoulders to prevent urine or faeces running back under the plaster.

2. Place an absorbent pad at the cast edge as an additional safeguard — this pad must be removed with the bedpan.

3. Position the bedpan by rolling the patient to the unaffected side and placing the pan so that the buttocks contact the rim of the utensil. Position pillows to support the back and limbs and roll the patient on to his back.

Care of the patient's skin

Good powers of observation are vital when caring for patients in plaster. All visible skin must be inspected daily for signs of abrasion or irritation. Immediately after plaster application, the nurse should ensure that the patient's fingers or toes are thoroughly washed so that this inspection can be carried out.

Chafing and irritation are particularly likely at cast edges. Fingers, lightly dusted with talcum powder, should be used to explore the skin as far as it is possible to reach. The exploration can reveal skin eruptions and is also useful in removing plaster crumbs and debris from the cast.

Inspecting the plaster involves more than merely looking at it. The experienced nurse uses her sense of smell as well as her senses of sight or touch. Learning to use the sense of smell discerningly takes time, but occasionally even an inexperienced nurse can locate the exact position of the musty odour which may be the only sign of a plaster sore. It is sometimes possible to detect the position of an area of necrosis by the temperature of the cast, as the plaster tends to become much hotter over an area that is beginning to discharge. Other areas which are commonly vulnerable are the heel of the 'good' foot, which is used by the patient to heave himself about in bed. The elbows receive a lot friction as the patient tries to see what is going on around him. These places can be easily cared for and therefore should never be allowed to get to the stage of skin breakdown.

Arm and leg plasters

The previous section was mainly concerned with the problems associated with care of patients in large casts. There are also some important points to note about the patient wearing an arm or leg plaster.

To prevent oedema following the application of an arm or leg plaster, it is usually necessary to support the extremity in an elevated position. If oedema occurs, the doctor may require the limb to be supported in a position equal to or higher than the level of the heart.

Full arm plasters should be supported in a sling when the patient is out of bed. The weight of an unsupported cast on the shoulder is considerable and will cause the patient discomfort. The patient in an arm plaster should also be reminded to exercise the shoulder joint several times daily to avoid unnecessary stiffness.

Long leg plasters must be supported on pillows when the patient is using a bedpan; otherwise, the patient will feel insecure and uncomfortable.

Care of the patient when the plaster is removed

Although a plaster cast looks clumsy and awkward, it is in fact a highly efficient fixation apparatus. The patient himself may not realize until the cast is removed just how efficient it was. This is a difficult time for the patient. He has tolerated the long weeks needed for healing to take place and at last the day he has been waiting for arrives. The bone has healed and the plaster can be removed. Now to his consternation he is suddenly aware of many aches and pains; even minute changes of joint position will cause acute discomfort. Joint structures and muscles that have become contracted are suddenly stretched. Circulation has become sluggish, and coldness, mottling and swelling often occur. The patient is frightened to discover that, although the primary problem was the hip, it is now the knee which gives rise to pain, and he will need physical and emotional help. Joints should be supported in a relaxed position and assurance given that with time and exercise function will improve.

When a plaster has been worn for a considerable time, the skin may become covered with a dense yellow scale. This is partly dead skin and partly skin exudates. It is usually considered unwise to try to soften this loosely adherent scale or to remove it forcibly, as this will cause rawness and bleeding. The scale can be cleaned away gently and gradually over a period of several days.

Traction

Traction means the action of pulling and it involves the opposition of forces of equal strength (Fig. 2.19A).

Figure 2.19B shows one method of exerting this pull, balanced traction, which is similar to a tug-of-war, or to a dog pulling on a hand-held lead. When the opposing forces are equal, neither side can win and the pull is balanced. This is the principle used when balanced traction is applied in the treatment of orthopaedic disorders. The pull in one direction is the patient's body weight; in the other it is a weight which exactly counterbalances the patient's weight.

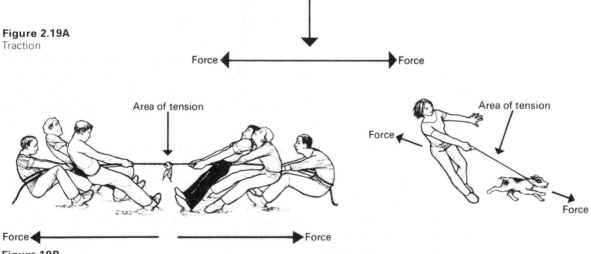

Figure 2.19A
Traction

Figure 19B
Examples of balanced traction

Neither of the methods of applying traction shown in Figure 2.20 would be practical, of course. In the first (A) the pulling forces would soon tire and have to release the pull. In the second (B) the area of tension is on the rope at the central pulley and in any case the patient would get tired and be unable to hold on to the rope. Various pieces of apparatus are therefore used so that the pulling force can be exerted on the appropriate bone or joint. For balanced traction these devices consist of:

1. A mechanism for attaching the patient to a length of cord.
2. A pulley or series of pulleys over which the cord can run.
3. A weight or several weights to counterbalance the patient's body weight.

Thus when the bed is tilted the pulley becomes the pivotal point. Gravity pulls the patient's weight in one direction but also acts upon the weight to exert the counter-pull (Fig. 2.21).

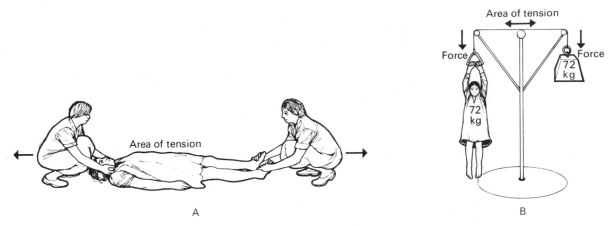

Figure 2.20
Traction: B Equal weights
A. Equal pull

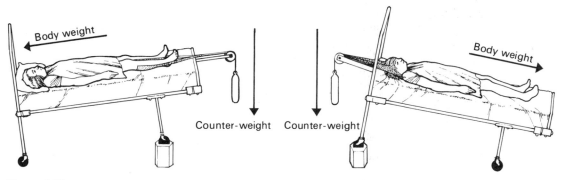

Figure 2.21
Traction: A Leg traction
B. Head traction

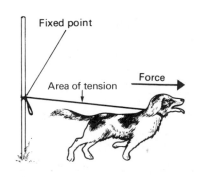

Figure 2.22
Fixed traction

Once the essential nature of traction as a system of counterbalancing forces has been grasped, it is easier to appreciate the several variations on a 'theme' which can be seen in orthopaedic practice. Balanced traction, as its name implies, is an exact counterbalancing of body weight to the pull of traction weights. Some systems increase the pull exerted by the weights by running the traction cords over a zig-zag arrangement of pulleys.

An alternative way in which the same objective can be achieved is by exerting a pull against a fixed point (fixed traction), as if a dog were pulling a lead attached to a post (Fig. 2.22). This situation can be imitated when applying traction to the upper or lower limb (Fig. 2.23). In the long term a splint is used, usually a Thomas splint (Fig. 2.24). The ring of the splint is gently pushed over the patient's leg until the ring impinges on the patient's ischial tuberosity. Then when the patient's leg is attached to the cords and the cords are secured to the W shaped bow at the lower end of the splint, the pull against the fixed point can be exerted.

Traction is used for a variety of purposes in orthopaedic work:

1. To realign fractured bone ends.
2. To realign joint surfaces which have become dislocated.
3. To overcome muscle spasm.
4. To correct deformity caused by shortened tendons or ligaments.
5. To immobilize joints.
6. To immobilize fractures.
7. To relieve weight-bearing stress on a joint.
8. To relieve pressure on a nerve or nerve root.

Traction may be of short or long duration. It will be of short duration, for instance, if the surgeon manipulates a fractured limb: this procedure is known as reduction. It will be of long duration if the surgeon chooses to immobilize a fractured shaft of femur by traction until the fracture has healed.

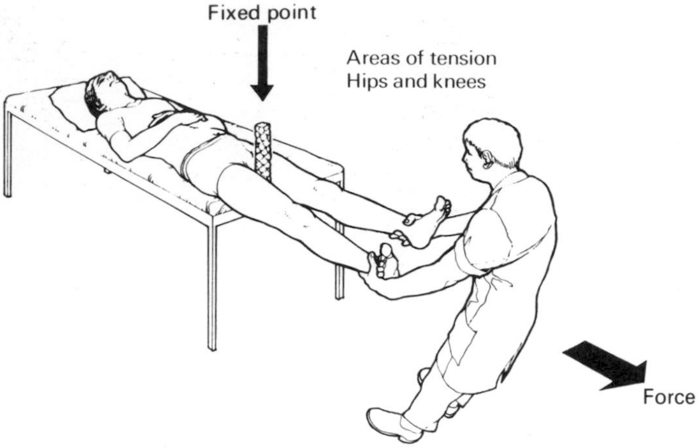

Fixed point

Areas of tension
Hips and knees

Force

Figure 2.23
Traction against a fixed point

Leather covered ring

Angle to
accommodate
greater
trochanter
of femur

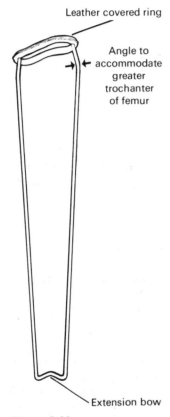

Extension bow

Figure 2.24
Thomas splint (for left
leg—front view)

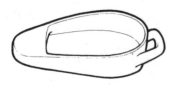

Figure 2.25
Slipper bedpan

Common methods of achieving traction

Skin traction
Traction is applied to the skin and thus indirectly to the skeletal system. Various tapes or bandages can be used to provide adhesion, allowing a pull to be exerted on the skin.

Skeletal traction
Traction is applied directly to the skeletal system using special appliances such as the Steinmann pin, Kirschner wire, or skull calipers of various makes.

Nursing care of patients on traction

Skill in the nursing care of patients on traction develops with knowledge and experience. Patients in plaster casts have their problems, but these are usually simpler than those of the patient on traction. The patient in a cast can be moved as often as required or desired for comfort or skin care without endangering the immobilized part. Patients on traction, on the other hand, usually have to be nursed in one position, commonly supine. The aim of good nursing is to keep the patient clean, comfortable and free from pressure sores or other complications of his enforced and prolonged recumbency, not the least of which may be boredom and depression.

Special thought must be given to make feeding and elimination as easy as possible. At first the patient will require assistance with feeding when lying flat. Later he will learn to feed himself if food is presented in a readily 'forkable' manner.

Certain appliances are of value in helping to overcome some of these problems. An overhead trapeze is an invaluable aid to mobility, and a sheep skin pad may help to protect sacral skin from pressure. A fracture bedpan, sometimes called a 'slipper bedpan' because of its shape (Fig. 2.25), is easier for the recumbent patient to use. Female patients often find a female urinal easier to use than a bedpan for micturition.

Ensuring the warmth and comfort of the patient on traction also requires some thought. The bed linen must often be put on in a special manner to allow the traction ropes to run freely or to accommodate a splint. This results in a series of very uncomfortable draughts for the patient. Use of warm socks and small extra blankets will help to prevent this discomfort. The patient feels exposed and vulnerable in the 'divided bed' that is necessary to accommodate traction. Normal briefs cannot be worn as they cannot be put on and removed due to the traction equipment. A special garment with side ties should therefore be provided for the patient's peace of mind. Prism spectacles (Fig. 2.26) can be used to make reading less fatiguing, and strategically positioned mirrors will help him to keep in touch with the activity around him.

Types of traction

Balanced traction
A state of traction can be achieved with a patient by using metal weights as the traction force and the patient's body weight as the counter-traction (Fig. 2.27). The degree to which the bed is elevated and the amount of weight applied will depend upon the weight

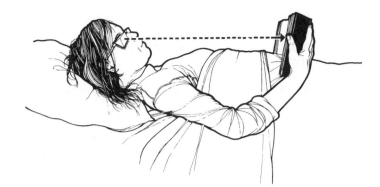

Figure 2.26
Patient using prism spectacles for reading

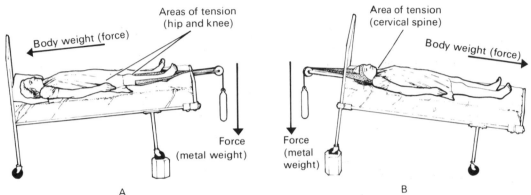

Figure 2.27
Balanced traction

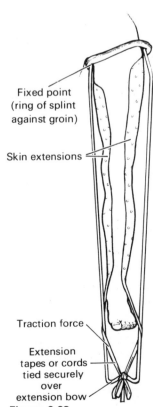

Fixed point
(ring of splint
against groin)

Skin extensions

Traction force

Extension
tapes or cords
tied securely
over
extension bow

Figure 2.28
Fixed traction (Note: the ring fits snugly into the groin, but the point of pressure (not shown) is the ischial tuberosity)

of the patient, but both must be sufficient to maintain a **balanced traction**. The patient must not slide up or be pulled down the bed by excessive weight in either direction.

There are certain points to note with balanced traction:

1. The patient is nursed in a supine position.
2. Bed elevation is maintained continuously.
3. Friction is reduced by ensuring that ropes run freely over pulleys.
4. Weights must hang free at all times.
5. No extra pillows are allowed as this increases friction and reduces traction.
6. Correct body alignment must be maintained at all times.
7. The patient must not be allowed to slip towards the head or foot of the bed.
8. The patient should be taught to move himself up the bed as and when required.

Fixed traction

An alternative method of achieving traction is to exert a pull against a fixed point. The axilla and ischial tuberosity are anatomical fixed points against which a pull may be exerted via a splint such as the Thomas leg splint (Fig. 2.28). Slings are used to support the leg in the splint, and pads are positioned to maintain the optimum position of the knee. As this splint is heavy, it is usual to arrange a system of pulleys and weights to counterbalance the weight of the splinted leg. This time the weights act as a device to aid the patient's mobility in bed and are not involved in the maintenance of traction.

There are certain points to note with fixed traction:

1. The ring of the splint must fit snugly against the ischium in order to maintain the traction. This will be achieved if the traction tapes are kept firmly tied over the extension bow at the lower end of the splint. Check twice daily.

2. The ring of the splint can exert pressure on the groin and cause tissue necrosis. To avoid this the nurse must: (a) keep the area clean and dry by 2-hourly attention, and (b) teach the patient to ease the tissue gently under the ring to a different position every hour or each time he feels discomfort, whichever is the more frequent.

3. The patient can be nursed in the sitting position with this type of traction, but he should lie flat for several hours each day to prevent hip contractures.

4. The patient should be taught how to use his arms and sound leg to increase his mobility in bed and to allow inspection of the vulnerable sacral area.

General observation of the patient on traction

1. Circulation — skin colour and joint mobility must be checked. Note any complaints of numbness, coldness or swelling of the extremity. Avoid pressure in the popliteal space.

2. Skin condition — check areas over Achilles tendon, heel, dorsum of the foot and sacral area. (Check groin and buttocks if fixed traction is being used.)

3. Body alignment and position of the extremity — is traction being achieved and maintained?

4. Counter-traction — is this efficient, or does the patient have to be regularly moved up the bed? If he does, increasing the tilt of the bed may improve matters.

5. Outer bandages and securing tapes — are these neatly and securely in position? Remove and reapply as required. (Note: The traction tapes and rubber foam bandages, should not be reapplied without specific instruction.)

6. Supporting pads and slings — are they correctly positioned to do the required job?

7. Prevention of deformity — have measures been taken to prevent foot drop, or hip flexion in the sitting patient?

8. Pressure — is there any pressure on the lateral aspect of the leg over the head of the fibula? Pressure here can damage the lateral popliteal nerve and so cause foot drop.

9. Comfort — traction should never be a source of discomfort for the patient. Listen carefully and investigate promptly every complaint.

10. Complications — hypostatic pneumonia is a constant threat to the patient, especially if he is elderly. Encourage deep breathing and regular coughing. Ensure adequate fluid intake.

General exercise of the joints and muscles not immobilized by traction is vitally important and the nurse plays a large part in this task by her teaching, encouragement and frequent reminders. Diversional therapy cannot be overemphasized since the orthopaedic patient, being closely confined to bed for an extended period, quickly becomes bored and depressed.

Application of principles

Throughout this chapter an attempt has been made to give broad outlines of some of the more important aspects of body mechanics related to function. It is to be hoped that the thinking nurse can apply these principles to a variety of situations and patients other than those with disorders of the locomotor system. Specific details of particular diseases and conditions have been deliberately avoided as the nurse needing a deeper knowledge would be advised to study a more specialized text in order to develop the art of orthopaedic nursing.

A knowledge and appreciation of the principles of orthopaedic care can serve the nurse well in her own life as well as in the treatment of her patients. Maintenance of a healthy musculoskeletal system is vital for everyone, not only those who have suffered injury or disease to bones or joints.

SUGGESTED ASSIGNMENTS

1. How would you attempt to maintain muscle tone in a bedfast or chairfast patient? How far could these measures be used by a relative caring for a patient at home?

2. Observe the nursing staff with whom you work for two spans of duty. List the number of occasions and the circumstances in which there is particular danger of backstrain.

3. For each patient in your care list the most likely complications which could be prevented by nursing measures. How would you put such measures into operation?

4. Examine the various types of chair (upright, wheel or easy) in the unit in which you are working. What alterations in design or size would be needed to ensure that all the patients who use them are comfortable and correctly supported?

5. What housing alterations or aids might be needed to help an active young married woman who, as the result of a road accident, is suddenly faced with permanent loss of power in one arm?

6. Prepare a list of conditions other than obvious bone and joint disorders, which have had an adverse effect on the mobility of patients you have nursed.

FURTHER READING

Apley A G 1977 A system of orthopaedics and fractures, 5th edn. Butterworth, London
Larson C B, Gould M 1978 Orthopedic nursing, 9th edn. Mosby, St. Louis
Pearson J R, Austin R T 1977 Accident surgery and orthopaedics for students. Lloyd Luke, London
Pollen A G 1973 Fractures and dislocations in children. Churchill Livingstone, Edinburgh
Powell M 1976 Orthopaedic nursing, 7th edn. Churchill Livingstone, Edinburgh
Roaf F R, Hodkinson L J 1979 Textbook of orthopaedic nursing, 3rd edn. Blackwell Scientific, Oxford
Rowe J W, Dyer L (eds) 1977 Care of the orthopaedic patient. Blackwell Scientific, Oxford
Webb J T 1977 Notes on orthopaedic nursing. Churchill Livingstone, Edinburgh

3. The Nervous System

In order to give nursing care to patients suffering from the effects of injury to, or disease of, the nervous system and, equally important, to appreciate the significance of observations which the nurse will be asked to make, an understanding of the structures involved and how they function is essential.

ANATOMY AND PHYSIOLOGY

Nerve tissue is made up of millions of nerve cells and their processes. These are the functional units of the nervous system and they are supported by a connective tissue called glia.

1. Neurones. These nerve cells vary in size and shape, each consisting of a cell body containing a nucleus imbedded in protoplasm. Processes arise from the cell, a number of short ones called dendrites and a long one called the axon or nerve fibre.

Impulses are received by the dendrites, transmitted to the cell body and conducted from the cell body by the axon.

The dendrites and axon have similar structures:

  a. A delicate central fibre called the axis cylinder.
  b. The myelin sheath composed of adipose tissue. A number of nerve fibres do not have a myelin sheath and are described as non-myelinated. In order that impulses may be transmitted along myelinated fibres the myelin sheath is absent at intervals and these spaces are known as the Nodes of Ranvier.
  c. The neurilemma is a delicate membrane surrounding the myelin sheath of the peripheral nerves only i.e. those found outwith the skull and vertebral column.

The myelin sheath has several functions:

  i. to protect the axis cylinder.
  ii. to act as an insulator.
  iii. to stimulate transmission of impulse through the nerve fibre (Fig. 3.1).

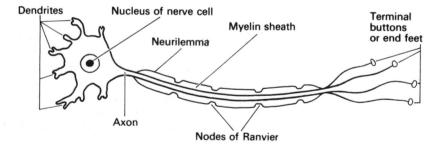

Figure 3.1
A neurone

2. The Glia This is a tissue, consisting of cells and fibres, found in the brain and spinal cord. There are three types of glial cells, astrocytes, oligodendrocytes and microglia. Their collective functions are to protect, support and nourish the neurones.

Nerve tissue has two properties.

Irritability. The ability to respond to stimulation which is partly electrical and partly chemical.

Conductivity. The ability to transmit an impulse.

Generation of a nerve impulse. The propagation of a nerve impulse is an electrochemical process. The nerve cell has a 'resting potential' of −70 millivolts (mV). The axon membrane separates the extracellular fluid (rich in sodium ions Na⁺) from the intracellular fluid (rich in potassium ions K⁺). In the resting state the axon membrane is relatively impermeable to sodium, and the 'sodium pump', a metabolic process, excretes any sodium entering the nerve cell. An impulse begins with the axon membrane becoming permeable to sodium ions, which then pass in. They take with them positive charges which alter the cell potential from −70mV to +40mV, and this change is termed an 'action potential'. Immediately following this an equal number of potassium ions leave the cell and the potential returns to −70mV thus restoring the electrical status quo. When the impulse passes, sodium is pumped out and potassium returns to the cell thus restoring the chemical status quo. These alterations in the state of the axon membrane are propagated along the nerve. A nerve impulse lasts about 1 millisecond during which the complete process occurs (Figs 3.2 and 3.3).

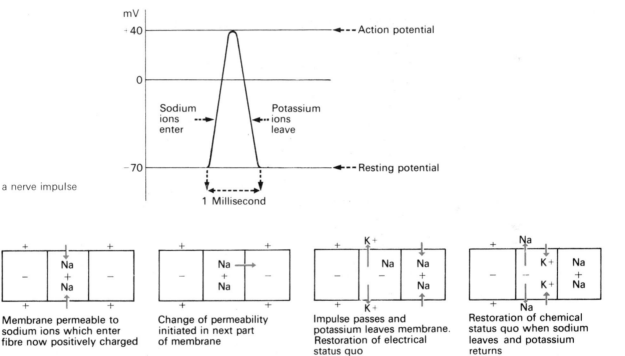

Figure 3.2
Generation of a nerve impulse

Figure 3.3
Transmission of a nerve impulse

Chemical transmitters and the synapse. There is no anatomical continuity between neurones. The axon of one neurone divides into small branches that terminate in small swellings called the terminal buttons or end feet. These lie in close proximity to the dendrites of the next neurone. The action potential of the cell i.e. +40mV is not strong enough to permit passage of impulse over this synapse and a chemical bridge is necessary. The terminal button manufactures and stores a chemical transmitter. There are a number of chemicals known to act as transmitters such as acetylcholine, noradrenaline and dopamine.

When an impulse arrives at the terminal button the chemical transmitter is released which excites the next neurone and initiates another impulse. The released chemical is then neutralised by enzymes which ensure that the synapse remains inactive prior to the arrival of another impulse. The synapses between neurones, and those between neurones and structures they supply, function in the same manner (Fig. 3.4).

Functionally, the nervous system can be divided into two parts:

1. **Somatic system** — this part is under voluntary control.

2. **Autonomic system** — controls smooth muscle, cardiac muscle and the secretory glands of the body.

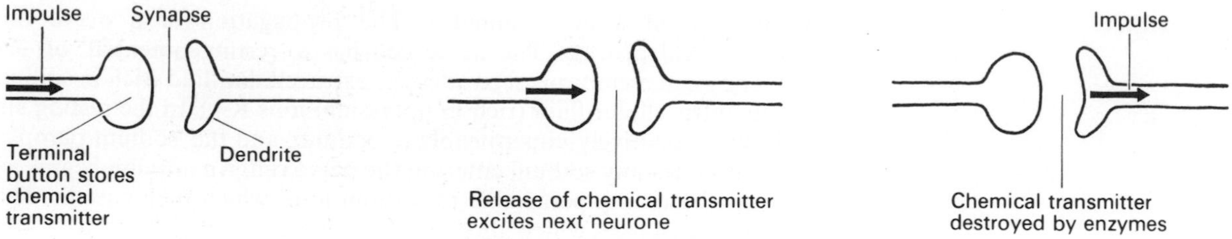

Impulse   Synapse

Terminal
button stores
chemical
transmitter

Dendrite

Release of chemical transmitter
excites next neurone

Impulse

Chemical transmitter
destroyed by enzymes

Figure 3.4
Chemical transmitter and a
synapse

The skull

The brain is contained within a rigid bone structure called the skull.

The skull is divided into three compartments: the **anterior**, **middle** and **posterior fossae** (singular: fossa, meaning, in Latin, a ditch).

Attached to the under surface of the skull is a white inelastic membrane called the **dura** (p. 73). Folds of this membrane, called the **tentorium cerebelli**, separate the anterior and middle fossae from the posterior fossa. Further folds of the membrane, called the **falx** (in Latin, a sickle), incompletely separate the anterior and middle fossae (Fig. 3.5).

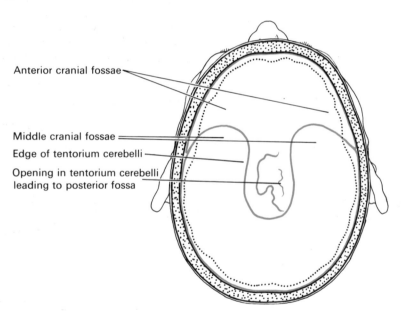

Anterior cranial fossae

Middle cranial fossae

Edge of tentorium cerebelli

Opening in tentorium cerebelli
leading to posterior fossa

Figure 3.5
Horizontal section of skull
showing cranial fossae

The brain

The brain can be anatomically divided into three parts: the **cerebrum**, the **cerebellum** and the **brain stem**.

The cerebrum

This forms the largest part of the brain and is divided by the falx into two hemispheres, the **left** and **right cerebral hemispheres**. The hemispheres are connected by a group of nerve fibres called the **corpus callosum** situated deep within the cerebrum. The cerebral hemispheres are divided into lobes — the **frontal, parietal, temporal** and **occipital lobes**. The lines of demarcation of these lobes are not exact.

The outer part is composed mainly of nerve cells (grey matter) and is called the **cerebral cortex**. The lobes are connected by **nerve fibres** or tracts (white matter). An important area situated within the cerebrum is the **internal capsule**. This consists of nerve fibres which either transmit nerve impulses from the body to the cerebral cortex (sensory) or from the cerebral cortex to the body (motor) (Fig. 3.6). A haemorrhage

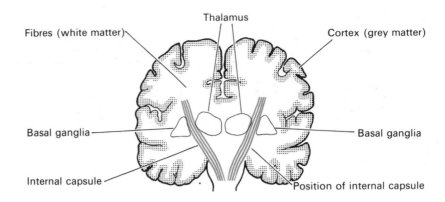

Figure 3.6
Coronal section of brain

within the internal capsule may interrupt the pathway of nerve impulses controlling voluntary movement, resulting in paralysis of muscles. Most cerebrovascular accidents (strokes) result from bleeding within the internal capsule.

The outer surface of the cerebrum consists of elevations called **gyri** (singular: gyrus) and of depressions called **sulci** (singular: sulcus). A well-defined sulcus, the **central sulcus**, separates the frontal from the parietal lobe. Immediately posterior to the central sulcus lies the **postcentral gyrus**, which is the site of the sensory cortex. Anterior to the central sulcus is the **precentral** gyrus, which is the site of the motor cortex (Fig. 3.7).

One cerebral hemisphere tends to be dominant, and in the right-handed person this is the left hemisphere. The left hemisphere controls movement on the right side of the body and the right hemisphere controls movement on the left.

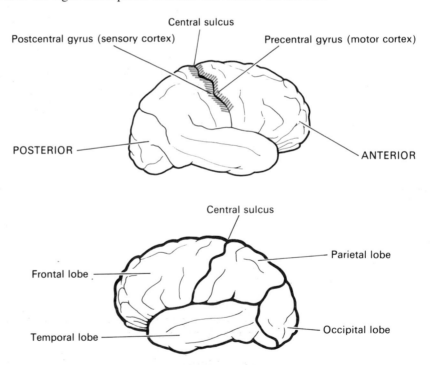

Figure 3.7
Cerebrum: right lateral view

Figure 3.8
Lobes of the cerebrum

The functions of the cerebrum can be subdivided according to the lobular divisions (Fig. 3.8).

The frontal lobes occupy the anterior fossa. The anterior portions are concerned with behaviour, learning, creative thinking, personality, emotional responses, memory and ethical values. The posterior portions initiate the motor function by which movement occurs in the opposite side of the body. The dominant hemisphere is responsible for speech.

The temporal lobes occupy the front portion of the middle fossa and receive impulses from the special senses of smell, taste and hearing. The temporal lobe of the dominant hemisphere is important for understanding the spoken word.

The occipital lobes occupy the rear portion of the middle fossa and are concerned with vision.

The parietal lobes lie behind the frontal, above the temporal and in front of the occipital lobes. Each receives sensory impulses from the skin, muscles, joints and tendons of the opposite side of the body. The cortex of these lobes can recognize the size, shape, texture and consistency of an object.

The cerebellum

This occupies the posterior fossa and lies below the occipital lobes from which it is separated by the tentorium. It consists of two hemispheres and a central section called the **vermis** (worm-like). The surface is composed of grey matter. The white matter under the surface presents a branched appearance called the **arbor vitae** (tree of life). Collections of nerve fibres called **cerebellar peduncles** (tracts) connect the cerebrum, cerebellum and brain stem (Fig. 3.9).

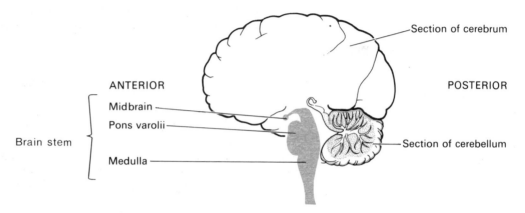

Figure 3.9
Cerebrum, cerebellum and brain stem: relationships

The cerebellum controls balance and co-ordination of voluntary muscle movements. Impulses are received from muscles and joints indicating their position in relation to the body, and impulses from the semicircular canals in the ears indicate the position of the head in space.

By influencing the contractions of skeletal muscles the cerebellum maintains balance and ensures smooth and precise actions.

The brain stem

This lies deep in the midline. It is an elongated structure which passes from the cerebrum through an opening in the tentorium called the tentorial hiatus and enters the posterior fossa where it connects with the cerebellum. Anatomically it can be divided into three parts (Fig. 3.9):

1. **The midbrain** lies below the cerebrum and is composed of two groups of nerve cells and nerve fibres called the **cerebral peduncles**. It is by means of these peduncles that nerve impulses pass from the cerebrum to the cerebellum and spinal cord, and from the cerebellum and spinal cord to the cerebrum.

2. **The pons varolii** lies below the midbrain and anterior to the cerebellum. It is composed mainly of nerve fibres which connect the two hemispheres of the cerebellum and allow communication between the cerebral cortex and the spinal cord.

3. **The medulla oblongata** lies below the pons varolii and is continuous with the spinal cord. The outer part consists of nerve fibres which run to and from the higher areas of the brain and the spinal cord. The inner part consists of nerve cells some of which act as relay stations for sensory nerves travelling to the cerebrum.

Deep within the medulla are groups of cells associated with involuntary reflex activities called the **vital centres**. These are:

The **respiratory centre** which controls the depth and rate of respirations.

The **cardiac centre** which controls the force and rate of contractions of the heart.

The **vasomotor centre** which controls the calibre of blood vessels, particularly arterioles.

This area also contains the reflex centres of coughing, sneezing, swallowing and vomiting.

Travelling from the medulla through the brain stem and up to the cerebral cortex is a network of nerve cells and their fibres. This network is called the **reticular formation**. If all sensory impulses reaching the body were sent to the brain it would be, literally, swamped. The function of the reticular formation is to determine which sensory impulses will be allowed to reach the cerebral cortex. A state of arousal within the cerebral cortex is activated by the reticular formation. Any factor which impairs the function of this network (for example, head injury) will prevent sensory information reaching the cerebral cortex and a state of unconsciousness will result.

Motor pathways

Although the motor pathways should be considered as an integrated system, it can best be understood if considered in two parts working in co-ordination:

1. The corticobulbar and corticospinal tracts collectively known as the *pyramidal tract*
2. All other pathways involved in motor activity are described as *the extrapyramidal tract*

1. *The pyramidal tract*

This pathway probably arises in many parts of the cerebral cortex, but predominantly within the motor area of the cerebral cortex of the precentral gyrus. Present are large pyramidal shaped cells — Betz cells — which are considered to give rise to the axons of the pathway. The fibres pass through the internal capsule to the mid brain. It is within the internal capsule that fibres pass through the pons varolii to the medulla. Within the medulla on each side of the midline is a ridge called The Pyramids. It was the presence of fibres in this area which gave rise to the name of pyramidal tract. During the passage through the brain stem, fibres are given off to the motor nuclei of cranial nerves. While all fibres will cross in the medulla to innervate motor nuclei on opposite side, there are instances where the fibre sends a branch to innervate the motor nuclei on same side as in the motor nucleus of the branch of the facial nerve controlling the upper part of the face. An appreciation of this will explain the following feature. If, for example, there is interference to the pathway from the left hemisphere affecting fibres to facial nerves, then paralysis of the right side of the face occurs. However, as the branch to the upper part of the face is also innervated by fibres from the pathway from the right hemisphere i.e. the same side, the muscles of the upper part of the face are not affected.

The components of tracks innervating the cranial nerve nuclei are called the corticobulbar tracts to distinguish them from fibres going to the spinal cord — the corticospinal tracts — but otherwise there is little else to distinguish them (Fig. 3.10).

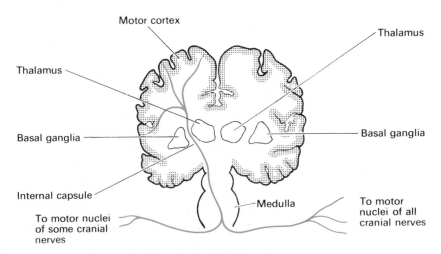

Figure 3.10
The corticobulbar tracts

Approximately 85 per cent of fibres of the corticospinal tracts cross within the medulla in the decussation of the pyramids to the opposite side then descend in the white matter of the spinal cord between the anterior and posterior columns of grey matter. The remaining fibres descend in the white matter between the anterior columns of grey matter and cross to the opposite side at the level of termination (Fig. 3.11). The corticospinal tracts terminate either

    a. Around Alpha cells in the anterior column of grey matter.
    b. Around an internuncial neurone which synapses with Alpha cells. Alpha cells innervate muscle fibres of voluntary muscles.

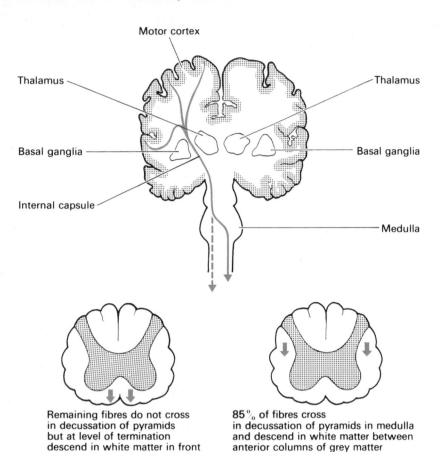

Figure 3.11
The corticospinal tracts

Remaining fibres do not cross in decussation of pyramids but at level of termination descend in white matter in front

85% of fibres cross in decussation of pyramids in medulla and descend in white matter between anterior columns of grey matter

2. The Extrapyramidal tract

In the past the extrapyramidal tract was thought to consist of all pathways excluding those of the pyramidal tract. However both anatomical and physiological separation are becoming increasingly more difficult and the tract has come to be considered as a functional rather than an anatomical unit. The tract is composed of fibres arising from:

    i. wide spread areas of the cortex but especially frontal and parietal lobes.
    ii. the cerebellum.
    iii. the basal ganglia.

The basal ganglia consists of several masses of grey matter embedded in the white matter of the cerebral hemispheres. The term 'basal ganglia' is used most frequently to denote motor nuclei that are closely related functionally.

The **corpus striatum** is the major centre in the extrapyramidal tract and is divided into the lenticular nucleus and the caudate nucleus. While the division is of secondary importance in respect of function an understanding of anatomical relationship is of value. The lenticular nucleus is wedge-shaped and about the size of a Brazil nut. The narrow part is called the globus pallidus (pale globe) and the lateral portion is called the putamen (Fig. 3.12).

The caudate nucleus consists of a head which tapers into a slender tail. The head bulges into the anterior horn of lateral ventricle and the first part of the tail lies along the floor of the lateral ventricle and then extends forward to the temporal lobe

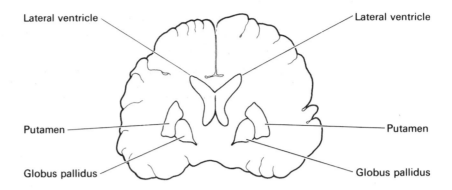

Figure 3.12
The lenticlear nucleus of the corpus striatum

Lateral ventricle — Lateral ventricle

Putamen — — Putamen

Globus pallidus — Globus pallidus

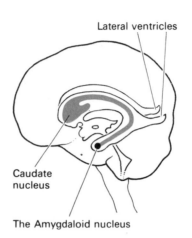

Lateral ventricles

Figure 3.13
The caudate nucleus

Caudate nucleus

The Amygdaloid nucleus

terminating at the amygdaloid nucleus. The caudate nucleus and amygdaloid nucleus have no functional relationship (Fig. 3.13).

There are many afferent and efferent intranuclear connections within the corpus striatum.

The particular contribution of the corpus striatum to motor function is poorly understood, but it is seen to participate in three ways:

a. it may provide for motor activity of an autonomic type including response to emotion.
b. to relay influence of cerebral cortex on voluntary muscles.
c. to exercise an influence on fibres of the pyramidal and extrapyramidal tracts.

Fibres arising from the cortex, cerebellum and basal ganglia form tracts which descend in the white matter of the spinal cord. The tracts terminate around Gamma cells in the anterior column of grey matter (Fig. 3.14).

The extrapyramidal tract exerts its influence by modifying the muscle fibres in the muscle spindle thereby modifying response to change in tension. Without such influence, normal smooth movements would be impossible and maintenance of posture and balance would be severely affected.

The final common pathway

The pyramidal pathways convey impulses to the large Alpha cells whose axons are distributed to muscle fibres of motor units. The extrapyramidal pathways convey impulses to the smaller Gamma cells whose axons are distributed to the muscle spindle in muscle fibres.

The alpha neurone is called the final common pathway.

Influences descending in pyramidal and extrapyramidal tracts constitute the *upper motor neurone.*

The alpha neurone or final common pathway constitutes the *lower motor neurone* (Fig. 3.15).

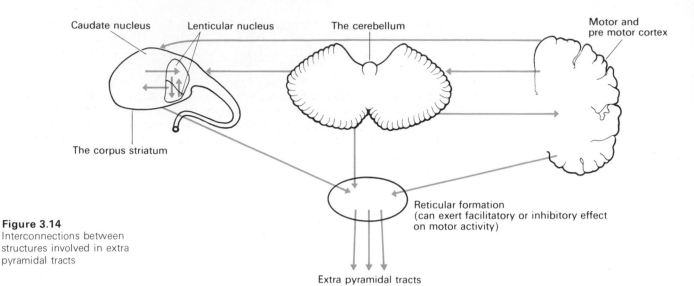

Figure 3.14
Interconnections between structures involved in extra pyramidal tracts

The sensory pathways

In order that we may be made aware of our internal and external environment, sensations must reach the sensory area of the brain. Sensory nerves bring such information from the skin and deeper structures.

Within the skin are four types of receptors which are sensitive to touch, pain, cold and heat. From the joint capsules, receptors convey information about position of joints in space, and from the muscle spindles information concerning degree of contraction of muscles. These nerves are called proprioceptors. The deeper structures also contain nerves transmitting sensations of pain.

The stimuli will either travel via the sensory cranial nerves (from the head) or the peripheral spinal nerves (from remainder of body).

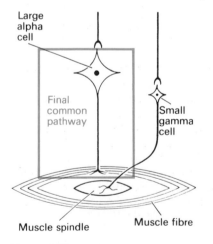

Figure 3.15
The final common pathway

Figure 3.16
Cross section of spinal cord

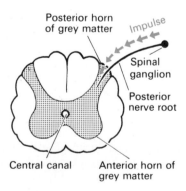

Sensory nerve cells arise in the spinal ganglia which lie outside the spinal cord and the nerve fibres travel to the posterior horn of grey matter in the spinal cord. The sensory fibres outside the spinal cord form the posterior nerve root and are separate from the motor fibres. When receptors are stimulated impulses are transmitted to the posterior nerve root and from there conveyed to the posterior horn of grey matter (Fig. 3.16).

The nature of the sensation being transmitted to the brain will determine the pathway taken.

The posterior tracts

Nerves conveying sensations of touch or proprioception (i.e. sense of position of joints and muscles) enter the posterior horn cells of grey matter. They ascend the spinal cord in the posterior column of white matter to the medulla. In the medulla they synapse with a second group of nerves which cross to the opposite side — sensory decussation —and travel to the thalamus. In the thalamus a synapse occurs with a third group of nerves which travel to the sensory area of the cortex (Fig. 3.17).

The anterior tracts
Nerves conveying sensations of pressure, pain and temperature enter the posterior horn cells of grey matter. They synapse with a second group of nerves which cross to the opposite side and ascend in the anterolateral columns of white matter to the thalamus. These fibres have already crossed and there is no decussation in the medulla. In the thalamus, a synapse occurs with a third group of nerves which travel to the sensory area of the cortex (Fig. 3.17).

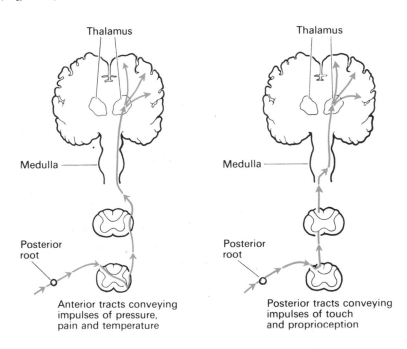

Figure 3.17
The sensory pathways

Thalamus

Thalamus

Medulla

Medulla

Posterior root

Posterior root

Anterior tracts conveying impulses of pressure, pain and temperature

Posterior tracts conveying impulses of touch and proprioception

Tracts which travel from spinal cord to thalamus are called the spinothalamic tracts, and those from thalamus to sensory cortex, the thalamocortical tracts.

The thalamus As already stated the term 'basal ganglia' is used most frequently to denote motor nuclei that are closely related functionally, and some of these nuclei have been mentioned when discussing the extrapyramidal tract. Another mass of nerve cells forming part of the basal ganglia is the thalamus. These are situated below the corpus callosum. All sensory impulses are conveyed to the thalamus which is thought to perceive sensation but is unable to discriminate between or interpret these stimuli. There may be some crude appreciation of sensation but this is debatable. If pain occurs, the thalamus has a 'perception of pain' but the cerebral cortex analyses information in terms of locality, intensity and nature of pain.

The meninges
These consist of three membranes which cover the brain and spinal cord (Fig. 3.18).

1. **The dura** (hard) is a white inelastic membrane consisting of two layers of fibrous tissue. The outer layer is attached to the under surface of the skull and the inner layer covers and protects the brain and spinal cord. It is the inner one which forms the tentorium cerebelli and falx.

Between the two layers are sinuses which allow drainage of venous blood from the brain. These are called the *venous sinuses*.

2. **The arachnoid** (spider-like) lies immediately under the dura and is a serous membrane. Web-like processes extend from the arachnoid to the third membrane, the pia. Separating the dura from the arachnoid is a potential space called the **subdural space**.

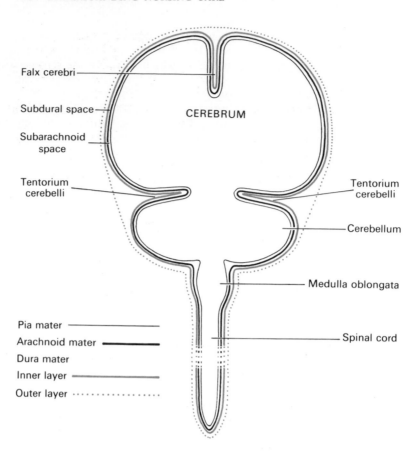

Falx cerebri

Subdural space

Subarachnoid space

CEREBRUM

Tentorium cerebelli

Tentorium cerebelli

Cerebellum

Medulla oblongata

Pia mater

Arachnoid mater

Dura mater

Inner layer

Outer layer

Spinal cord

Figure 3.18
The meninges

3. **The pia** (tender) is a delicate membrane which is firmly attached to the brain and consists mainly of small blood vessels.

Between the arachnoid and pia is a space called the **subarachnoid space**, which is filled with **cerebrospinal fluid (CSF).**

The ventricles

At the centre of the cerebrum are two irregular-shaped cavities, one in each hemisphere. These are the **left** and **right lateral ventricles**. Each lateral ventricle communicates with the third ventricle via an opening called the **interventricular foramen**. The third ventricle communicates with the fourth ventricle via a canal called the **aqueduct of the midbrain**, which lies between the medulla and cerebellum. The fourth ventricle is continuous with the central canal of the spinal cord.

Formation, circulation and absorption of CSF

Cerebrospinal fluid is formed from the blood by the action of vascular processes called choroid plexuses which are found in the lateral, third and fourth ventricles. It is a modified form of plasma consisting of water, protein, glucose, minerals and a few lymphocytes.

The circulation of CSF commences in the lateral ventricles from where it flows into the third ventricle, through the interventricular foramen and then into the fourth ventricle via the aqueduct of the midbrain. It leaves the roof of the fourth ventricle by two openings called the **medial and lateral foramina** and enters the subarachnoid space. As the fourth ventricle is continuous with the central canal of the spinal cord, cerebrospinal fluid also flows into the central canal (Fig. 3.19). It is absorbed back into the venous circulation through projections in the arachnoid called arachnoid villi to the jugular veins and back to the heart. Any obstruction within the ventricular system will result in impairment in flow of CSF, the ventricles will dilate and intracranial pressure will increase.

The composition of CSF is standard but changes occur in disease.

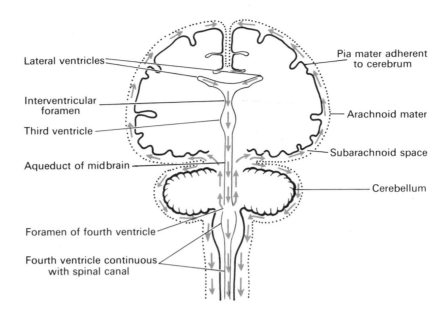

Figure 3.19
Flow of cerebrospinal fluid
(CSF)

The pressure range is 60 to 180 mm of water, the specific gravity of water being identical to that of CSF. Examination of this fluid can therefore be an important aid in diagnosis.

The cranial nerves

Arising from the brain are 12 pairs of cranial nerves (Table 3.1). Some are sensory, some motor and some consist of both sensory and motor fibres. To avoid confusion it should be mentioned that certain cranial nerves carry fibres from the autonomic system, but the cranial nerves, in themselves, form part of the somatic system.

The spinal cord

The spinal cord, a direct continuation of the medulla oblongata, lies within the vertebral canal and, like the brain, is surrounded by the meninges. The spinal cord extends from the first cervical to the first or second lumbar vertebra. The cord is divided into segments, 8 cervical, 12 thoracic, 5 lumbar, 5 sacral and 1 coccygeal. The centre of the spinal cord contains **grey matter**, composed of nerve cells, grouped in the shape of an H, surrounded by **white matter** (nerve fibres) arranged in tracts. In the centre of the spinal cord is the **central canal**, a continuation of the fourth ventricle. This canal is normally obliterated in whole or in part. The posterior limbs of the H are known as the **posterior horns** and the anterior limbs as the **anterior horns** of grey matter (Fig. 3.20).

The anterior horns contain the cell bodies of the lower motor neurones. They receive voluntary motor impulses from the motor cortex of the brain via the upper motor neurones, which descend in the lateral columns of the spinal cord as the **pyramidal or corticospinal tracts** (Fig. 3.21). The axons of the lower motor neurones leave the spinal cord by the anterior nerve roots and reach the organ innervated by the peripheral nerves. The transmitted substance released at nerve endings is acetylcholine. The posterior horn cells receive sensory impulses from the periphery via the peripheral nerves and the posterior nerve root. Thus the spinal cord conveys motor impulses from the brain and sensory impulses to the brain via tracts of white matter. Thirty-one pairs of spinal nerves arise from the spinal cord and emerge from the vertebral canal through the intervertebral foramina (Fig. 3.22).

A motor response to a sensory stimulus, which occurs without reference to the brain is called a reflex response; the withdrawal of a limb from a painful stimulus, coughing and the tendon reflexes are examples. If the tendon of the quadriceps muscle is stretched by tapping with a tendon hammer, the sensory stimulus passes centrally in the peripheral nerve and posterior nerve root and activates the anterior horn cells. They respond by passing motor impulses to the quadriceps muscle via the anterior roots and

Table 3.1
The cranial nerves

Number	Name	Type	Function
1	Olfactory	Sensory	Convey sense of smell.
2	Optic	Sensory	Convey sense of vision
3	Oculomotor	Motor	Control muscles which move eye up, in and down Carry **parasympathetic** fibres which constrict circular muscles of iris
4	Trochlear	Motor	Control muscles which move eye downwards and outwards
5	Trigeminal	Mixed	Sensory: convey sensations of pain, temperature and pressure from head and face Motor: innervate muscles of mastication
6	Abducent	Motor	Control muscles which move eye outward
7	Facial	Mixed	Sensory: convey perception of taste from anterior two-thirds of tongue Motor: control muscles of face Carry **parasympathetic** fibres which stimulate salivary and lacrimal glands
8	Acoustic (2 parts): — Cochlear — Vestibular	Sensory	Cochlear: convey perception of sound Vestibular: fibres from semicircular canal of ear convey impulses to cerebellum and assist in maintaining body equilibrium
9	Glosso-pharyngeal	Mixed	Sensory: convey perception of taste from posterior third of tongue and sensation from soft palate and tonsils Motor: innervate muscles of pharynx and control swallowing Carry **parasympathetic** fibres to parotid glands
10	Vagus	Mixed	Sensory: convey impulses from respiratory and digestive structures and back of ear. Motor: control voluntary muscles of pharynx and larynx. Individual groups of **parasympathetic** fibres: 1. stimulate peristalsis and control secretions from digestive tract, liver, gall-bladder, pancreas and kidneys 2. control constriction of bronchi and bronchioles 3. decrease rate and force of heart beat
11	Accessory	Motor	Control sternomastoid and trapezius muscles Fibres travel with vagus nerve to supply muscles of pharynx and larynx
12	Hypoglossal	Motor	Control muscles of tongue

peripheral nerve causing the muscle to contract. This is an example of a simple segmental reflex arc (Fig. 3.23). More elaborate reflex actions may involve many segments of the cord at many different levels.

Although the spinal cord ends at the level of the first lumbar vertebra, the spinal meninges extend as low as the second sacral vertebra. The spinal nerves arising from the lower end of the cord hang down within the theca until they leave at their appropriate levels (theca, space containing CSF formed by the meninges). These nerve fibres form the **cauda equina**, so called because they resemble a horse's tail.

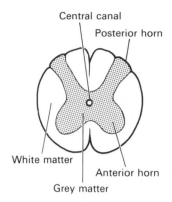

Figure 3.20
Section through spinal cord

Central canal
Posterior horn
White matter
Anterior horn
Grey matter

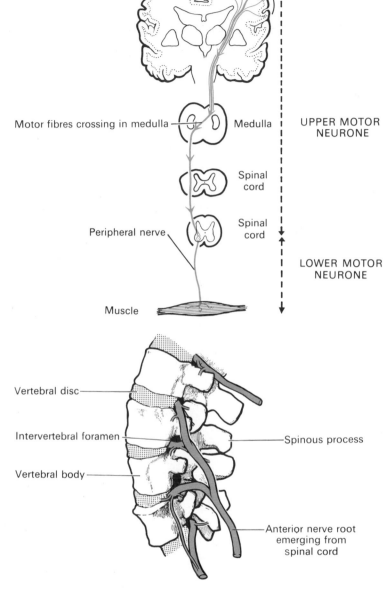

MOTOR CORTEX

Motor fibres crossing in medulla — Medulla

UPPER MOTOR NEURONE

Spinal cord

Spinal cord

Peripheral nerve

LOWER MOTOR NEURONE

Muscle

Figure 3.21
Pyramidal tract

Vertebral disc

Intervertebral foramen

Vertebral body

Spinous process

Anterior nerve root emerging from spinal cord

Figure 3.22
Spinal nerves emerging through intervertebral foramina

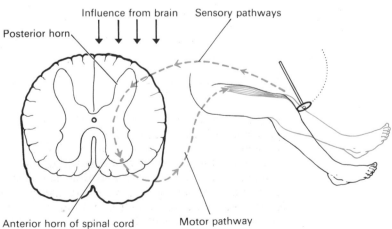

Influence from brain   Sensory pathways

Posterior horn

Anterior horn of spinal cord   Motor pathway

Figure 3.23
Simple segmental reflex arc (knee jerk)

The autonomic system

The spinal cord also transmits autonomic nervous impulses. They are called autonomic because they are not subject to voluntary control. The autonomic nervous system consists of two parts:

1. A sympathetic component
2. A parasympathetic component.

Sympathetic nerve fibres

These leave the cord with the motor fibres between the first thoracic and second lumbar segments. They soon leave the motor fibres and join the sympathetic chain, branches of which go to the blood vessels, air passages, digestive tract, bladder and bowel. The sympathetic system is particularly active in states of stress and fear. A chemical transmitter substance, noradrenaline, is released at sympathetic nerve endings causing the pupils to dilate, the heart to accelerate, skin and blood vessels to constrict thus increasing blood pressure.

Parasympathetic nerve fibres

These leave the central nervous system with some of the cranial and sacral nerves. The cranial outflow includes the vagus nerve, which supplies most of the internal organs. This system is sometimes called the 'emptying system' as it speeds up digestion of foodstuffs and plays an important part in defaecation and micturition. The parasympathetic activating substance is acetylcholine.

In most cases the actions of the sympathetic and parasympathetic nerve fibres are mutually antagonistic, circumstances determining which action will predominate at any given time.

An anterior and two posterior spinal arteries extend the length of the cord getting additional supply from branches of the aorta (Fig. 3.24). The anterior artery gives off branches which encircle the cord anastomosing with the posterior spinal arteries. At various intervals another branch leaves the anterior spinal artery and supplies the substance of the cord.

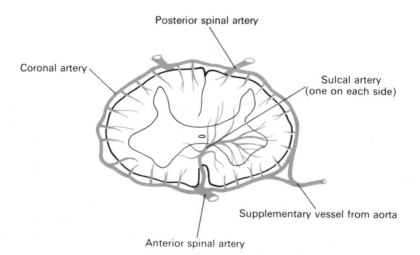

Figure 3.24
Segment of spinal cord: blood supply

DISORDERS OF THE NERVOUS SYSTEM
Head Injuries

Head injuries are usually caused by either the head coming to a sudden stop after travelling at a considerable speed (someone falling from a height and coming to an abrupt halt on reaching the ground) or an object travelling at speed striking the head (a metal fragment from a bomb explosion).

A series of events can then occur.

There can be a fracture of the skull either at the point of impact or at a point distant from it. If a blood vessel is ruptured blood will escape and result in the formation of a blood clot between the skull and the dura. Movement of the skull may separate the dura from the brain and cause rupture of blood vessels passing between them. This is an **extradural haemorrhage** (Fig. 3.25A).

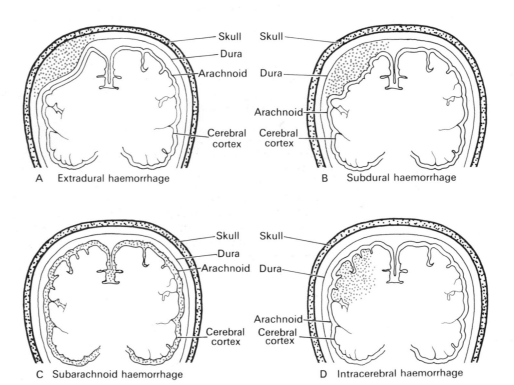

Figure 3.25A–D
Types of intracranial haemorrhage

Although the skull comes to a halt, the brain continues to travel within it. The brain strikes one side of the skull then moves in the opposite direction to strike the other side. This is known as the **contra coup** (opposite to blow) injury and as a result both sides of the brain suffer.

Several injuries can result from this movement of the brain:

1. Blood vessels passing from the cerebral cortex to the dura may rupture resulting in a **subdural haemorrhage** (Fig. 3.25B).
2. Any ruptured blood vessel on the surface of the brain or passing through the subarachnoid space may bleed into the subarachnoid space resulting in a **subarachnoid haemorrhage** (Fig. 3.25C).
3. The force may be sufficient to cause tearing of blood vessels within the brain resulting in an **intracerebral haemorrhage (**Fig. 3.25D).
4. The brain may be bruised; this is called **contusion**. If the brain is bruised, swelling can occur resulting in an increase in intracranial pressure.
5. Movement of the cerebrum can cause a transient distortion of the brain stem which results in loss of consciousness. This is known as **concussion**. If damage is slight then loss of consciousness will be temporary; if severe then a state of prolonged loss of consciousness will result.

As the maximum damage to the brain always occurs at the time of the accident, an improvement in the patient's condition will normally follow unless recovery is complicated by a rise in intracranial pressure.

Investigations

Two techniques used routinely as an aid to diagnosis of the damage sustained following a head injury are:

Echoencephalography

This utilizes sound as a basis. Ultrasonic impulses from a machine called an ultrasonic diasonoscope are directed through the patient's skull. The bones of the skull and the midline structures of the brain act as reflectors and will reflect a number of these impulses back to their initial source. These reflected impulses are seen on a screen and can be photographed. Any shift in the midline structures of the brain from, say, the pressure of a blood clot, will be demonstrated (Fig. 3.26).

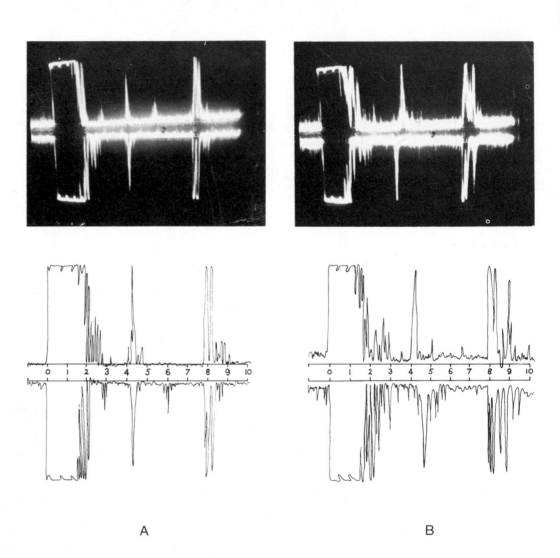

A   B

Figure 3.26
Echoencephalogram
A. Normal B. Midline
shift to left

The advantages of this procedure are that no special preparation of the patient is necessary and it is rapid and safe.

Angiography

This entails the injection of a radio-opaque contrast medium into the carotid artery or the vertebral artery during which radiographs are taken. The films will demonstrate the cerebral arteries and returning venous circulation. Any abnormalities can then be localized.

If the patients' condition allows, the procedure is explained and written permission is obtained. If it does not, written consent of the next of kin is obtained.

A sedative may be given on the evening prior to the angiography and, if a general anaesthetic is to be used, no fluid or food is given during the 6 hours prior to the procedure.

On return from the X-ray department the patient is placed in the recumbent position for 24 hours. If a general anaesthetic has been given, the patient is placed in the lateral position until fully conscious. The routine observations following general anaesthesia are maintained.

Rarely do complications arise, but the nurse must be aware of two possible major problems.

A haematoma may occur at the site of the injection and, if sufficiently large, will compress the oesophagus and trachea. The nurse must observe the patient's neck for evidence of swelling; this, and any difficulty experienced in breathing or swallowing, must be reported.

Spasm of the cerebral arteries or oedema may occur giving rise to an increase in intracranial pressure. The clinical features of this condition are described under observations (p. 84). Fortunately these complications are very unusual.

Types of head injury
The severity of a head injury is greatly influenced by age. A small child can have a serious fall with little or no effects, while in the elderly a slight bump can lead to severe intracranial damage.

Head injuries may be divided into two main groups:

Closed — the skull may be fractured but the meninges remain intact.
Open — the skull is fractured and the meninges and brain are exposed.

The types of fracture are:

Simple — no break in the skin (Fig. 3.27A).
Compound — the scalp is breached (Fig. 3.27B).
Comminuted — the bone is broken in several places (Fig. 3.27C).
Depressed — a piece of bone is driven inwards (Fig. 3.27D).

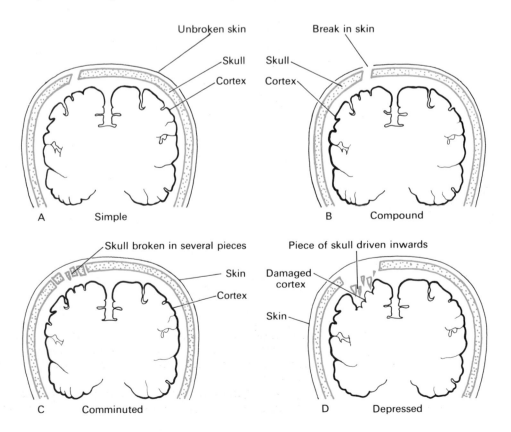

Figure 3.27
Fractures of the skull

It is the site of the fracture which is important rather than the fracture itself. Two areas are of particular importance:

If the frontal bone is damaged and there is a breach in the dura, CSF can escape via the frontal sinus from the nose. This is called **rhinorrhoea**.

If the fracture occurs at the base of the skull and the petrous bone, which contains the middle ear, is damaged, a breach in the dura will result in an escape of CSF from the ear. This is called **otorrhoea**.

The nurse must remember to observe the nose and ears and report any discharge immediately. If such a discharge is observed, under no circumstances should the nurse attempt to stop the flow by plugging either the nostrils or ears as this may result in infection from the back flow of CSF being introduced into the subarachnoid space. The orifice should be covered with a sterile dressing until the patient is seen by a doctor.

Intracranial bleeding

Bleeding may occur outside the dura, extradural haemorrhage; under the dura, subdural haemorrhage; or into the cortex of the brain, intracerebral or subarachnoid haeomorrhages.

Extradural haemorrhage

Haemorrhage may result from injury or, in some instances, from disease (p.79). This occurs most commonly following injury to the temperoparietal region of the skull because of the large number of blood vessels in that area, but it can also occur following injury to any area. The onset of clinical features will depend on the site of impact and the degree of haemorrhage.

If haemorrhage is mild to moderate, the patient may or may not become unconscious at the time of injury, but as the clot formation increases in size an impairment in the conscious level will occur. If the middle meningeal artery is ruptured the result is the very rapid formation of a blood clot with a correspondingly rapid impairment in the conscious level.

Other features that may occur depend on the site of injury; they include headaches, neck stiffness, vomiting, paralysis of one side of the body and an increase in the size of the pupil of the eye on the side of bleeding.

The urgency of immediate surgical treatment is dependent on the clinical findings made on admission. X-ray of the skull and echoencephalography may be carried out, but the surgeon would not allow these diagnostic procedures to delay operation in a case of urgency. The patient is taken to the operating theatre where hair is shaved from the area considered appropriate. The scalp is incised and a hole made in the skull and widened by means of a burr. When the clot formation has been confirmed the exposed piece of bone can be removed. The clot is evacuated by suction and the bleeding vessel controlled by diathermy. The dura can then be opened to ensure there is no bleeding below this level. A drain is placed in position and the scalp incision closed with silk sutures.

Ideally, the patient should be transferred from the operating table to his bed as this will avoid unnecessary movement on his arrival back in the ward.

Following the removal of the clot and relief of pressure on the brain there may be a rapid improvement in the level of consciousness.

Subdural haemorrhage

This can range from an acute type, which usually occurs following a blow of considerable violence when bleeding is severe, to a chronic type, which follows an injury of milder degree when bleeding occurs slowly. Clinical features may be evident within the first few days or may not appear until weeks after the injury. These features include headaches increasing in intensity, drowsiness, changes in normal pattern of behaviour and confusion. If the motor cortex is involved then paralysis of one side of the body will occur. Pressure on the cerebral cortex will lead to fits. There is one classic feature — namely, the variations which occur in the levels of consciousness. The patient may be alert and talking but within a short time may become drowsy and uncommunicative. He is, however, easily aroused and will then appear as alert as before.

As this condition does not demand the same degree of urgency as an extradural haemorrhage, an X-ray of the skull will be taken to determine the site of any fracture.

An echoencephalography and angiography are also carried out.

The operative measure is to evacuate the clot and control any bleeding vessels. The technique is similar to that described for extradural haemorrhage.

Intracerebral and subarachnoid haemorrhages

As most haemorrhages occurring in the cortex result in bleeding into the subarachnoid space producing a subarachnoid haemorrhage, the two conditions can be discussed together. The amount of blood found in the subarachnoid space is determined by the degree of injury to the cortex or the size of the torn blood vessel passing through the subarachnoid space itself.

The clinical features will depend on the severity of damage and the resulting haemorrhage. These range from headaches, neck stiffness, rise in temperature, irritability and photophobia (dislike of bright light) to progressive impairment of the conscious level.

Examination of CSF for evidence of blood is the diagnostic aid used in this condition. The procedure is called a **lumbar puncture** (p.114).

In most cases, apart from a period of rest in bed, no specific treatment is necessary. There is no procedure which will hasten the reabsorption of blood from the subarachnoid space. The patient's recovery is spontaneous.

In the remainder of cases where there is delay in recovery and definite clinical features are present such as weakness of voluntary muscles of one side of the body (hemiparesis) and impairment of conscious level, surgery will be contemplated. An angiography will be carried out to determine the site of the haemorrhage.

If only a small area of the cortex is involved the clot can be aspirated through a burr hole in the skull. If, however, an extensive area of the cortex is involved then the skull will be exposed, a piece of bone removed and the clot evacuated. Any bleeding vessels will be controlled and the bone opening will be closed.

Nursing observations

The following are the observations the nurse must make and record as part of her total care of the patient.

Level of consciousness

There is no doubt that the level of consciousness is the most important sign of an improvement or deterioration in the condition of the head injury patient. To assess this the nurse must have a standard of levels of consciousness. The following is an accepted standard:

Level 0 — Fully conscious and well orientated but may suffer amnesia regarding the accident.

Level 1 — Fully conscious but suffers from confusion at times. This is more common in the elderly patient who can answer personal questions but is unaware of immediate surroundings.

Level 2 — Drowsy but can be roused to answer questions, then quickly falls asleep again.

Level 3 — Not answering questions but obeying simple commands.

Level 4 — Responds to painful stimuli. There are two types of response here and it is important that the nurse can distinguish them. In the first, only the limb that is being subjected to the painful stimuli is withdrawn. In the second, all limbs react and there is an increase in the rate of respirations. This indicates damage to the brain stem and the patient's prognosis is most unfavourable.

Level 5 — Deeply unconscious and there is no response to painful stimuli.

Limb movement

If the area of the brain responsible for movement of voluntary muscles is impaired by pressure then a weakness or paralysis of muscles on the opposite side of the body will occur.

When it is due to contusion at the time of injury paralysis results immediately but progressively improves. If it is due to pressure from an extradural or subdural haemorrhage the paralysis can be established by the vigour with which the patient withdraws the limb from painful stimuli.

Pupillary reaction
The reaction of the iris of the eye to light can indicate displacement of the brain due to pressure. It should be remembered that all smooth muscle is normally in a state of partial constriction. If the eye is exposed to the bright light from a torch, the parasympathetic fibres travelling within the third cranial nerve will cause further constriction of the iris and the pupil will become smaller.

If the brain is displaced the only escape valve is through the tentorial hiatus. The brain squeezes through and displaces the third cranial nerve, which ceases to function (Fig. 3.28). As parasympathetic control is lost the iris will relax and the pupil will dilate.

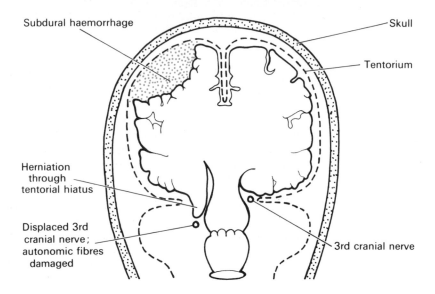

Figure 3.28
Displacement of brain

The significance of this observation is that the greater the amount of brain squeezed through the tentorial hiatus, the greater the pressure brought to bear on the reticular formation of the brain stem. It will be remembered that the reticular formation activates a state of arousal in the cerebral cortex which affects the level of consciousness.

The nurse should make the following observations regarding iris reaction of both eyes:

Are both reacting briskly to light?
Is one reacting more sluggishly than the other?
Is one pupil larger than the other?
If so, is it still reacting to light or has reaction ceased?

The nurse must always remember to ascertain if the patient has a glass eye or contact lens: failure to do so has led to unnecessary anxiety in the past!

Features of increased intracranial pressure
In a rigid container such as the skull, an increase in volume will result in an increase in pressure. If the contents are semisolid (as is the brain) and an increase in pressure arises, the contents will flow out.

If for any reason there is an increase in volume within one of the fossae of the skull, such as a clot of blood or a tumour, the pressure within the fossae will rise and the semisolid brain will flow out. This will eventually result in compression of the brain stem with a resulting disturbance in function.

Irrespective of the cause of increased intracranial pressure the nurse should be able to recognize certain features:

Headache, particularly on waking in the morning.
Blurring of vision.
Nausea accompanied by vomiting.
A slowing of the pulse rate.
A rise in the systolic blood pressure.

Slowing and irregularities of respiration. If the brain stem is damaged the respirations become periodic. The patient will take a few rapid breaths and then stop breathing completely. After a few seconds he will begin breathing again.

An impairment of the conscious level.

The vital signs

The frequency of observation of temperature, pulse, respirations and blood pressure will depend on the individual patient and his injury. In the initial acute stage or immediately after surgery, observations are made every 15 to 30 minutes. As the patient's condition improves these observations can be made at less frequent intervals. Any change, sudden or gradual, must be reported as complications may be averted or treated by prompt intervention.

Nursing care

The principles of nursing care are basically the same in all classifications of head injuries.

Respiratory function

Maintenance of a clear airway is of prime importance and takes precedence over all other care. Depression of respiratory function is the commonest cause of deterioration in the unconscious patient. It can be the result of several factors. The jaw tends to fall downwards and the tongue backwards, thus blocking the upper part of the respiratory tract. Because the cough and swallowing reflexes are not functioning, secretions from the mouth and pharynx trickle down into the trachea. These secretions, and secretions formed in the bronchi, which are not cleared can block the lower respiratory tract. Another hazard facing the patient is that blood from the mouth and any vomitus can be inhaled into the respiratory tract. If the nurse observes the following rules the risk of respiratory difficulties for the patient will be greatly diminished.

Dentures should be removed and placed in the appropriate receptacle. The patient should be placed in the semiprone position, which can be maintained by placing a pillow under the lower part of the chest to prevent him falling forward; if the upper leg is flexed and a pillow placed between the legs he will not fall backwards (Fig. 3.29). A waterproof square covered by a disposable towel should be placed under the patient's head. This will protect bedding should vomiting occur. The lateral positions can be used as an alternative. The patient's position should be altered every 2 hours to help ventilation of both lungs. The changing of position requires at least two nurses — an individual nurse should never attempt it on her own.

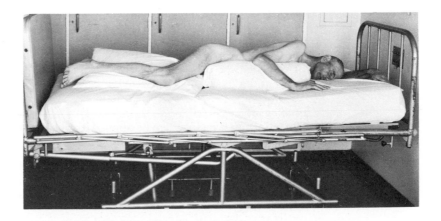

Figure 3.29
Unconscious patient in semiprone position

Observation should be made of the skin for evidence of cyanosis which might indicate blockage within the respiratory tract. The respirations should be observed for any change which might suggest difficulty in breathing.

Although correct positioning will do much to ensure drainage of secretions, it is often insufficient. Excessive secretions can be aspirated by using a suction machine and catheter. The catheter is connected to the tubing from the suction machine, inserted gently into the mouth and directed to the pharynx. Suction is then applied and the secretions aspirated. A fresh catheter is then connected to the suction machine and gently inserted into each nostril to allow for aspiration of secretions. While a soft rubber catheter is ideal in that it lessens the risk of injury to the mouth, it does tend to curl before reaching the pharynx and a polythene catheter is more effective. This procedure requires considerable practice before skill is attained and should not be delegated to a nurse inexperienced in the technique unless under supervision. It is less distressing for the patient if this procedure is carried out at frequent intervals of short duration; prolonged exposure to aspiration technique at lengthy intervals should be avoided. An oral airway may be introduced to assist in maintaining effective respiratory function. If so, it is important that the nurse realizes that the airway can become plugged with mucus; it must be removed when oral hygiene is being carried out and a fresh airway inserted.

Despite maintenance of correct position of the patient and adequate aspiration there are situations where respiratory embarrassment is such that other techniques must be employed. An endotracheal tube can be introduced or a tracheostomy performed (Ch. 6).

Care of the skin

The conscious patient confined to bed can do one of two things if he becomes aware of discomfort. He can change his position in bed or, if unable to do so, he can inform the nursing staff of his problem. The unconscious patient can do neither. Here, an awareness of the patient's needs by the nurse is of the utmost importance.

Changing the patient's position in bed has already been mentioned in maintaining adequate respiratory function. It also serves the double purpose of ensuring that one area of the body will not be subjected to the harmful effects of pressure over a prolonged period. Routine care of skin and pressure areas (Ch. 14) is particularly important as the patient's skin is in constant danger of contamination from vomit, urine and faeces; these contaminants should be removed at once and the area washed. Any soiled linen must be removed and clean linen supplied. A bed-bath should be given each day. Any evidence of reddening or an actual break in the continuity of the skin must be reported at once. The special care necessary if pressure sores occur is described in Chapter 14.

Under no circumstances should hot water bottles be placed in the bed of an unconscious patient, because of the danger of burns from direct contact or from water escaping unnoticed from the bottle. The nurse should also ensure that the patient's finger- and toe-nails are cut and filed. Unless contraindicated, the hair should be brushed and combed and arranged in an attractive style.

Care of the mouth

In many instances the unconscious patient tends to breathe through his mouth, which will become excessively dry. It may also become heavily coated with mucus. If an oral airway is *in situ*, it is removed, the oral cavity gently but thoroughly cleaned every 2 hours and a fresh airway inserted.

Feeding

The following principles can be applied in considering the safest method of feeding the patient:

1. If the patient is conscious with both cough and swallow reflexes present he may be fed by the normal oral route.

2. If the patient is unconscious but cough reflex is present then feeding by nasogastric route is used.

3. If the patient is unconscious and both cough and swallow reflexes are absent intravenous feeding is essential.

Feeding by intravenous route

Various regimes may be advocated. Table 3.2 shows preparations totalling 5828 kJ which, if infused over a 24-hour period, will meet the patient's basic kilojoule requirements.

The specific responsibilities of the nurse in the care of the patient are as follows.

Prior to the start of the infusion the site chosen must be shaved of hair and thoroughly cleaned. Strict observance of an aseptic technique must be given by both the doctor commencing the infusion and the nurse assisting. The infusion site must be inspected regularly for signs of inflammation. If for any reason blood or plasma are transfused (Ch. 8) the infusion apparatus must be changed before feeding recommences. The addition of any supplements (such as vitamins) to the infusion flask must be kept to a minimum as this will increase the risk of introducing a contaminant to the sterile solution.

Table 3.2
An intravenous feeding regime

Preparation	Volume (litres)	Constituents	Kilojoules supplied	Advantages	Disadvantages
Intralipid 20%	$\frac{1}{2}$	Soya beans 10% Glycerol 2·5%	4200	Contains essential fatty acids and phosphorus; neutral pH.	Expensive
Aminoplex 14	1	Synthetic amino acids	1428		
Glucose 50%*	$\frac{1}{2}$		4200	Normal physiological substrate essential for cerebral metabolism.	Viscid and an irritant to veins. Must be given via large central vein. Hyperglycaemia with excessive loss of water in urine. Insulin must be given to ensure effective metabolism.
Normal saline 0·9%	$\frac{1}{2}$			Isotonic solution	

Potassium 1·5 g added to each flask.
Parentrovite (vitamin B complex) given every second day.

* Fructose 20% can be substituted for glucose 50%. It is less irritating and can be infused via a peripheral vein. Less water is lost in the urine. It does, however, carry risk of causing lactic acidosis and must be used with caution.

Observations should be made to ensure that the rate of infusion is as prescribed and care taken that the flask is not allowed to empty completely before being changed. Should a flask empty, under no circumstances must it be replaced with a full flask until the doctor has examined the infusion tubing to see if air has entered. Fluid running through tubing which contains air will force the air into the venous circulation and expose the patient to the risk of formation of an air embolus.

Fungal infections are not uncommon and the application of an antifungal agent to the infusion site is advised.

The amount of fluid given from any flask should be recorded on the patient's fluid balance chart after the fluid has been infused.

Feeding by nasogastric route (Fig. 3.30)
The most important point to remember is that the unconscious patient must be nursed in either the lateral or semiprone position. Then, if vomiting of food occurs, the patient can maintain a clear airway. Ideally a disposable polythene catheter should be used. This is firmer than rubber and therefore easier to pass into the stomach. It also has the advantage of being less irritating to tissues than rubber and diminishes the volume of secretions.

The nostrils should be cleaned of any dirt or secretions. The upper third of the catheter should be lubricated avoiding the orifice of the catheter. It should then be inserted into a nostril and gently guided into the stomach. If the nurse experiences any resistance to the passage of the catheter force should not be used as this may result in damage of the delicate turbinate bone. The other nostril can be used or the catheter

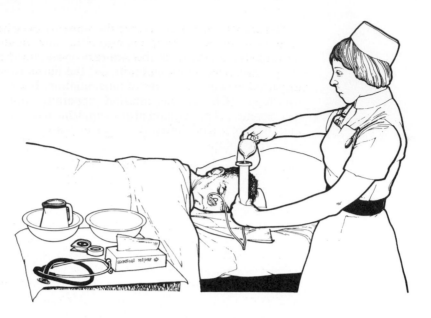

Figure 3.30
Nasogastric feed

passed by the oral route. The nurse can satisfy herself that the catheter has not entered the respiratory tract by carrying out the following observations:

1. Looking for any evidence of cyanosis which would indicate respiratory embarrassment.
2. Listening for the sound of expirations whistling through the tube.
3. Making sure any aspirate obtained from the tube shows an acid reaction on litmus paper, indicating gastric contents.

The practices of placing the open end of the catheter in a bowl of water to see if bubbles appear, and of injecting water down the tube, which, if in the respiratory tract, will result in the patient coughing, are not recommended.

A spigot should be placed in the open end of the catheter. The catheter should then be brought across the cheek and behind the ear where it is secured by a piece of tape.

Before administering a feed the total contents of the stomach should be aspirated, measured, and the amount of aspirate recorded on the fluid balance chart. This will indicate how effectively the feed is passing from the stomach to the small intestine. If feeds are continued without assessing emptying ability of the stomach, the patient may regurgitate food which may then be inhaled. As the aspirate contains important electrolytes most of it should be returned to the stomach. If the amount of aspirate indicates that previous feeds are not being passed effectively, then medical advice should be sought.

The following regime is an example of one commonly used:

Water 15 ml hourly for 4 hours.
Water 30 ml hourly for 4 hours.
Water 60 ml hourly for 4 hours.
Milk 30 ml and water 30 ml hourly for 4 hours.
Milk 60 ml and water 30 ml 2 hourly for 4 hours.
Milk 90 ml and water 60 ml 2 hourly for 4 hours.
Milk 120 ml and water 90 ml 2 hourly for 4 hours.

If at the end of this 28-hour period the patient has tolerated the gradual increase in amount, an instant breakfast food product 120 ml and water 90 ml should be given 2 hourly for the following 24 hours.

Special feeds consisting of milk, eggs, Casilan and a vitamin syrup are prepared by the dietician. Usually the total feed for 24 hours is sent to the ward and this must be kept in the refrigerator to prevent the growth of bacteria. This special feed 120 ml and water 90 ml can be given 2 hourly for an indefinite period.

Drugs should, if possible, be given in liquid form. Powders or crushed tablets should be dissolved in a quantity of water from the diet allowance and given following the feed.

The part of the catheter entering the nose should be kept free from crust formation by the application of a lubricant. The catheter should be removed and a fresh one introduced into alternate nostrils every fourth day. Changing of the catheter should always take place immediately before a feed and following aspiration of stomach contents.

Observations of vital signs

The frequency with which these observations are made depends on the patient's condition and can range from 15-minute to 4-hourly intervals. Irrespective of the time interval the nurse should remember the following points.

As all patients who have sustained a head injury will suffer a degree of shock, the skin will tend to be cold and clammy.

The **hypothalamus**, a group of cells within the cerebrum forming part of the autonomic nervous system, may be damaged. As one of the functions of the hypothalamus is the control of body temperature, damage to it can result in marked variations in temperature during 24 hours. The patient may develop a chest infection with a resulting elevation of temperature. Infection entering the subarachnoid space will result in meningitis with an accompanying elevation of temperature. These changes will not always be apparent if the axillae or groins are used as the site for placing the thermometer. The nurse should therefore always use the rectum to register changes in temperature. It should be noted that, while in most patients evidence of a chest infection would indicate the use of semirecumbent or upright position, in the unconscious patient following head injury no change can be made from recommended positions.

The rate, rhythm and volume of the pulse and respirations should be observed and any change, no matter how slight, must be reported.

The absence of a pulse beat can prove frightening to a young nurse who may immediately assume that arterial circulation has ceased. While this may be the case, it is not necessarily true. The fluctuation between systolic and diastolic pressure gives rise to the pulse beat. If no difference existed between systolic and diastolic pressures there would be no evidence of a pulse beat but circulation of blood would still be adequate.

Accuracy in recording blood pressure is essential (Ch. 7). The sphygmomanometer should be placed at a level corresponding to the level of the patient's heart and not on a table top well above the level of the recumbent patient.

The importance of observing pupillary reaction to light has already been discussed (p. 84). The patient should be informed of the procedure. Both eyes should be opened and the pupils observed for size and equality. The beam from the torch should then be directed on the pillow near the patient's head and gradually brought over the patient's face and finally to the eyes. Under no circumstances should the beam be directly focused on the eyes because, if there is existing damage to the eyes or surrounding tissue, a sudden involuntary closure of the eyelids can result in a haemorrhage. Light directed on one pupil should result in both pupils becoming smaller. The reaction should be tested with the light being directed into one eye, then, after allowing a short interval of time for the pupils to return to their original size, the procedure should be repeated with the light being gradually directed into the other eye. The observations should then be recorded and any change reported at once.

Care of the eyes

If unconsciousness results from an organic cause the corneal reflex is absent. As the secretion of tears is diminished and the patient cannot close the eyelids completely, the eye is exposed to irritation by dust particles and to excessive dryness. Regular observations should be made for evidence of inflammation; neglect can result in ulceration of the cornea (Ch. 12).

Crusts on the eyelids or eyelashes should be gently removed with sterile cotton wool balls soaked in warm normal saline. Each eye is treated separately using a fresh cotton wool ball for every application to the eye. Then each eye is gently irrigated with warm normal saline and a drop of castor-oil is instilled into the lower conjunctival sac. The oil has a soothing effect on irritated tissues. The eyelids are gently closed and can be maintained in position by applying a small strip of tape or micropore over the eyelid and cheek. Great care must be taken when removing this strip as the delicate skin below the eye can be easily damaged. Eye shields made of X-ray film can be used to cover the eyes and afford protection from dust or other harmful substances.

Observations of limb movement

As noted earlier, the patient's response to painful stimuli helps determine his level of consciousness. However, the nurse should approach this method with some thought for the patient and should seek guidance as to what is permissible. For example, forcible twisting of the patient's earlobe, which can result in damage to the skin, is not permissible.

The observant nurse can notice other signs which indicate a change in the patient's level of consciousness. Does he respond to a sudden, loud noise in the ward? When his position is being changed does he resist in any way? Has he himself altered the position in which he was last placed? Does he respond to any form of care being given? When performing any task the nurse should always ask first for the patient's co-operation. If, for example, the nurse is about to observe pupillary reaction to light she should ask the patient to open his eyes and not assume that he cannot. At a certain stage he may do so or may show signs that he is trying, if not succeeding.

Nurses unfamiliar with the neurosurgical unit often become unnecessarily distressed if a previously quiet, unconscious patient becomes noisy and confused. They tend to assume that this indicates a further complication in the patient's condition. A period of disorientation is, however, quite normal as the patient's level of consciousness improves and should be observed with joy rather than consternation.

Care of the urinary bladder

The unconscious patient usually suffers from incontinence of urine with the resulting increased risk of contamination of the skin. The nurse can help reduce this risk by offering the patient a bedpan or a urinal at regular intervals. It is important to remember that although the patient is unable to communicate his needs, he may be aware of his immediate environment, and it is possible to establish a bladder training regime. By observing the times at which the patient voids urine the nurse can plan the times at which to offer the bedpan or urinal.

Obviously contamination of the skin and bed linen will occur and the regime itself can be time-consuming, but the advantages to the patient cannot be overemphasized.

If bladder training is not possible, male patients may be kept dry by the use of Paul's tubing. A suitable length of the tubing is cut and one end is placed over the penis and secured if necessary with a strip of Micropore. The other open end is introduced into a urinary drainage bag which is secured by a holder to the bed below the level of the patient. To avoid irritation to the skin from the tubing a protective layer of petroleum jelly should be applied to the penis prior to application of the tubing.

The practice of placing a urinal *in situ* is to be discouraged. The patient is exposed to the dangers of damage to the surrounding skin from pressure by the urinal and contamination of the skin by spillage of urine.

Catheterization of the urinary bladder should not be contemplated unless absolutely necessary. It carries the grave danger of introducing infection into the urinary tract and adding a further embarrassment to the patient's chances of recovery. The following situations would, however, necessitate catheterization:

Development of retention of urine.

Administration of a diuretic such as mannitol (by intravenous infusion) in the treatment of cerebral oedema will result in a vast diuresis and an accurate record of the urinary output is essential.

If catheterization is carried out, a form of tidal drainage is desirable:

To prevent contamination of the skin with urine.

To produce regular emptying of the bladder and obviate the necessity of repeated catheterizations.

To assist in maintaining normal tone of bladder muscle.

To reduce the risk of infection.

To treat infection by the introduction of an irrigating antiseptic solution.

To reduce the exposure of the patient to physical and mental distress.

Care of bowel function

The principle of offering the patient a bedpan is equally applicable here. Constipation or impaction of faeces can be avoided by the administration of an enema every third day.

Care of the joints

Prolonged immobilization will result in a stiffening of the joints, often in an abnormal position. This complication can be avoided by ensuring that all joints are put through their full range of movements several times each day. The nurse can complement the work of the physiotherapist by performing these passive exercises at appropriate times during the day, for example following the patient's daily bed-bath. It is important, however, that the nurse is shown the correct method of carrying out these exercises by the physiotherapist before attempting to put them into practice. An overvigorous movement of the limbs of an unconscious patient can result in a tearing of associated muscles.

Reduction and control of temperature

A slight elevation of temperature is common in most patients following head injury and is not of any particular import. However, if the elevation is above 38°C it would suggest either infection or damage to the heat-regulating centre in the hypothalamus. The main danger is that this temperature elevation will increase the amount of oxygen required by the brain but, as there is not a corresponding increase in volume of air reaching the lungs, the volume of oxygen will not meet its needs. The result is a deterioration in the patient's level of consciousness. The nurse can employ the following techniques to reduce and control the patient's temperature.

The patient should be naked, a cradle placed in the bed and a sheet loosely draped over him. As far as possible a calm, noise-free atmosphere should be ensured. An electric fan can be placed next to the patient and cool air directed over his body.

Unless contraindicated the fluid intake should be increased. This decision, of course, would rest with the doctor.

If the mechanism of sweating is absent, tepid sponging can be carried out thus allowing the loss of heat from the body by evaporation. If, however, the patient is sweating, the sweat must be removed from the skin by frequent sponging. Sweat allowed to remain on the skin will quickly cool and if the patient starts to shiver there will be a further elevation in temperature. Observations and recordings of temperature should be made every half hour.

Postoperative nursing care

The care necessary following surgery to evacuate an intracranial haematoma is basically the same as for the unconscious patient (p. 85). If a drain has been left *in situ* the amount and colour of drainage is observed and recorded. The dressing is inspected for staining and repacked with sterile material as required. The initial dressing should not be disturbed until removal of the drain, usually 48 hours following surgery. The surgeon may wish to carry out this procedure himself. The fresh dressing is not disturbed until the removal of sutures within 5 to 7 days.

The patient may experience a period of disorientation about the third postoperative day. The nurse must ensure that he does not disturb or remove the dressing. In certain instances a form of restraint may be used, such as application of splints to the arms, but this can result in the degree of disorientation becoming more marked and should never be employed without the written permission of the surgeon in charge.

The formation of crusts on the scalp can be dealt with following removal of sutures. A liberal application of petroleum jelly should be gently massaged into the scalp and the head covered with a towel arranged as a turban. The following morning the scalp should be shampooed and crusts can easily be removed. The female patient may well be self-conscious about her shaved head, and encouraging her to wear a wig or an attractively designed head scarf will do much to lessen her anxiety.

Treatment of fracture

If the patient has sustained a simple fracture no specific treatment is required. If it is a compound fracture, the scalp laceration is sutured and a course of antibiotic therapy is begun. A comminuted or depressed fracture can be dealt with following admission; however it is more common for the surgeon to wait until the patient has made a complete recovery from the effects of his head injury. Therefore treatment for this type of fracture usually takes place about 6 months following the injury.

The patient is readmitted to the neurosurgical unit. X-rays of the skull are taken to determine the site and the extent of the fracture. The patient is taken to the theatre where the scalp is shaved and then infiltrated with a local anaesthetic. The scalp is incised and bone fragments removed. Any blood clots or dead tissue are removed by suction. The bone defect can be closed in several ways: by utilizing fragments of bone that were removed or by inserting bone grafts or specially moulded plastic or metal caps. The scalp is then closed by sutures, and further X-rays are taken.

The postoperative care of the patient follows a pattern identical to that already described.

The course of head injuries

Fortunately most patients make a spontaneous recovery and can return to their homes and occupations with little if any change in their previous pattern of living. However, there are others who will suffer from some disturbance which may or may not be due to an organic condition. Only a brief summary will be given, as the number of disturbances which can arise are too varied to be dealt with here.

Post-traumatic epilepsy
This is divided into two stages:

1. **Early epilepsy** Occurs 1–7 days following initial injury and usually takes the form of focal seizure (see p. 101). Commonly follows a depressed fracture or an intracranial haematoma. Approximately 25 per cent of patients will develop status epilepticus (see p. 100). Anticonvulsant drugs are prescribed for 12 months to 18 months.
2. **Late epilepsy** This usually occurs about 12 months following initial injury, but, in a small number of cases, the first seizure may be delayed for 4 years. This commonly takes the form of a psychomotor seizure (see p. 102), and unfortunately tends to persist. Anticonvulsant drugs are prescribed for 18 months to 2 years.

Brain stem injury
The effect varies according to the degree of trauma. The patient may remain in a state of unconsciousness for months or years. If the injury is less severe the ability to balance and walk may be impaired.

Headaches
These may arise from the patient's anxiety on return to the outside world, particularly if he has difficulty in concentrating or remembering. Headaches can also result from scars on the scalp, but this is not common.

Severe brain damage
This can result in a deterioration in both patterns of behaviour and intellect.

The postconcussion syndrome
Although organic damage may have occurred this can be classified as a neurotic condition. The disturbances the person complains of are far in excess of any which might arise following minimal organic damage. The symptoms are constant headaches, impairment of memory, intolerance of noise, fear of traffic and crowds, inability to sleep and vertigo. The patient may complain of a sensation of fear if placed in a situation similar to that experienced prior to his injury. The exact cause of this condition is still being debated, but it is most commonly seen in patients of previously low intelligence.

Post-traumatic vertigo
In this condition the patient feels either that he is spinning round or that his immediate external environment is spinning around him. He usually falls to the ground but there is no impairment of his conscious level. These attacks can persist for months following the initial injury but recovery will eventually take place.

Rehabilitation

It is generally accepted that the most important aspect in ensuring an adequate regime of rehabilitation is the nurse's approach to her patient. She must at all times display a cheerful, optimistic outlook on the patient's eventual ability to cope after leaving hospital. She must not, however, fall into the trap of being oversympathetic to any impairment of function experienced by the patient. A patient suffering from the postconcussion syndrome (p. 92) would play unmercifully on this well-meant but misguided approach.

It is most important that the patient should be allowed to develop both his physical and his mental capabilities to their fullest extent before leaving hospital. This aspect of care is not normally carried out in the acute neurosurgical unit. Following gradual ambulation the patient is transferred to a rehabilitation unit. The following members of the health team then have specific responsibilities for ensuring an adequate rehabilitation regime.

The **physiotherapist** begins active exercises which the patient must continue until recovery of impaired voluntary muscles has been achieved or no further improvement is anticipated.

The **speech therapist** deals with any speech defect which had arisen following injury.

The **social worker** collects information regarding the patient's home circumstances and any financial problems likely to arise during the period prior to the patient returning to work.

The **rehabilitation officer**, by co-ordinating with the social worker, physiotherapist, speech therapist, doctor and educational psychologist, determines whether the patient can return either to his former job or to a modified form of it. If not, suitable training is given which will prepare the patient for work geared to his needs.

The patient's own **doctor** is informed of the extent of injury sustained and the treatment given. He can then decide what further medical care is necessary from him. This may require the services of a district nurse who co-ordinates with the family doctor.

Education of the patient's family is vital. They must have a clear understanding of any deficits from which the patient is suffering or may suffer. Guidance should be given as to how they can best offer support during any difficult times. This will go far in preventing misunderstanding and a possible breakdown of relationships within the family circle.

Finally, the period of rehabilitation should not be hurried. If the patient is allowed to develop a sense of physical well-being there is less likelihood of a neurotic breakdown.

If the patient is a child the problems of rehabilitation are minimal. The main concern is that the child will overtire himself by too much activity. The parents should be advised to ensure that the child has regular rest periods. The family doctor will decide when attendance at school is permissible and this is better done in gradual stages — a few hours for the first week, then half a day for the following week and finally full attendance.

In all cases arrangements should be made for the patient to visit the out-patient department to see the surgeon 3 months following discharge from hospital.

Tumours

Tumours arise in the following areas:

1. The brain tissue.
2. The meninges.
3. The skull.
4. Peripheral and cranial nerves.

The brain tissue

a. Astrocytomas

These arise in the astrocytes and while occasionally they may be of a benign nature they are mostly malignant. They may occur in any age group and are the commoner type of brain tumour.

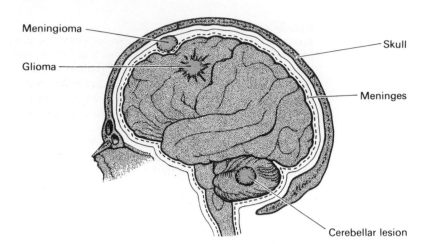

Figure 3.31
Common brain tumours

b. Ependymomas
Most occur in children from 8 to 15 years of age. The tumour usually arises in the floor of the 4th ventricle but may arise in the posterior end of the 3rd ventricle or at the cerebellopontine angle.

c. Oligodendrogliomas
These arise in the cerebral hemisphere and may infiltrate and become adherent to the dura mater. They occur mainly in adults.

d. Medulloblastomas
These arise in the vermis of the cerebellum and are highly malignant. They invade the 4th ventricle thus obstructing the flow of cerebrospinal fluid. The tumour may spread to the 3rd ventricle and seeding may occur in the subarachnoid space. Occasionally metastases occur in bones and lymph nodes. The tumour is more common in boys between the ages of 6 and 10 years. The anticipated life span is 1 to 2 years. It can occur in adults when seeding is not a feature and therefore the prognosis is more favourable.

The meninges

Meningiomas
These tumours usually arise from a small area of the dura mater, and are essentially benign tumours. They are most common in adults especially middle-aged women.

The skull
Primary tumours of the skull are very rare and may be benign (osteomas) or malignant (sarcomas)
   Secondary tumours of the skull are more common and arise as metastases from a primary growth in thyroid gland or bronchi.

Peripheral and cranial nerve tumours

Benign tumours may arise from peripheral and cranial nerve sheaths. A common example is an acoustic neuroma, a benign tumour of the eighth cranial nerve.

Features of intracranial tumours
The combination of headaches, vomiting and papilloedema known as 'the Classical Triad', is the most characteristic presentation of a tumour, although tumours may be present when the classical triad is absent.

Headaches
There is controversy over the cause of headaches. The two theories put forward are that they result either from a stretching of the dura mater or from abnormal tension in the walls of blood vessels.

Vomiting
This is due to interference to the reflex centre of vomiting in the medulla.

Papilloedema
The raised pressure of cerebrospinal fluid within the subarachnoid space is communicated to fluid within the optic nerve. As a result there is interference to the venous return and the optic disc swells and retinal veins distend.

Investigations

Plain skull X-rays
These may be helpful because a tumour may cause bone erosion. In a few instances a meningioma may invade the bone causing *hyperostosis*.

Spine and chest X-rays
These may demonstrate erosion of bone and may show a primary lesion such as a bronchogenic carcinoma (Ch. 6, p. 209).

Computerized axial tomography (CAT) or Electro medical industry (EMI) Scan
This is a non-invasive X-ray procedure which allows the densities of a transverse slice of the brain to be seen by producing an image at any given level. Any abnormality such as a tumour can therefore be detected. The scanner (Fig. 3.32) employs conventional X-rays but instead of using a film a computer reproduces a picture. While no specific preparation is necessary for this procedure, it is important that the patient remains still during the scan which takes about four minutes. It therefore may be necessary for a sedative or a general anaesthetic to be given. Occasionally the radiologist may inject intravenously an iodine contrast medium to enable some tumours to be more readily demonstrated.

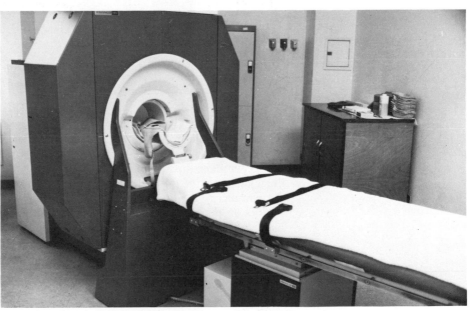

Figure 3.32
EMI scanner

Angiography
This may occasionally be undertaken to demonstrate the abnormal blood supply in tumours. Space occupying lesions may show displacement of the blood vessels (pp. 80–81).

Radio-isotope scanning
This procedure may be used in centres where computerized axial tomography is not available. A radioactive isotope is given intravenously, usually technetium (Tc^{99M}) pertechnetate. Any disturbance within the blood brain barrier allows this radionuclide to pass through and accumulate in the oedema around the space occupying lesion. The

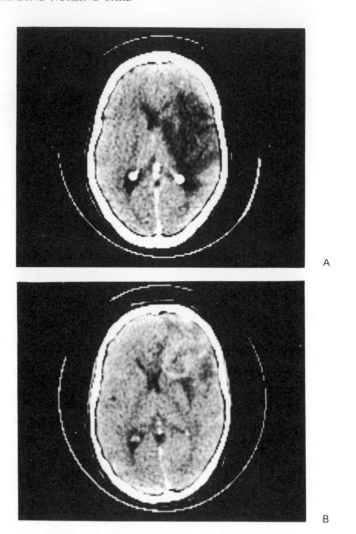

Figure 3.33
Two different scans showing
A   an infarct
B   a tumour.

patient preparation is minimal. An oral dose of 200 mg of sodium or potassium perchlorate is given 1–2 hours prior to intravenous injection. This drug stops the uptake of the isotope in the thyroid gland and empties the choroid plexus which would also accumulate the isotope. The examination is performed about 60–90 minutes after the injection of the isotope. The head is scanned using a rectilinear scan which detects the gamma rays emitted by the isotope. This can record the concentration of the isotope as dots on paper or a polaroid film. A gamma camera may also be used.

Cranial nerve examination
Examination of the cranial nerves may demonstrate abnormalities. Tumours involving the optic nerve pathway may produce a visual field defect. Hearing tests may be given to test the cochlear component of the acoustic nerve. The vestibular component is tested by irrigating the auditory canal with ice cold water. If there is no nystagmus or nausea, the vestibular function is impaired.

Treatment and nursing care
Surgical excision of the tumour is the main aim although this is not always possible without causing disastrous neurological deficits; there is no justification for complete removal at the expense of disabling the patient totally. Biopsy of the lesion may be undertaken for histological report only. If the lesion is contained within a lobe of the brain, it may be possible to perform a lobectomy without further damage to functional areas. A subtotal removal of the tumour will reduce the size of the lesion and thus relieve the intracranial pressure for a time. Cystic tumours if accessible can be drained and completely removed. If *craniotomy* has been performed, routine postoperative care is given (p. 91). The patient will be nursed as any unconscious patient until fully

recovered from the anaesthetic (p. 85). The nurse should in addition pay particular attention to neurological assessments (p. 83) and record her observations half hourly for 24 hours at least. Many tumours are highly vascular and therefore some bleeding may occur postoperatively causing an extradural or subdural haematoma (p. 82). Serial observations lead to the detection of this complication and allow measures to be taken to obviate their dangerous effects. As far as his condition allows the patient may be mobilized around the second post operative day and encouraged to carry out everyday tasks for himself.

Posterior fossa operations may be performed to excise cerebellar tumours, or acoustic neuromata. In general the postoperative care is the same as that following craniotomy. In addition because of the possibility of swelling around the brain stem the respirations should be recorded quarter hourly and any fall below ten breaths per minute should be reported to the medical officer.

Management of cranial nerve palsies

Cranial nerve palsies may be present preoperatively or may occur as a result of posterior fossa exploration in an attempt to remove the tumour. The fifth, seventh, eighth, ninth and tenth cranial nerves are the ones usually involved (Table 3.1, p. 76).

One or more nerves may be affected.

Trigeminal Nerve (fifth) dysfunction will cause sensory loss to one side of the face and eye. This anaesthetic eye is now much more liable to injury and it is necessary therefore for the nurse to protect it. Initially postoperatively a protective celluloid eye shield may be placed over it. Condensation occurring inside the shield will keep the eye moist and should only be removed to renew the dressing around the shield. If eye care is required, great care is taken to keep the eye tightly closed so that the cotton wool does not separate the eyelids and come in contact with the insensitive cornea. If the patient cannot feel dust he will not blink and therefore tears will not be produced to wash away any foreign substances. Protection must also be given to the patient prior to discharge. This may take the form of wing pieces fitted to plain glass spectacles or to the patient's own spectacles. These must be worn on all occasions when out-of-doors and in all circumstances where dust may go into the eye. The patient should be taught how to inspect and clean his eye, and to report to the doctor, should inflammation occur.

The *facial nerve* (*seventh*) may also be damaged. The motor component supplies the muscles of the face. Incomplete eyelid closure if combined with fifth nerve paralysis may further complicate the care of the anaesthetic eye. A tarsorrhaphy (p. 409) may be performed as a temporary or permanent measure. Here the outer margins of the upper and lower eyelids are sutured together. The tarsorrhaphy suture line is kept clean of discharge and crusts using sterile cotton wool balls soaked in normal saline, swabbing from the inner canthus out. Sutures are removed around the 14th day.

Damage to the ninth and tenth nerves, the *glossopharyngeal* and the *vagus* may cause swallowing difficulties. Instructions may be given that no oral fluids be given until the nerves are tested and proved to be functioning normally. Nurses may observe that the patient has difficulty in swallowing his own saliva and therefore requires gentle suction to alleviate his distress. A facial nerve palsy resulting in drooping of the angle of the mouth, combined with ninth and tenth damage will add to the patient's troubles. If swallowing is a problem, feeds will have to be given by other routes, for instance via a nasogastric tube (pp. 87–88) or by jejunostomy (Ch. 5). These cranial nerve palsies may not be present at the time of operation and indeed may only occur as the lesion enlarges. The nursing care of patients with space occupying lesion will depend very much on the symptoms occurring at that time.

Treatment of hydrocephalus

Hydrocephalus may occur at any time due to blockage of the cerebrospinal pathways by tumour invasion or by pressure and can be relieved by the insertion of a ventriculoperitoneal or atrial shunt (p. 122). Routine postoperative care should be instituted. Transient adynamic ileus may occasionally be a complication of peritoneal placement of tubing and the nurse should be aware of the clinical features of this. (Ch. 5, p. 189).

Radiotherapy is often combined with surgical treatment. This regimen will be started after the sutures are removed and the wound is well healed, and may continue over a period of four to six weeks. Life expectancy following radiotherapy may be increased from months to years depending on the grade of the tumour. Since a medulloblastoma metastasizes into the cerebrospinal fluid the spinal cord may also be irradiated as well as the cerebellum and fourth ventricle.

Patients undergoing radiotherapy are often extremely tired and may feel worse during the weeks of treatment. Bone marrow is irradiated therefore the patient's white blood cell and platelet counts fall, sometimes dramatically, requiring temporary cessation of treatment. This low count makes the patient very susceptible to minor infections and clotting defects. Nausea and vomiting may accompany radiotherapy. Patients should be encouraged to eat and drink small appetizing meals and plenty of high calorie drinks should be provided; anti-emetics may be administered prior to food. If the salivary gland is in the field of radiation production of saliva may be diminished and loss of taste may occur. Citrus sweets can be given to stimulate production and help maintain a moist mouth. When the spine is also irradiated, constipation may result and routine mild laxatives may overcome this. Patients should be made aware of the possibility of epilation and to avoid some of the embarrassment the patient and relatives are encouraged to choose a wig prior to surgery.

Skin reactions and care
Some redness and flaking of the skin, similar to sunburn, may develop but application of creams is not encouraged except on medical instructions. Washing of the area is permissible but the patient should be careful not to rub off the radiotherapy markings. If patients are treated with fast neutron therapy, (Cyclotron) they will develop marked skin reactions which heal four to six weeks following treatment if careful skin care is given. The skin reaction progresses from erythema to dry desquamation and occasionally to moist desquamation. Crusting and pigmentation may occur on healing. Epilation may be permanent.

Dry desquamation. Keep dry and exposed to the air if possible. Do not attempt to pick off the crusts.

Moist desquamation Use normal saline or sterile water to clean the area and apply Graneodin ointment sparingly. If possible expose to the air. If a dressing is necessary choose a non-adherent dressing with micropore strapping which should be applied outside the treatment area.

Graneodin ointment may be used where crusting is heavy or the skin itchy. The following preparations are contraindicated:

Eusol (Edinburgh University Solution of Lime).
Zinc and castor oil ointment.
Silver nitrate.
Acriflavine.
Oily and occlusive dressings.

Patients are reviewed weekly while the reaction is minimal.

Drug therapy
Some drugs may be given at different times during the progress of the tumour. Dexamethasone for instance helps to control the oedema that surrounds the tumour thus reducing the intracranial pressure. Cytotoxic therapy may be given in an attempt to destroy the cancer cells but because of difficulty in crossing the blood brain barrier, these drugs have not proved really effective.

Continuing care
Continuous support must be given to the patient's family from the time of diagnosis and especially in the terminal stages of the patient's illness. The patient should be encouraged to go home for short periods of time and good liaison with the community services is essential for this to work well. Relatives should be made aware that they can communicate with the hospital staff for advice or a 'chat' when the patient is at home and that readmission can be easily arranged. As the patient's condition deteriorates he should be kept comfortable and free of pain. Relatives should be encouraged to visit whenever they wish and help nurse their relative if they desire to do so. This may help relieve some feelings of guilt which may be present at not looking after the patient at

home. The hospital chaplain may be involved with the relatives throughout the care of the patient. Terminal care of a child is also discussed (Ch. 15, p. 542).

Epilepsy

The production by the brain cells of stronger than normal electrical impulses will result in the condition of epilepsy. It can be divided into two main types:

1. Idiopathic.
2. Symptomatic.

Idiopathic
There is no apparent organic damage to account for the onset of epileptic attacks. They usually start in the early years of life and take the form of major attacks (grand mal) or minor attacks (petit mal). If both parents in a family suffer from epilepsy, there is an increased risk of their children suffering from this condition.

Symptomatic
Here there is organic damage to justify the attacks. Mention has already been made of post-traumatic epilepsy following a head injury, but any type of injury to or disease of the brain may trigger off such attacks. There are four main types of attacks: major (grand mal), Jacksonian, focal and psychmotor.

The grand mal seizure
   1. **The aura.** This is an hallucination which may take any of the forms mentioned in Chapter 16. It may or may not occur, but if it does it will only last for a short period. The value of the aura is that it can indicate to the doctor the area of the brain in which the abnormal, electrical discharge commences.
   2. **The tonic phase.** The patient emits a cry and falls unconscious to the ground. All muscles contract. The cry is from air being forced from the lungs through vocal cords which are contracted. The teeth are clenched and the tongue may be bitten. As the muscles involved in respiration are affected the patient will become cyanosed. The arms are flexed and the legs are extended. This phase will last 5 to 20 seconds.
   3. **The clonic phase.** The muscles contract and relax intermittently, sometimes violently. There may be incontinence. If the tongue has been bitten there will be evidence of bloodstained saliva. This phase usually lasts for about 2 minutes.
   4. **The postepileptic coma.** The muscles relax and the respirations become stertorous. Flushing of the face will also be observed. This period of coma may last for only a short interval or may continue for several hours.
   5. The patient's level of consciousness improves and he then passes through a transient period of disorientation.
   6. This is followed by a period of normal sleep.

In most instances the patient will awaken from this period of sleep fully recovered from the seizure. However, he may experience a period of postepileptic automatism. During this period he will carry out certain actions of which he is totally unaware. These actions may be harmless in themselves, such as wandering aimlessly about the ward or moving pieces of furniture. However, the nurse must remember that the patient can become acutely suicidal or homicidal during this phase and may be a danger to himself, other patients and staff. It must be emphasized that patients suffering a grand mal seizure do not necessarily pass through all the phases described. Some may only experience aura and tonic phases and then recover. There is no hard and fast rule.

Nursing care
The immediate nursing care necessary will be determined by the actual number of phases of the seizure through which the patient passes.

   1. **The aura.** The patient should be laid on the floor. Dentures should be removed and a rolled handkerchief placed between the teeth. As the aura may not occur or may be of

short duration, it may not be possible to carry out all the treatment recommended. Under no circumstances should any attempt be made to force the mouth open to insert a gag once the tonic phase has commenced. Because of contraction of muscles any such attempt can result in damage to the jaw muscles, fracture of the lower mandible or damage to teeth.

2. **The tonic phase.** The patient should be moved from any immediate danger such as an open fire or articles of furniture. Tight clothing at neck, chest or waist should be loosened and shoes removed.

3. **The clonic phase.** The convulsive movements of the limbs should not be restrained. Ideally the nurse should guide the movements of limbs thus reducing the risk of injury by sudden contact with a hard object.

4. **The postepileptic coma.** The patient can now be transferred to his bed. Maintenance of a clear airway is the prime duty of the nurse, and correct positioning of the patient is essential. Removal of excessive secretions from the mouth and pharynx should be carried out. If contamination of the skin by urine or faeces has occurred, soiled clothing must be removed and the skin cleansed.

5. Reassurance should be given during the transient period of disorientation.

6. The importance of careful observation for evidence of postepileptic automatism cannot be overstressed. The nurse can usually distinguish this from a normal awakening in that the patient will display a staring, vacant expression and will experience difficulty in orientating himself to his immediate and familiar surroundings. It may be necessary for the nurse to employ restraint in order to prevent the patient injuring himself or others.

Long-term treatment

The long-term treatment consists of drug therapy for a period of several years following the last seizure. Some physicians advocate maintaining drug therapy for the remainder of the patient's life. As this therapy in many instances will begin while the patient is in hospital, it is imperative that he realizes fully the importance of taking his drugs at the prescribed times. There is no problem when the administration of drugs is the responsibility of the nursing staff. The danger arises when the patient returns home, where he may either take his drugs at irregular times or, worse, discontinue his therapy. Unpalatable as it may be, the patient must be made to understand the absolute necessity of taking his drugs with clockwork regularity and, irrespective of how well he may feel, the importance of continuing to take them until told by his doctor that he may stop. While the support of relatives is no doubt of value, the onus should always be placed on the patient and not on them.

The action of anticonvulsant drugs is to decrease the excitability threshold of nerves and reduce the production of abnormal electrical impulses. The action of such drugs is enhanced when given in combination with phenobarbitone.

The following are examples of drug regimes:

Sodium valproate 600–2400 mg daily

or

Phenytoin 300 mg daily
Ethosuximide (Zarontin) 250 mg daily

If the cause of the seizure is symptomatic and conservative treatment is proving inadequate with the patient exposed to frequent seizures, surgery may be considered for two reasons:

1. The removal of a space-occupying lesion, for example a benign tumour.
2. The excision of scar tissue formed as the result of a head injury.

Status epilepticus

Recovery from a grand mal seizure will usually leave the patient well for a period before another attack. However, the patient may pass from one seizure directly into another without regaining consciousness. The most common cause for this condition is the abrupt stoppage of anticonvulsant drug therapy and usually occurs a few days following the discontinuation of drugs.

The respiratory embarrassment which accompanies the seizures results in insufficient oxygen reaching the brain and damage to cells. There will also be a marked elevation in body temperature. Unless this condition is treated promptly the patient will eventually die from exhaustion.

The nurse should approach the treatment of her patient bearing three important facts in mind:

1. The seizures must be controlled.
2. The patient is unconscious.
3. Steps must be taken to reduce and control the patient's temperature.

As care of the unconscious patient and reduction and control of temperature have already been described on page 91, only control of seizures will be discussed here.

There are various forms of treatment employed to control seizures but only one will be discussed here. The important point to recognize is the vital necessity for prompt action irrespective of the form it may take.

The patient is usually given an initial dose of Diazepam (Valium) 10–15 mg by intravenous route. An intravenous infusion of normal saline to which Diazepam (Valium) 40 mg is added may then be commenced. The rate of flow varies and is determined by the patient's response to treatment. If the seizure persists an anaesthetist may administer Thiopentone by intravenous route. If this form of therapy is prolonged the anaesthetist may find it necessary to employ the use of assisted ventilation. Following recovery of the patient an oral anticonvulsant drug regime is established.

The petit mal seizure

This seizure comes under the heading of idiopathic epilepsy and usually begins in the early years of life. It consists of a transient loss of contact with the child's immediate external environment and does not display the features of convulsions or incontinence. The child usually suffers from frequent attacks during his waking day. The attack can take different forms — a sudden cessation of speech in mid-sentence lasting a few seconds, then a resumption of speech; a momentary halt in walking; or merely a vacant, staring facial expression. The danger of such seizures is that they may endanger the child if they occur when the child is, say, crossing a busy road or in the bath. Fortunately petit mal seizures rarely continue beyond puberty and are well controlled by drug therapy. The following are examples of drug regimes:

Sodium valproate 600 mg–2400 mg daily

   or

Phenytoin 300 mg daily
Ethosuximide (Zarontin) 250 mg daily

Either regime should be maintained for a minimum period of 2 years following the cessation of seizures.

The Jacksonian or focal epileptic seizure

This type of focal seizure was described by John Hughlings Jackson. Convulsions occur in the muscles of one area of the body and spread to other muscles on the same side of the body. They may cease there or they may spread to muscles on the opposite side of the body, resulting in a loss of consciousness.

It should be appreciated that other types of focal seizures occur in which there is no spread of convulsions from the initial area of muscle involved. Such attacks are always indicative of a cerebral lesion and are therefore symptomatic in cause.

If the lesion lies in the sensory part of the cerebral cortex, the sensations experienced by the patient will be determined by the area involved.

If the lesion is localized to an area of the brain which would permit removal without causing the patient future intractable disability then surgery is contemplated. Otherwise the patient is given the same drug therapy as for grand mal seizures.

The psychomotor seizure

The classical feature of this seizure is an alteration in the pattern of behaviour. The patient carries out a series of actions of which he is unaware at the time and, if questioned about them later, will not remember. These actions may be perfectly acceptable socially or they may be antisocial. If antisocial they tend to be embarrassing to the observer rather than harmful. The area of the brain involved is the temporal lobes.

Treatment consists of surgery in carefully selected cases and the commencement of anticonvulsant drug therapy.

Nursing observations

Apart from providing the immediate necessary treatment, the nurse can be of inestimable value to the doctor in reaching a diagnosis if she has made certain observations during a seizure.

Most units dealing with patients suffering from epilepsy have a printed sheet of appropriate questions which the nurse should answer. It is essential that the nurse completes this form at the earliest opportunity as she may find it difficult to remember specific details later. She should not, however, attempt to fill in any part of the questionnaire during the seizure as her full attention must be given to the nursing care of her patient.

The following is a typical list of questions:

What was the time of the attack?
What was the frequency in relation to previous attacks?
What activity was the patient engaged in prior to the attack?
Did he appear calm or upset?
Did he experience an aura? If so, what form did the hallucination take?
Did he emit a cry?
Did he fall?
Did he appear to lose consciousness? If so, how long did it last?
Was there a phase of muscle rigidity?
Was there a phase of muscle convulsions?
If convulsions occurred where did they start?
Did they spread to any other areas of the body?
Was he incontinent?
Was there any change in skin colour?
Was there evidence of bloodstained saliva?
In the case of the female patient is there a relationship between the onset of a seizure and the onset of menstruation?
What was the patient's pattern of behaviour following recovery?

Investigations

Since epilepsy is, in itself, a symptom, the aim of investigations is to determine a cause. If no cause can be identified the condition is classified as idiopathic epilepsy. The following investigations are those normally carried out.

The doctor obtains a detailed medical history of the patient and his family. Particular note is made of any history of previous seizures experienced by the patient or any member of his family.

If the patient has suffered a seizure in the presence of a witness, a detailed account of observations made is of inestimable value.

The patient is subjected to a thorough physical and neurological examination.

X-rays of the skull are taken to detect any fractures or obvious focal lesions.

A specimen of venous blood is obtained and examined for the spirochaete which causes syphilis; the patient may have cerebral syphilis, which would account for the seizures. A double check can be made by examining a specimen of cerebrospinal fluid for the spirochaete.

The cerebrospinal fluid is also examined for pathogenic organisms causing meningitis, since a complication of this inflammatory disorder is epilepsy.

The level of sugar in the blood is estimated (normal is 70–180 mg per 100 ml of blood). If this level rises above 200 mg per 100 ml of blood, seizures can occur.

The urine should be tested for the presence of albumen. If there is a high level of albumen in the urine, the fits may be associated with renal disease.

Electroencephalography

This is a recording on graph paper of the electrical activity of the brain. Electrodes are attached to areas of the scalp by means of a special harness or by collodion. Wires lead from the electrodes into a machine called an electroencephalograph. The electrodes transmit electrical activity from the brain through the wires to the electroencephalograph. Here they are amplified and traced by a mechanical pen on to the graph paper.

The patient is informed of the procedure. Ideally anticonvulsant drugs should be stopped 48 hours prior to the test, but as this will expose him to the danger of status epilepticus it is not commonly done. The patient's hair should be shampooed to remove grease which would interfere with the transmission of impulses through the electrodes. If the patient is a child a sedative is usually prescribed to ensure that he will not become restless during the procedure.

The test is normally carried out in a semidarkened room free from noise or unnecessary movements. The patient is either seated in a chair or placed in the recumbent position on a couch. The electrodes are applied and he is advised to close his eyes and to relax. This prevents movements which would result in an incorrect tracing. The recordings may continue from 30 to 60 minutes. At intervals the recordings are stopped and the patient is allowed to move to prevent him from becoming unduly tense or fatigued.

Any abnormalities can be accentuated by making the patient breathe more deeply and at a faster rate for a few minutes (hyperventilation). The principle here is that, as carbon dioxide is washed out of the lungs, the level of carbon dioxide in the blood falls. Carbon dioxide is carried in the blood as carbonic acid and as the level falls the blood becomes more alkaline. This increased alkalinity stimulates the activity of the brain cells. Apart from feeling tired following this prolonged procedure, the patient should not suffer from any after-effects.

It must be stated that, although patients suffering from epilepsy may present abnormal tracings, many do not. A **normal tracing**, therefore, does not indicate an absence of epilepsy. On the other hand, an **abnormal tracing** can be obtained from a person with no history of epilepsy. It will be appreciated that an electroencephalography is not the most reliable of aids to diagnosis.

Rehabilitation

The greatest disservice the nurse can render her patient during his period of rehabilitation is to adopt an overprotective attitude towards his illness. If by her approach she convinces him he is unwell or 'different' from other people, he will soon feel unwell and different, and nothing is more likely to inhibit his prospects of a good recovery. She would be guilty of an equal injustice, however, if she did not make clear to him that certain restrictions are necessary. The following guidelines should prove of value in this aspect of patient care.

The importance of the patient taking his drugs at the prescribed times has already been discussed. The nurse should emphasize that, provided the drugs are taken, the patient will remain as healthy as anyone else and can live a useful and active life. She must inform him of any possible side-effects of the drugs and avoid any undue alarm on his part.

Apart from the fact that excessive smoking will increase the likelihood of a seizure, there is the added danger of the patient being burned should he be smoking prior to the onset of a seizure, especially if he is in bed. He should be advised to cut his cigarette consumption to a minimum and only to smoke when in company.

A patient in the U.K. should be made aware of the existence of the British Epilepsy Association from whom he can obtain an identity card stating that he suffers from epilepsy. If he carries this card with him at all times it will ensure that, if a seizure does occur outside his home, prompt and correct treatment can be given and his family will be informed.

The patient should be encouraged to participate in sports, as the more active he is, the less chance there is that he will have a seizure. The importance of avoiding extremes of physical and emotional excitement should be mentioned as they can result in an excessive degree of fatigue. Also, any sports which carry a special risk should be discouraged, such as swimming, cycling or mountain climbing.

Because alcohol increases the sedative effect of phenobarbitone it must be avoided.

If he knows of any circumstances which have led to the occurrence of an attack, these should obviously be avoided.

A shower is preferable to a bath. An electric razor for shaving is recommended. The bathroom door should never be locked.

A firm pillow should always be placed under his head. If he has a seizure while asleep and his face is turned towards the pillow he will not suffocate. He should never be aroused suddenly from a state of sleep.

The patient should be advised that before beginning a meal he should cut large portions of food into small pieces. Then, should a seizure occur while he is eating, he will not choke on a large piece of food.

He must be strongly discouraged from driving a car. It should be pointed out that he would be placing other road users, both drivers and pedestrians, at considerable risk. He would personally run the risk of possible injury and would be faced with both legal and insurance liabilities.

His family must be educated as to the nature of his condition. Guidance must be given in the immediate action necessary if a seizure occurs at home. They must be made aware of the restrictions the condition imposes on him. They should of course be reassured that if he adheres to the advised regime and they do not adopt an overprotective attitude, all will be well.

The patient should be advised to visit his own doctor at regular intervals. His doctor can then assess the effectiveness of the drug therapy and if necessary alter the dosage or refer him to the appropriate out-patient department.

The biggest problem the patient faces is that of employment. It may be that the position previously held is no longer suitable, for instance, if sharp tools or machinery were used. In other cases the work may be suitable but the employer reluctant to accept anyone with a history of epilepsy. There is a small percentage of patients who, because of very frequent seizures, are too incapacitated to work and they unfortunately remain permanently unemployed.

In the majority of cases there are three main avenues by which the patient can obtain employment.

The disablement resettlement officer has the responsibility to assess the patient's capabilities. He then approaches selected employers and endeavours to arrange a trial period of work. After a suitable lapse of time he will visit the employer to see how the patient is coping. The results are in many instances most encouraging. Sheltered employment can be obtained in one of the Remploy factories situated throughout the U.K. These factories employ handicapped persons in jobs which are within their ability. A percentage of the vacant posts are made available to patients suffering from epilepsy. Also, the patient can enter an industrial rehabilitation unit.

As the prejudice of many employers lessens, the opportunities for finding suitable work increase. This in turn is resulting in a decrease in the number of patients suffering from feelings of apathy, depression and a tendency to seizures due to an inability to secure employment.

Cerebrovascular accident

The main blood flow to the brain is from two internal carotid arteries and two vertebral arteries (Fig. 3.34). The vertebral arteries converge around the pons varolii to form the basilar artery, which in turn gives off the two posterior cerebral arteries. The internal carotids also give off branches, the two anterior cerebral arteries, joined together by the anterior communicating artery. The middle cerebral artery also leaves from the internal carotid. The posterior cerebral arteries communicate with the internal carotids through the posterior communicating arteries. This arrangement is in the form of a circle called the Circle of Willis (Fig. 3.35). Normally, blood within the circle does not mix, that is basilar blood does not mix with blood from the internal carotids, but in disease a good cross circulation may develop and be all important for brain function.

Aetiology Three main lesions, excluding trauma, may alter the blood supply within the brain. All are vascular in origin damaging nervous tissue by oxygen depletion. Cerebrovascular accident (stroke) is the term given to this damage.

1. Cerebral thrombosis

Here atheromatous changes associated with arteriosclerosis occur within the cerebral circulation (Ch. 7) eventually causing complete blockage of the vessel lumen. This depletes the oxygen supply to the part of the brain supplied by the diseased vessel. Death of tissue, or infarction, may occur. The clinical features vary depending on:

1. The site of infarction.
2. The extent of vessel blockage.

Cerebrovascular accident from thrombosis is regarded as a disease of the elderly. Gradual occlusion causes a progressive deterioration in the patient's condition. Signs and symptoms occur and diminish with no lasting effect, but recur at intervals.

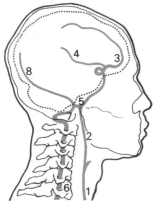

1. Common carotid artery
2. Internal carotid artery
3. Anterior cerebral artery
4. Middle cerebral artery
5. Posterior communicating artery
6. Vertebral artery
7. Basilar artery
8. Posterior cerebral artery

Figure 3.34
Arterial blood supply to brain: lateral view

Figure 3.35
Circle of Willis: basal view

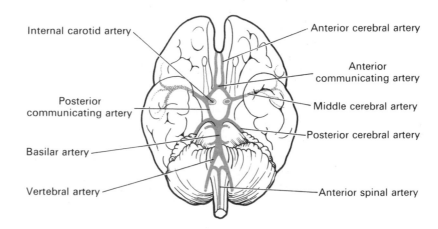

Eventually, when the blockage becomes complete, deficits become permanent. Occlusion may affect any of the vessels of the circle of Willis, but most commonly the internal carotid and middle cerebral arteries. These supply the motor and sensory areas and internal capsule within the temporal and frontal lobes. The presenting feature is usually a hemiplegia. If the dominant hemisphere is affected (containing the speech centre), the patient may also have speech problems, such as expressive dysphasia.

2. Embolism

An embolus may also block cerebral blood vessels. In this case blocking occurs suddenly, the embolus having broken off, say, from vegetations around diseased heart valves such as those which occur in subacute bacterial endocarditis. Occasionally a thrombus may give off multiple emboli.

3. Haemorrhage

Primary intracerebral haemorrhage associated with arteriosclerosis and hypertension is almost always fatal. Patients are usually deeply comatose on admission. Subarachnoid haemorrhage may be due to an aneurysm or an arteriovenous malformation. There is spontaneous rupture of the aneurysm (weakness in the wall of an artery) into the subarachnoid space. Aneurysms tend to occur at the bifurcation of vessels within the circle of Willis. All age groups are affected. Rupture occurs suddenly and often at rest. There is intense headache, vomiting, photophobia and neck stiffness. There may be loss of consciousness and paralysis depending on the affected area. Untreated aneurysms may rebleed within 14 days causing further damage.

Recently it has been found that the use of an antifibrinolytic agent can decrease the risk of rebleeding. This is given initially intravenously and then orally preventing fibrinolysis of the thrombus in and around the aneurysm. This drug therapy is maintained until the time of surgery. The use of this drug allows a longer period of time to be spent on investigations and assessment prior to surgery.

In all three types if loss of consciousness extends over 48 hours the prognosis is poor. Care of the unconscious patient has already been given (pp. 85–91).

Investigations

Echoencephalography, lumbar puncture and angiography are performed. *Scan*, using radioactive isotopes, is injected into the venous circulation. As the isotopes break down they give off radiation which can be detected and measured. Brain tumours have a higher uptake of radioactive material. Occasionally tumours bleed giving features similar to cerebral thrombosis. Scanning is one means of investigating this problem.

Treatment and nursing care

If possible aneurysms are treated surgically by application of a clip to the aneurysm neck and/or wrapping the aneurysm with muslin.

The usual postoperative care is given. However, the patient requires constant care for at least 24 hours with temperature, pulse, respiration and blood pressure assessments being performed every 30 minutes, as well as assessment of conscious level. Any deterioration in conscious level, limb movements or pupillary reaction should be reported and, if necessary, specific treatment given. Deterioration may indicate:

1. **Cerebral vessel spasm.** A mild hemiparesis may become severe. Intravenous dextran 40, 500 ml daily, may improve this situation. Dextran is of low molecular weight which helps reduce erythrocyte 'sludging' when cerebral blood flow is slow.

2. **Oedema of cerebral tissue.** The aim of treatment is to reduce the water content of the brain. A solution with a high osmotic pressure given intravenously will attract fluid to itself from the tissues, including brain tissue. As the blood volume increases a diuresis is inevitable. Such a solution is mannitol which, when given quickly, is very effective.

Steroids such as dexamethazone may also be given for their anti-inflammatory properties, thus restricting the development of oedema. Dexamethazone acts slowly and may therefore be combined with mannitol.

3. **Haematoma formation.** Pressure from the clot may alter conscious level. Surgical intervention may be required to evacuate it.

The rehabilitative treatment for hemiplegia is identical irrespective of the cause.

Nursing a patient with hemiplegia

The aim in the treatment of this patient is to achieve as much independence as possible. The earlier treatment begins, the greater the extent of recovery. Therefore as soon as the patient is conscious rehabilitation should begin. This is a team effort that relies on the knowledge of physiotherapists, occupational and speech therapists, medical and nursing staff and the patient's family, who should be helped to understand the patient's problems and capabilities.

Care begins before the patient is mobilized. Initially efforts are directed at preventing hypostatic pneumonia while the patient is unconscious by removing any secretions, while conscious by encouraging deep breathing and expectoration.

The paralysis is at first flaccid but often becomes spastic as tone returns. Positioning, therefore, is important and paralysed limbs should be supported on pillows in a natural position to prevent contractures. The toes tend to point down, a position which, if uncorrected, allows foot drop to develop, which later makes walking impossible. The foot should therefore be propped up. The hand may tend to become tightly clenched but the use of a foam roll will keep it in a grasp position, help to prevent deformity and promote the return of normal function.

Each joint is moved through its painless range at least twice daily. The patient is encouraged to use his 'good' limb to move his paralysed limb whenever possible. As the patient improves, active exercises are given which require the patient's fullest co-operation; problems may arise if there is intellectual or speech impairment. The active exercises may become difficult due to spasticity and may have to be modified; for instance, a flexed knee helps reduce spasticity while the patient lifts his paralysed arm above head level using his good arm. It is essential for him to learn trunk control, and initially the patient may be taught how to turn in bed. Once this is achieved the patient is promoted to pushing himself up or down the bed, then to sitting on the edge of the bed, then getting out and standing up.

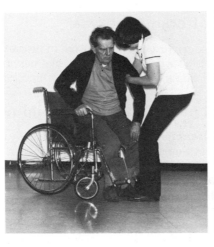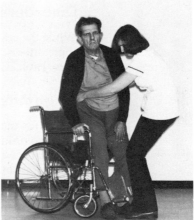

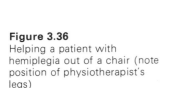
Figure 3.36
Helping a patient with hemiplegia out of a chair (note position of physiotherapist's legs)

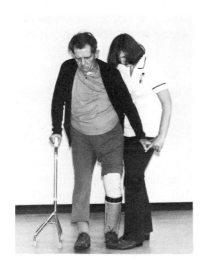
Figure 3.37
Walking with the aid of a tripod and a physiotherapist

Standing is important. The patient tends to neglect the paralysed side and requires constant reminding. The nurse, too, must think of the patient as a whole and not concentrate on a specific weakness. When the patient gets out of bed or up from a chair, the nurse should have her foot in front of the patient's weak foot, her knee acting as a lever maintaining pressure on the patient's knee to keep it straight (Fig. 3.36). The nurse is a 'crutch' to the patient and once balance is achieved walking can begin. The patient may have a tripod and should be taught: 'Tripod forward followed by good leg, then weak leg forward'. The nurse will be at the weak side and, if necessary, may help the weak leg forward by lifting it onwards with her own foot (Fig. 3.37).

As soon as the patient achieves this goal, further independence must be gained, for instance, getting from a bed to a chair.

Occupational therapy
This should also start early to avoid overdependency of the patient. While still in bed the patient should be encouraged to wash and feed himself and be provided with aids designed for the task, such as special cutlery (knife and fork or spoon and fork combined) and non-slip mats for crockery and basins. Although these devices will improve the patient's morale when used successfully, much encouragement and practice is needed.

As the patient makes progress, ordinary daily activities like dressing will be taught and practised. Success here and the gradual return of independence help the patient to look to the future with optimism. When he is able, the patient will go to the occupational therapy department and be taught simple cooking, washing, ironing, getting in and out of the bath, and so on. Tasks like woodwork or knitting may be given to strengthen weak muscles.

Speech therapy
The patient's ability to speak, but not necessarily to think rationally, is affected if there is paralysis of the dominant hemisphere of the brain. His speech may be unintelligible and it may be difficult for an inexperienced person to realize that intelligence is not affected. A code for certain expressions like 'yes' and 'no' should be established as early

as possible to reduce the very great frustration the patient will feel because of his inability to communicate normally. It would be additionally demoralizing for a person so afflicted to be treated other than as an intelligent adult. The speech therapist has a very important contribution to make, sometimes in partnership with an occupational therapist who may be helping the patient to relearn writing.

Prior to discharge the occupational therapist, physiotherapist and medical social worker pay a home visit to assess if help is needed and what alterations are required, such as putting up handrails, removing loose carpets, introducing 'meals on wheels'.

Even after discharge treatment continues. The patient may attend a medical rehabilitation centre. Previous skills and interests may be utilized here if the patient must change his occupation.

Disorders of cranial nerves

While the cranial nerves may be involved in diseases associated with other structures, there are disorders specific to certain cranial nerves, and only those will be described (See Table 3.1 for cranial nerves and their functions).

Trigeminal neuralgia (5th cranial nerve)

The cause of this condition is not known. It usually occurs in middle and late life and is more common in women. The main symptom is an acute episode of severe pain which commences at a specific point of the face and then radiates through the affected area. The distribution of pain will depend on the division of the trigeminal nerve affected. Most frequently pain is localized initially to the second (maxillary) division but will in time spread to the first (ophthalmic) and third (mandibular) divisions. The pain is almost always confined to one side of the face. Although each acute episode may only last for seconds, the pain will persist for days or weeks and will increase in intensity. Attacks may be precipitated by food or fluids at extremes of temperature, exposure of face to cold wind, or touching a particular point of face, gums or teeth (trigger points).

Treatment and nursing care

During acute phases the aim of treatment is relief of pain by administration of drugs. A drug which is proving particularly beneficial is Carbamazepine (Tegretol).

Sedatives may be ordered to ensure adequate sleep.

Relief from pain can also be achieved by the injection of alcohol into the affected division of the trigeminal nerve. The relief from pain may last for several months and treatment can be repeated.

However the only permanent cure lies in cutting the sensory root of the trigeminal nerve. Unless the three divisions are involved, a partial section is performed thus sparing divisions unaffected. As the after effects of this surgery are permanent, i.e. sensation of stiffness and numbness of affected area, it is recommended that surgery should always be preceded by an injection of alcohol. In this way the patient can be acclimatized to the permanent sequelae.

Prior to surgery, the patient should be mobile unless this is contrindicated. Exposure to draughts or inclement weather should be avoided. As chewing may trigger off an attack of pain, food should consist of semisolids and fluids given at room temperature. If pain still occurs a nasogastric infusion of nutrients may be commenced. The tube should be passed via the nostril on the unaffected side of face. As any form of pressure can trigger off an acute episode of pain, the patient may neglect to wash his face, shave or brush his teeth. The nurse must encourage the patient to perform these daily activities in spite of possible resulting discomfort. The face cloth should be of a soft material and water for washing or mouth rinsing should be lukewarm.

If the patient is a woman, it is of particular importance that the minimal amount of hair is shaved from her head. Remaining hair should be secured in an attractive style away from the site of operation. This attention may help to maintain morale.

The immediate preoperative care is as for any operation requiring a general anaesthetic. The operation for trigeminal root section is performed using an extradural approach and is a relatively safe procedure. Immediate postoperative care is as for any operation under a general anaesthetic. Specific observations should be made for any sign of facial weakness when the patient closes his eye or smiles, for evidence of facial oedema or the appearance of sordes. The patient is confined to bed for 24 hours following recovery from anaesthetic. When the patient realizes that eating is no longer accompanied by pain ensuring an adequate intake of nutrients ceases to be a problem. However, as there is now absence of sensation on the affected side of the mouth, the patient should be reminded to chew food on the opposite side to prevent biting of the inside of the cheek. Hot food or fluid must be avoided to prevent burning of desensitized tissue. The patient must be told that he will no longer be aware of particles of food left in the mouth and a mouth rinse is essential after every meal.

If the ophthalmic division of the trigeminal nerve has been sectioned, anaesthesia of the cornea on the affected side will result following surgery. A Bullar shield will be fitted over the affected eye to protect it against entry of foreign bodies. If the patient wears spectacles, he will be visited by an optician who will fit a shield over the spectacle frame. It is vitally important that the patient is educated in the care of his eyes prior to discharge. He will be told that he will not feel particles entering the eye nor will debris be washed away by tears. He must therefore protect the eye, by wearing the special shield supplied on all occasions when out of doors and in any circumstances where debris may enter eye such as attending to a coal fire, sweeping or polishing. He must never rub the eye with fingers or handkerchief. If any discharge does develop he should use a small piece of moist cottonwool and wipe from outer surface of the lids while eye is closed. The eye should not be irrigated nor should drops or ointment be instilled. If inflammation of the eye does develop he must report at once to his doctor. His doctor will receive details of surgery performed from the surgeon and will be aware of possible complications to his patient.

Another form of treatment which may be considered is stitching the eyelids together by means of nylon suture — a tarsorrhaphy. No anaesthetic is required as the area is already insensitive. The suture is removed in approximately 14 days after which closure of the eye is usually secure.

The patient will be discharged about 7 days following surgery.

Facial paralysis— Bell's palsy (7th cranial nerve)

The cause is thought to be a viral infection. Another theory is that it is caused by a local ischaemia and oedema. The initial symptom is a feeling of discomfort behind an ear, which within hours is accompanied by a complete flaccid paralysis of the affected side of face. The patient is unable to close the eyelid, raise the eyebrow, smile or show his teeth and the mouth is displaced towards the unaffected side. As a result of these features the patient presents a grotesque appearance. (Fig. 3.38). He experiences difficulty in swallowing food or fluid and loses sense of taste on affected side of tongue.

In the majority of cases the muscles regain their tone within 3–4 weeks and complete recovery can be anticipated in 3–4 months. However, in a minority of cases recovery may take 6–12 months and may not be complete.

Treatment and nursing care
The aim of treatment is the prevention of complications. Massage and electrical stimulation (faradism) may be used to stimulate and maintain muscle tone. Vasodilating drugs may improve circulation of blood supply to the affected area. Steroids have been prescribed to reduce oedema of the nerve. The use of a facial sling aids in preventing stretching of the weakened muscles, and by improving lip alignment, it facilitates eating (Fig. 3.39).

A malleable wire splint may be used to support the patient's mouth on the affected side. One end of the splint is hooked into the angle of the mouth and the other end is secured behind the ear. The wire is flesh coloured which reduces any embarrassment to the patient. The aim of nursing management is also towards alleviation of patient's disabilities and prevention of complications. The patient should be instructed to chew food on the unaffected side to prevent biting of cheek. Hot food or fluid must be avoided to prevent burning of insensitive area of mouth. As patient will be unaware of particles of food left in an insensitive area, a mouth rinse is essential after every meal. As difficulty on swallowing and partial loss of taste are particular features of this condition, anorexia can be prevented by ensuring that meals are small, attractively presented and of a

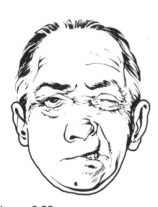

Figure 3.38
Bell's palsy

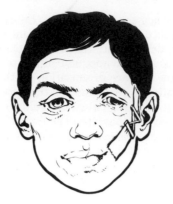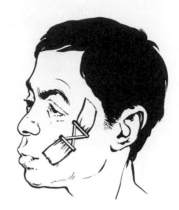

Figure 3.39
Facial sling

semisolid and fluid consistency. Eye care is the same as that described in trigeminal neuralgia.

As the patient will react emotionally to his appearance, the nurse must adopt a positive attitude to a possible recovery. The patient's relatives and friends should be advised to adopt a matter of fact acceptance of his disabilities. Such steps should help to minimize adverse emotional reactions.

If recovery is not complete, the patient will be told of the possibility of anastomosis of the facial nerve with the eleventh and twelfth cranial nerves or alternatively of plastic surgery.

Ménières syndrome (8th cranial nerve) As this condition affects the acoustic nerve which is involved in both hearing and balance, it has been described in another chapter (see p. 438).

Parkinson's disease

The cause of this condition has not been determined. Research has proven that approximately 80 per cent of dopamine the chemical transmitter in the brain is concentrated in the corpus striatum. In Parkinson's disease the level of dopamine in the corpus striatum is markedly reduced. Research has also shown that the level of the chemical transmitter acetylcholine within the nervous system is increased.

The symptoms of Parkinson's disease are caused by this imbalance of chemical transmitters. The patient presents a characteristic rigidity of movement and appearance. (Fig. 3.40). When walking, short steps are taken and these become increasingly more rapid and outwith the patient's control (propulsion). The arms do not swing as they normally do while walking but remain pressed to the sides. All movements take longer to perform and, as the disease progresses, chewing, swallowing, speaking and writing become more difficult. Due to impairment of facial mobility the patient will present a mask-like appearance which does not alter in response to emotion. As the patient's ability to swallow becomes impaired he will drool saliva. Tremors may occur in any part of the body but are most noticeable in the hands. (Fig. 3.41). Involuntary movements of the fingers have been given the name of 'pill rolling'. (Fig. 3.42). The patient may display an apparent inability to use a limb which is not affected by rigidity or tremor (Bradykinesia). Tremors may disappear when the patient is engaged in purposeful activity involving the affected limb, but become exaggerated when activity involves other limbs. Emotion may also exaggerate tremor. Sometimes the disease is associated with intellectual deterioration and/or hypertension.

Treatment and nursing care
The introduction of certain drugs has revolutionized the treatment of patients suffering from Parkinson's disease enabling many to resume their activities of daily living within a short period of time. The aims of treatment are to increase the level of dopamine in the nervous system and reduce the level of acetylcholine in the nervous system. The level of dopamine is increased by the oral administration of levodopa, the precursor of dopamine. The problem is that very large doses have to be given as most of the drug is destroyed before reaching the nervous system. This difficulty has been remedied by the

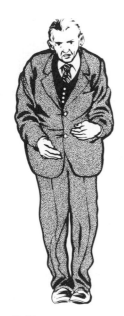

Figure 3.40
Parkinsonism

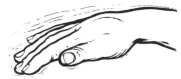

Figure 3.41
Tremor

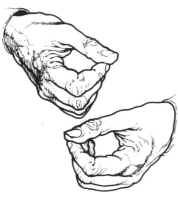

Figure 3.42
Pill rolling'

introduction of a drug containing levodopa and carbidopa (Sinemet). Carbidopa inhibits the enzyme which is responsible for the breakdown of levodopa in the tissue, thus ensuring that most of the levodopa administered will reach the nervous system. Levodopa is effective in reducing rigidity but not tremor.

The level of acetylcholine is reduced by the oral administration of an anticholinergic drug; the two most commonly used are benztropine (Cogentin) and benzhexol (Artane). Anticholinergic drugs are effective in reducing tremor. A combination of both types of drugs are therefore necessary to combat the cardinal symptoms.

Administration of levodopa may cause hypotension, nausea, vomiting, anorexia and delusions of persecution.

Anticholinergic drugs may produce the side effects of nausea, constipation, blurred vision, tachycardia and loss of concentration.

Drooling of saliva is reduced by administration of benzhexol. Amphetamine sulphate may be prescribed to produce a sense of euphoria.

The patient is normally admitted to hospital for 2 to 3 weeks until stabilization of drug therapy is achieved. He must be kept as active as possible and encouraged to maintain his independence. Sitting upright in bed is discouraged as the patient tends to slide down so he should be seated in a chair and supported by pillows. The nurse should ensure that he has a plentiful supply of tissues to cope with excessive salivation. The diet should be light and semisolid, and additional fluids should be given to compensate for that lost in saliva. Drugs are given in five small doses daily immediately following meals; this has been found to reduce the incidence of nausea. Regular observations must be carried out for signs indicating side effects to drug therapy. The blood pressure must be recorded four hourly with the patient in recumbent and upright positions. As delusions of persecution are a possible side effect the nurse must realize that a display of aggression towards her by the patient is outwith his control. Her reaction must be one of firm but sympathetic understanding of her patient's needs. The patient's tremor can be made less obvious if he or she is allowed to carry something for example a newspaper or a handbag. A programme of physical therapy is essential and will involve the physiotherapist, the nurse and the patient's relatives. Specific exercises have been designed to improve efficiency of muscles and prevent deformities and they will be demonstrated to the nurse and the relatives by the physiotherapist so that all parties will play a role in the rehabilitation programme. In particular, the patient must be encouraged to perform again and again any motor activity that he finds especially difficult. The use of zips rather than buttons will make dressing or undressing that much easier. Walking aids are of little value, but the trolley type of Zimmer is helpful in some cases. The patient and his family must be informed of the nature of illness in order that they are best prepared to participate in the programme of treatments.

While all patients who suffer from Parkinson's disease can be helped by stereotaxic surgery, the best postoperative results occur in patients who are deteriorating slowly, those who present with unilateral rigidity and tremor, and when surgery involves the non-dominant hemisphere of the cerebrum. Surgery involves the introduction of an electrode or cannula through the brain to selected areas of the basal ganglia which are then destroyed. In most cases the rigidity and tremor are markedly reduced if not completely abolished. Ideally the patient should be nursed prior to and following surgery by the same team of nurses. This helps to ensure that any alteration, no matter how slight, in the patient's condition is noted and recorded. As most if not all patients are apprehensive regarding the outcome of surgery and require support in adjusting to their improved capabilities, the presence of familiar faces following surgery is invaluable. An assessment of the patient is made by the surgeon, the psychologist, the physiotherapist, the speech therapist and the charge nurse. This is essential as comparisons will be made following surgery. The patient's hair is shaved off and his scalp washed and dried. Base line recordings are made of temperature, pulse, respirations and blood pressure. Surgery is performed under local anaesthetic. It is essential that the vital signs (p. 85) are observed and recorded every 15 minutes following surgery. Haemorrhage may occur as a result of the introduction of electrode or cannula and the nurse must be vigilant in her observations for signs of increased intracranial pressure. (see p. 84). As drug therapy is discontinued, albeit for a very short time, there is a risk of oculogyric crisis (deviation and fixation of the eyes) (Fig. 3.43) occurring, and the nurse must report this at once. The patient may develop a

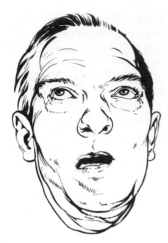

Figure 3.43
Oculogyric crisis

hemiplegia but can be reassured that this is of a temporary nature. Normally the patient is confined to bed for 24 hours following surgery. The aim of treatment now is to encourage the correct use of limbs which have regained function and to correct posture and gait. The patient is usually discharged in 5 days.

Multiple sclerosis

This is the most common disease affecting the nervous system. The cause is unknown. The myelin sheath of the neurone disintegrates and, as a result, the nerve is no longer able to conduct impulses correctly. This is followed by an impairment of function of the area supplied by the nerve. As the disease affects nerves throughout the brain and spinal cord the patient can present a variety of signs and symptoms. The disease is characterized by periods of remission and relapse of symptoms over a period of months or years.

The usual mode of onset is a partial paralysis of one limb. The paralysis disappears after a time only to return. Visual disturbances include blurred vision, double vision and nystagmus (involuntary and repetitive movement of eyeballs). There may be an increased frequency of micturition or a retention of urine. Retention of urine can lead to the formation of calculi and/or a urinary tract infection. Constipation and impaction of faeces is a common problem. The patient may complain of a sensation of tingling, numbness, burning, dampness or coldness of the skin. He may experience difficulty in identifying parts of his body — 'altered body image'. Tremor of a limb while in motion may be observed 'an intention tremor'. Irregular and jerky movements (ataxia) of the lower limbs may be present. The patient may have difficulty with articulation of words (dysarthria) and in the latter stages of the disease he may have a peculiar staccato voice or sometimes scanning of speech. The patient's mood may swing from one of elation to one of depression.

Factors which are known to worsen symptoms temporarily are smoking, excessive fatigue, hot baths, exposure to sunlight, vaccinations and menstruation.

Treatment and nursing care

The aims of treatment are to assist the patient in achieving his maximum physical capacity and optimum psychological adjustment to his condition. If patient suffers double vision (diplopia), an eye patch can be worn and his head positioned to make the best use of remaining vision. If partially sighted his ability to read can be enhanced by use of large print books, talking book or magnifying glass. The patient's name can be entered in the register for the blind or partially sighted. The handicap accompanying tremor may be reduced by the use of lead shot wrist bands and by positioning the patient's elbows between the chair and his body. A wing chair and high backed wheel chair should be provided for maximum comfort. At meal times the patient should be given his own table. A feeding cup with lid should be provided, forks should be avoided and if possible food which can be picked up with the fingers should be served. Smoking should be permitted only when a member of staff or a relative is with the patient as a cigarette may be dropped with disastrous results. If the patient has speech problems, the nurse should phrase sentences so that patient need only reply 'yes' or 'no' and should resist the temptation to complete the sentence for patient, or to anticipate his requests. If speech is non-existent, a communication chart and, if the patient can write, a scribble pad and pencil should be provided. Physiotherapy is necessary to strengthen non-affected muscles and to ensure maximum use of those weakened by the disease. Adequate support of paralysed limbs is essential especially if paralysis is flaccid. Flat heeled shoes should be worn and aids such as calipers, tripods, Zimmer and wheel chair provided as required. The occupational therapy department will supply bath aids. The application of ice to limbs gives sufficient relief from spasms to enable limbs to be put through a full range of movements. The stimuli provoking spasm can be reduced by using a cage to relieve the weight of bed clothes, ensuring bladder and lower colon are emptied of contents and observing measures necessary to prevent any breaks in the continuity of the skin. The use of drugs such as Diazepam and Nitrazepam aid in reducing spasms.

The patient should be encouraged to void urine every two hours. Tapping over the bladder area and applying pressure over the suprapubis may help in initiating micturition. If the problem is increased, frequency of micturition the use of Paul's tubing, incontinence pads, incontinence pants and uridoms must be considered. As a last resort catheterization of the urinary bladder will be necessary if the patient's skin is becoming damaged by incontinence of urine. The patient should be encouraged to defaecate at the same time each day, preferably after breakfast. Senokot should be given on two evenings a week followed by a sodium phosphate enema; manual evacuation of faeces may be necessary. Oral fluids should be in excess of 3 000 ml per day. If the sensory pathways are involved certain precautions are necessary to prevent injuries, for example the temperature of the bath water must be determined, the patient should avoid direct heat from a fire, hot water bottles should not be used. Stockings should be intact and free fitting, and protective felt boots provided. If a plastic foot-drop splint is used the area under the splint should be observed for signs of pressure. Constant visual reassurance regarding the size, shape and position of limbs and body is the only support the nurse can offer the patient who suffers the distressing symptom of altered body image. Patients who have an altered body image and a paralysis require frequent change of position when in bed.

Prior to the patient's discharge from hospital action should be taken to ensure that his home circumstances are as ideal as possible. Patient may attend a day centre and when at home receive visits from district nurse and health visitor. The local authority social work department may be able to give assistance such as the services of a house help, meals on wheels or Aids to Daily Living (Ch. 20). His house may require alterations, perhaps to allow a wheelchair to be used, or it may be possible to arrange for ground floor accommodation. Financial help in the form of a heating allowance, mobility allowance and attendance allowance are entitlements in the United Kingdom.

The patient's family may become exhausted as a result of caring for him at home and the patient can be admitted to hospital to allow the family to have a period of rest.

The life expectancy of a person with multiple sclerosis is 15 to 20 years. Death is usually due to renal failure, bronchopneumonia or involvement of vital centres within the brain.

Spinal lesions

Spinal lesions can result from pathology within the cord (intrinsic — for example demyelinating) or outside the cord (extrinsic). Extrinsic pathology may lie within or without the meninges.

Causes of spinal lesions
These are given in Table 3.3.

Table 3.3
Causes of spinal lesions

Cause		Example
Congenital		Spina bifida
Acquired	1. Traumatic	Fractures Dislocations Gunshot and stab wounds.

	2. Infective
	  a. Acute
	
	  b. Chronic
		
		Abscess
		Poliomyelitis
		Syphilis

	3. Neoplastic
	  a. Benign
	  b. Malignant
	    i. Primary
	    ii. Secondary
		
		Neurofibroma
		
		Ependymoma
		Deposits from breast cancer.

	4. Degenerative	Cervical spondylosis. Prolapsed disc.

Note: This table does not include demyelination since the aetiology is unknown.

General features of spinal lesions

The features depend on the level and severity of the lesion but usually all functions of the cord — motor, sensory, and autonomic — are affected to a greater or lesser degree. The motor signs depend on whether the upper or lower motor neurone, or both, are involved (Fig. 3.21, p. 77). Damage to the upper motor neurone will result in spastic weakness and increased reflexes below the level of the lesion. Lower motor neurone damage presents as profound muscle wasting, flaccid weakness and depressed or absent tendon reflexes at the level of the lesion.

Different sensory tracts convey different types (modalities) of sensation, pain, temperature, touch and proprioception. The type of sensation lost will depend on the tract or tracts affected. If sensory roots are affected all form of sensation will be impaired.

Since the spinal cord ends at the level of the first lumbar vertebra, any lesion below this level, such as protrusion of a lumbar intervertebral disc, can only produce root lesions resulting in lower motor neurone weakness and impairment of all forms of sensation.

Investigations

Plain X-ray

This is the simplest form of investigation and may demonstrate fractures, dislocations and carcinomatous deposits in the vertebrae. Secondary deposits invading the vertebral column tend to arise from a primary carcinoma of the breast, kidney or prostate. Osteophytes (bony outgrowths) and narrowing of the intervertebral disc spaces are often demonstrated on X-ray in cases of cervical spondylosis.

Lumbar puncture

Since the spinal cord is encased within the meninges it is possible to obtain a sample of cerebrospinal fluid by lumbar puncture.

Lumbar puncture may be necessary for one of the following reasons:

1. To estimate CSF pressure (occasionally to remove some CSF to reduce the pressure) and to demonstrate any blockage of the subarachnoid pathways.

2. To obtain CSF for diagnostic purposes, say, for confirmation of a subarachnoid haemorrhage or meningitis. Immediately after subarachnoid haemorrhage the CSF is bloodstained. After a time is becomes xanthochromic (yellow in colour) due to the breakdown of red blood cells. In meningitis the CSF may be turbid. If meningitis is suspected a specimen of CSF will be sent to the laboratory for estimation of cell, protein, chloride and glucose content, culture of organisms and antibiotic sensitivity tests. CSF stagnating below a spinal block may be yellow in colour and will have an increased protein content.

3. To instil drugs in cases of infection.

4. For contrast radiography. A contrast medium, such as air for outlining the ventricular system or a dye for spinal myelography, may be injected.

The nurse can do much to alleviate the anxiety of the patient by explaining the lumbar puncture procedure to him. Usually the lumbar puncture is performed with the patient in the left lateral position. The legs are drawn up and flexed on the abdomen, the head and neck are flexed towards the chest wall. This flexes the vertebral column separating the vertebral spines so as to facilitate entry of the lumbar puncture needle. The nurse should hold the patient in this position during the procedure (Fig. 3.44). The level chosen is usually the space between the second and third or third and fourth vertebrae. As the spinal cord ends above this level there is no risk of damage to the cord.

As one of the indications for lumbar puncture is to estimate CSF pressure a calibrated manometer can be fitted to the spinal needle. Normally CSF pressure varies from 60 to 180 mm of water and is affected by pulse and respiration. The flexed position also increases the pressure; therefore, the pressure should be measured with the patient in a relaxed position after entry of the lumbar puncture needle. Increased pressure may be due to a space-occupying intracranial lesion such as an abscess, neoplasm or blood clot, brain swelling or hydrocephalus.

If blockage of CSF pathways is suspected, Queckenstedt's manoeuvre may be performed (Fig. 3.45). This shows whether or not there is an unobstructed CSF

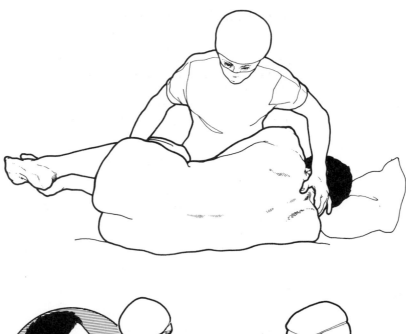

Figure 3.44
Positioning patient for lumbar puncture

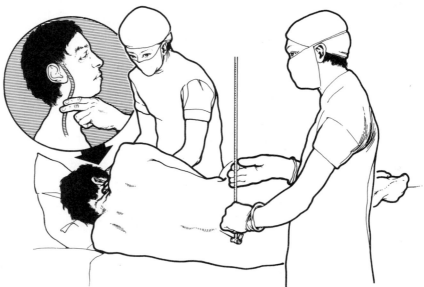

Figure 3.45
Queckenstedt's manoeuvre

pathway between the lumbar and intracranial subarachnoid space. The nurse will be asked to compress both jugular veins; if done correctly this causes no discomfort. Pressure on the jugular veins causes an increase in the intracranial venous sinus pressure. This pressure rise is transmitted to the CSF in the subarachnoid space. If there is no subarachnoid blockage, there is free rise and fall of the CSF in the manometer. If there is a partial blockage there may be a sluggish rise and fall, and in complete blockage pressure on the jugular veins will cause no rise in the CSF pressure.

Following lumbar puncture the patient is nursed flat or head down for 24 hours. This should lessen the likelihood of headache which may result from removal of CSF from the subarachnoid space, or later leakage of CSF following withdrawal of the lumbar puncture needle. If headache is severe, analgesics may be prescribed. Some patients may have difficulty in micturition because of their unaccustomed position. If so it may be permissible to allow the patient up to use a commode. The decision is the doctor's and will depend on the patient's condition. If there is any indication of increased intracranial pressure a close watch must be kept on conscious level, pupils, pulse, respiration rate and blood pressure (vital signs). In extreme cases where there is great pressure increase the sudden reduction of pressure may cause part of the temporal lobe to slip through the tentorial hiatus and impact against the brain stem or may cause the cerebellum to be pushed into the foramen magnum. This causes deterioration in conscious level and alteration in vital signs and may cause respiratory arrest.

Myelography

This consists of injecting a radio-opaque iodine substance which is heavier than CSF. The patient is placed on a tilting X-ray table. A lumbar puncture is performed, a quantity of CSF is withdrawn and a smaller quantity of contrast medium is injected into the subarachnoid space. Since this is heavier than CSF, by tilting the X-ray table it can be made to run along the whole spinal subarachnoid space, outlining any abnormalities.

Irregularities of the theca or spinal block will be observed using the X-ray image intensifier and X-ray films can be taken of the level. The dye is removed following the procedure and the patient is nursed flat for the following 24 hours. The care is the same as for lumbar puncture.

A water soluble dye may demonstrate more clearly the outline of the nerve roots and could be used in preference to the iodine dye. The patient sits upright for six hours following this and then may be allowed up. The upright position is used following radiculogram as occasionally the water soluble dye may act as an irritant to the cord and brain.

Traumatic spinal lesions

Fracture or dislocation of the vertebral column may damage the spinal cord in several ways:

1. Concussion.
2. Contusion.
3. Laceration.
4. Compression.
5. Damage to blood supply.

Clinical features depend on the level and severity of the lesion. If the whole of the cord is damaged there will be complete paralysis and loss of sensation below the level of the lesion. A thoracic or lumbar lesion will result in paralysis of the lower limbs (**paraplegia**). A cervical lesion results in paralysis of all four limbs (**tetraplegia**) (Fig. 3.46). In both paraplegia and tetraplegia the autonomic system is also involved so that bladder,

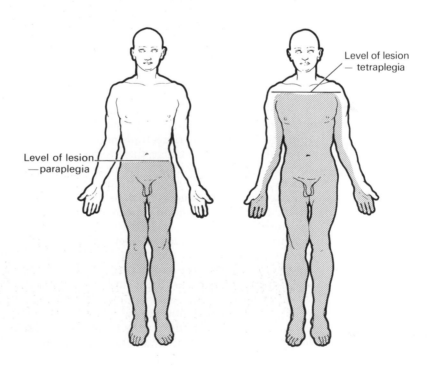

Figure 3.46
Left: Paraplegia
Right: Tetraplegia

bowel, vasomotor and sexual functions may be lost. Lesions of the conus and nerve roots result in paralysis of the lower motor neurone type.

Paraplegia and tetraplegia

At the time of injury the patient presents with a flaccid paralysis. Autonomic control is lost resulting in retention of urine and faeces. Sympathetic paralysis results in postural hypotension, troublesome at the stage of mobilization. A patient with a high cervical lesion has respiratory problems, since the diaphragm is paralysed. Diaphragmatic breathing is preserved in lower cervical lesions because the diaphragm is controlled by the phrenic nerve derived from cervical segments three, four and five.

Nursing a patient with paraplegia

The treatment of spinal injury in the acute phase aims at stabilization of fractures. reduction of dislocations and prevention of further complications such as pressure sores, limb contractures and urinary tract infections.

Initially the aim is to correct spinal deformity by positioning, which is most conveniently achieved by nursing the patient on a Stryker frame (Figs. 3.47 and 3.48).

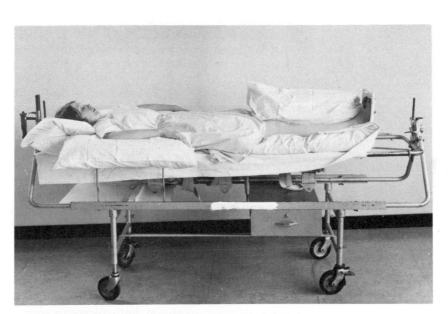

Figure 3.47
Patient on a Stryker frame

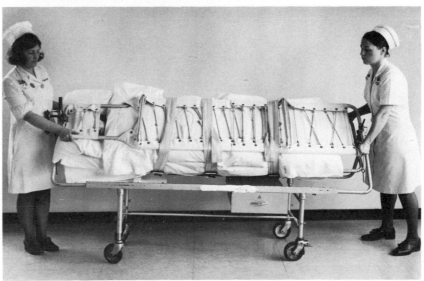

Figure 3.48
Turning a patient on a Stryker frame

This treatment will not undo cord damage but it will lessen the risk of further damage. The patient is nursed on the frame on a layer of pillows suitably placed to maintain his spine in the best position (usually hyperextension) for correction of the deformity. He should be turned every 2 hours. Only two nurses are required for this procedure. The patient may be nursed on the frame for 8 to 12 weeks.

Alternatively, the patient may be nursed on a Stoke Egerton or an ordinary hospital bed on pillow packs. The Stoke Egerton bed operates electrically and turns the patient from one side to the other. Pillow packs are disposed so that the bony prominences (sacrum, trochanters, heels and shoulders) are supported. Pillows should be placed under and between the legs to avoid pressure on the condyles of the knee and the malleoli of the ankles. The disadvantage of nursing a patient on a bed as opposed to a frame is that, four or five nurses are required to lift and turn the patient in 'one piece', maintaining proper alignment of the vertebral column.

Care of the skin

Due to his lack of sensation the paraplegic is not aware of discomfort. The nursing staff must turn the patient every 2 hours to relieve areas of prolonged pressure, thus minimizing the risk of pressure sores. The skin should be inspected at every turn and any area which is red or broken should be relieved of pressure until healed. The skin is kept clean by daily baths and by washing the pressure areas more often if necessary. Even when artificial methods are used to relieve pressure, for example a ripple mattress (a device which constantly redistributes the patient's weight), turning should not be omitted — such devices are no substitute for regular turning. Sheets must be kept dry, crumb- and wrinkle-free. Hot water bottles or electric blankets should never be placed in the bed since the patient can be burned without experiencing any discomfort. (There is great temptation to use them as paralysed extremities are very cold.) For the same reason, once mobilized the patient must be warned against sitting too close to fires, radiators or unlagged hot water pipes; handling hot water taps; using too hot water; and so on. The slightest break in the skin may take a long time to heal. A high protein diet and correction of anaemia, if present, are necessary if sores are to heal.

Care of limbs

In upper motor neurone lesions, return of reflex activity and tone is usually noticeable about 6 weeks after injury causing the flaccid paralysis to become spastic. In a conus or cauda equina lesion the legs and bladder remain flaccid since it is the lower motor neurones which are damaged. With return of reflex activity the patient may develop flexor or extensor spasms. Untreated spasms may give rise to permanent deformities of the limbs due to contractures of the muscles. Contractures can be prevented by careful positioning in bed and by putting the joints through their full range of movements twice daily. The patient may be nursed face down if he has severe flexor spasms. Pressure sores tend to increase spasm. Antispasmodics such as baclofen (Lioresal) and diazepam (Valium) may be of considerable value in the control of spasm.

Care of the urinary bladder

Renal failure is a common cause of death in paraplegics. Initially the bladder is flaccid. Overdistension must be avoided either by continuous bladder drainage or intermittent catheterization. Strict aseptic technique must be practised.

In upper motor neurone lesions, if the continuous method is being used, when reflex activity returns (or in any case in 6 weeks), the catheter is clipped and released at 2-hourly intervals. The patient may have a bizarre sensation of bladder fullness or he may experience headache, flushing or sweating. The catheter is withdrawn and attempts made to initiate reflex bladder evacuation by stimulating 'trigger spots' — tapping over the lower abdomen or rubbing the vulval area. If reflex evacuation is achieved, an injection of a drug such as carbachol is given resulting in further voiding. The residual urine is measured by reintroducing the catheter. Subject to obtaining satisfactory residuals (less than 60 ml) the catheter is left out for progressively longer periods and may eventually be dispensed with altogether, as indeed may the carbachol injections.

The patient should endeavour to empty his bladder regularly, say, every 2 to 4 hours, before the onset of sensations of fullness, headache or sweating. Great patience and perseverance are necessary to achieve such automatic bladder function. It may take many months, but it is a worthwhile achievement since bladder emptying is likely to be fairly complete. It is also more socially acceptable.

In conus and root lesions the bladder remains flaccid and autonomous bladder emptying may be achieved by straining and suprapubic compression. These patients tend to have greater residuals and are therefore more prone to infection. Surgery may be necessary to achieve relaxation of the internal and external sphincters. If neither automatic nor autonomous bladder function is achieved an in-dwelling catheter will be necessary, carrying with it a higher risk of infection and calculus formation.

Once the initial oliguria of the first fortnight has passed a high fluid intake (3–4 litres) must be encouraged. Catheters are changed daily at first, then at longer intervals. Permanent in-dwelling catheters are changed monthly, and urine is sent for culture regulaly. A concentration of organisms of 10^6/ml or greater is usually treated irrespective of whether or not there is constitutional upset. Organisms of lesser concentration require no treatment, unless there is systemic upset.

It is important to assess renal and bladder function at regular intervals after discharge from hospital. The procedures undertaken include intravenous pyelography, measurement of residual urine volumes, estimations of blood urea, creatinine and serum electrolytes.

Care of bowel function

Digital evacuation is performed initially by the nursing staff. Once the patient is mobilized he is taught to transfer to the toilet seat from his wheel-chair and to evacuate his own bowels by straining or by digital evacuation. Digital check should always be carried out to ensure that the rectum is emptied. Laxatives and/or suppositories may be necessary as may periodic enemas.

Sexual function

Although this aspect of paraplegia is very rarely raised by the patient it is nevertheless a cause of anxiety to many.

Females. Paraplegic women can conceive and bear children normally. They do not, however, have the normal sensations of sexual intercourse.

Males. Some men with upper motor neurone lesions may get reflex erections but of those only a few ejaculate, so that the chances of fathering a child are remote. During intercourse the female must be the active partner. In conus or root lesions erection and ejaculation are impossible.

A group entitled SPOD (Sexual Problems of the Disabled) has recently been set up by the National Fund for Research into Crippling Diseases, to study and to give advice on this difficulty. Information is available from the Committee on Sexual Problems of the Disabled, 49 Victoria Street, London SW1.

Mobilization

Transfer from a Stryker frame or pillow packs is usually possible 8 to 12 weeks after injury. Gradually the number of pillows under the head and shoulders are increased. Due to sympathetic paralysis patients with high lesions frequently suffer from dizziness and fainting attacks and it may be some time before they can tolerate the upright position. When the patient can sit upright he is supported with his legs over the edge of the bed and taught sitting balance in front of a long mirror. He is then transferred to a wheel-chair. Dependent feet may develop oedema and to alleviate this condition elastic stockings may be necessary. In the physiotherapy and occupational therapy departments, the patient is taught feeding; toilet and dressing procedures; transfer from bed to chair, chair to toilet seat; and so on. In transfer the weight is taken by the arms, and upper limb musculature must be developed to enable the patient to do these manoeuvres. In the wheel-chair the patient sits on a 5–10 cm foam cushion and is advised to raise his buttocks off the cushion every 15 minutes to lessen the risk of ischial pressure sores.

Excessive reflex sweating is common. Sheepskin seat covers are useful to absorb sweat.

Rehabilitation

Rehabilitation starts from the moment the patient is diagnosed as paraplegic. The patient may find it very difficult to accept that he may never walk again. He may be very depressed, frustrated and aggressive. The aggression is a defence mechanism and may be directed towards members of staff or close relatives. It is a way of getting rid of pent-up emotions. Psychological support from the whole team is necessary. Relatives also require help and advice. The medical social worker can help with financial problems as well as by assessing the home situation with the occupational therapist. Change of accommodation may be necessary. The living room, bedroom and bathroom should be on ground-floor level. Doors may need to be widened, ramps provided at outside doors, furniture rearranged and even kitchen fittings lowered.

The disablement resettlement officer can arrange for assessment, retraining and placement in suitable employment. He can also arrange for the provision of a special car and an allowance.

Ideally the district nurse is invited by the ward team to visit the patient in hospital in order to become familiar with the patient and any special care necessary.

The patient should not be without his hobbies, relaxations and pastimes. In hospital the patient should be encouraged to engage in swimming, archery, table tennis, and so on, all of which strengthen arm muscles, as well as providing the stimulus of competitive sport.

At the end of the patient's stay in hospital — amounting to a year or more — it is hoped the patient will have gained some measure of independence and that he will again be integrated in home and society.

Spina bifida

Neural tube defects comprise a large percentage of congenital abnormalities, the most common in Great Britain being spina bifida. This defect is subdivided into:

1. Spina bifida occulta

2. Spina bifida cystica

    a. meningocele

    b. myelomeningocele

There is failure of the vertebral arch to close in the midline (Fig. 3.49) thus allowing meninges or meninges and cord to prolapse through the gap. These defects can occur anywhere within the vertebral column, the most common site being in the lumbosacral area. The vertebral arch normally closes by the twelfth week of gestation.

Spina bifida occulta This as the term implies is a hidden lesion. Detailed examination of the new born infant (p. 512) may enable the midwife or doctor to detect this. There may be a slight dimpling of the skin and a tuft of hair may be present. A slight gap may be felt on palpation of the vertebral spines. Spina bifida occulta is usually of no significance and may not produce neurological symptoms. Occasionally, however there may be an underlying sinus leading to a lipoma or demoid cyst. This may become infected or the nerve roots may be compressed by the lesion. Surgical exploration and excision usually gives good results.

Spina bifida cystica *a. Meningocele.* In this abnormality the meninges herniate through the gap and lie on the surface of the back. The skin may not cover the defect completely. The middle is usually translucent and cerebrospinal fluid can be seen. There is danger therefore of the meningocele rupturing and greater risk of meningitis occurring prior to surgery. (Fig. 3.50).

b. Myelomeningocele. This is by far the commonest and most serious type of spina bifida. As well as meninges herniating, the spinal cord and nerve roots are also contained in the sac, and are adherent to it. Again skin covering is imperfect often consisting of a thin arachnoidal membrane with an even greater risk of rupture and infection. A myelomeningocele involving the lumbosacral region causes a flaccid paralysis of legs, bladder and bowel. Fig. 3.51 (Fig. 17.11, p. 514).

Treatment and nursing care
Aspects of nursing care include prevention of infection, maintenance of body temperature and careful observation of bladder and bowel function. Closure of the

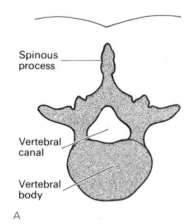

Spinous process

Vertebral canal

Vertebral body

A

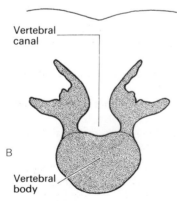

Vertebral canal

B

Vertebral body

Figure 3.49
Spina bifida
A. Normal vertebra
B. Failure of neural arch to close

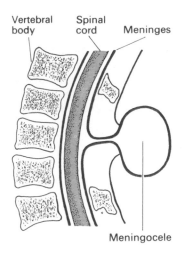

Figure 3.50
Meningocele

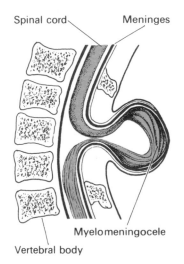

Figure 3.51
Myelomeningocele

defect will be carried out as early as the child's general condition permits, should operation be the course decided upon. The infant is nursed without clothing in an incubator, in the prone position. This allows maximum observation of the baby and prevents pressure on the lesion. The area is covered with a sterile non adherent dressing or sterile gauze soaked in sterile normal saline. This is replaced with aseptic technique as often as is necessary. Changing of napkins should be carried out as often as required with careful cleansing and drying of the skin each time, avoiding, as far as possible, contamination of the lesion. If paralysis is present careful observation on bladder and bowel emptying is necessary. Compression of the bladder may be required to avoid overdistention. Dribbling incontinence is often a problem pre and post operatively and the skin requires to be kept clean and dry.

Surgical closure of the lesion aims at separating any neural tissue from the sac and after exploration of the canal replacing it into the spinal canal. The lesion is then closed by direct closure or by a rotation skin flap. It is not always possible to improve motor or sensory function and the infant may remain paralysed requiring careful skin, bladder and bowel care.

A child with spina bifida may have other complications, such as scoliosis and talipes; closure of the spina bifida cystica may be first of many operations. Permanent dribbling incontinence causing excoriation may require a urinary diversion, a ureterostomy, to avoid skin breakdown.

The parents should be made aware that long periods of hospitalization may be required. Through counselling sessions they should be fully informed of the implications of this handicap. Advice can be given of the practical and supporting help provided by listed charitable organizations principally the Spina Bifida and Hydrocephalus Society, The Disabled Living Foundation and Riding for the Disabled.

Hydrocephalus

This condition is caused by a gradual accumulation of cerebrospinal fluid with associated dilatation of the ventricular system. The condition occurs in combination with spina bifida cystica which may be present at birth or develop following closure of the lesion. Other causes include aqueduct stenosis, closure of the aqueduct between the third and fourth ventricle and complications from an accidental or non accidental injury. Measurement of the occipital—frontal circumference is carried out and an increase above the normal limits may indicate the presence of hydrocephalus.

Other signs of developing hydrocephalus are:

1. A tense and bulging fontenelle. Increase in CSF pressure displays the suture lines thus allowing the head circumference to increase and a normal slack fontenelle to become tense.

2. The scalp veins become engorged due to interference with intracranial venous drainage.

3. The infant may also develop 'sunsetting' of the eyes. This occurs with midbrain compression impairing upward and outward gaze (Fig. 3.52).

4. As the intracranial pressure increases the infant shows signs of irritability and malnutrition due to reluctance to feed and projectile vomiting.

These clinical features occur before drowsiness and other neurological deficits as the intracranial pressure is temporarily relieved by the increasing head circumference. Should hydrocephalus develop later in life after closure of the anterior fontenelle, e.g. following subarachnoid haemorrhage or be secondary to a space occupying lesion then the clinical features are of raised intracranial pressure. (p. 84).

Investigation
Computerized axial tomography will be performed which may demonstrate enlargement of the ventricular system (p. 95).

Treatment and nursing care
Preoperatively the infant is given good nursing care to prevent skin breakdown, by changing position frequently. Areas at risk are in the parietal regions of the skull, upper and lower limbs which may require to be wrapped in cotton wool if the baby is very

irritable, to prevent excoriation due to hyperactivity. Nasogastric tube feeding may be necessary to prevent further malnutrition and to ensure adequate fluid intake.

A shunt procedure is the operation of choice. This consists of diverting the CSF from the lateral ventricles to another area where it can be absorbed. Commonest is the ventriculoperitoneal shunt (Fig. 3.53), the distal end is placed in the subphrenic space, or the ventriculo-atrial shunt (Fig. 3.54), the distal end of which is threaded into the internal jugular to the right atrium. The valve used in the shunt system is either the Pudenz (Fig. 3.55) or Spitz-Holter.

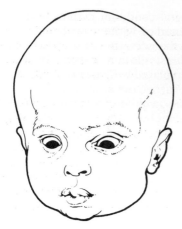

Figure 3.52
'Sunsetting'

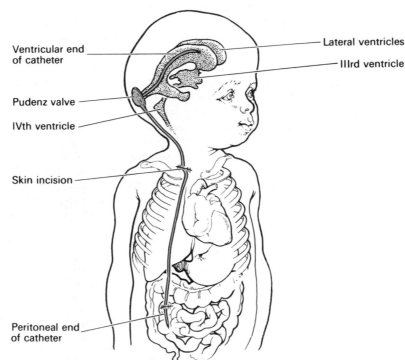

Figure 3.53
Ventriculoperitoneal shunt

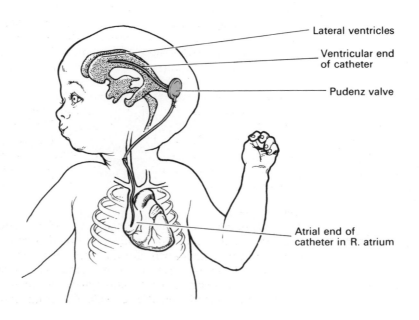

Figure 3.54
Ventriculo-atrial shunt

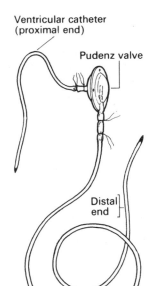

Figure 3.55
Pudenz valve

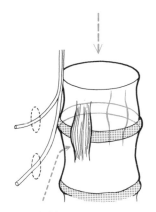

Figure 3.56
Normal lumbar vertebrae and
intervertebral discs

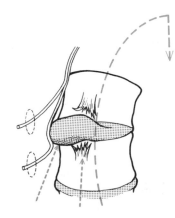

Figure 3.57
Prolapsed lumbar intervertebral
disc

Postoperatively the child is observed carefully for signs of shock or haemorrhage, the incision being checked for leakage of spinal fluid. Record of TPR are maintained and deep breathing encouraged. The child is positioned on the side opposite to operation to prevent pressure being applied to the valve. Accurate recordings of intake and output should be maintained, the child occasionally requiring intravenous fluids and nutrition.

The anterior fontenelle should be observed for bulging or excessive depression indicating an ineffective or an overactive shunt. The shunt valve is not pumped routinely. Continuing care includes the teaching of the parents to recognize complications that may arise at any time e.g. the shunt system may become blocked, kinked or as the child grows the tubing requires lengthening. Very quickly the child will develop raised pressure, becoming irritable and drowsy. The effectiveness of the shunt system can be judged by medical and nursing staff. A valve that is difficult to depress indicates the distal end is blocked, whereas a valve that remains concave indicates ineffectiveness of the ventricular end.

Gradually the nurse can teach the parents to feed, hold and bathe their baby, to express his bladder, aid him in his bowel evacuations, exercise his limbs, pump his shunt (if necessary) and to recognize the early signs of raised intracranial pressure. By encouraging them to take an active part in looking after their baby they will learn to feel confident in their own abilities to provide him with adequate care in spite of his physical handicap.

When the infant is feeding well, the shunt is working satisfactorily, and when medical and nursing staff feel that the parents are able to meet his needs, he will be discharged home. Before doing so, the community nursing services must be contacted and also the family general practitioner. They should arrange to visit as soon as the baby arrives home, so that they can give assurance to the parents, that they can be contacted if difficulties arise.

Close supervision of the child's growth and developmental progress is made by the paediatrician and psychologist, and guidance and support given to the parents to help them understand the severity of the problem, the consequences of surgical treatment and the future for their child.

Prolapsed lumbar intervertebral disc

The spinal cord is enclosed within the neural arch of the vertebral column. The vertebrae are movable bones held in their respective positions by ligaments placed around the vertebral column, which limit to a certain extent the possible movements of individual vertebrae. Between each vertebral body is a cartilaginous intervertebral disc held in place by a fibrous band, the annulus fibrosis, which also holds the vertebrae together. The vertebral column as a whole has a variety of movements — flexion, extension, rotation and lateral flexion. The majority of these movements, however, occur in the lumbar region because the rib cage reduces thoracic movement; therefore the lumbar area carries the total weight of the body and any object the person may carry. Figure 3.56 shows normal lumbar vertebrae and intervertebral discs.

Aetiology

In more than half the cases of disc protrusion there is a history of trauma, either direct or indirect, which places a strain on the spinal ligaments and annulus causing laxity so that the disc extrudes. The lumbar levels affected are usually lumbar 4 (L4) and lumbar 5 (L5) or lumbar 5 (L5) and sacral 1 (S1). When a disc prolapses it compresses the spinal nerve leaving from the intervertebral foramen below (Fig. 3.57). Therefore a disc protrusion between L5 and S1 compresses the first sacral nerve.

General features

The patient may have had backache or sciatic pain on and off for years due to increasing pressure on the lumbar or sacral nerves. Acute lumbar disc protrusion occurs suddenly: the patient lifts an object awkwardly and feels something 'give' in his back. Initially he may be unable to straighten up and feels a shooting pain down his leg. This pain is termed sciatica. Scoliosis may develop in an attempt to ease the pain, the spine flexing towards the affected side. Coughing and sneezing increase the pain.

The distribution of pain depends on the affected nerve. In fifth lumbar nerve compression, the pain radiates along the back of the thigh and leg crossing into the foot towards the great toe, whereas pressure on the first sacral nerve causes pain in the lateral aspect of leg and foot and into the small toe. Since it is a lower motor neurone lesion there may be minimal wasting and motor power loss of the muscles affected.

Investigations
1. General examination may reveal a scoliosis.
2. Straight leg raising increases pain due to stretching of the sciatic nerve.
3. Pain can also be induced by pressing the appropriate intervertebral space.
4. Plain X-rays may show narrowing of the disc spaces, and myelography (p. 116) should demonstrate disc prolapse.

Treatment
If treated conservatively with bed rest, traction and analgesics most lesions resolve. Some, however, require surgical excision if the pain persists or a neurological deficit develops for example due to compression of the nerves to the bladder and bowel. A laminectomy is performed in which the lamina of the neural arch is removed and the prolapsed disc excised.

Pre- and postoperative general care is the same as for any operation. In turning the patient from side to side it is usually easier and less traumatic for the patient if he is rolled face down instead of on to his back. The problem of difficulty in micturition may arise, and a careful note should be made of the amount of urine passed. If the disc prolapsed centrally on to the cauda equina, compressing nerves to the bladder, the problem may have existed preoperatively and will not resolve immediately postoperatively. In this case the care is as for paraplegia until tone has been recovered (p. 117).

Depending on the surgeon, the patient is mobilized in 1 to 3 days and physiotherapy is begun. The patient is taught to reuse weakened muscles to maintain correct posture and to lift objects correctly. Sutures are removed 7 to 10 days postoperatively.

SUGGESTED ASSIGNMENTS

1. Patients who have suffered severe brain damage due to head injury may have both behavioural and intellectual deterioration. In a young child this will present an educational problem.
   a. List the difficulties which you think the child's teacher might encounter.
   b. When a suitable opportunity arises, ask a teacher involved in the education of such children what problems he or she encounters.
   c. Now compare these with your previously prepared list and note the validity of your comments.

2. Paralysis of the dominant hemisphere of the brain may affect the individual's ability to understand the spoken word and/or to express himself orally. This defect is one of the commonest sequelae to a cerebrovascular accident.
   a. Keep a written account of how you have attempted to communicate with a group of patients suffering from dysphasia.
   b. When given the opportunity, discuss your methods with patients who have recovered from this disability.
   c. From the comments given, evaluate how effective your methods have been.

FURTHER READING

Bickerstaff E R 1978 Neurology, 3rd edn. Hodder and Stoughton, London
Carini E, Owens G 1978 Neurological and neurosurgical nursing, 7th edn. Mosby, St. Louis
Hooper R 1969 Patterns of acute head injury. Arnold, London
Kemp R 1963 Understanding epilepsy. Tavistock, London
Purchese G 1977 Neuromedical and neurosurgical nursing. Bailliere Tindall, London
Van Zwanenberg D, Adams C B T 1979 Neurosurgical nursing care. Faber, London

4. Nutrition

This chapter provides the essential information on the subject of nutrition that will enable the nurse to meet the dietary needs of her patients and herself. An understanding of the functions of the components of a normal diet will enable the nurse to be aware of the logic behind therapeutic modifications of diet and to understand the effects of toxicity or deficiency on a patient's physical and mental well-being.

Some knowledge of physiology, and the ability to use it as a source of information, is assumed. The kilojoule (kJ) will be used as the unit of energy throughout.

Energy is produced as the result of the metabolism of proteins, carbohydrates and fats, and in dietetics it is measured in kilojoules. A joule is an electrical unit of energy or heat which is generated by a current of 1 ampere, acting for 1 second, against a resistance of 1 ohm ($= 10\,000$ ERG). A kilojoule is therefore this amount of energy $\times 1000$. Table 4.1 gives the practical equivalents used in dietetics.

Table 4.1
Practical kilojoule (kJ)/calorie equivalents

Kilojoules	Calories
4·2	1
17	4
37	9
4000	1000
8800	2100
10 500	2500
11 500	2750
12 500	3000
14 750	3500
15 750	3750
16 750	4000
17 850	4250

NUTRITION IN HEALTH

What is nutrition? It is the provision of the essential ingredients for cell metabolism of an organism. This is achieved by a series of complex activities — ingestion, digestion, absorption, assimilation and excretion. All must be taken into consideration when dietary decisions are made, either by the individual or for him. Each must function normally, and any interference with the function of any one of these activities will necessitate dietary modifications. These may be merely the manner of presentation or may involve adjustments to specific components of the diet.

'**Diet**' means the total solid and liquid intake (with the exception of drugs) for any individual, fit or ill. The term is frequently misused to describe only intake which differs from the normal.

'**Balanced diet**' is the term used to describe intake in which each nutrient is in adequate quantities for the body's needs, with no excesses being either stored or wastefully excreted.

The choice of dietary components depends on many variables:

1. The age of the individual certainly affects dietary presentation, the presence or absence of teeth being an important factor at both ends of the age range.

2. Personal taste, which may be fairly rigid in the very young and the elderly, may place restrictions on the variety and nutritional value of meals.

3. Physiological factors, such as the immature digestive tract of the young child and the decreased sensitivity of the taste buds and sense of smell in the smoker and the elderly, will affect selection.

4. Economics plays a large part in food choice, as does the availability of a variety of foodstuffs. Inability to shop in the cheaper supermarkets because of lack of time, the distance, or a person's physical incapacity may reduce choice in two ways: the small local shops may have a narrower range of goods, and many articles may be more highly priced, putting them beyond the means of the shopper.

5. Cooking facilities, especially those available in many single-person accommodations, will certainly increase the likelihood of the selection of prepared foods. These usually cost more, thus militating against wide variety and possibly affecting the nutritional value of the diet as a whole.

6. Cookery skills affect the economics, appearance and digestibility of the prepared meal, as well as determining selection for others.

7. Climate affects choice — by its relation to the availability of food at reasonable cost — and also affects presentation, cold foods being more desirable in hot weather and vice versa.

8. Custom, for instance the Scottish high tea habit, religious observances, etc., may affect the choice of food and, in some instances, the total nutritional value of an individual's diet.

The constitutents of a balanced diet are:

> Proteins.
> Carbohydrates.
> Fats.
> Mineral salts.
> Vitamins.
> Roughage.
> Water.

Each will be discussed separately below and, where appropriate, some approximate figures to meet daily requirements will be given. A more detailed description of the digestive processes than that given in the ensuing sections may be found in any textbook of applied human physiology. The **energy requirements** are dependent upon age, sex, size, amount of activity and climate, which are interdependent variables. Table 4.2 gives some commonly accepted levels for various groups of individuals.

Table 4.2
Daily energy requirements

Activity level	Men (kJ)	Women (kJ)
Sedentary	10 500	8800
Moderately active	12 500	10 500
Active	14 750	12 500
Very active	17 850	15 750
Pregnant (last 3 months)		11 500
Lactating		12 500

Proteins (Fig. 4.1)

These complex substances are composed of **carbon, hydrogen, oxygen, nitrogen, sulphur** and **phosphorus**; rich sources are lean meat, fish, egg whites, cheese, milk, pulses, nuts and cereals. Digestion occurs as a result of their combination with gastric, pancreatic and intestinal enzymes, which break down the complex protein into a number of different amino acids; in this form they can be absorbed across the wall of the small intestine.

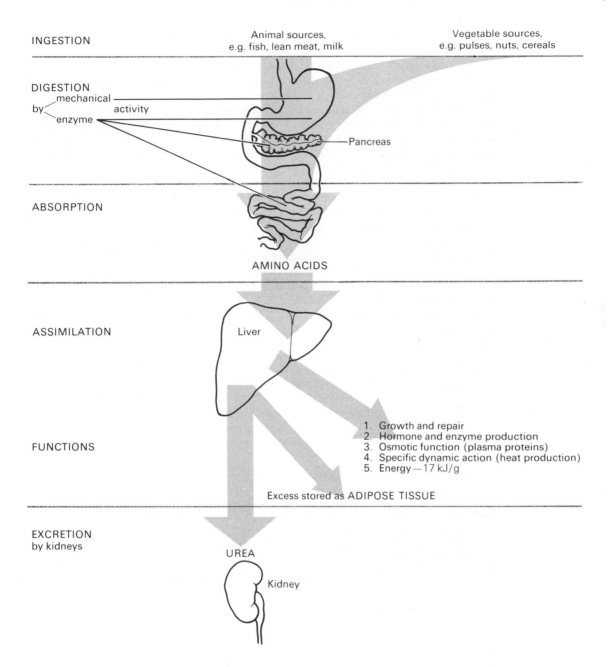

INGESTION — Animal sources, e.g. fish, lean meat, milk — Vegetable sources, e.g. pulses, nuts, cereals

DIGESTION
by mechanical activity
enzyme
Pancreas

ABSORPTION

AMINO ACIDS

ASSIMILATION
Liver

FUNCTIONS
1. Growth and repair
2. Hormone and enzyme production
3. Osmotic function (plasma proteins)
4. Specific dynamic action (heat production)
5. Energy—17 kJ/g

Excess stored as ADIPOSE TISSUE

EXCRETION
by kidneys

UREA
Kidney

Figure 4.1
Proteins

In the liver, various amino acids are combined to form complex molecules required by the body, or are synthesized into other amino acids not available in the diet. Any excess over need is taken up by the liver; the nitrogenous substances are formed into urea and excreted by the kidneys, the remainder of the molecule being oxidized to form carbon dioxide (excreted by the lungs) and water (excreted by the kidneys). If oxidization does not occur, conversion into carboyhdrate can take place. As a result energy can be produced or, alternatively, the carbohydrate can be converted into fats which are stored as adipose tissue.

Classification
Proteins are classified according to their biological value:

1. Those of animal origin, which contain all of the essential amino acids, are called first class proteins. The essential amino acids are those which the human liver cannot synthesize and which must therefore be taken in through the diet.

2. Those of vegetable origin usually contain only some of the essential amino acids. A diet which contains no animal protein is regarded as deficient.

Functions of proteins

1. Proteins provide basic materials for growth, maintenance and repair of body tissues. As all cells have a protein component, the dietary needs are increased during periods of growth, or following injury (including surgical wounds) when repair with new cell formation is required. The healthy adult requires approximately **55 to 85 g per day**, or 10 per cent of total energy intake. The amount of protein in dairy products is variable, but the following approximations may be helpful: one large egg 7 g (mainly in the white); two slices of lean meat 35 g; one average helping of macaroni cheese 20 g; 500 ml of milk 20 g. More detail of this and other components discussed below may be obtained from specialist dietetic texts. The growing child needs about five times this amount in proportion to his body weight.

2. Proteins are constituents of all hormones and enzymes.

3. Proteins are the source of the blood proteins and cells that have a vital function in immune response mechanisms and in maintaining the osmotic pressure within the circulation.

4. Proteins have a specific dynamic action by which the metabolic process produces more heat from the same quantity of food (without alteration in thyroid function). This is of importance in cold climates, where a diet high in protein plays a significant role in maintaining an adequate body temperature.

5. In the absence of an adequate total intake of kilojoules or any excessive protein intake over need, energy and heat will be produced by *gluconeogenesis* in the liver. Energy yield: 17 kJ per g.

Proteins are the only dietary sources of nitrogen. The body is said to be in nitrogenous equilibrium, or **nitrogen balance**, when the nitrogen intake equals the nitrogen lost in the excreta over a measured period of time.

When the intake of nitrogen is greater than the amount excreted, the individual is described as being in a state of **positive nitrogen balance**. Positive nitrogen balance is necessary for normal growth; growth will be stunted if a child's nitrogen intake does not exceed his nitrogen loss — hence the statement made earlier that the proportion of dietary protein to body weight for a growing child should be five times greater than the proportion for an adult.

If the intake of nitrogen is less than the output, the person is said to be in a state of **negative nitrogen balance.** An inadequate intake of protein, and therefore of nitrogen, may have many causes including economic: most protein foods are more expensive than carbohydrates. Excessive loss of protein from the body may result from pathological conditions, such as burns (Ch. 14) or some renal diseases (Ch. 9). Protein deficiency results in poor healing of wounds, muscle wasting with subsequent loss of power, oedema due to changes in osmotic pressure resultant upon loss of plasma proteins, and an increased vulnerability to a cold environment and possibly also to infection. The low-protein diet of many elderly people in Great Britain is partially responsible for the increasing number who become victims of *hypothermia* each winter.

From this discussion, it can be seen that the nurse has a responsibility to ensure an adequate protein intake to maintain her own health and resistance to infection. Also she must endeavour to assist her patients, who are often anorexic, to ingest a suitably presented form of protein to meet the demands of their individual circumstances.

Carbohydrates (Fig. 4.2)

These are composed of **carbon, hydrogen** and **oxygen** in variable proportions; the more carbon molecules present, the more complex the substance and consequently the longer it takes to break down and become available for absorption. Sources are all cereals and their manufactured products, pulses, root vegetables including beetroot, cane sugar and anything to which it has been added, honey, fruits and milk.

Digestion begins in the mouth for cooked starches only; the breakdown of uncooked starch commences in the small intestine due to the activity of pancreatic and intestinal enzymes which also act on the cooked starches until a simple molecular form is reached, which can be absorbed through the mucosa of the small intestine. If required immediately, glucose is metabolized in the cells (the presence of insulin being necessary to enable it to enter the cell) and heat and energy are produced, water and carbon

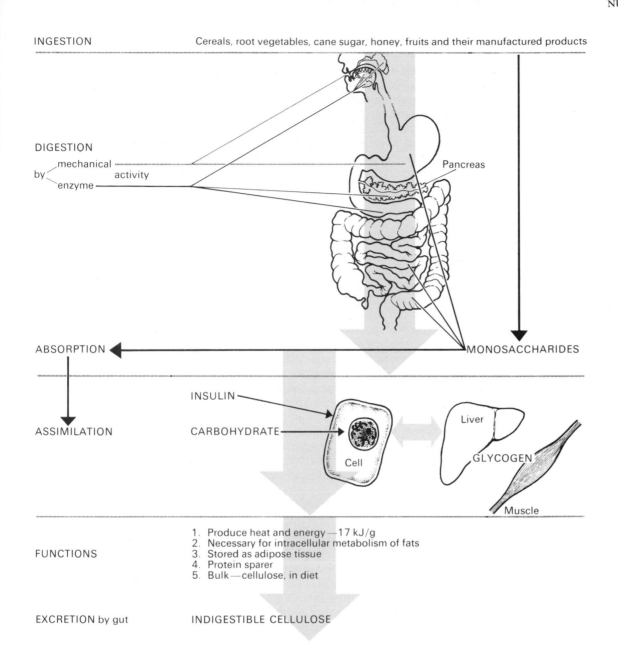

INGESTION   Cereals, root vegetables, cane sugar, honey, fruits and their manufactured products

DIGESTION
   by mechanical   activity
       enzyme   Pancreas

ABSORPTION   MONOSACCHARIDES

ASSIMILATION
                    INSULIN
                    CARBOHYDRATE   Liver
                                        Cell   GLYCOGEN
                                                Muscle

FUNCTIONS   1. Produce heat and energy—17 kJ/g
                    2. Necessary for intracellular metabolism of fats
                    3. Stored as adipose tissue
                    4. Protein sparer
                    5. Bulk—cellulose, in diet

EXCRETION by gut   INDIGESTIBLE CELLULOSE

Figure 4.2
Carbohydrates

dioxide being the waste products. If not required for immediate energy needs, glucose can be converted into glycogen and stored as such in the liver and muscles or converted into fat stores. Because glycogen can be converted rapidly back into glucose, eating can be discontinuous and even fairly prolonged fasting can be undertaken without impairment of mental function. The brain, although only one-fiftieth of total adult weight, utilizes one-fifth of all absorbed glucose and appears to acquire all its energy from this source and not from fat sources. Any ingested carbohydrate which is not broken down into glucose will be excreted as waste (see Roughage, below).

Classification
Classification of carbohydrates is by molecular complexity.
   Monosaccharides are simple sugars and are the form in which carbohydrates are absorbed into the bloodstream through the gut wall. Glucose (from honey), fructose (from fruits) and galactose (from milk) are monosaccharides; carbohydrates which arrive in the stomach in this form will be absorbed through the stomach wall, the only

energy sources except alcohol which are, and thus provide a useful source of 'instant energy'.

Disaccharides are more complex, being two molecules combined together, therefore requiring a one-stage breakdown process before absorption can occur. Lactose (from milk) and sucrose (from cane sugar) are common dietary sources.

Polysaccharides are very complex molecules, requiring prolonged digestive processes before the monosaccharide form is reached. Many forms are not broken down in the human alimentary tract and are not therefore available for energy (see Roughage, below). Main forms of polysaccharides are starch, glycogen and cellulose; readily available sources are cereals, pulses, liver, root and leafy vegetables.

Functions of carbohydrates

1. To produce heat and energy when combined with oxygen in the cell. Energy yield: **17 kJ per g**.

2. To participate in the intracellular metabolism of fats.

3. To form adipose tissue which protects organs and insulates the body from cold. The greater proportion of subcutaneous fat in women compared with men offers them protection from exposure to adverse weather conditions.

4. To act as a protein sparer: insufficient intake of carbohydrate will result in utilization of protein for energy with a subsequent impairment of specific protein function. This role is of special significance in untreated diabetes mellitus (Ch. 11), when cells (though not the body as a whole) are starved of carbohydrate, resulting in the muscle wasting and weakness of which the patient complains. It is also the reason why patients suffering from acute glomerulonephritis (Ch. 9) are normally given 100 g of carbohydrate daily. It is common practice for these people to be advised to restrict their fluid intake to 500–600 ml of water each day and to reduce protein drastically. Some carbohydrate must be taken to meet energy needs. In its absence body protein would be converted to supply energy and consequently nitrogenous wastes would be produced, so defeating the aim of the regime. Subsistence on a diet containing no protein, restricted water and a small quantity of carbohydrate should result in a fall in blood urea and at the same time decrease the load on renal function. This regimen is only suitable for short periods.

5. To provide roughage (see below).

The average daily requirement of carbohydrate is about 55 per cent of total energy intake, usually **400 to 500g per day**. Of particular importance to those with a tendency to be overweight, it is worth noting that one rounded teaspoonful of white sugar contains 8 g of carbohydrate; one average slice of fruit cake 20 g; a slice of bread 10 g. Because the sources of carbohydrates are usually the cheaper foods, hungry people and adolescents who seem never to be satisfied generally 'fill up' on them. This may develop into undesirable eating habits which are hard to change when activity decreases. The excess is then stored as fat and the process leading to obesity starts (p. 146).

Inadequate intake of carbohydrate may produce ketosis (p. 132) from incomplete fat metabolism. This produces symptoms of nausea, impairment of mental function and confusion as a result of neuronal deprivation; muscle wasting and weight loss as a result of utilization of proteins and fats for energy; and general lassitude due to inadequate catabolism and energy production. The mechanism of hunger usually prevents these symptoms from becoming severe, as a meal or a snack would normally be taken to raise the blood sugar and replace the glycogen stores which are being utilized to maintain an adequate blood glucose level. It should be remembered, however, that many patients are required to fast for prolonged periods for diagnostic or therapeutic purposes. Postoperative nausea may be due as much to an overprolonged preoperative fast (plus operation time itself) as to any anaesthetic drug or operative manipulation that has been involved. A low blood sugar also prolongs the period, and increases the severity, of postoperative hypotension and increases the risk of infection. Unless specifically requested, the preoperative fasting period should not exceed 6 hours.

Many patients are also maintained for some days on intravenous therapy, which may incorporate only low concentrations of dextrose solutions as sources of energy. Two litres of 5 per cent dextrose will yield rather less than a quarter of the normal carbohydrate intake; this takes no account of other energy sources which would normally be ingested nor of the patient's energy requirements.

The nurse herself may have noticed that, when hungry, she is less efficient, less able to respond rapidly to changing situations, more easily tired and less tolerant with her patients. If both nurse and patient are irritable, interpersonal relationships may suffer.

Fats or lipids (Fig. 4.3)

These are composed of **carbon, hydrogen** and **oxygen** in complex molecules. Sources are cream, butter, cheese, fat meat, oily fish, some fruits for instance nuts and olives, and some vegetable sources such as sunflowers and corn. These last are common sources of cooking oils.

Digestion of fats begins in the small intestine where bile and lipase, a pancreatic and intestinal enzyme, emulsify the dietary fat into fatty acids and glycerol. These are converted into triglycerides in the cells of the wall of the small intestine and are then absorbed into the lacteals, thence to the lymphatic system and general circulation.

The liver then combines each triglyceride molecule with a protein molecule to form a lipoprotein, which is more readily transported round the body. In adipose tissue, fats are stored as triglycerides, the conversion process requiring the presence of carbohydrate in the cell. The protein molecule is now available for other purposes. The energy needs of the body are met by utilization of fatty acids, the form in which triglycerides are mobilized from adipose tissue. Deposits of adipose tissue are in a continuous state of change. Energy needs are met from these stores and not from circulating fat. If energy needs become greater and the dietary intake of carbohydrate is not increased, no further deposition of fat occurs and the rate of mobilization of the stored fat accelerates. This is the rationale behind the management of obesity.

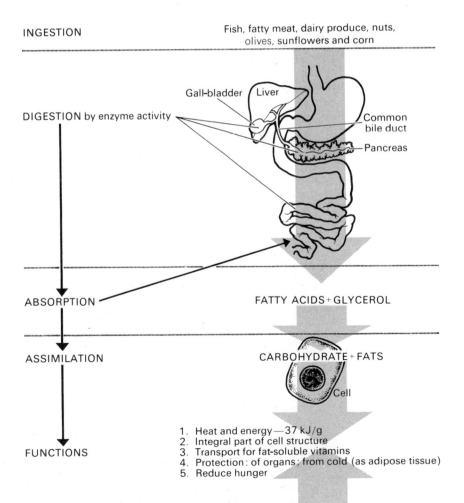

Figure 4.3
Fats

Classification

Lipids, when metabolized, fall into three groups:

1. The **triglycerides**, including fatty acids, may be stored in the body; they are sources of energy and fulfil a protective function.

2. The **phospholipids** are an integral part of cell structure and circulate in the blood; in the latter situation they are a means of transport for fatty acids.

3. The **sterols**. Cholesterol, the more important, is concerned with the transport of fatty acids; ergosterol has a role in vitamin D synthesis. The androgenic hormones and adrenocortical hormones are closely related to this group (hence the name steroids).

Functions of fats

1. To produce heat and energy. Fats yield **37 kJ per g** and therefore permit large increases in total energy intake without creating too much bulk or the need for frequent ingestion. The complete metabolism of fats in the cell is dependent upon the presence of an enzyme produced during carbohydrate metabolism. In the absence of this enzyme the incompletely metabolized products of fat, called ketoacids, are released into the circulation causing acidosis and nausea. If very large quantities of ketoacids are circulating, coma may ensue. These ketoacids are excreted by the kidneys and can be found in the urine of persons who are incompletely metabolizing fat for any reason, by testing for ketones using the appropriate reagent.

It can be appreciated that any condition in which the body is unable to metabolize carbohydrate, either because it is not being ingested, as in anorexia nervosa, or because it is unable to enter the cell, as in diabetes mellitus, will affect the metabolism of fat.

2. To form an integral part of cell structure.

3. To transport fat-soluble vitamins.

4. To protect organs and insulate the body by contributing to the formation of adipose tissue.

5. To add palatability to the diet and, by reducing the speed of gastric emptying, to increase the time available for mechanical digestion and the absorption of any glucose and water present through the gastric mucosa. By reducing the rate of gastric emptying, fats maintain the state of *satiety*, reduce the desire to eat again and therefore reduce the total energy intake and subsequent risk of obesity. Approximately 30 per cent of the total energy intake is in the form of fat: **80 to 100 g per day**. This apparently large amount is easily ingested, if it is realized that one small pat of butter yields 8 g of fat; one slice of bacon 16 g; one large egg (mainly the yolk) 6 g; a portion of herring or mackerel 15 g; 20 peanuts 9 g.

Mineral salts

These are widely distributed in the body, forming approximately 4 per cent of total body weight, and are found in considerable variety and proportion. They are present as simple elements — salts or electrolytes — and have general functions related to:

1. The skeleton, of which they form 45 per cent.

2. The body fluids, in which the electrolytes maintain the osmotic balance between the intracellular and extracellular fluids.

3. The acid-base balance of the body: many of the complex salts are capable of absorbing acids to maintain the blood within the range of pH 7·2 to 7·4.

Some minerals are found in quantity and must therefore be ingested in quantity; these are sodium, potassium, calcium, iron, chlorides, magnesium, phosphorus and sulphur. Traces of iodine, copper, zinc, fluoride, cobalt and manganese are also found, but assessment of intake is rarely necessary as a normal diet would include adequate quantities.

Sodium

Functions of sodium

1. To give, with calcium, rigidity to bone.

2. To exert an osmotic effect by its presence, as an electrolyte, in the extracellular fluids.

3. To assist in maintaining the acid-base balance in the body. The salts of sodium which influence this balance are sodium bicarbonate, sodium carbonate and sodium phosphate.

4. To make the diet more palatable.

This last 'asset' results in the daily ingestion of about 20 g per day, but health could be maintained adequately if intake was **2 to 5 g per day**. Sodium is readily available in fish, meats and nearly all manufactured foods, is used as a preservative and is freely added to food as a condiment at table or in cooking.

In health, sodium imbalance rarely occurs because the excess intake is excreted by the kidneys and the necessary quantities are retained as a result of the action of aldosterone on the renal tubules. In occupations where severe sweating occurs, such as mining or smelting, fluid replacement without additional sodium will produce sodium depletion.

Conditions in which aldosterone activity is impaired, for instance Addison's disease (Ch. 11), or in which excessive sodium is lost, as in diarrhoea and vomiting, result in loss of sodium from the circulation with subsequent hypotension, muscle cramps, weakness and collapse. (It should be remembered that the heart is a muscular organ whose efficiency is dependent upon the concentrations of sodium and potassium on either side of the cell membranes.) Sodium retention causes oedema due to the increased osmotic pressure in the extracellular fluid. If sodium intake is reduced, the amount of water retention possible must also be reduced. As oedema is a feature of congestive cardiac failure and as it can be seen that the average daily intake of this mineral far exceeds need, the simple measure of restricting added salt in cooking and at table, combined with the avoidance of foods preserved in salt, may greatly influence the patient's progress.

Potassium

Aldosterone influences the excretion of potassium by the kidneys and a daily intake of **2 to 5 g** of potassium is adequate. Fish, meat, vegetables and some fruits, especially citrus fruits and grapes, are rich sources of this mineral. Pathological conditions attributable to inadequate potassium intake are unknown.

Functions of Potassium

1. To maintain osmotic balance between intracellular fluid (in which it is present in relatively high concentrations) and extracellular fluid.

2. To exercise an important role in muscle contraction (notably the heart) and nerve conductability.

Retention of potassium may occur as a result of renal disease, or Addison's disease; a raised serum potassium level is a characteristic feature of these conditions. The nurse should appreciate the need to discourage the intake of fruit juices by such patients and seek alternatives to meet their fluid needs. Depletion of body potassium, from diuretic therapy, severe diarrhoea with desquamation of intestinal mucosa, diabetic (hyperglycaemic) coma, or inability to absorb potassium due to prolonged use of liquid paraffin as a laxative will cause potassium to leave the cells and enter the circulation, thus giving rise to high serum potassium levels. Muscle cramps and cardiac irregularities will ensue. It is important to note that rapid changes in serum potassium levels, which can occur, for example, when infusing potassium in intravenous solutions, can cause severe cardiac arrhythmia or sudden death due to ventricular fibrillation. As the nurse is responsible for the regulation of the rate of intravenous infusions within the time span ordered by the medical staff, she should be aware of the special dangers of irregular flow when potassium is added to the fluid and avoid them.

Calcium

Calcium is absorbed in the gut, stored in the bones and excreted by the kidneys under the control of parathormone. This is activated by a negative feed-back mechanism; when the serum calcium level drops, the hormone is released and raises the serum calcium by (a) increasing absorption, (b) increasing solubility of the stored calcium in bone so that it enters the circulation and (c) reducing excretion.

Functions of calcium

1. Calcium forms a major part of bones and teeth (Fig. 4.4). Its presence is especially important during their formation in fetal life and childhood, and for their subsequent maintenance and repair.
2. It maintains neuromuscular stability.
3. It is essential for the clotting mechanism of blood (see Ch. 8).

Daily requirements are **1g per day**, but this should be exceeded during pregnancy and childhood. Sources are milk, cheese, eggs, cereals, soft-boned fish (for instance, pilchards, of which the bones are eaten) and green vegetables.

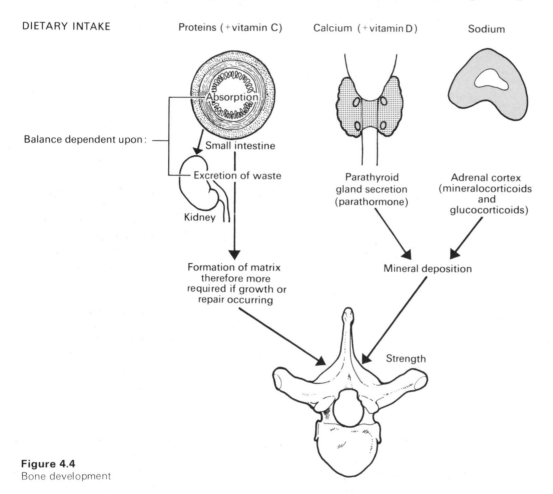

Figure 4.4
Bone development

Deficiency may result from a poor diet or failure to absorb calcium adequately from the gut. Absorption of calcium is increased in the presence of proteins and vitamin D, whilst unabsorbed fatty acids and phytic acid (a compound of carbohydrate metabolism) hinder calcium absorption. The deficiency produces rickets, osteomalacia, tetany and bruising. Tetany may be the first evidence of the accidental removal of one or more of the parathyroid glands during surgery of the thyroid gland, with consequent reduction in parathormone secretion (see Ch. 11).

Retention of calcium results from a parathyroid tumour, which continues to secrete parathormone despite a high serum calcium level causing renal calculi, dental caries and osteomalacia. The clotting mechanism is not affected (except possibly in the newborn producing haemolysis), as the amount of calcium required is not quantitative for this function and clotting will occur provided the serum calcium level is not **below** normal levels.

Iron

This is necessary for the formation of haemoglobin (Fig. 4.5). Normal daily requirements of **12 mg** should be increased during pregnancy; women during their menstrual years should ensure that this level is maintained. Red meat, liver, egg yolks, oatmeal, pulses, green vegetables and chocolate are rich sources; two slices of calves' liver yields 9 mg of iron; an average portion of spinach 2 mg; 100 g of dark chocolate 4 mg. The absorption of iron is increased in the presence of proteins and vitamin C, whereas oxalic acid (found in rhubarb) and phytic acid (see above) interfere with its absorption.

Deficiency due to failure of absorption, lack of adequate intake or excessive loss results in *hypochromic microcytic* anaemia. Female nurses should recognize the need to maintain an adequate iron intake so that deficiency is avoided with its consequent fatigue, loss of efficiency and accident proneness. The frequency with which iron-deficiency anaemia is found in the elderly, who form an increasingly large proportion of the patient population, should be borne in mind when planning nursing care, with particular reference to the problems of wound healing and the prevention of trauma.

Chlorides, magnesium, phosphorus and sulphur

These are present in quantity in all living matter and therefore do not present a dietary problem.

Of the trace elements mentioned above, the role of two is of special significance to certain social groups.

Iodine

This mineral is found in seafood and in vegetables grown near the sea. It is a constituent of the thyroid hormones and is therefore concerned with general metabolism. Before the development of rapid and refrigerated transportation methods, land-locked areas such as Derbyshire and Switzerland had a restricted supply of this mineral, and iodine deficiency with simple goitre formation resulted. To overcome the problem, iodine was added to all table salt by the processors, but this practice is no longer necessary.

Fluorine

This mineral may play a valuable part in the prevention of dental caries (and the resultant digestive problems of poor mastication) because of its role in the formation of bone and dental enamel. It is found naturally in many areas of the world in drinking water, and can be added artificially to promote dental health. Such mass medication is not acceptable in some societies, and in some areas weekly mouthwashes with fluoride solutions for schoolchildren are substituted.

Vitamins

These are classified according to source, that is fat-soluble and water-soluble vitamins. The fat-soluble vitamins are A, D, E and K; the water-soluble vitamins are the B complex group and vitamin C. Utilization of vitamins is affected by various factors: the availability of the substance (it may be present but in an unabsorbable form) or the inability to digest the fats in which the fat-soluble vitamins are found. Some substances in food, termed **antivitamins**, may be taken up by the body and may block the activity of the true vitamin at its site of action in enzyme systems. Another factor is the availability of **provitamins**: these are substances which can be converted by the body into specific vitamins. Finally, the gut normally contains bacterial flora capable of synthesizing significant amounts of some vitamins.

Fat-soluble vitamins

Vitamin A (chemical name: retinol)

The provitamin carotene is found in plants; it is responsible for the red or yellow colouring but is also found in green leafy vegetables in association with chlorophyll. The conversion of carotene into vitamin A occurs in the walls of the small intestine; large amounts of the provitamin are required to produce relatively small quantities of vitamin A. The vitamin itself is only available from animal sources such as liver, dairy produce and fatty fish, especially the oils derived from their livers. (Vitamin A is stored in the liver.) Vegetable oils, except red palm oil, are devoid of vitamin A. In Great

Britain, margarine, which is made from vegetable oils, has vitamin A added to it, making it a dietary source of the vitamin.

Vitamin A is essential for night vision, being a vital component in the formation of rhodopsin (visual purple), which is present in the rods of the retina (which are responsive to dim light). The condition of epithelial tissue is also adversely affected by a deficiency of this vitamin. This is most noticeable on the scleral conjunctiva, where heaps of dried epithelial cells result in xerophthalmia (and permanent scarring may leave the patient blind); similar lesions block the sweat glands of the skin.

The average daily requirement of **750 µg** retinal equivalents (2500 *iu*) is readily available in a normal diet containing reasonable helpings of vegetables and dairy produce. Children and pregnant and lactating women should receive supplements of this vitamin, but care should be exercised in dosage, as it is not soluble in water and excesses will not therefore be excreted by the kidneys but will be stored in the liver. Toxicity can result producing symptoms of anorexia, dry irritant skin, coarse, sparse hair, *exostoses* of the long bones and sometimes hepatomegaly.

Vitamin D$_2$ (calciferol) Vitamin D$_3$ (7 dehydrocholesterol)

Calciferol can be manufactured by irradiating ergosterol, which is found in fungi and yeasts, with ultraviolet light. It can therefore be used as a therapeutic tool.

Vitamin D$_3$ is formed by the action of the sun's rays on 7 dehydrocholesterol, which is found in adipose tissue, including subcutaneous fat. Man acquires it directly through his skin; dietary sources are fish-liver oils and dairy produce.

Its function is to facilitate and promote the absorption of calcium and phosphate from the gut, so making them available for bone formation. It is stored in adipose tissue, and there is evidence to suggest that bile and fatty acids are necessary to enable the absorption of the vitamin from the gut to take place.

Deficiency results in rickets or osteomalacia, and it is therefore termed the 'antirachitic' vitamin. Daily requirements range between **2.5 µg and 10 µg (100 iu and 400 iu)**. Healthy adults eating a good mixed diet should not require supplements; children and pregnant women, especially if the dietary sources are barely adequate, should be given cod-liver oil. It is of therapeutic value in increasing the absorption of calcium, even if malabsorption syndrome or hypoparathyroidism are the cause of low serum calcium levels.

Calciferol poisoning is possible. Nausea and vomiting, thirst, diarrhoea, irritability and coma may occur, with calcium deposits in the blood vessels and many organs. The addition of vitamin D to powdered milk preparations, in view of earlier weaning practices, is no longer routine.

Vitamin E (the tocopherols)

This group of substances is found in all foodstuffs known to be eaten by man, the richest sources being vegetable fats. They appear to have a controlling effect on the metabolic rate of cells and, in conjunction with vitamin A, slow down the oxidation process by which fats become rancid.

The value of vitamin E in man's diet is doubtful, though in other mammals its withdrawal has been shown to have an adverse effect on male sterility. Deficiencies in humans are not recognized, the average Western diet giving **20 mg per day**.

Vitamin K (phytomenadione)

This substance is essential for the normal formation of prothrombin in the liver. It is present in fresh dark-green leafy vegetables such as spinach, kale and nettles and also in cauliflower. *Escherichia coli* in the bowel are known to synthesize this vitamin, but the biological value of this process is questioned. Deficiency is unknown in health. As for all fat-soluble vitamins, however, it is first necessary to absorb the fat carrier, which must have been ingested. Thus patients suffering from malabsorption syndrome and those with liver disease have a tendency to bleed. The risk of postoperative haemorrhage following surgical treatment of obstructive jaundice is reduced by preoperative vitamin K therapy. The implications of this for nurses observing such patients should not be overlooked. The therapeutic use of this vitamin, usually in water-soluble form as Konakion, has a place in the treatment of the bleeding diseases of the newborn, malabsorption syndrome and as an antidote to anticoagulant drugs.

Water-soluble vitamins

The B complex group of vitamins is generally found in the same dietary sources, but each vitamin has a specific chemical makeup and specialized function. The sources are germ and husk of cereals, yeast, dairy produce, liver, meat, pulses and green vegetables.

Vitamin B_1 (thiamin)

This vitamin must be present for the complete metabolism of carbohydrate. The brain acquires all its energy from carbohydrate sources. It is therefore the organ most affected by thiamin deficiency, symptoms being caused by deterioration of cerebral function. The deficiency does, however, have an adverse effect on all tissues, producing a condition known as beriberi. This is not a disease of famine but the result of a poorly balanced diet. It is necessary to ingest **0·4 mg** of thiamin for every 4200 kJ of intake. Nursing mothers require a slightly higher proportion. Because it cannot be stored, there must be adequate amounts in each day's diet; one small slice of liver would provide 70 μg of thiamin. Excess, being water soluble, is excreted by the kidneys.

Vitamin B_2 (Riboflavin)

This vitamin has an active role in cell metabolism. As a result, chronic deficiency from childhood will be demonstrated in stunted growth. The vitamin is found in high concentration in tears and appears to play a major role in maintaining healthy corneal cells, which depend on the intracellular oxidation (as the cornea is not vascular) provided by riboflavin. Deficiency results in the cornea becoming vascularized to meet its oxygen need; stomatitis and cheilosis are also found. Daily needs are **1 to 2 mg**; one small slice of liver would produce 1280 μg of riboflavin.

Vitamin B_3 (niacin, nicotinic acid, nicotinamide)

Essential for tissue oxidation, a deficiency of this vitamin produces a severe condition, pellagra, involving skin lesions (dermatitis), gastrointestinal disturbances (especially persistent diarrhoea) and mental changes (dementia). Average requirement is **10 mg per day** which would be provided by one small slice of liver; an average portion of peas yields 2163 μg of this vitamin. There are no toxic effects of this vitamin, though the side-effects of peripheral vasodilatation have promoted its use in circulatory disorders such as chilblains.

Vitamin B_6 (pyridoxine)

This vitamin plays an important role in the metabolism of amino acids; in infants whose brain cells are developing rapidly a deficiency has been known to be a rare cause of convulsions. As a **trace** of the vitamin is all that is required, deficiency in otherwise healthy adults is rare.

Vitamin B (folic acid)

When metabolized, this vitamin provides a base for essential components of the red blood cells and other cells. A deficiency causes *megaloblastic anaemia*. The deficit may be due to insufficient intake, impaired absorption or increased demands, as in pregnancy. The daily requirement of **traces** of folic acid is readily met by a good mixed diet; in pregnancy a daily supplement should be given; it also has a therapeutic value in the management of megaloblastic anaemias of infancy and pregnancy and those associated with the malabsorption syndrome.

Vitamin B_{12} (cyanocobalamin) (Fig. 4.5)

This is the 'extrinsic factor' which is not manufactured by the body but absorbed from the gut if combined with the intrinsic factor produced by the oxyntic cells of the stomach. Thus persons who do not produce this factor suffer from pernicious anaemia. So too will some patients whose stomachs have been partially removed. This severe disease responds readily to small doses of cyanocobalamin, which has to be given intramuscularly. Without it, the red blood cells do not mature, are less efficient and are more readily destroyed. Only a **trace** is required per day; it is stored in the liver and in muscle tissue.

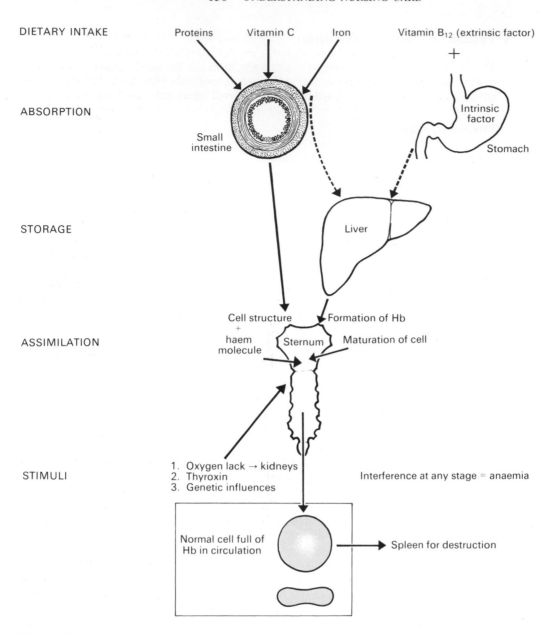

DIETARY INTAKE — Proteins   Vitamin C   Iron   Vitamin B$_{12}$ (extrinsic factor)

ABSORPTION — Small intestine   Intrinsic factor   Stomach

STORAGE — Liver

ASSIMILATION — Cell structure + haem molecule   Formation of Hb   Sternum   Maturation of cell

STIMULI —
1. Oxygen lack → kidneys
2. Thyroxin
3. Genetic influences

Interference at any stage = anaemia

Normal cell full of Hb in circulation   →   Spleen for destruction

Figure 4.5
Erythrocyte and haemoglobin formation

Vitamin C (ascorbic acid)

This vitamin is found in citrus fruits, currants, root and green vegetables. Requirements of **30 to 70 mg per day** must be met to avoid the condition known as scurvy. One small orange will provide approximately 50 mg of ascorbic acid. Vitamin C is necessary for the formation of the matrix of connective tissue and the integrity of capillary walls. Scurvy is characterized by gingivitis, a condition in which the gums bleed very readily. Minute perifollicular haemorrhages occur in the skin and the hairs cork-screw from their follicles as a result of heaps of keratin-like material on the surface. The haemorrhages later become petechial (Ch. 8) in type, followed by the appearance of large spontaneous bruises. Anaemia (and listlessness) are common — a result of increased haemolysis.

A reduced dietary intake over time may have an adverse effect on wound healing.

Roughage

Cellulose is one of the three most important polysaccharides in man's diet, the other two being glycogen and starch. Like the others, it is formed from several glucose molecules linked together, but man is unable to break this down and so it remains undigested within the lumen of the gut. It forms the bulk of faeces and plays an important role in stimulating peristalsis. The highly refined diet of the Western world, low in roughage, is thought to be a significant factor in the high incidence of diverticulitis. A chemical product of cellulose, **methyl cellulose**, which is inert, tasteless and bulky because of its hygroscopic action, is used therapeutically to increase the bulk of ileostomy excretions; it can also be given to persons prescribed weight-control diets to reduce hunger pangs.

Water

All plant and animal life is composed of a high proportion of water. The maintenance of water balance depends on intake, the various means by which fluid is lost from the body and the controls. Intake is regulated by the thirst mechanism, which is activated by a series of neurosecretory mechanisms that monitor the osmolality of the blood. When thirsty, fluids are taken into the body and the antidiuretic hormone from the posterior pituitary is released to increase the reabsorption of water from the distal convoluted tubules of the nephrons.

Fluid is lost from the body in measurable quantities via the kidneys and in the faeces. Insensible loss through the skin can become an important mechanism in maintaining fluid balance if the environmental or body temperature is raised; water vapour is also lost in expiration.

Control of fluid loss is exerted mainly in the kidney, but the formation of urine, which is a means of excreting many waste products, requires a sufficient intake of fluid to dilute the waste products adequately.

PREPARATION AND CARE OF FOOD

Cooking

Cooking of food by any method may change the nutritional value by rendering some components less absorbable or by splitting coarse fibrous coatings, such as are found on pulses and cereals, enabling the digestive enzymes to act upon the starch and protein they contain. Meat fibres are converted into gelatin — tougher (that is, more fibrous) meat takes longer to reach this stage. Meat tenderized in this way is more readily digested.

The method of cooking used may destroy some of the nutritional value of food; minerals and water-soluble vitamins may be lost in large quantities when the cooking water is discarded — hence the value of steaming or using minimum quantities of water when cooking vegetables. The loss that results from washing rice in societies where it forms a major part of the diet is sufficient to cause beriberi.

The most easily destroyed nutrient is ascorbic acid. Its decomposition occurs as a result of oxidation. The process is more rapid in the presence of heat, enzyme action, alkalis, traces of copper and free access to atmospheric oxygen. As storage in the body is not possible, care must be taken to protect sources of this vitamin from copper cooking pots, prolonged cooking, 'keeping warm' (even standing in strong sunlight) or standing uncovered.

Obviously cooking may increase the nutritional value of a diet. Salt may be added to enhance flavour and other additives may increase palatability so that intake is encouraged. Using oils for frying increases the vitamin and energy intake. For oedematous patients it may be necessary to use salt substitutes in cooking and at table, and alternative methods of food preparation must be practised if the obese individual is to lose weight.

By producing and maintaining a temperature high enough to kill micro-organisms, cooking serves a preservative and protective function. But this asset can be negated by careless food handlers with unclean personal habits or by using dirty equipment or inappropriate storage methods.

Storage

Storage methods are geared to the prevention of contamination by vectors and to the provision of an environment in which micro-organisms will not multiply (Ch. 1).

Preservation

Refrigeration (short term) and freezing (longer term) are suitable for many foods and do not adversely affect nutritional value. It is important to note the advice of manufacturers regarding the maintenance of equipment and the length of time for which specific foods may be stored. Once defrosted, frozen foods are subject to the same deterioration and contamination risks; usually they may not be refrozen.

Canning of goods, whole or evaporated to reduce bulk, involves an airtight container which is then sterilized by heat. Provided the tin is undamaged and the canning process is carried out correctly, goods preserved in this way retain their food value almost indefinitely. If the tin is damaged, micro-organisms can enter; if the sterilization process fails, any micro-organisms in the tin will multiply producing gases and the 'blown' tin.

Smoking, pickling and salting all produce environments not conducive to growth and multiplication of micro-organisms. Drying is an effective means of preservation since all living organisms require water to sustain life; however, storage in a safe place is necessary to avoid contamination from mice and rats.

DIETARY MODIFICATIONS

Under certain circumstances it may be necessary to adjust the intake of one or all the components of the balanced diet to meet changes in body needs. The presentation of the diet may be modified in infancy, childhood and old age. Modifications may be necessary to meet changing physiological needs in healthy individuals or the changes arising from pathological processes.

PHYSIOLOGICAL CHANGES INFLUENCING NUTRITIONAL NEEDS

Infancy and childhood

The rate of growth of all tissues demands a large supply of proteins for cell structure, calcium for bones and iron for the formation of large numbers of red blood cells to provide oxygen for the anabolic process. Vitamin supplements, notably of vitamins A and D, may be of value, especially in deprived areas.

Adolescence

During adolescence the increased energy needs must be met as well as the protein and mineral needs for the final growth spurt. The temptation is to increase the carbohydrate content of the diet on the grounds of economy. Although understandable, this solution increases the problem of teenage acne and may initiate obesity or promote the liking for sweet things, which will persist when physical activity decreases.

Adulthood

Women, because of their physiology, are prone to iron deficiency anaemia throughout their menstruating years. The use of the contraceptive pill, with the resulting reduction in menstrual flow, and the smaller average family size, with less strain being placed on a woman's iron stores, have reduced the severity of the problem but not its frequency in society as a whole.

During pregnancy, the needs of the developing fetus will be met at the expense of maternal needs, especially of the minerals iron and calcium. A diet rich in these should be advised and iron and folic-acid supplements supplied to meet the high demands for these by the fetus.

During lactation, large quantities of nutrients are lost from the maternal stores. However, in the latter stages of pregnancy a woman increases her deposits of adipose tissue and does not need to 'eat for two' in terms of carbohydrates and fats. Proteins must be ingested in large quantities, however, since they cannot be stored. Equally, calcium and vitamins must be taken in, either from the diet or from supplements. An adequate fluid intake is also necessary if the needs of the thirsty baby are to be met satisfactorily.

Dietary modifications for milk-fed infants

The nutritional needs of infants, whose intestinal tracts are immature, are met by feeding with milk. **Human milk** will meet the needs of the normal baby without modification, and other milks can be altered to make them suitable. **Goat's milk**, because of its fine curd and small fat molecule, is easily digested by babies. However, a fresh supply is not readily available and the evaporated and dried preparations are expensive and difficult to obtain. **Cow's milk** is the most freely obtainable source for infant feeding. It can be used fresh (boiled), or is available in a variety of dried and evaporated milk preparations. It is necessary to dilute this milk to reduce the high protein and mineral salt content and to add sugar to increase ite energy value. Dried milk preparations, if reconstituted exactly as directed, take these considerations into account.

SOME PATHOLOGICAL STATES INFLUENCING NUTRITIONAL NEEDS

Modifications to diet will be necessary if pathological processes interfere with the ability to digest, absorb, assimilate or excrete all or any components of the normal balanced diet. An understanding of the physiology of digestion and absorption and of the assimilatiom and excretion processes and their controls, together with a comprehension of the nature of the various pathological processes (such as inflammation or tumours), will ensure that the nurse sees the specific modification of the intake as a logical part of a patient's therapy.

Diseases requiring dietary modification as part of therapy are discussed in the relevant chapters for example, see diabetes mellitus in Ch. 11.

Pathological conditions in the young child in which dietary modifications are therapeutic require **special milk preparations** to meet specific needs. Many firms produce various suitable products, available by prescription only. Some examples are given in Table 4.3.

Table 4.3
Special milk preparations

Type or preparation	Name	For treatment of:
Low protein	Prosparol	Renal disease
Low sodium	Edosol	Cardiac failure
Low calcium	Locasol Low Calcium Milk Food	Hyperparathyroidism
Low lactose	Galactomin Nutramigen Low Lactose Milk Food	Galactosaemia
Low phenylalanine	Minafen Lofenalac Cymogram Albumaid	Phenylketonuria
Soya bean	Allergillac Velactin	These are free of milk proteins and suitable for treating children who seem allergic to caseinogen and lactalbumen
Low fat	Snow Queen (Alfonal) Cow and Gate Separated	Obesity

SOME RARE CONDITIONS OF CHILDHOOD
Phenylketonuria

This is a condition in which, due to a genetic defect, the enzyme necessary to convert phenylalanine, a protein substance, to tyrosin is missing. The blood levels of phenylalanine rise above the normal 1 to 2 mg/ml and these high levels damage the developing brain, resulting in severe mental retardation. Though a rare condition (1 in 10 000 births) and incurable, it is possible by dietetic means to prevent the brain damage, which only occurs once milk feeding is established and consequently high levels of phenylalanine enter the blood.

Diagnosis

Early diagnosis is essential. This is made by estimating the level of phenylalanine in the infant's blood, usually between the seventh and tenth day of life. (A minimum of 48 hours must have passed since the commencement of milk feeding.) This blood test is called the Guthrie test.

Treatment

Treatment is aimed at keeping the blood level of phenylalanine below 5 mg/100 ml and is achieved by feeding the baby with a low phenylalanine preparation (Minafen). Change to mixed feeding of non-phenylalanine foods and Cymogram usually occurs early, since the milk preparations have an unpleasant taste and smell. Regular Guthrie tests are the most reliable monitor of the child's condition, but a quick estimation can be made by testing the urine with Phenistix for the presence of phenylpyruvic acid, which will occur if the blood level of phenylalanine rises above 15 mg/100 ml. Ingenuity on the part of the mother and encouragement and support from medical and nursing staff are necessary to ensure that the child takes his diet. The management of the diet requires expert advice, as the number of proprietary foods, such as soups, to which protein substances have been added is enormous and limits choice. It is very expensive.

It is possible that only the developing brain of the young child is vulnerable to the effects of high phenylalanine levels, and therefore a gradual return to a more normal food intake may be possible once the child is about 10 years of age. The major practical difficulty in testing this theory lies in the inability to measure reliably intellectual ability. Mental deterioration, should it occur after the introduction of normal diet, is likely to be slow. It may, therefore, be impossible to diagnose before irreversible damage has occurred.

Cystic fibrosis

Clinical features

The baby with this condition may present before 3 months of age suffering from 'failure to thrive', or 'malabsorption syndrome'. He is likely to be irritable, pale in appearance, with a ravenous appetite and yet static weight or actual weight loss, abdominal distension and offensive, fatty stools. The condition is caused by a **genetic defect** which results in the absence of the pancreatic enzymes, amylase, lipase and trypsin. Digestion is impaired, absorption cannot take place and the child is hungry. He will also exhibit signs of calcium and vitamin deficiency.

Diagnosis

It is important that other causes of malabsorption are excluded, and the nurse plays a vital role in assisting in various diagnostic tests. A **sweat test**, in which a piece of filter paper is placed on a carefully cleaned part of the child's arm or thigh and enclosed by a polythene square, may be carried out. It must be kept in place for half an hour, and is then sent for estimation of sodium content. Sweat from a child with this condition will contain an abnormally high level of sodium (above 60 mEq/litre). **Stool collections** will be required, and great skill is necessary to achieve this from such a young baby; they are sent for estimation of fat content and tryptic activity. A **jejunal biopsy**, obtained by passing a Crosby capsule (see p. 160) via the mouth into the jejunum, requires great patience from nursing staff as the child must be fasted prior to this test and prevented from pulling the tube up before it reaches the jejunum. In order to get the tube to pass through the pylorus, the child must lie on his right side. X-rays will be taken at intervals until the desired site is reached. The biopsy material is sent for estimation of tryptic activity. This test may take many hours.

Management
Once diagnosed, the management of this condition is to replace the missing enzymes by using Pancrex, which can be sprinkled on to food, and by dietary modification. This involves a low fat diet, as the digestion and absorption of proteins and carbohydrates are reduced in the presence of much fat in the intestines. Alfonal and the Cow and Gate Separated Milk preparations both provide a fat content of 0·1 per cent. It is necessary to increase protein and carbohydrate intake to meet energy needs, and the fat-soluble vitamins A, D and possibly K must be given as water-soluble supplements. Unfortunately, the other aspect of this disease, the viscosity of mucus, especially in the respiratory tract, is less easily managed. These patients suffer from recurring, severe respiratory infection and most die in their early teenage years.

Coeliac disease

This condition results from undue sensitivity of the mucous membrane of the small intestine to gluten. Gluten is the protein found in wheat and rye. The inflammatory reaction produces a massive secretion of mucus which interferes with the absorptive processes, particularly of fat, but also of minerals, vitamins, proteins and carbohydrates. If untreated, the villi of the small intestine become flattened, decreasing the available absorptive surface and aggravating the degree of malabsorption. Diagnosis is established by jejunal biopsy (p. 160).

Clinical features
The symptoms usually appear in the early years, once a good mixed diet has been established, but may occur in adults. The child is small for his age, has a poor appetite and distended abdomen. He passes large, pale, offensive stools, and suffers from iron-deficiency anaemia.

Treatment
A gluten-free diet will be effective within a few weeks but presents numerous practical problems. Gluten-free flour is available for making bread, cakes, biscuits, pastry, etc. at home; it must also be used in preparing any food that would normally contain ordinary flour. It may be possible to arrange for a local baker to make a batch of gluten-free bread, which can then be frozen and used as required. Many proprietary products contain gluten, including sauces, soups and puddings, and must be avoided.

This dietary modification is palatable and does not present as great a problem in some ways as the management of phenylketonuria. It is, however, expensive, and may need to be continued for life, as it is doubtful if complete recovery ever occurs. Cautious additions of gluten to the diet may be permitted after a long symptom-free period (usually taken as a minimum of 5 years after diagnosis) and the effects assessed.

Anaemia and vitamin deficiencies should be corrected by giving iron and vitamin supplements as necessary.

DISEASES OF MALNUTRITION

Malnutrition — or bad nourishment — is a term which describes a range of pathological conditions whose causal factors are related to an intake of food (or its availability in the body) which is unsuited to the body's needs. The treatment, therefore, is concerned with establishing the cause and applying dietary modifications as appropriate.

The deficiency diseases are conditions in which one particular dietary component is available in insufficient quantity; the disorders in this group commonly found in Great Britain are discussed below, but others of significance elsewhere are kwashiorkor and scurvy. Subnutrition is another aspect of malnutrition, in which one or more of the major energy providing foods is inadequate; examples are anorexia nervosa (see below and Ch. 16), those suffering from malabsorption syndrome (see p. 167), or starvation. A major nutritional disorder in which excessive amounts of food (principally carbohydrates) are ingested is obesity (see below).

It should not be thought that these three groups are mutually exclusive. Persons suffering from subnutrition may well be more profoundly affected by one specific deficiency which general re-feeding will not rectify. It is also not uncommon for obese people, whose dietary intake is often grossly distorted, to suffer from a deficiency disease, usually iron deficiency anaemia.

Rickets

This disease of calcium and phosphorus metabolism results from an insufficient intake or synthesis of vitamin D and, additionally, inadequate calcium in the diet. Increasing costs of the foods which would supply these nutrients and overcrowding in industrial cities, combined with diets high in cereals and low in milk and milk products, have produced an increased incidence particularly among immigrant populations.

Clinical features
The growth rate of the child is greater than the speed at which he can form bone, and hard bone produced by adequate quantities of mineral deposits is not achieved.

Lack of calcium also affects muscle tone and the child is restless, pale and flabby. He has a distended abdomen (due to weak abdominal muscles and intestinal fermentation from the high carbohydrate content of the diet) and tends to sweat excessively, especially over the scalp. The normal milestones of sitting up, crawling, standing, walking and eruption of teeth are delayed; the 'soft' teeth are vulnerable to caries and the 'soft' bones to deformity once weight-bearing occurs. Deformity of the chest is accompanied by both a prominent sternum and spinal deviations; in the female, pelvic deformities may cause serious difficulties later at childbirth.

Delayed milestones, a fretful, sweaty baby and poor dietary history, combined with radiological evidence and a raised serum alkaline phosphatase level, will establish the diagnosis. Early recognition and treatment will prevent irreversible bony deformities.

Treatment
Treatment depends on establishing an adequate intake of calcium in the diet and a therapeutic dose of vitamin D. This ranges from 1000 to 8000 *iu* daily and should be continued until the serum alkaline phosphatase level returns to normal, after which the vitamin D dose should be gradually reduced to the prophylactic level of 400 *iu* daily. It can be given as cod-liver oil, halibut-liver oil or calciferol, depending on the quantity which would be required to give the prescribed dose. It is important to improve the environment of the child; often he is overdressed and his mother may need tactful education to allow him to be outside in the sunshine as much as possible and to continue the improved diet once he appears well. It is in this area that the nurse in the community can play a vital role, as well as by noting any early symptoms.

Osteomalacia   (Fig. 4.6)

This is the adult counterpart of rickets. Calcium and vitamin D are deficient with a resulting failure to lay down calcium in the organic matrix of bone; therefore the ratio of calcium phosphate to matrix is reduced. In Eastern countries it occurs in women who live on a high cereal diet with little milk, who rarely go out into the sunshine and who by repeated pregnancies (and lactation) are depleted of calcium. In Western societies it is more common as a secondary feature of chronic renal disease or some form of malabsorption.

Clinical features
Bone pain and tenderness may be prominent and the gait is uneven due to pain in tarsal and metatarsal joints. Spontaneous fractures may occur, and iron deficiency anaemia is usually present. Diagnosis is made on clinical evidence — the radiological appearance of generalized rarefaction and the presence of pseudofractures, which are pathognomonic of osteomalacia.

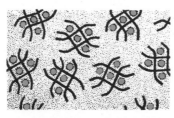

NORMAL   Collagen fibres } equal proportions
Calcium deposits }

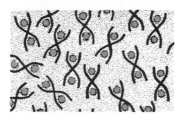

OSTEOPOROSIS   Normal ratio collagen:calcium
but BOTH reduced

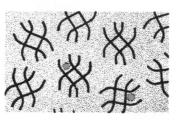

Figure 4.6
Osteoporosis and osteomalacia

OSTEOMALACIA   Collagen normal but
reduced calcium

Treatment

Treatment is based upon dietary correction or the addition of calcium lactate to the diet in countries where dairy produce is not readily available. Vitamin D in doses up to 50 000 *iu* daily must be given. Bony deformities do not respond to medical treatment and will require surgical correction.

Osteoporosis   (Fig. 4.6)

In this condition, which is the most common nutritional bone disease found in clinical practice, there is atrophy of bone leading to a reduction of the total quantity of bone. Thus the ratio of calcium phosphate to matrix is normal. It may be localized as a result of inflammation or neoplasm or, more commonly, immobilization. Hence the bedridden, the elderly, the patient whose movement is reduced by pain (as in rheumatoid arthritis) or splinting will be prone to this condition. The importance of early mobilization, active (and where necessary passive) physiotherapy and adequate pain relief should be noted as a part of nursing care, especially of the elderly.

Generalized osteoporosis is associated with the reduction of androgen formation and occurs more commonly in women and at an earlier age due to the abrupt nature of the menopause. Malnutrition, with associated abnormal protein metabolism, and endocrine disorders such as Cushing's syndrome, thyrotoxicosis and acromegaly exacerbate the condition. Corticosteroid therapy over prolonged periods is also associated with this condition. Osteoporosis in the young is generally found in conjunction with hypofunction of the gonads.

Diagnosis and treatment

Diagnosis is made on the history and radiological appearances. Blood chemistry is all normal. Treatment is aimed at:

1. Relieving pain, which may be severe and incapacitating.
2. Preventing deformity, especially of the spine, which may damage the cervical, thoracic or lumbar nerves.
3. Reducing the demineralization of bone by increasing mobility.
4. Enhancing the opportunities for adequate bone formation by a good mixed diet, rich in calcium and protein.

Supplements of calcium and vitamin D may help. The administration of hormones (oestrogens, androgens and other anabolic agents) leads to the relief of pain and an increased sense of well-being. There is no evidence that any of the above measures increases the amount of bone laid down, but it appears that the progress of the disease is arrested.

Prevention

Prevention is the important factor, as this is a slowly progressive disease. An active life and a well-balanced diet which includes a pint of milk daily would be the appropriate approach. As advancing years are associated with the onset of many chronic conditions which affect appetite and mobility, their adequate management and the appreciation of these factors in the patient's future well-being will reduce the degree of osteoporosis from which the elderly may suffer.

Anorexia nervosa (Fig. 4.7A)

This condition, in which anorexia is conditioned by an hysterical reaction, may be a grave threat to life. Although refeeding will result in weight increase, it is generally agreed that this is an illness primarily of psychological origin.

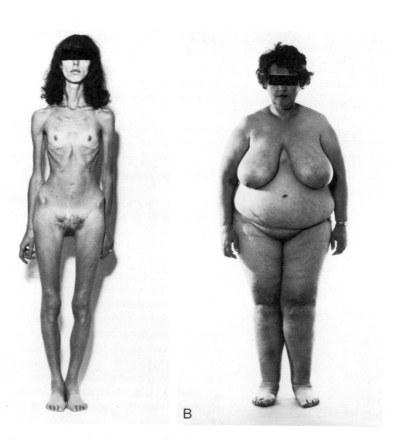

Figure 7
A. Anorexia nervosa
B. Obesity

A   B

Obesity (Fig. 4.7B)

Obesity is the most common disease of malnutrition in the Western world. It results from ingesting more energy foods than are required for the energy expenditure; the excess is stored as fat. The term obesity is generally applied if the individual's weight is 10 per cent in excess of the standard weight shown in Table 4.4. (The weights shown in this table include an allowance of 7 to 9 lb for men and 4 to 6 lb for women, to take account of clothing worn when weighed.)

Table 4.4
Desirable weights of adults according to height and frame (*from* Macleod J. 1977 Davidson's Principles and Practice of Medicine, 12th edn. Churchill Livingstone, Edinburgh)

Height without shoes			Desirable weight in kilograms and pounds (in indoor clothing), ages 25 and over					
			Small frame		Medium frame		Large frame	
metres	ft	in	kg	lb	kg	lb	kg	lb
				Men				
1·550	5	1	50·8–54·4	112–120	53·5–58·5	118–129	57·2–64	126–141
1·575	5	2	52·2–55·8	115–123	54·9–60·3	121–133	58·5–65·3	129–144
1·600	5	3	53·5–57·2	118–126	56·2–61·7	124–136	59·9–67·1	132–148
1·625	5	4	54·9–58·5	121–129	57·6–63	127–139	61·2–68·9	135–152
1·650	5	5	56·2–60·3	124–133	59 –64·9	130–143	62·6–70·8	138–156
1·675	5	6	58·1–62·1	128–137	60·8–66·7	134–147	64·4–73	142–161
1·700	5	7	59·9–64	132–141	62·6–68·9	138–152	66·7–75·3	147–166
1·725	5	8	61·7–65·8	136–145	64·4–70·8	142–156	68·5–77·1	151–170
1·750	5	9	63·5–68	140–150	66·2–72·6	146–160	70·3–78·9	155–174
1·775	5	10	65·3–69·9	144–154	68 –74·8	150–165	72·1–81·2	159–179
1·800	5	11	67·1–71·7	148–158	69·9–77·1	154–170	74·4–83·5	164–184
1·825	6	0	68·9–73·5	152–162	71·7–79·4	158–175	76·2–85·7	168–189
1·850	6	1	70·8–75·7	156–167	73·5–81·6	162–180	78·5–88	173–194
1·875	6	2	72·6–77·6	160–171	75·7–83·5	167–185	80·7–90·3	178–199
1·900	6	3	74·4–79·4	164–175	78·1–86·2	172–190	82·7–92·5	182–204
				Women				
1·425	4	8	41·7–44·5	92–98	43·5–48·5	96–107	47·2–54	104–119
1·450	4	9	42·6–45·8	94–101	44·5–49·9	98–110	48·1–55·3	106–122
1·475	4	10	43·5–47·2	96–104	45·8–51·3	101–113	49·4–56·7	109–125
1·500	4	11	44·9–48·5	99–107	47·2–52·6	104–116	50·8–58·1	112–128
1·525	5	0	46·3–49·9	102–110	48·5–54	107–119	52·2–59·4	115–131
1·550	5	1	47·6–51·3	105–113	49·9–55·3	110–122	53·5–60·8	118–134
1·575	5	2	49 –52·6	108–116	51·3–57·2	113–126	54·9–62·6	121–138
1·600	5	3	50·3–54	111–119	52·6–59	116–130	56·7–64·4	125–142
1·625	5	4	51·7–55·8	114–123	54·4–61·2	120–135	58·5–66·2	129–146
1·650	5	5	53·5–57·6	118–127	56·2–63	124–139	60·3–68	133–150
1·675	5	6	55·3–59·4	122–131	58·1–64·9	128–143	62·1–69·9	137–154
1·700	5	7	57·2–61·2	126–135	59·9–66·7	132–147	64 –71·7	141–158
1·725	5	8	59 –63·5	130–140	61·7–68·5	136–151	65·8–73·9	145–163
1·750	5	9	60·8–65·3	134–144	63·5–70·3	140–155	67·6–76·2	149–168
1·775	5	10	62·6–67·1	138–148	65·3–72·1	144–159	69·4–79	153–174

Based on weights of insured persons in the United States associated with lowest mortality (*Statist bull Metrop Life Insur Co* 40. Nov.–Dec. 1959)

Associated factors

There are many factors which may affect the regulating mechanism of appetite and produce obesity;

1. **Age and sex.** In childhood the sex ratio of obese subjects is equal. After puberty, obesity is much more common in women, especially after pregnancy and the menopause.

2. **Pregnancy.** Part of the weight gain during pregnancy is due to an increase in adipose tissue which serves as a store against the demands of lactation. This may not be lost after the baby is born or weaned, and with each subsequent pregnancy, the woman's weight at the time of conception will be greater than on the previous occasion.

3. **Economics.** Most cheap meals are formed largely of carbohydrates. These satisfy the appetite less readily than protein and fatty foods, so an increased quantity is eaten — hence the greater number of obese people in the lower economic groups.

4. **Eating habits.** Many obese people are nibblers, and people concerned with food preparation are particularly vulnerable. Obese people appear to be stimulated to eat more by habit than in response to stomach contractions due to hunger.

5. **Physical activity.** Scientific advances, which have provided mechanized household equipment and transport, enable work to be done without as much energy expenditure as in the past. The advent of sedentary leisure occupations like the cinema, television and radio, and our growing cities which discourage walking as an occupation, all increase the likelihood of obesity.

6. **Psychological factors.** Unhappy people may find solace in overeating and consequently become obese. On the other hand, there are many obese men and women who appear to lead happy, full lives.

7. **Genetics.** Although genetic factors may play a part, it is probable that environmental factors are more important, such as family custom and eating habits.

8. **Endocrine factors.** Many endocrine diseases are associated with weight gain, but it is unlikely that they are a cause of obesity.

9. **Overfeeding in childhood.** Fat babies tend to become fat adults. Fat cells which are formed in early childhood tend to refill rapidly, even after dieting has reduced their size. These unfortunates fight a constant battle against becoming overweight.

Consequences of Obesity

Why treat obesity? The reduction of body weight will not remove any of the causative factors, but the obese person will feel better, look better and survive longer if his weight is reduced to the standard for his height and build.

Aesthetic considerations, which mean that the obese person finds it difficult to dress well and look attractive, may add to the burden of mechanical disabilities from which obese people suffer.

Mechanical problems result from the excessive weight the skeleton is being asked to support and transport. Flat feet and osteoarthrosis of the knees and hips are common. Muscular tissue is infiltrated with fat, giving rise to uterine prolapse, abdominal herniae and varicose veins. The deposition of excessive amounts of fat in the subcutaneous tissues around the rib cage interferes with its free movement, giving rise to recurrent chest infections.

Many **metabolic disorders** are associated with obesity: diabetes mellitus, gout, atherosclerosis and cholelithiasis are all more common in overweight people. Patients with these disorders are also prone to their complications — peripheral neuropathy, hypertension, and cerebrovascular accidents.

Cardiovascular problems, especially angina, are more common among the obese because of the increased amount of effort required to move an overweight body. The coronary arteries will have atheromatous plaques, and cardiac failure occurs.

Generally speaking, obese people are **more accident prone** than persons of normal weight. The excess tissue prevents a good grip and the obese person readily drops things, spills kettles of boiling water or trips over things. Because of his increased bulk and tendency to mechanical disorders the obese person cannot rapidly avoid danger as can other people. Finally, the complications of obesity, combined with slow wound healing, make the obese patient a **poor anaesthetic and surgical risk.**

All these factors mean that the expectation of life for the obese individual is reduced. A man of 45 years who is 11 kg above standard weight has a reduced life expectancy of 25 per cent.

Management

The nurse can play a vital role in the management of obesity both in hospital and in the community. Primarily, the patient must be motivated to lose weight and to maintain a standard weight once it is achieved. This motivation may be based on very individual factors, but every effort must be made to reinforce it and to support the patient with advice and encouragement during the times when the goal appears more remote.

It is important that the members of the patient's intimate circle do not sabotage these efforts, either psychologically (the husband who says he likes his wife plump) or physically by encouraging the ingestion of prohibited foods. Another vital factor in successful weight reduction is that the supervisors have a realistic goal in time and make sure the patient is aware of it. Other factors, such as the need to recognize that the initial dramatic weight loss will not be repeated each week and that premenstrual tension and fluid retention may temporarily increase weight despite adherence to the dietary regime, should be explained so that the patient is not unnecessarily depressed by temporary set-backs and abandons treatment.

Because the cause of obesity is an increase of food intake over energy expenditure, the aim of treatment is to change eating habits, so that weight is lost, and to increase the amount of exercise. This will permit a reasonable energy intake while still achieving the primary objective.

Although small amounts of excess adipose tissue can be lost by 'crash' dieting, this method is unsuitable for the obese person. The diet must be sufficiently satisfying to ensure that the ill-effects of *ketosis* or excessive tiredness do not occur, which would interfere with daily activities, impair interpersonal relationships and reduce motivation to the point where the attempt at weight reduction is discontinued. The diet must be flexible to allow variety and economic food buying, and also to reduce the temptation to cheat. Each failure makes further attempts less likely to succeed.

To avoid these complications and to allow a sufficiently prolonged period under close supervision for habit changes to take place, it is wise to allow the patient a diet which provides between **4000 and 4500 kJ per day**. The average middle-aged housewife requires about 9250 kJ per day, and would then be short of approximately 5000 kJ per day, which she will obtain from her adipose tissue. A weekly weight loss of approximately 1 kg is possible on this regime (based on the physiological fact that the energy value of adipose tissue is approximately 31·5 kJ per g) and should be the aim.

To attempt to change habits outside the normal environment is short-sighted — the patient is best treated in an out-patient setting. Education and support in practical and psychological terms form the basis of success. It is often helpful to make a graph on which the patient's progresss can be charted; if the gradations on the ordinate are fixed so that even a small weight loss looks significant, it has a good psychological effect, even for those patients who know and understand exactly the ruse that has been practised!

The balance of the diet is altered to meet the physiological needs. The carbohydrate intake is reduced to 100 g per day. This reduction appears very drastic to the patient, since overindulgence in these foods is the most common cause of obesity. Protein intake of 60 g per day is adequate for the patient's needs and negates the argument often raised in defence of obesity, that reducing diets are expensive. If these two components are taken in these quantities, only 40 g of fat may be ingested if the total energy intake is not to exceed that stipulated.

Because this is a new pattern of behaviour for the patient, it is desirable that energy-producing constituents in the diet be weighed in the early stages. The amount of time spent on explanation and discussion of a suitable dietary regime is never wasted. Frequent discussion of difficulties and repetition of advice and encouragement are all worthwhile. It may be helpful to reduce salt intake, especially during the premenstrual period; vitamin supplements should not be necessary, as most vegetables supply few kilojoules and can therefore be taken freely. Iron supplements may be worthwhile: most obese patients are middle-aged women who also tend to be slightly anaemic.

Although the control of diet is the corner-stone of treatment, other factors can influence its success. An increase in daily exercise is desirable, and walking (often the most strenuous activity possible for obese people) requires a steady energy output. A minimum of 3 miles a day should be encouraged. **Regular daily exercise** is more valuable and less dangerous than spurts of intense activity at intervals.

Exercise in combination with a low carbohydrate intake is effective in increasing weight loss for two reasons. Firstly, an increase in energy demands requires the mobilization of triglycerides from the fat stores; secondly, because of the reduced carbohydrate intake, the ability to convert lipoproteins into triglycerides and store them is reduced. The use of skin calipers to measure this reduction in skin fold thickness is only valid if practised by an expert, using the same area of tissue on each occasion.

Drug therapy as an adjunct to diet has some place, especially in the treatment of the relapsed obese person. How much of the effect is psychological and how much physiological is difficult to say. In some cases the side-effects of drugs make them unsuitable for the patient. The addictive properties of amphetamines have led to their withdrawal, but there are other anorectic agents available. Metformin, for example, is particularly suited to the needs of the obese diabetic patient, since it is thought that this drug (one of the biguanide group) increases the uptake of glucose in muscle. Another drug which has undergone successful controlled trials is fenfluramine: it is thought that this drug increases the breakdown of fat and decreases the synthesis of trigly-cerides, thus reducing the fat depots. All drugs should be used with caution and their use does not obviate the need for strict adherence to the dietary regimen.

The role of surgery in the treatment of obesity is doubtful. It is possible that operations on the small intestine which involve bypassing segments of the gut and so reducing the absorptive surface available may be of value. Such procedures, however, neither treat the cause of obesity nor bring about the necessary long-term changes in eating habits. Only in severe, intractable cases, and with due consideration of the special risks of surgery to which obese persons are vulnerable, should such measures be considered.

Overeating destroys more than hunger — efforts to sustain and encourage those who endeavour to apply the remedies and avoid destruction are more than gratifying.

SUGGESTED ASSIGNMENTS

1. Make a poster suitable for a group of 13-year-olds to illustrate the composition of a balanced diet.

2. Discuss the factors concerned in selection of a balanced diet; relate these to conditions in your locality.

3. What dietary advice would you give to a recently widowed, elderly man?

4. A child of 6 months is diagnosed as suffering from coeliac disease. What advice and practical support would you offer his family in the immediate and long-term future?

5. A 45-year-old woman is 155 cm tall and weights 100 kg.
How would you establish her standard weight? How would you assist her to achieve and maintain this?

FURTHER READING

Beck Mary E 1977 Nutrition and dietetics for nurses, 5th edn. Churchill Livingstone, Edinburgh
Craddock D 1973 Obesity and its management, 2nd edn. Churchill Livingstone, Edinburgh
Macleod J (ed) 1977 Davidson's principles and practice of medicine, 12th edn. Churchill Livingstone, Edinburgh
McLaren D S 1976 Nutrition and its disorders, 2nd edn. Churchill Livingstone, Edinburgh
Ministry of Agriculture Fisheries and Food 1975 Manual of nutrition. HMSO, London

REFERENCE ONLY

Davidson Sir Stanley, Pasmore R. Brock J F, Truswell A S 1979 Human nutrition and dietetics, 7th edn. Churchill Livingstone, Edinburgh
Passmore R, Robson J S 1976 A companion to medical studies, 2nd edn. Blackwell Scientific, Oxford, vol 1

5. The Gastrointestinal Tract and the Abdomen

Many gastrointestinal disorders when diagnosed can be cured or controlled by dietary or drug therapy without the patient having to be hospitalized. Therefore it is likely that the nurse in training may only care for these patients when they have been admitted to hospital during an acute exacerbation of a gastrointestinal disorder or when complications require surgical correction.

ANATOMY AND PHYSIOLOGY

The gastrointestinal tract

The gastrointestinal tract is a muscular tube about 9 metres in length (Fig. 5.1). It includes the mouth, pharynx and oesophagus, which lead to the stomach. From the stomach it continues as the duodenum, jejunum and ileum, known collectively as the **small intestine**. It proceeds as the caecum, ascending, transverse, descending and sigmoid colon known collectively as the **large intestine**. The tube continues and becomes the rectum, then ends as the anal canal. The tract is under autonomic nervous control, is lined throughout with mucous membrane (Fig. 5.2) and is constructed in such a way that the different parts can play their separate roles. The various glands associated with the tract are the salivary glands, the pancreas and the liver. These glands empty their secretions into the tract and are necessary for its proper functioning. The functions of the gastrointestinal tract are the **ingestion, digestion** and **absorption** of

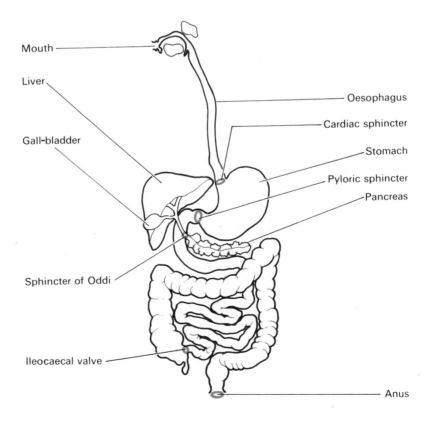

Figure 5.1
The gastrointestinal tract

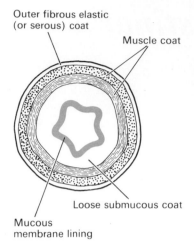

Outer fibrous elastic
(or serous) coat

Muscle coat

Loose submucous coat

Mucous
membrane lining

Figure 5.2
Cross-section: gastrointestinal
tract

food, and the **elimination** of semisolid waste. The various sphincters of the tract enable the timely passage of intestinal content.

When food is ingested the action of the teeth, tongue and muscles in the sides of the mouth reduce it to small particles. This chewing action stimulates increased flow of saliva containing the enzyme amylase and digestion begins. The food is formed into a soft bolus which can be swallowed. It passes through the cricopharyngeal sphincter down the oesophagus into the stomach by peristatic movement. The oesophago-gastric sphincter prevents regurgitation of food and gastric acid into the oesophagus.

The stomach is the expanded part of the tract and the oesophagus enters its upper end just below the diaphragm. The stomach has three zones: the fundus, the body and the antrum. The parietal cells producing acid and the chief cells producing pepsin are concentrated in the fundus and body of the stomach. The antrum secretes alkaline mucus and the hormone gastrin. There are two phases. Initially, the vagus nerve stimulates the flow of gastric secretion in response to the sight, taste and smell of food. This is the **cephalic phase.** When food passes into the antrum the hormone gastrin is released into the blood and further stimulates gastric secretion. This is the **gastric phase.**

The action of the gastric muscles and secretions reduces the food to a semisolid, partially digested state called **chyme.** This is stored in the stomach before passing through the pyloric sphincter into the small intestine at a rate which will allow further digestion and absorption. Intestinal secretion and hormones are produced when chyme enters the duodenum. The hormones stimulate the secretion of pancreatic enzymes, cause contraction of the gall-bladder and relaxation of the sphincter of Oddi. Bile from the liver which has been stored in the gall-bladder flows into the duodenum along with the pancreatic enzymes, and the further breakdown of fat, carbohydrate and protein occurs. The food is now in a fluid alkaline state. Once this stage is reached the absorption of chemicals and nutrients can take place across the specially constructed walls of the small intestine into the blood. Residue passes on through the ileocaecal valve into the large intestine. Large quantities of water are absorbed mainly through the walls of the caecum and ascending colon. By peristalsis the residue then moves through the transverse to the sigmoid colon where further water absorption takes place. This gives the residue, faeces, its normal semisolid consistency. The entry of faeces into the rectum causes the desire for defaecation and there is relaxation of the internal anal sphincter. After the first few years of life the external anal sphincter comes under voluntary control, and defaecation occurs at will.

Accessory organs

The salivary glands
Saliva is a thin watery solution containing salts and an enzyme called amylase which splits cooked starch. It is produced by three pairs of salivary glands: the parotid, the submandibular and the sublingual, whose ducts open into the mouth. There is a continuous flow of small amounts of saliva which cleanses and lubricates the mouth and tongue. In response to the sight, smell, taste or thought of food an increased amount of saliva is produced. The mechanical breakdown of food which is then mixed with saliva in the mouth is the start of the process of digestion.

The pancreas
The pancreas is a large gland which has an exocrine and endocrine function. The exocrine or external secretion of the pancreas contains the enzymes **trypsinogen, amylase** and **lipase** and alkaline salts. When acid chyme enters the duodenum the hormone secretin is released to stimulate and maintain the secretion of pancreatic juice into the duodenum. Its function is to neutralize the acid from the stomach and to continue the digestion of protein, carbohydrate and fat. The endocrine or internal function of the pancreas is the production of the hormones glucagon and insulin which circulate in the blood and regulate carbohydrate metabolism (Ch. 11).

The liver, biliary tract and gall-bladder
The liver is the largest gland in the body and is indispensable to life. One of its many functions is the production of **bile** (Fig. 5.3). The liver is composed of a large number of lobules from which pass small bile ducts. These unite with similar ducts to form the

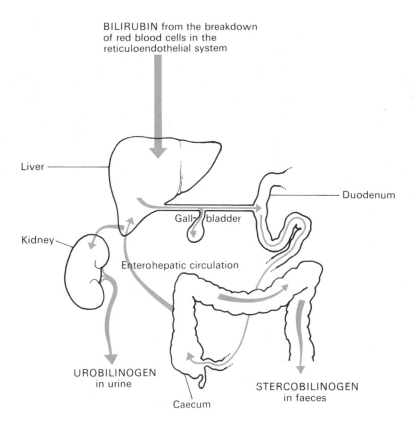

Figure 5.3
The formation and excretion of bile

largest hepatic ducts. The bile secreted by liver cells passes from the hepatic ducts to the cystic duct and is then stored and concentrated in the gall-bladder. When fatty foods are present in the duodenum the hormone **cholecystokinin** causes contraction of the gall-bladder and relaxation of the sphincter of Oddi. The bile then passes down the bile duct and enters the duodenum along with the pancreatic secretion. One of the functions of bile is emulsification of fats by the bile salts. It also provides a means of excreting the pigment bilirubin, an end-product of the breakdown of red blood cells.

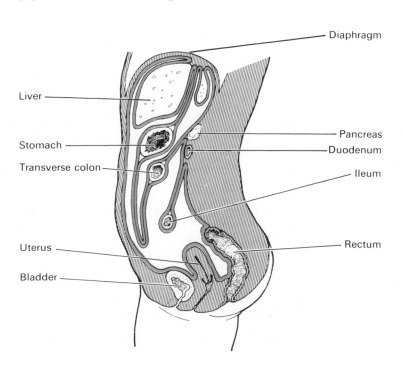

Figure 5.4
The peritoneum

After the absorption of nutrients and chemicals from the intestinal tract into the blood, it is transported via the portal vein to the liver. There some substances are altered, some stored and others passed into general circulation to reach the tissues of the body.

The peritoneum

The stomach, small and large intestine, liver, pancreas and gall-bladder are contained in the **abdominal cavity**. The peritoneum, the serous membrane which lines the cavity, covers and supports the abdominal viscera (Fig. 5.4). The **peritoneal cavity** is the potential space between the two layers of peritoneum.

The blood vessels and nerves to the small and large intestine are supported by thickened folds of peritoneum called the mesentery, the transverse mesocolon and pelvic mesocolon. The large fold in front of the abdominal viscera is the omentum. This supports blood and lymph vessels and is capable of isolating infection within the peritoneal cavity.

Further support for the abdominal viscera is provided by the muscles of the anterior abdominal wall, the pelvic muscles and the diaphragm.

AETIOLOGY

Aetiology of disease varies from one level of the tract to another and it is not proposed, therefore, to provide a comprehensive list of influencing factors. The following points are of particular relevance.

Diet

As discussed in Chapter 4, dietary imbalance may occur in a variety of ways and may cause disturbance of gastrointestinal function.

Poor food hygiene

This, and deficient sanitation, are associated with poor social conditions, overcrowding and lack of health education. Inflammatory gastrointestinal infections are, however, still relatively common in affluent communities where there is little excuse for laxity in standards of cleanliness. Fashionable restaurants and, even more regrettably, hospital kitchens are among the offenders.

Psychosocial factors

The influence of **emotional** factors on gastrointestinal tract disorder is universally accepted. Anxiety and continuous tension can predispose to mechanical upsets such as acute vomiting and diarrhoea. The incidence of structural breakdown as in peptic ulceration is high in people subject to stressful conditions.

Cigarette smoking and the **ingestion of alcohol** tend to aggravate, complicate and predispose the individual to certain gastrointestinal disorders, especially malignant disease and peptic ulceration.

GENERAL FEATURES OF DISORDER

The patient's history and symptoms are of particular importance since the signs of gastrointestinal disorder are relatively few.

'**Indigestion**' is a collective term used by patients to describe many of their symptoms. True indigestion, as found for example in pancreatic insufficiency when there is failure to produce the necessary digestive enzymes, is very rare.

'**Dyspepsia**' is also a collective term used, it must be admitted, by medical and nursing staff, to describe almost any type of abdominal discomfort associated with the taking of food. It is better to use more specific terms.

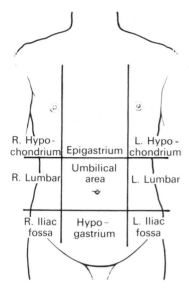

Figure 5.5
Regions of the abdomen

R. Hypo-chondrium | Epigastrium | L. Hypo-chondrium

R. Lumbar | Umbilical area | L. Lumbar

R. Iliac fossa | Hypo-gastrium | L. Iliac fossa

Pain

Pain is the most common symptom. It is caused by either:

1. Strong contractions of smooth muscle, giving rise to colic such as intestinal or biliary colic.
2. Inflammation of the peritoneum as in appendicitis.
3. Stretching of the capsule of a viscus when the organ within becomes swollen, as in hepatitis.

The character of the pain may vary and patients may differ in the description of their pain; these varying accounts can be misleading. Nonetheless, the site of the pain is of significance and the nurse should be able to report whether it is, for example, epigastric, umbilical or hypogastric (Fig. 5.5). Symptoms of local or generalized rigidity or tenderness are commonly associated with abdominal pain.

Another related phenomenon is that of referral of pain from the diseased area to some distant region. The mechanism of this is not quite clear.

The nurse should note the degree and the duration of pain, its relationship, if any, to meals and whether or not the taking of food aggravates or relieves pain.

Flatulence

Under normal circumstances ingested air is rapidly eructated from the oesophagus and stomach. In some conditions, such as pyloric stenosis, the patient may complain of excessive amounts of 'wind' which may also be foul smelling. Gas accumulating in the colon whether ingested or resulting from imperfect digestion is passed via the rectum.

In the postoperative patient gas cannot be eructated normally and some passes into the intestines. It becomes trapped, causing distension of the upper colon, and discomfort results. It will only be relieved when the patient becomes mobile. Therefore, it is important to ensure some movement even when the patient continues to rest in bed.

Heartburn

This is a sensation of burning behind the lower end of the sternum and is often accompanied by regurgitation of fluid into the pharynx. The causes are many but the burning sensation suggests gastric acid reflux at the lower end of the oesophagus.

Alteration in eating habits

The desire to eat (appetite) is often diminished. This loss of appetite is known as **anorexia** and will result in weight loss. Persistent refusal to eat for psychological reasons is termed **anorexia nervosa** (Ch. 4). Some patients may omit certain items of diet in the belief that they disagree with them. This is characteristic of people suffering from peptic ulceration who may, as a result, develop signs of nutritional deficiency. Such deficiencies may also arise from persistent vomiting.

Nausea

The feeling of sickness is experienced mostly in the epigastrium. The accompaniment of salivation, sweating and pallor usually indicates that vomiting is to follow.

Vomiting

This is a reflex act caused by a wide variety of stimuli, too many to list comprehensively. They include unsuitable food, many systemic diseases and psychological disorder. The reflex can to some extent be suppressed by taking deep breaths through the mouth or by holding the breath.

Alterations in bowel habit

These are manifest by diarrhoea or constipation due to altered peristalsic activity. However, they may or may not have an underlying organic cause. Dietary indiscretion or deficient food hygiene play an important part in the disorganization of gastrointestinal tract function, hence the importance of health education in the community.

Diarrhoea
   Acute diarrhoea may be due to infection or overindulgence in fatty foods.
   Chronic diarrhoea is a common symptom of a large number of diseases, particularly those affecting the colon, such as ulcerative colitis.

Constipation
   Acute constipation is likely to be organic in origin; it is present, for example, in intestinal obstruction.
   Chronic constipation is often due to faulty eating or toilet habits. In hospital the usual practice is to record the number of bowel movements a patient has each day. Abnormalities of stools must be noted and reported with care.

Intestinal haemorrhage

Melaena, blood in stools, and haematemesis, blood in vomitus, are extremely serious symptoms indicative of some structural erosion within the gastrointestinal tract. Such symptoms always merit immediate investigation.

Dysphagia

This is the term used to describe difficulty in swallowing. It is a symptom of many disorders, including painful conditions of the mouth and throat, compression of the oesophagus — for example by an enlarged thyroid gland — and a growth or disease of the oesophagus itself, in particular from carcinoma and inflammatory conditions.

   As can be seen, many symptoms of gastrointestinal disorder cause both acute physical distress and social embarrassment; therefore, mental depression is a common sequel.

INVESTIGATIONS

Gastrointestinal studies tend to be exhausting and very lengthy. Patients already fatigued by disease processes require the utmost consideration and care when undergoing investigation.

Analysis of gastric content

Gastric aspirate
This is obtained by using a radio-opaque Levin tube passed through the nasal cavity into the antrum of the stomach. The position of the tube should be checked by the accepted method in the ward, for example, by using litmus paper. Some doctors like to check the position fluoroscopically.

   Intubation is usually performed in the early morning following an 8- to 10-hour fast. In the normal fasting subject the amount of gastric-secretion rarely exceeds 100 ml. Volumes in excess of this amount occur in gastric hypersecretion, pyloric obstruction and duodenal regurgitation.

Gastric acid secretion
Definite variations in hydrochloric acid content are present in some diseases; therefore the quantitative assessment of gastric acid secretion is of diagnostic importance.

   The patient is fasted overnight and left to rest in bed in the morning. A Levin tube is passed, its position checked and the fasting juice aspirated. With the patient lying comfortably in the left lateral position gentle suction is applied to the tube to provide continuous aspiration. After 1 hour this resting juice is collected and a gastric stimulant is given. The most suitable gastric stimulant is pentogastrin (Peptavalon), a synthetic polypeptide structurally related to gastrin. It is given subcutaneously in a dose of 6 μg per 1 kg body weight. The gastric juice is then collected for 1 hour. The volumes are measured, the juice titrated and the output of acid calculated. The results are of value in deciding the type of surgery needed.

The total absence of hydrochloric acid is termed achlorhydria and is uncommon except in patients with pernicious anaemia or in those who have undergone extensive gastric surgery.

Collection of stools

Stool collections for 3 or 5 days may be ordered in the event of suspected malabsorption syndromes, especially in cases of steatorrhoea, which indicates abnormal fat digestion. Faecal fat estimations are made while the patient's daily fat intake is being controlled by the dietician.

Radiology

Plain films

Supine and erect films of the abdomen are indicated in cases of suspected intestinal obstruction or ileus in order to demonstrate distended loops of bowel and fluid levels. Free gas may be seen under the diaphragm following perforation of a duodenal ulcer, or indeed any part of the alimentary tract. Gallstones and renal stones may sometimes be demonstrated on plain films.

Barium meal

The main indications for this examination are suspected gastric or duodenal ulcer, gastric carcinoma and hiatus hernia. The examination is normally carried out in the morning and it is essential that the patient should have had nothing to eat or drink since the previous evening. The mucosa of the oesophagus, stomach and duodenum are coated with barium and the lumen distended with air. The patient is then positioned by the radiologist and X-ray films taken under television control to demonstrate any lesions that may be present. Many radiologists give 20 mg i.v. Buscopan (hyoscine-N-butylbromide) in order to make the stomach and duodenum hypotonic during the examination. This may cause some blurring of vision and the patient should be told not to drive a car until this effect, which usually lasts for less than an hour, has worn off.

Small bowel barium studies

This technique may be used to investigate suspected malabsorption, Crohn's disease or tumours of the small bowel. The preparation of the patient is the same as for a barium meal. Some radiologists give the barium by mouth taking frequent X-ray films until the whole small bowel has been examined whilst others prefer to intubate the duodenum with a special nasogastric tube and instil the barium into the small bowel. Most examinations should be completed within an hour using modern rapid transit barium.

Barium enema

The purpose of this examination is to demonstrate polyps and tumours of the colon, diverticular disease and ulcerative and Crohn's colitis. These lesions are shown by coating the mucosa with barium and distending the lumen of the colon with air. X-ray films of the colon are taken in various positions as determined by the radiologist. In order to carry out a satisfactory barium enema the colon must be completely free of faeces. The bowel may be prepared either with water washouts or with an enema containing a colonic activator such as veripaque (dihydroxyphenylisatin). 3 g of veripaque are mixed with 1½ litres of warm water and this is run into the colon at least one hour before the barium examination. The patient spends the interval between the preliminary cleansing enema and the barium enema in the toilet in order to ensure complete evacuation of the colon. There is no need to fast the patient for this examination.

Sinography

A sinogram may be helpful in demonstrating the site and extent of a sinus track or fistula between the bowel and abdominal wall. For this procedure a fine Portex or Foley catheter is introduced down the sinus track and a water soluble contrast medium injected. X-ray films are taken when the full extent of the sinus or fistula has been demonstrated.

Cholecystography and cholangiography

Oral cholecystography is indicated if gallstones are suspected. The patient is given a light meal the night before the examination. The contrast medium is taken by mouth in tablet form and thereafter the patient is given nothing to eat or drink until after the X-ray examination the following morning.

If the gall-bladder fails to concentrate the contrast then an **infusion cholangiogram** may be performed in an attempt to show the gall bladder and bile ducts. While the intravenous infusion of the contrast medium is in progress the nurse should observe the patient for any sign of an allergic reaction.

During cholecystectomy most surgeons routinely perform **operative cholangiography** in theatre to make sure that there are no residual stones in the bile ducts.

If the patient is jaundiced the oral and intravenous contrast media will not be excreted by the liver. In such cases the biliary tract may be outlined by **percutaneous transhepatic cholangiography** which involves passing a thin needle through the skin and into the liver under local anaesthesia. Contrast medium is injected into the bile ducts to show the cause and site of the obstruction. After such an examination the patient is usually given a broad spectrum antibiotic; regular checks on the pulse and blood pressure are made by the nurse as the examination carries a small but definite risk of biliary peritonitis, intraperitoneal bleeding and ascending cholangitis.

An alternative method of examining the biliary tract is by **endoscopic retrograde cholangiopancreatography**. At this examination a fine catheter is passed into the bile ducts through a fibreoptic endoscope under X-ray control and contrast medium injected to outline the bile ducts. This examination has the added advantage that the pancreatic duct can also be X-rayed following cannulization and the injection of contrast medium.

Arteriography

This is occasionally of value in demonstrating vascular abnormalities of the alimentary tract and tumours of the liver and pancreas. The examination is performed by passing a catheter from the femoral artery into the aorta and taking rapid serial films following the injection of contrast medium. Following the examination regular checks should be made to ensure that there is no bleeding from the puncture site in the femoral artery and the pulse and blood pressure should also be checked regularly by the nurse.

Ultrasonography

Detail of the anatomy of the liver, gall bladder, bile ducts and pancreas can now be demonstrated by means of ultrasound examination. This examination, which is described more fully on page 331, has the advantage that it is non-invasive and is therefore without risk to the patient. No special preparation or after care is required except that patients for gall bladder examination should fast.

Nursing care

The nurse can be of great assistance when an ill patient is being X-rayed, particularly if an intravenous infusion is being administered. The patient will also require help and support when turning into the various positions required by the radiologist and radiographer.

Endoscopy

Endoscopy is the examination of the inner lining of an organ, such as the colon or stomach, by direct vision using a special illuminated tube or fibreoptic instrument.
The procedure may be:

1. Diagnostic, to observe, photograph and obtain a biopsy of tissue.
2. Therapeutic, for example, to dilate strictures or remove foreign bodies.

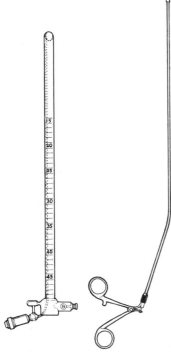

Figure 5.6
Left- Oesophagoscope
Right: Oesophageal biopsy
forceps

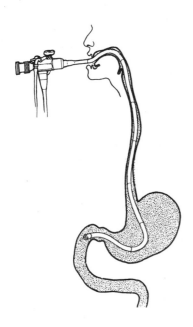

Figure 5.7
Oesophago-gastro-
duodenoscope in use

Preparation of the patient
This varies according to the organ which is to be examined and the type of anaesthesia required. Upper endoscopy involves the use of a local anaesthetic throat spray but general anaesthesia may be necessary for patients who are very apprehensive or unable to co-operate.

In some instances, for example during oesophagoscopy, the patient is unable to speak. Although the procedure may not be painful it is uncomfortable and can be alarming. Therefore the patient should be given an explanation of the preparation and procedure necessary for his examination.

Patients who are to have upper endoscopy carried out fast for at least six hours prior to examination. Five minutes before the procedure begins the throat is sprayed with local anaesthetic, Diazepam 20 mgs is given intravenously, and if the patient is under 60 years of age Buscopan is also given.

Oesophagoscopy
Oesophagoscopy is the examination of the oesophagus using a metal oesophagoscope (Fig. 5.6) or a fibreoptic instrument which is passed through the mouth and down the oesophagus to the cardiac sphincter. The nurse should stay with the patient and hold his hand as this is his only way of communicating when the instrument is being passed. Any sudden movement at this stage could damage the oesophagus.

Bouginage. Dilatation of oesophageal stricture can be carried out via an oesophagoscope. The patient is prepared as for upper endoscopy. Graduated dilators (ranging in size from 21 mm to 45 mm) are used.

Because of the risk of trauma, after care of the patient is extremely important. Frequent observation of pulse and blood pressure is carried out for the first 12 hours. Initially the patient is given nil orally, but mouthwashes during this time will be greatly appreciated. After approximately six hours the patient may be given sips of water, iced, but previously boiled. If tolerated, free fluids are introduced. Following examination by the physician a soft diet may be recommended.

Gastroscopy/duodenoscopy
Gastroscopy is the examination of gastric mucosa using a flexible fibreoptic instrument (Fig. 5.7). It can be controlled so that it is possible to examine the pylorus, duodenum or postoperative reconstruction. Biopsy can be obtained under direct vision.
After care of patients having upper endoscopic examination
When the procedure has been completed the patient must not eat or drink until his swallow reflex has recovered from the local anaesthetic, usually in about 4 hours. In the few days following he may be hoarse or complain of a sore throat; this can be relieved with warm gargles. Patients who are investigated as out-patients should be allowed time to recover before being escorted home by a friend or relative.

Proctoscopy
This is the examination of the anus and rectum using a metal or plastic proctoscope which is about 8 cm long and 2 cm in diameter. The patient is allowed a light breakfast on the morning of the test. Preparation of the rectum varies; patients who are not suspected of having inflammatory disease may be ordered a small enema to clear faecal matter which would obscure the examiner's view of the rectal mucosa. For this examination the patient is helped into the left lateral position with his knees drawn up. He should be adequately covered. The nurse should help him maintain this position and encourage him to relax by taking deep breaths.

After examination the patient is allowed to rest.

Sigmoidoscopy
The examination of rectal and sigmoid mucosa using a sigmoidoscope, which is a metal tube 25 cm long and 1·5 cm in diameter, is called sigmoidoscopy. Preparation for this examination is as for proctoscopy. The patient is examined in the knee-chest or left lateral position; though uncomfortable, the procedure should not be painful. During sigmoidoscopy air may be pumped into the colon to distend the lumen and allow a better view of the mucosa. This may cause pain; therefore the nurse should observe the patient carefully since he may feel faint.

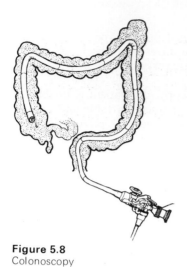

Figure 5.8
Colonoscopy

After this tiring examination the patient is allowed to rest and have a light meal, especially if he is an out-patient.

Colonoscopy
This examination (Fig. 5.8) is gradually replacing sigmoidoscopy mainly due to the versatility of the fibroscope which allows an extended view to the level of the caecum. Preparation of the patient may, in some circumstances, need to be more extensive and include colonic washout. It may be performed under general anaesthesia.

Biopsy
Removal of a small portion of tissue for microscopic examination is termed biopsy.

A biopsy of the small intestine can be taken using the Crosby capsule. This apparatus consists of a small hollow capsule with a side hole; inside there is a circular, spring-loaded blade. The capsule is attached to a long thin polythene tube. When suction is applied to the tube mucosa is pulled into the side hole of the capsule and the spring-loaded blade severs the trapped tissue.

Preparation of the patient involves fasting overnight and receiving an explanation of the procedure. On the day of the examination the patient is asked to swallow the capsule. This can be made easier if he sits in the upright position. The doctor may prescribe a drug such as Maxolon to stimulate peristalsis and prevent nausea. The time taken for the capsule to reach the small intestine depends on motility and the state of the pyloric sphincter. When the capsule reaches the antrum (estimated by markings on the tube) the patient is asked to lie in the right lateral position for 2 hours. The presence of bile-stained duodenal juice in the tube indicates entry of the capsule into the duodenum. The position is checked fluoroscopically before the biopsy is taken. The capsule is withdrawn, opened and the tissue carefully removed. The apparatus is checked to ensure that it is complete.

Biopsy of the small intestine may be necessary during the investigation of malabsorption syndrome.

DISORDERS OF THE ORAL CAVITY

Glossitis, inflammation of the tongue, in acute and chronic forms is frequently caused by deficiency of substances essential for the metabolism of healthy cells such as iron and vitamins of the B group (Ch. 4). The shiny, smooth and often painful tongue is due to the surface being denuded of papillae. Chronic inflammation leads to leukoplakia characterized by snowy-white patches on the tongue and sometimes on cheeks and gums. Painful, tender fissures develop later and become sites of chronic infection or malignant changes.

Halitosis (offensive breath) may result from dental disorders or the excretion of odour from the gastrointestinal tract or lungs. In addition to its clinical significance it is socially embarrassing.

Stomatitis or inflammation of the mouth appears in many forms. The commonest type is thrush.

Thrush (moniliasis)

This condition occurs readily in infants (Ch. 17) and the fungus is easily transmitted by inadequately sterilized feeding bottles or poor hygiene of nursing or medical staff. In adults it occurs either during debilitating illnesses when resistance to infection is low, or in those receiving corticosteroid or antibiotic therapy when normal bacterial flora are diminished.

Clinical features
The yeast-like fungus, *Candida albicans*, forms ivory-white patches on the mucous membrane of the mouth, tongue, palate or pharynx. These patches coalesce to form an easily detached membrane which, when wiped off, leaves a bleeding excoriated surface. The membrane is easily recognized when examined under a microscope.

Treatment
The condition is uncomfortable rather than painful. Two-hourly mouth care is carried out very gently using weak solutions of sodium bicarbonate. An oral suspension of nystatin may be prescribed; this is applied locally by being held in the mouth for several minutes. Fruit juices are most useful in stimulating the flow of saliva to cleanse and bathe the mouth.

As the condition is easily transmitted the patient's feeding utensils are reserved for his use only and are sterilized afterwards.

DISORDERS OF THE OESOPHAGUS
Oesophagitis

Any substance causing injury and irritation to the oesophageal mucosa produces oesophagitis.

Corrosive poisons
The consequences of wittingly or unwittingly ingesting corrosive substances are dramatic. Severe burning sufficient to cause collapse is felt throughout the length of the oesophagus. The mucosa becomes ulcerated.

Treatment
This involves identifying the poison and giving oral preparations immediately to neutralize the effect. The healing process produces scar tissue which may result in oesophageal narrowing and stricture formation.

Foreign bodies
Almost any small object may be swallowed by a young child, irritate the mucous membrane and produce pain. Obstruction by a radio-opaque foreign body such as a fish bone is readily seen on X-ray examination, but other materials may not show up at all. Oesophagoscopy is carried out to locate and remove the foreign body.

Oedema
Swelling resulting from mucosal trauma may cause temporary oesophageal stricture and accompanying dysphagia. A soft diet and a plentiful fluid intake must be encouraged until the swelling subsides and normal diet can be resumed.

Reflux oesophagitis
This may occur in an acute form after repeated vomiting. However, inflammation caused by regurgitated gastric acid secretion quickly decreases as the vomiting subsides and the associated pain disappears. In some conditions, such as hiatus hernia, reflux of gastric juice occurs repeatedly causing chronic irritation, ulceration, eventual stricture formation and dysphagia in several cases.

Stricture formation
This may follow ingestion of corrosive poisons or foreign bodies or a severe case of reflux oesophagitis. After inflammation and oedema have settled, the resulting stricture is amenable to dilatation (see bouginage, p. 159).

Hiatus hernia

The diaphragm has several openings through which herniation of abdominal viscera into the thorax can occur. The commonest and most important is the oesophageal hiatus.

Aetiology
Age is important, for hiatus hernia is commoner in middle and later life, probably because muscle tone diminishes with age and the hiatus becomes more lax. The condition occurs more frequently in women. Increased intra-abdominal pressure in pregnancy and obesity predisposes to it, as do some chest deformities, for instance

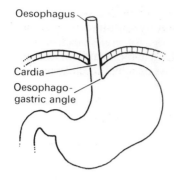

Oesophagus

Cardia

Oesophago-
gastric angle

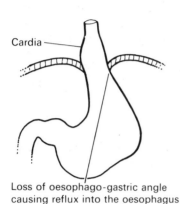

Cardia

Loss of oesophago-gastric angle
causing reflux into the oesophagus

Figure 5.9
Top: Normal
Bottom: Hiatus hernia

those associated with kyphosis. In children the condition is due to congenital short oesophagus.

Clinical features

In adults hiatus hernia may be symptomless if the cardiac sphincter remains in a normal position (Fig. 5.9 *top*).

After taking food, a feeling of substernal discomfort may be experienced owing to distension of the hernial sac. Heartburn is the cardinal symptom and is typically associated with any change of posture which increases intra-abdominal pressure, for example stooping, lifting or straining. Patients tend to be awakened from sleep and pain is only relieved by sitting upright. A feeling of food sticking in the oesophagus is a common complaint. Regurgitation of food into the mouth occurs unexpectedly, especially during exercise immediately after a meal.

Careful enquiry into the patient's history and a clear description of the site and character of the pain and its relationship to posture make diagnosis almost certain. A barium meal examination will demonstrate the hernia (Fig. 5.9 *bottom*) and on oesophagoscopy the inflammatory changes characteristic of reflux oesophagitis can be seen.

Complications which may arise are peptic ulceration within the hernial sac or, more rarely, bleeding.

Treatment

The majority of middle-aged patients respond well to medical treatment. In obese patients reduction of weight with consequent reduction in intra-abdominal pressure relieves symptoms. Similarly the hernias of pregnancy disappear after parturition.

Prevention of reflux at night is assured if patients are encouraged to sleep in a semiupright position with the head of the bed raised on blocks. Tight clothing should not be worn. A bland diet is advised, and during acute stages antacid medications are given frequently for the immediate relief of heartburn and to protect the inflamed oesophageal mucosa from further damage by gastric acid.

Persistent oesophagitis and the intractible pain associated with ulcer and stricture formation are only relieved by surgery. The purpose of surgery is to reduce the hernia, strengthen the hiatus and restore the oesophago-gastric angle.

Achalasia (cardiospasm)

This is the condition of deranged oesophageal motility. As a result of this nervous disturbance, the cardiac sphincter fails to relax and allow entry of food into the oesophagus. Progressive dysphagia with persistent vomiting are the outstanding symptoms. Treatment involves selective division of the sphincter muscle (Heller's operation).

Carcinoma of the oesophagus

This malignant growth, occurring usually in middle-aged or elderly patients, produces a progressive dysphagia.

Clinical features

At first, difficulty is experienced when swallowing solids. Finally even fluids cannot be tolerated, with resultant dehydration, wasting and anaemia from lack of nourishment. The constant regurgitation is distressing and carries the risk of aspiration pneumonia. The stricture is demonstrated on barium swallow X-ray and diagnosis of malignancy is confirmed by oesophagoscopy and biopsy examination. Pain is a late symptom.

Treatment

Radiotherapy is effective in causing regression of the tumour.

Oesophagectomy, a severe mutilating operation, involves removing a large section of the oesophagus and anastomosing the remainder to the stomach below.

Palliative therapy. The aim of palliative treatment is to provide the patient with adequate nourishment. Because of the stricture, it is often impossible to pass a nasogastric tube into the stomach. It is sometimes possible to pass a tube such as an *MB tube* through the growth to allow partial freedom from dysphagia. Failing this a gastrostomy is performed: a small opening is made into the stomach and a catheter is inserted for feeding purposes.

DISORDERS OF THE STOMACH AND DUODENUM

Incapacitating conditions of the stomach and duodenum are common in the Western hemisphere and, since they often affect people in their middle years, they have important social and economic implications.

Gastritis

Inflammation of the mucous membrane lining of the stomach is termed gastritis.

Acute gastritis generally results from some gross dietary indiscretion or ingestion of contaminated food. In most cases the intestine is also inflamed (gastroenteritis).

Chronic gastritis presents a more serious clinical problem and is likely to be encountered in patients who habitually enjoy highly seasoned foods, overindulge in alcohol or have a raised acid secretion. Symptoms are similar to those of peptic ulceration and the patient is treated medically as for this condition.

Peptic ulceration

The term peptic ulceration refers to an ulcer formed on any mucosal surface exposed to the irritating effects of gastric hydrochloric acid and the enzyme pepsin.

Aetiology
The areas affected are the lower end of the oesophagus, when it is subjected to acid reflux, the stomach and the duodenum. Peptic ulcers may occur in areas brought into contact with gastric juices following gastric surgery. The incidence of ulcer disease is lower in women than in men and this apparent immunity is increased during pregnancy. It is possible, therefore, that hormonal substances increase normal mucosal resistance. Heredity is a well-recognized factor as is the association of peptic ulcer with patients in blood group O. It is also recognized that emotional factors play an important part in the development of an ulcer.

The ingestion of alcohol and certain types of food as well as cigarette smoking tend to aggravate ulcers.

Clinical features
Pain and discomfort, often described as burning in character, are usually felt in the epigastric region and at specific times in relation to meals. Localized tenderness and rigidity are felt directly over the ulcer site. Food eases the pain caused by most peptic ulcers but relief is more lasting in the case of duodenal ulcer. Vomiting is likely when pain is severe and always affords some measure of relief. If appetite remains good weight loss in uncommon. heartburn is experienced in most cases.

Ulcers may be acute or may follow a chronic course with the patient complaining of long-standing but intermittent dyspepsia. These recurring attacks, often preceded by emotional stress, tend to become more frequent and severe before the patient seeks medical advice.

Investigations
Diagnosis is usually made on barium meal examination which shows an ulcer crater.

Gastroduodenoscopy may be performed to confirm the presence of an ulcer and, more important, to determine whether the lesion is malignant or benign. A biopsy is therefore taken during endoscopy.

Gastric secretion tests are carried out: normal acid levels are usually found in patients with gastric ulcer, while excessive amounts may be found in those with duodenal ulcer. A finding of achlorhydria excludes the possibility of simple peptic ulcer. Examination of faeces may reveal the presence of occult blood.

Course and complications

The uncontrolled symptoms of peptic ulceration affect the patient's life at home and at work. From time to time he will have acute exacerbations of the disease and complications may arise. Common complications are:

1. **Pyloric stenosis**. The formation of scar tissue and of inflammation around the pyloric sphincter may cause delayed emptying of the stomach resulting in stasis of gastric content.

2. **Perforation** of an acute or chronic ulcer (p. 165) will allow the irritating gastric or duodenal content to drain into the peritoneal cavity resulting in peritonitis (p. 184).

3. **Haemorrhage**. Severe haemorrhage occurs if the ulcer erodes a large blood vessel producing the alarming symptom haematemesis.

4. **Malignancy**. There is the risk of malignant changes occurring in chronic gastric ulceration (p. 166).

Treatment and nursing care

Medical treatment

The aims of medical treatment are the relief of symptoms, the healing of the ulcer and the prevention of complications.

1. **Bed rest**, whether at home or in hospital, is the single most effective part of patient care. Ambulation is allowed for toilet or bathing purposes only; otherwise, the patient must be afforded all the physical and mental rest possible in order to relieve pain and hasten the healing process. Since stress is a contributory factor in the hypersecretion of acid the patient is advised to avoid anxiety; sedatives may be prescribed for the very anxious person.

2. Bland, small, frequent meals may be prescribed — some authorities consider them a means of neutralizing gastric acid. Although a particular **dietary regime** may ease the patient's pain there is no evidence that any specific diet assists healing. The continuing presence of occult blood in faeces proves this point.

3. **Drug therapy** plays an invaluable role in treatment by neutralizing and inhibiting acid output and reducing spasm and inflammation.

Antacids such as aluminium hydroxide or magnesium trisilicate can be taken between meals to neutralize gastric acid and relieve pain. These preparations must be fast-acting, harmless, palatable and — above all — cause no interference with bowel function or the acid-base balance of the body.

Anticholinergic drugs depress gastric motility and acid secretion by inhibiting the vagus nerve stimulus. Prescribed in addition to diet and antacid therapy, drugs such as propantheline (Probanthin) help to prevent pain, particularly during the night. Carbenoxoline (Biogastrone), an oral preparation derived from extract of liquorice, is found to have some effect on ulcer healing in the ambulant patient. It is thought to reduce inflammation around the ulcer.

4. Since there is evidence to suggest that cigarette smoking inhibits healing, **smoking is discouraged.**

Healing takes 4 to 6 weeks according to the initial severity of the condition. However, at the end of a week following medical treatment symptoms should subside; gradual return to normal activity is then permitted. Thereafter, management involves the prevention of recurrence. Regular, non-irritating meals with interjacent milk drinks are recommended and the avoidance of alcohol, cigarette smoking and stress situations are advised.

Unfortunately, there is no sure means of maintaining healing or preventing relapses, therefore surgery is recommended when medical treatment fails, when complications occur or when there is any suspicion of malignant change.

Surgical treatment

The aim of surgical treatment, for those who do not respond to medical treatment, is the reduction of acid secretion. This may be achieved by diminishing vagal stimulation to the parietal cells of the stomach by severing some branches of the vagus nerve, (highly selective vagotomy) (Fig. 5.10 *left*). Another means of reducing acid production is by removing the antrum, the gastrin-secreting area of the stomach, by performing antrectomy (Fig. 5.10 *right*).

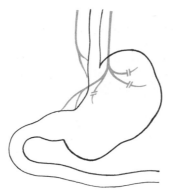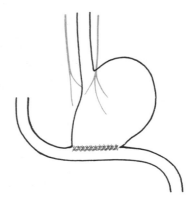

Figure 5.10
Left: Highly selective Vagotomy
Right: Antrectomy

Postoperative complications. Following gastric surgery, the majority of patients can again enjoy normal digestive function and good health. Regular out-patient examination is advised, however, to detect and treat any late postoperative complications. These include:

Nutritional disorders. The alimentary canal has considerable adaptive powers following surgery, but sometimes, because of gastric resection, food is not prepared properly for its onward passage through the tract. Also, when a drainage procedure has been carried out, unprepared food may leave the stomach at a rapid rate. Undigested food cannot be absorbed and deficiency diseases with weight loss will result.

Anaemia. This is a late complication associated in particular with partial gastrectomy. The anaemia may be due to malabsorption of iron or failure to produce the intrinsic factor.

Dumping syndrome. The usual complaint is of epigastric fullness, giddiness and extreme fatigue occurring during a meal or immediately afterwards and when the patient is in an upright position. It is probably due to the sudden distension of the jejunum. The symptoms are eased if the patient eats dry meals, avoids hot fluids and rests immediately after eating. Explanation of symptoms does much to allay the patient's anxiety. If symptoms do not subside corrective surgery may be necessary.

Perforated peptic ulcer

This is an abdominal emergency of sudden onset and with early signs of acute peritonitis. Perforation of the ulcer allows gastric contents to drain into the peritoneal space. It may also erode a blood vessel and cause severe haemorrhage.

Clinical features
The patient is pale, tense and afraid to move because of the intense pain. Respirations are shallow and rapid. The abdomen is held rigid and does not move on breathing. The pulse is rapid and of poor volume.

The patient complains of severe, generalized, abdominal pain which may be referred to his shoulders because of the presence of gas and irritant fluid under the diaphragm. Haematemesis will indicate erosion of a major blood vessel.

Investigations
The patient's history is important: he may already be known to have a peptic ulcer. X-ray of the abdomen in the supine and erect positions will show air under the diaphragm in most cases.

Nursing observation and records
Pulse and blood pressure.
Degree of pain and signs of circulatory collapse.

Treatment and nursing care

Pain is relieved and the patient prepared for surgery to repair the perforation and control bleeding.

A nasogastric tube is passed to aspirate gastric contents before and after the operation. Intravenous infusion is started to replace fluid, electrolyte and blood loss. The operation is usually a simple closure of the perforation and ligation of the eroded blood vessels.

In the postoperative period gastric suction and intravenous infusion are continued until the patient is free of pain, has no abdominal distension and no signs of toxaemia. Antibiotics may be prescribed if chest infection or peritonitis complicate the postoperative period.

There is usually a dramatic improvement in the patient's general condition. If this is maintained oral fluids and then light diet can be introduced about the fourth day after surgery. Stitches are removed and the patient is allowed home about the tenth day.

Because of the possible recurrence of complications most patients are reviewed at a later date for elective surgery. This may be vagotomy and gastroenterostomy for duodenal ulcer or partial gastrectomy for gastric ulcer.

Gastric carcinoma

Carcinoma of the stomach is the commonest malignant tumour of the gastrointestinal tract.

The condition is commoner in men than in women and mostly occurs in middle age. The cause is unknown but the incidence of malignant change is greater in those patients who have a previous history of chronic gastritis and peptic ulceration.

Clinical features

Early symptoms of dyspepsia, usually vague, are readily dismissed and the patient may seek medical advice only when the tumour is advanced and there are signs of extensive spread. Epigastric pain resembling that of peptic ulcer but lacking the characteristic relationship to meals may occur alone or accompanied by nausea, vomiting, anorexia, weight loss and constipation. An abdominal mass easily palpable suggests an advanced unresectable tumour. Gastrointestinal bleeding is a feature found in one-third of patients. Coffee-grounds vomiting and melaena indicate a slow but constant ooze of blood from the lesion. Anaemia is always present.

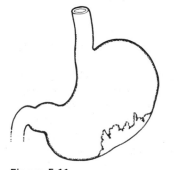

Figure 5.11
Defect in the stomach outline indicative of malignant tumour

Investigations

Diagnosis is confirmed by a combination of radiology, gastroscopy and biopsy. Barium meal examination shows a filling defect caused by the tumour (Fig. 5.11).

Treatment

Management of gastric carcinoma is by immediate surgery where possible and involves either partial or total gastrectomy. When the growth is widespread no resection may be attempted, but accessible areas of tumour may be removed thereby affording considerable symptomatic relief from obstruction and haemorrhage. Radiotherapy is of little value in these circumstances.

DISORDERS OF THE SMALL INTESTINE

Regional enteritis (Crohn's disease)

This is a non-specific inflammatory process affecting the whole thickness of the intestinal wall. It may occur in single or multiple segments and most commonly affects the ileum. There is thickening of the submucosa, ulceration and hypertrophy of the muscle wall causing narrowing of the lumen of the intestine. As the ulceration heals, scar tissue formation prevents absorption of nutrients and also causes strictures. The inflammatory process may affect the mesentery and lymphatic system in the area.

The disease usually occurs between the ages of 20 and 30 years. It affects men and women equally and may take the form of an acute or chronic illness.

Clinical features

The patient with chronic regional enteritis has a history of general ill health, weight loss and anaemia. Intermittent colicky pain associated with diarrhoea may occur three or four times daily. The stools often contain mucus, pus and undigested food; there can be fistula formation and intestinal obstruction. In acute regional enteritis, the patient has severe abdominal pain low on the right side. He may have a moderate fever and mild diarrhoea.

Investigations

A barium meal and follow-through X-ray will show the areas of the small intestine that are affected. A barium enema is also performed to assess any involvement of the colon.

Nursing observations

Temperature, pulse, respiration and blood pressure.
Fluid intake and output.
Character and frequency of diarrhoea.
Early signs of intestinal obstruction, such as abdominal distension, pain, vomiting and dehydration.

Course and complications

The inflammatory and fibrotic changes in the mucosa of the small intestine prevent the normal absorption of fat and protein. This causes deterioration in the patient's general health. Oedema and congestion can result in adhesions between loops of bowel or other abdominal organs and lead to the formation of fistulae or abscesses. Intestinal obstruction may occur due to strictures caused by adhesions or narrowing of the small intestine lumen.

Treatment and nursing care

The patient has a chronic debilitating disease and will require sympathetic nursing care to help him accept this and adjust his way of living. General health can be improved by attention to diet, which should be bland, high calorie and high protein with iron and vitamin supplements. During an acute phase the patient is nursed in bed. He may require intravenous replacement of fluids and electrolytes if diarrhoea becomes a problem. Steroid drugs may be prescribed to reduce acute inflammation during relapses. Antibiotic therapy will be prescribed if there are signs of infection and abscess formation. Antispasmodic drugs will help to relieve pain associated with diarrhoea.

Although treatment is essentially conservative, complications such as intestinal obstruction, abscess or fistula formation will require surgery. Grossly affected segments can be excised leaving as much normal intestine as possible for the absorption of nutrients.

Rehabilitation and community care

Because the patient has a chronic illness a great deal of support is required. Patient and family should be educated in maintaining nutrition. Ideally the help of a dietician to explain the preparation of special diets and supplements should be made available. Although the patient should be encouraged to become employed, within the limitations imposed by the illness, financial support may be needed — particularly to help finance the diet required to maintain his general health.

Malabsorption syndrome

The term can be applied to any disorder of the gastrointestinal tract which impairs the digestion and absorption of one or a number of nutritional substances. However the term usually refers to conditions where there is multiple malabsorption. The conditions may be grouped in the following way:

Incomplete digestion — from either a lack of pancreatic enzymes, as in pancreatitis, or absence of bile salts due to biliary tract obstruction (p. 180). It may also be the result of gastric surgery such as gastrojejunostomy when chyme leaves the stomach and enters the jejunum without being mixed with the enzymes and bile salts in the duodenum.

Impaired absorption — caused by either inflammatory conditions of the small intestine, such as regional ileitis (p. 166), or bacterial invasion of this part of the tract, which is usually sterile. It may occur as a result of gastric surgery, for example in the blind end of the duodenum following some types of gastrectomy.

Congenital malformation of the mucosal lining of the small intestine, as in coeliac disease, will reduce the area and ability of the small intestine to absorb.

Clinical features

Signs of malnutrition — glossitis, anaemia, weight loss and bone disease — are evident. There may be abdominal distension and the patient often complains of diarrhoea with pale, bulky, offensive stools.

Investigations

The patient's history of any previous gastrointestinal surgery.
Barium meal and follow-through X-ray.
Biopsy of small intestine (p. 160).
Faecal fat estimations.
Glucose tolerance test.
Blood levels of various substances, such as urea.
Urine collection.

Treatment

This depends on the cause of malabsorption. Surgery may be necessary to relieve biliary tract obstruction and to correct the blind loop following gastric surgery. Specific treatment will be required for conditions such as regional ileitis, pancreatitis and coeliac disease.

Intestinal obstruction

Intestinal obstruction develops when the contents of the gastrointestinal tract cannot pass through the lumen of the small or large intestine. This may be caused by mechanical, adynamic or vascular disorders of the tract.

There are three categories of mechanical obstruction:

1. Extramural obstruction caused by pressure outwith the wall of the intestine.
2. Mural obstruction caused by an abnormality of the intestinal wall causing narrowing of the lumen.
3. Intraluminal obstruction due to tumour or foreign body within the lumen of the intestine.

Extramural obstruction is most commonly caused by the formation of adhesions following surgery or inflammatory disease. These strands of tissue may constrict the intestine or provide a focus for rotation or kinking of the gut; this condition is called volvulus. Another cause of obstruction may be that part of the intestine becomes trapped within a hernial sac. Pressure exerted on the wall of the intestine by tumour in an adjacent organ could occlude the lumen so causing obstruction.

Mural obstruction may result from the healing and scarring process of some inflammatory disease or from malignant growth within the wall of the intestine causing narrowing of the lumen.

Intraluminal obstruction may be caused by a bolus of meat or fruit, a large gall-stone or by tumour within the lumen of the intestine.

Adynamic **obstruction** results from any condition which impairs peristalsis; severe pain or handling the intestine during surgery can result in paralysis of the intestine.

Vascular disease of the mesentery such as mesenteric embolus will prevent adequate blood supply to a segment of the intestine causing loss of function.

Obstruction causes distension of the immediately proximal part of the intestine. This is due to the accumulation of gas derived from swallowed air (which is normally passed through the tract) and produced by bacterial decomposition of stagnant intestinal content. The pressure exerted by the accumulated gases stops the absorption of fluids and electrolytes from the lumen of the gut.

Clinical features

Symptoms vary according to the level at which the obstruction has occurred. High obstruction in the small intestine will produce symptoms more rapidly than obstruction lower down the intestinal tract. The four classical features are pain, vomiting, abdominal distension and constipation.

Pain. The first reaction of the intestine to obstruction is to produce more and more powerful contractions, hyperperistalsis, which causes waves of abdominal colic. In obstruction of the small intestine the waves of pain occur every two to three minutes: in the large intestine every ten to twenty minutes.

Vomiting. As time passes the affected intestine becomes weak and distended by the collection of fluid. When the fluid level reaches the stomach the patient begins to vomit: at first stomach contents, bile-stained fluid and later, faeculent fluid.

Distension. The exhausted distended intestine becomes adynamic and distension increases.

Constipation. As a result of hyperperistalsis the patient may have diarrhoea, but as the adynamic state is reached there will be absolute constipation and absence of flatus.

The patient appears pale, tense and afraid. Signs of dehydration such as thirst, dry furred tongue are apparent.

Investigations

Physical examination, auscultation of the abdomen may elicit hyperactive bowel sounds.

X-ray of the abdomen with the patient in the erect and supine position will show gas patterns and fluid levels.

Observations and records

Temperature, pulse, respiration and blood pressure.
Fluid balance.
Amount of pain.
Character of vomitus.

Course and complications

The patients general condition deteriorates rapidly. Gross dehydration may lead to peripheral circulatory failure. The accumulation of gas produced by bacterial decomposition of stagnant intestinal content causes increased distension. This prevents the absorption of fluids and electrolytes. The affected part of the intestine may become necrotic if its blood supply becomes strangulated. Due to the increasing pressure there is the possibility of perforation of the intestine.

Treatment and nursing care

A combination of conservative and surgical treatment is employed to relieve obstruction, correct dehydration and electrolyte imbalance and remove the cause.

A nasogastric tube is passed to enable the gastric content to be removed. This will relieve vomiting and prevent aspiration pneumonia (Ch. 6). The amount and nature of the aspirate must be recorded. Intravenous infusion of fluid electrolytes and plasma are necessary to correct dehydration which may have reduced the blood volume. Pain relief will allow rest and lessen apprehension. Emergency surgical treatment may be required to remove the cause of obstruction when there is risk of strangulation.

Obstruction of the small intestine can be relieved by the release of strangulation or adhesions and, if necessary, resection and anastomosis of the necrotic segment or excision of the tumour. This will restore continuity and allow normal flow of intestinal content. Postoperative management is explained on page 188.

Obstruction of the large intestine is usually treated in three stages:

1. Decompression of the intestine by temporary colostomy (p. 173). In some cases resection of the cause of obstruction, for example carcinoma of the colon, may be done at the same time.

2. Resection of the cause of obstruction a few weeks after the decompression operation. The patient's general condition can be improved in the time before resection (p. 176).

3. Closure of colostomy at a later date when healing of the resection is satisfactory.

DISORDERS OF THE LARGE INTESTINE

Appendicitis

This is an inflammatory condition of the appendix. The cause has not yet been defined but it may result from obstruction of the appendix lumen by hardened faeces or a foreign body. The obstruction impairs circulation and results in lowered resistance to organisms normally present in the bowel such as *E. coli*. The condition is more frequent in males and usually occurs in older children and young adults.

Clinical features

There is sudden onset of pain in the umbilical area, anorexia, nausea and vomiting. The pain then becomes sharp in the area halfway between the umbilicus and the right ileum. These symptoms, occurring suddenly in an otherwise healthy person, are typical of acute appendicitis. There may also be a moderate rise in temperature and a change in bowel habit.

Investigations

Abdominal palpation may elicit other symptoms such as guarding and tenderness in the right lower abdomen. rectal examination is carried out. It may produce pain in response to pressure high on the right of the rectum.

Nursing observations and records

Records of temperature, pulse and respiration are kept by the nurse. The general condition of the patient and the degree of pain he has should be observed and recorded. Any changes in his condition must be reported promptly.

Course and complications

As the disease progresses, abscess formation may occur around the appendix and in the pelvis. Total obstruction of the appendix will result in its becoming gangrenous and then rupturing. This will cause generalized peritonitis.

Treatment and nursing care

When appendicitis is suspected, the patient is admitted to hospital immediately. He will be confined to bed until investigations and observations have been made. An operation may be required shortly after admission, and for this reason the patient is given nothing to eat or drink. A nasogastric tube may be passed and intravenous infusion started. The patient is given frequent mouth care and helped into a comfortable position in bed. If the patient is a child the doctor will inform the parents and request their permission to operate, once the diagnosis has been confirmed.

The appendix is usually removed through a small incision in the right side of the lower abdomen. Drains are inserted only when there is evidence of abscess formation or if the appendix has ruptured.

Following surgery, the symptoms disappear and normal bowel function soon returns. Fluids and food can then be given as desired. The patient is allowed out of bed the day after operation. Moving out of bed and standing can cause anxiety and wound pain. The nurse who is helping the patient at this time should therefore assess his condition before encouraging him to take short walks. Early discharge from hospital may be arranged if home circumstances are suitable and community care is available. Provision is made for the removal of sutures in the patient's own home or in the out-patient department. Normal activity should be resumed within 2 to 4 weeks.

When it has been necessary to insert a wound drain, the patient should be nursed in an upright position to encourage free drainage. The character and amount of drainage should be observed and dressings changed when necessary. The patient should have plenty of fluids and may be given antibiotics. Attention to skin and mouth will help to make the patient comfortable. He will be discharged from hospital when he has recovered from the acute phase of his illness and is able to be up and about. If necessary, dressings can be changed by the community nurse or the patient's own doctor.

Ulcerative colitis

Ulcerative colitis is an inflammatory disease of unknown origin involving the mucosa and submucosa of the large intestine. The incidence is highest among young adults, especially young women. Although the cause is unknown, it is thought that psychological factors play a part in the disease process.

Initially, the mucosa of the rectum and the sigmoid colon becomes swollen and congested. The mucosa bleeds easily and patchy ulceration occurs where the mucous membrane has been eroded. The condition may spread to other regions of the colon and may involve the caecum. The disease is progressive with periods of remission and of acute exacerbation.

Clinical features

The onset is insidious with abdominal discomfort, mild diarrhoea, blood in the stools and possibly anal excoriation. The symptoms then become more defined with loose stools and frequent urgent discharge of blood and mucus. In the acute stage, the patient has pain, weight loss, fever and general debility. The profuse diarrhoea causes severe fluid and blood loss. The patient, understandably, may display signs of emotional disturbance and depression.

Investigations

Examination by direct vision of the rectum (proctoscopy) and the sigmoid colon (sigmoidoscopy), during which a biopsy of mucous membrane can be obtained.

Barium enema to assess the extent of ulceration.

Haematological examination to assess haemoglobin, electrolyte and protein loss.

Nursing observations and records

Degree of anxiety and mental stress.

Accurate records of fluid intake and output.

Stools — amount, frequency, consistency and presence of blood or mucus.

Course and complications

At first only inflammatory changes occur; ulceration follows later. In the chronic condition the thickened oedematous mucosa may undergo changes which produce pseudopolyps. The continuous healing process and formation of scar tissue cause loss of both elasticity and absorptive capability of the colon; secondary infection may supervene. The loss of fluid, electrolytes, blood and protein from the colon into the faeces causes dehydration, anaemia and weight loss.

The spread of infection from the colon to the systemic and portal circulation causes bacteraemia and toxaemia. The muscle coat of the colon is affected only when secondary infection occurs. This causes loss of muscle tone and leads to fissure formation, dilatation of the colon and risk of perforation. Malignant changes and tumour formation may occur when the disease is long standing and severe.

Treatment and nursing care

The aims of nursing care during an active phase of the disease are to understand and support the patient during this exhausting illness and to ensure the provision of adequate rest, warmth and nutrition. The patient will require meticulous attention to his personal hygiene and should be nursed in a well-ventilated environment.

Medical treatment

Distressing diarrhoea can be controlled by drugs which will slow down the hyperactive colon. The addition of bulk such as bran or cellulose to the diet will reduce the amount of fluid loss. Anaemia and loss of protein can be corrected by giving the patient a high protein diet with iron supplements. Losses during an acute exacerbation may require blood replacement and intravenous infusion to correct the electrolyte balance.

Anti-inflammatory drugs such as Salazopyrin can be given in tablet form during periods of remission to prevent relapse. In severe cases cortisone may be prescribed and can be given in several forms — orally, by intramuscular injection, or by local application using suppositories and retention enemata.

A sympathetic, hopeful attitude towards the anxious and depressed patient will improve morale considerably. He can then be helped to recognize and cope with any emotional stress which may have caused the exacerbation of the disease.

It is important that the patient and his relatives are made aware that the condition will not be cured but only alleviated when the patient returns home. They should be guided in how to maintain good nutrition and helped to understand the disease and accept the patient's behaviour. The anxious patient will require encouragement to continue a fairly normal life between active phases of the disease. Socioeconomic problems may be solved with the help of a medical social worker thus relieving these causes of anxiety. Careful follow-up of the individual as an out-patient is essential because of the possibility of malignant changes in the colon. Early detection of other complications may prevent them from reaching serious dimensions.

Surgical treatment
Surgery will be indicated if medical treatment fails to control the symptoms. Recurrent acute exacerbations may make life intolerable for the patient. The operations which may be performed are subtotal colectomy or total colectomy with establishment of an ileostomy (p. 177). The patient is admitted to hospital and specific preparation is given to help him accept that he will have a permanent stoma. Many of the patients are from a fairly young age group. Their age and the relief obtained from the distressing symptoms of ulcerative colitis allow them to adapt to the situation and resume their normal place in society.

Diverticular disease

A diverticulum is a herniation of the mucosa through the muscle wall. Muliple diverticula (Fig. 5.12) may occur anywhere in the gastrointestinal tract. It is an acquired condition mainly affecting the colon. **Diverticulosis** only implies that diverticula exist. When diverticula become inflamed because of faecal impaction and infection, the condition is known as **diverticulitis** (Fig. 5.13). It is considered a deficiency disease of Western civilization where the diet has become refined and of low residue. The lack of bulk in the diet requires increased pressures in the colon to transport faeces. This increase in pressure is thought to be the cause of herniation through the muscle coat.

Clinical features
Diverticulosis may be asymptomatic or there may be some history of dyspepsia and change in bowel habit.

Diverticulitis causes lower abdominal distension and pain. There may be recurrent attacks of acute pain and fever with a history of increasing constipation.

Investigations
Barium enema.
Sigmoidoscopy.

Nursing observations and records
Stools frequency, consistency and appearance.
Temperature, pulse and respiration.

Course and complications
Diverticulitis may resolve spontaneously, leaving only mild symptoms, or it may progress to an acute stage. In the acute phase the swollen and thickened colon becomes adherent to nearby structures with the possibility of formation of fistulae between colon and bladder or vagina. Peritonitis can occur following the formation of pericolic abscess or by performation of the diverticulum. The lumen of the colon may become narrowed resulting in intestinal obstruction.

Treatment and nursing care
A mild form of the disease can be treated at home. The patient is given advice on the prevention of constipation and the constituents of diet that can help this condition. The ingestion of unrefined foods and plenty of fluids and the addition to foods of bran or a

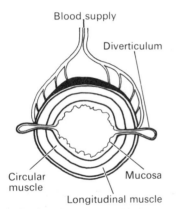

Figure 5.12
Cross-section of the colon showing diverticula

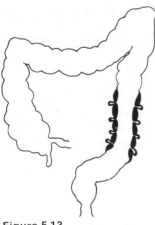

Figure 5.13
Narrowed lumen of the colon caused by diverticulitis

cellulose product are advised since they add bulk to the diet. Antispasmodic drugs may be prescribed to relieve pain.

During an acute attack, the patient may be nursed in hospital because of the need for early recognition of the dangerous complications. While the patient has pain and pyrexia, he requires bed rest. During this time a fluid diet is given. Parenteral antibiotic drugs may be prescribed to control infection and inflammation. When the patient has recovered from the acute attack, he can resume the treatment advised for the mild condition.

Recurrent exacerbations of this disorder can distress and debilitate the patient and for this reason elective surgery may be advised. If an operation is decided on, the patient is prepared for surgery (p. 176). The diseased part of the colon is excised and continuity re-established by joining the two ends of healthy colon. This operation is known as a colectomy.

Patients with complications such as intestinal obstruction and perforation require immediate surgery. A temporary colostomy will be made to relieve obstruction (Fig. 5.14 — stage 1). This will divert the faecal stream away from the grossly affected section of the colon. A second operation will be performed later when the patient's general condition has improved and there has been time for the preparation of the colon for surgery. At this point, a colectomy will be performed (Fig. 5.14 — stage 2). When this has healed satisfactorily, a third operation will allow the colostomy to be closed (Fig. 5.14 — stage 3).

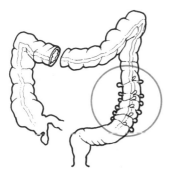

Stage 1

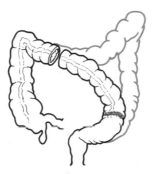

Stage 2

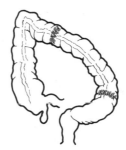

Stage 3

Figure 5.14
Stage 1: Temporary colostomy
Stage 2: Resection of the affected area of the colon
Stage 3: Closure of colostomy

Hirschsprung's disease

This is a congenital condition caused by abnormal nerve fibres and the absence of ganglion cells in the mesenteric and submucosal plexus of the colon. This abnormality always involves the distal end of the rectum and extends proximally for varying lengths. Two types are described: short segment Hirschsprung's disease when the area of aganglion cells extends from the internal anal sphincter to the mid-sigmoid region of colon; long segment Hirchsprung's disease when the area of aganglionosis may involve the entire colon and may extend into the small intestine. The result is failure of the affected segment to maintain peristalsis. Contents of the colon do not pass through the affected segment and this causes distension of the normal colon.

Clinical features
The condition is first noticed by the absence or delay in the normal passage of meconium shortly after birth and loose stools during the early weeks of life. During the first year of life there is abdominal distension and severe constipation with passage of small, ribbon-like stools. The condition may be severe enough to cause anorexia, vomiting and intestinal obstruction.

Investigations
X-ray of abdomen and small barium enema.
Rectal examination. Rectal manometry.
Biopsies of rectum and colon to establish the level at which normal nerve cells are present.

Nursing observations and records

The passage of meconium (or its absence) at birth and the character of subsequent stools should be noted and recorded. Weight should be recorded regularly. Signs of dehydration and abdominal distension should be looked for specifically.

Course and complications

The condition causes chronic, severe constipation and abdominal distension. The child fails to thrive and may develop acute intestinal obstruction.

Treatment and nursing care

Some infants require surgery for the relief of intestinal obstruction within days of birth. A temporary colostomy is made; fluid and electrolyte balance is maintained during the 24 hours following surgery by intravenous infusion via a scalp vein. Nutrition is then re-established by slow introduction of oral feeding. Careful observation and recording of fluid intake, fluid output and faecal output is important. The skin around the colostomy must be kept clean and dry to prevent excoriation. At this stage the mother can be involved in the care of her child. Practical experience, and education in the care of her child's colostomy and nutritional needs, should enable her to manage confidently when the child is discharged from hospital. Major surgery to resect the affected segment of colon will be delayed until the child is about 18 months of age. Children with less severe symptoms can be managed by observation and regulation of bowel habit by diet, aperients and enemata if necessary.

Follow-up

Regular health and developmental assessment should be carried out by a paediatrician. Support and education in nutrition and stoma care should be provided as the needs arise.

Carcinoma of the colon and rectum

A carcinoma of the large bowel is a malignant tumour arising from the mucous membrane. There is no known cause of malignant tumours, but benign polyps and ulcerative colitis are predisposing factors in some instances. Carcinoma may occur anywhere in the large colon although it is most commonly found in the caecum, sigmoid colon or rectum. The tumours are usually slow growing. They may be either (1) the polypoid type which projects into the lumen of the colon or (2) the annular type which grows around the lumen, causing a stenosing ring-like stricture (Fig. 5.15).

The spread of carcinoma is usually by direct invasion or by the lymphatic and venous drainage of the colon. Tumour cells are carried to the liver via the mesenteric and portal veins then into the circulation to produce secondary metastases elsewhere. There is increasing incidence of tumour with age: it is most common over the age of 50.

Clinical features

Carcinoma causes symptoms which differ according to the site of the tumour.

A tumour in the caecum or ascending colon is usually polypoid. There the colon is wider and the faeces more fluid so that obstruction rarely occurs. The symptoms of the patient are usually anaemia, melaena as a result of gradual bleeding from the tumour surface.

In the sigmoid colon there is a high incidence of the annular type of tumour. The resulting stricture leads to partial obstruction which causes alternating constipation and diarrhoea with abdominal pain. Accompanying the change in bowel habit may be rectal discharge with blood and mucus. Complete obstruction can occur due to total occlusion of the lumen by tumour or by the impaction of faeces above the tumour.

A tumour in the rectum also gives rise to changes in bowel habit and the passage of blood and mucus per rectum. In addition the patient has a constant feeling of fullness in the rectum. A patient in the advanced stages of the condition may show signs of intestinal obstruction, perforation or complications arising from secondary metastases.

Investigations

Barium enema.
Rectal examination.
Colonoscopy

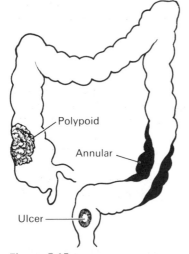

Figure 5.15
Types of carcinoma of the colon and rectum

Nursing observations and records

Bowel habit.
The presence of blood and mucus or occult blood in stools.
Fluid intake and output.
Signs of dehydration, abdominal distension and haemorrhage.

Course and complications

Obstruction of the flow of fluids and nutrients will prevent absorption and cause abdominal distension because of accumulation above the level of the obstruction. Eventually there will be copious vomiting of the intestinal content producing dehydration and loss of nutrients. The patient will appear very debilitated and in great pain.

Treatment and nursing care

Surgical removal of the tumour following early diagnosis gives good results. The operation, called a colectomy, consists of resection of the tumour and the adjacent lymph nodes and restoration of the continuity of the colon. In low rectal or advanced tumour of the sigmoid colon, removal of the anal canal, rectum and sigmoid colon is necessary. The open end of the remaining colon is brought to the surface of the abdomen and an artificial anus established — that is, a permanent colostomy.

The success of the surgery depends very much on meticulous preoperative preparation of the patient (p. 176). Special care must be taken to ensure that the colon is cleansed by colonic lavages; it is customary to administer antibiotics during the 5 days prior to surgery. Peristalsis is inhibited for about 48 hours after surgery, and if faecal matter has not been removed the normal absorption of water in the colon will cause the faeces to become hard. When peristalsis returns, this hard mass above the site of the operation may tear the suture line and cause a leak into the peritoneum.

If there is intestinal obstruction the colon cannot be cleansed, making a preliminary operation necessary to relieve the obstruction. The patient will have a temporary colostomy which may be closed at a later date when his general condition allows the appropriate surgical procedure to be performed.

Haemorrhoids

The term haemorrhoids refers to dilatations of the terminal parts of the haemorrhoidal veins lying in the submucosa of the upper anal canal. They are classified as first, second and third degree. First degree haemorrhoids project into the lumen of the anal canal and become congested during defaecation. Second degree haemorrhoids are larger and tend to prolapse. Third degree haemorrhoids are completely prolapsed (Fig. 5.16). Both men and women can be affected by this painful condition. The predisposing factors are thought to be conditions which obstruct the haemorrhoidal venous drainage, such as chronic constipation and pregnancy; haemorrhoids may be secondary to tumours in the pelvis or rectum.

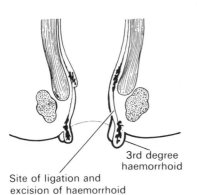

3rd degree
haemorrhoid

Site of ligation and
excision of haemorrhoid

Figure 5.16
Haemorrhoids

Clinical features

The first symptoms of haemorrhoids are local discomfort, prolapse and rectal bleeding during defaecation. With second and third degree haemorrhoids, the patient experiences pain, bleeding and anal discharge which causes pruritus. He may suffer from anaemia due to slow loss of blood over a period.

Investigations

History of bowel habit and physical examination.
Digital examination of anal canal and rectum.
Proctoscopy and sigmoidoscopy.

Course and complications

Congested, prolapsed haemorrhoids can become thrombosed and cause the patient great distress. Third degree haemorrhoids, which have prolapsed through the external anal sphincter, become oedematous and strangulated. This very painful situation completely incapacitates the patient as he is unable to walk or sit down.

Treatment and nursing care

The kind of treatment given depends on the severity and cause of the symptoms. In less severe conditions advice should be given to the patient about diet and regulation of bowel habit — to avoid straining at defaecation. Careful and frequent anal cleansing will help prevent pruritis. Rest in bed, local heat or hot baths can alleviate the pain caused by difficult defaecation.

Second degree haemorrhoids can be treated by injection therapy. A sclerosing agent such as 5 per cent phenol in oil is injected into the submucosa around the haemorrhoid; the resulting inflammatory reaction causes fibrous changes which obliterate the veins.

Third degree haemorrhoids are treated by surgical excision with ligation; this operation is called haemorrhoidectomy. The patient is prepared for anaesthesia and operation in the usual way.

During the first 24 hours after surgery, careful observation of pulse and blood pressure is necessary. Haemorrhage may result from a slipped ligature and the blood loss will be concealed if it gathers in the anal canal.

Patients often have severe pain following haemorrhoidectomy. This can be relieved by careful positioning and support in the most comfortable position possible and by giving prescribed analgesic drugs. On the day after surgery, the patient is usually allowed out of bed; he may have supervised warm baths and may use a bidet to ensure cleanliness and to relieve pain.

If spontaneous bowel action does not occur an aperient may be given on the third evening after surgery. Following each bowel action the area is cleansed as noted above and, if necessary, a dressing is applied and held in place with a T bandage.

The patient may be anxious about the first bowel action and needs careful nursing as he may suffer considerable pain and feel faint. The passage of a stool of normal consistency following haemorrhoidectomy prevents stricture of the anal canal.

Follow-up

When discharged from hospital, the patient is advised to avoid constipation by taking a diet with adequate roughage and fluids. He may be given a mild aperient to be taken until regular bowel habit has been established.

Nursing care of the patient undergoing surgery of colon or rectum

Preoperative management

In addition to the routine physical and psychological care necessary before any operation, those who are to have surgery of the colon or rectum need special care to provide the best possible conditions for the process of healing. This objective may be achieved by ensuring that no faecal matter remains in the colon and by reducing the number of bacteria present.

During the 4 days before operation, the patient is given a high protein, low residue diet with plenty of fluids. The surgeon may want colonic lavages and a broad spectrum antibiotic to be given preoperatively. The patient and his relatives will require explanations of the operation and its attendant procedures. They should be allowed to express their anxieties and should be helped to come to terms with them.

On the day of operation, a nasogastric tube is passed allowing aspiration of the intestinal fluids and gases, which will accumulate due to the inhibition of peristalsis. This inhibition is the result of anaesthesia and of the handling of the intestine during surgery and usually persists for 24 hours after operation. To prevent damage to the bladder, a self-retaining catheter is inserted to allow free drainage of urine.

Special psychological preparation is of great importance for those patients who are having surgery which results in the formation of an opening from the intestinal tract on to the abdominal wall (colostomy [Fig. 5.17] or ileostomy [Fig. 5.18]).

The surgeon will explain the operation and its consequences to the patient. It is then the nursing staff's responsibility to give the patient concerned the opportunity to ask questions. Issues such as diet, sport, the reaction of a partner, holidays may cause the individual concern. At this stage it may be possible to introduce the patient to the stoma care nurse, a clinical specialist, or to a representative of the Colostomy/

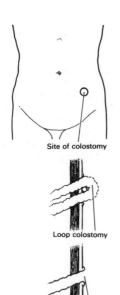

Site of colostomy

Loop colostomy

End colostomy

Figure 5.17
Colostomy

Ileostomy Association. Many areas prefer to invite the patient to discuss forthcoming self management with a former patient who is coping with a stoma successfully; if possible, patient and visitor should be matched for age, social group and sex. A selection from the various appliances available may be demonstrated, the patient being allowed to examine and handle these.

Careful preparation at this stage goes a long way to helping the patient come to terms with his stoma postoperatively. Emphasis is placed on the improved quality of life.

Operations on the colon and the rectum

Right hemicolectomy (Fig. 5.19A)
Restoration of continuity by anastomosing ileum to transverse colon.

Left hemicolectomy (Fig. 5.19B)
Restoration of continuity by end-to-end anastomosis between transverse colon and rectum.

Abdominoperineal excision of rectum (Fig. 5.19C)
Establishment of permanent colostomy in left iliac fossa.

Total proctocolectomy (*Fig.* 5.19D)
Excision of anus, rectum and colon. Establishment of ileostomy.

A stoma made in the terminal part of the ileum which is brought to the surface of the

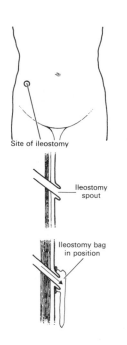

Figure 5.18
Ileostomy

Site of ileostomy

Ileostomy spout

Ileostomy bag in position

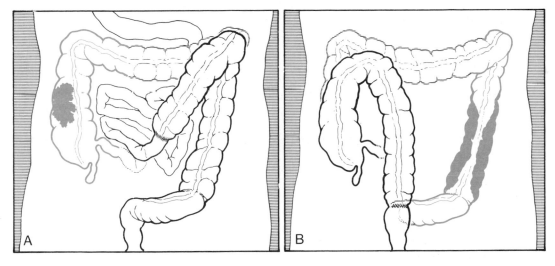

Figure 5.19
A. Right hemicolectomy and ileotransverse anastomosis
B. Left hemicolectomy
C. Exclusion of rectum and formation of colostomy
D. Proctocolectomy and formation of ileostomy

abdominal wall is known as an ileostomy. This can be a temporary or permanent means of draining the small intestine when there is disease of the colon.

Postoperative management

In the postoperative period, routine care is given with, in addition, observation of the stoma. It is important to notice if the circulation appears adequate and if there are signs of prolapse of the stoma into the abdominal cavity. At this time, there is very little intestinal activity with very small amounts of altered blood and mucus being discharged. When peristalsis does return the discharge is fluid and profuse. A well-fitting appliance is necessary to prevent excoriation of surrounding skin. Careful cleansing of the skin around the stoma and the application of a specially formulated adhesive to prevent leakage from the appliance are of great importance. Excoriation of the skin will cause the patient pain and distress. Whenever the patient's general condition allows, he should be gently encouraged to become involved in the care of his stoma.

Ileostomy

The particular problems associated with an ileostomy are caused by the normally semifluid contents of the small intestine. An ileostomy bag must be worn continuously and must be close-fitting to prevent the effluence coming in contact with surrounding skin as this would cause gross excoriation. Regulation of an ileostomy is difficult but the consistency can be varied by diet and the use of hydrophilic colloids. Before being discharged from hospital the chosen long-term management should be established, Careful follow-up is necessary to provide support and advice on diet, skin care and appliances.

Bacillary dysentery

Dysentry is an inflammatory disease of the colon and rectum which may be caused by bacterial or protozoan infection. Bacillary dysentery results from infection by *Shigella* organisms. The mucosa of the colon becomes inflamed and oedematous with superficial ulceration. The spread of infection is by personal contact or by food contaminated from unwashed hands. It is therefore possible to have an epidemic of the disease in large communities where sanitation is inadequate. The incubation period is between 1 to 7 days. The health authorities must be notified of any incidence of the disease.

Clinical features

The symptoms vary in severity from mild diarrhoea lasting about 3 days to a grossly debilitating illness. In the acute form the patient is febrile, dehydrated and has generalized abdominal pain with incontinence of blood-stained stools.

Investigations

Bacteriological examination of stools and rectal swabs.
Blood culture.

Nursing observations and records

Stool content and frequency.
Signs of dehydration.
Fluid intake and output records.

Course and complications

It is possible for some people to become carriers of the disease after complete recovery from an attack. A carrier, although symptomless, can spread the disease to others.

Treatment and nursing care

During a mild attack the patient can be nursed at home. He is advised to take plenty of fluids, drugs may be prescribed to control diarrhoea and antibiotic therapy instituted to suppress infection. He must be made aware of the need to prevent spread of the infection. Careful cleansing of the lavatory and handwashing after defaecation are essential.

A severe attack requires efficient barrier nursing. The patient is admitted to hospital for bed rest during the acute stage. Loss of fluids and electrolytes resulting from profuse diarrhoea can be replaced by intravenous infusions. Specimens of stool should be sent promptly for examination and should be collected with due precaution against spread of infection. The appropriate antibiotic therapy can then begin. Although symptoms subside and the patient recovers he cannot be declared free from infection until three consecutive stool cultures are negative.

DISORDERS OF THE LIVER

Viral hepatitis

Inflammation of the liver is known as hepatitis and the most common cause is viral infection. Normal liver cells take in bilirubin from the plasma; the cells then conjugate and excrete it into the biliary ducts (Fig. 5.3, p. 153). Inflamed liver cells are unable to carry out this function properly so that an excess of unconjugated bilirubin is left circulating in the blood, producing prehepatic jaundice. Failure to excrete bilirubin into the biliary ducts causes stasis within the liver and an excess of conjugated bilirubin in the circulation. This results in jaundice with symptoms similar to obstruction of the biliary tract.

There are two types of viral hepatitis — infective and serum.

Infective hepatitis

This is the most common liver disorder in Great Britain and other Western countries. The source of the virus is the human blood and faeces of an already infected person or healthy carrier of the disease. The incubation period is 10 to 40 days. The disease can be transmitted by ingestion of contaminated food or water; when the virus reaches the intestine it is absorbed into the blood. There is a higher incidence of the disease among children and people living in crowded communities where epidemics are more likely to occur.

Clinical features
There is a period of up to a week during which the patient complains of general malaise and experiences anorexia and low-grade fever. After this period jaundice appears from the increased levels of bilirubin in the blood and may become very marked within a few days. Urine becomes darker and stools paler in colour. The liver is tender and may become slightly enlarged. At this stage there may be a slight prolongation of prothrombin time. The course of the disease is 3 to 6 weeks. Some patients find that pruritis causes considerable discomfort.

Acute inflammatory changes may occur in the liver and result in liver cell necrosis, but usually the patient recovers completely.

Investigations
Examination of serum, for example, levels of bilirubin.

Treatment and nursing care
Treatment is aimed at resting the liver and supporting its function during the period of natural recovery. The patient can be managed at home and should be kept at rest until the serum bilirubin levels fall. No special dietary regime is thought necessary but the daily intake should include adequate protein and glucose. Alcohol, which, in health, is detoxicated by the liver, must be avoided for 6 months. Jaundice is usually present for 2 to 6 weeks; the patient can resume normal activities about 3 weeks after jaundice has faded. In patients who have jaundice due to intrahepatic cholestasis the jaundice persists for 7 to 20 weeks. A diet high in protein and low in fat is usual with vitamin K supplement. A common sequel to the disease is posthepatitis syndrome. The patient complains of malaise, is easily tired, has mild anorexia with fat intolerance and some

depression. This may be related to other postviral infection syndromes such as that following influenza. No special treatment is required but the patient should be reassured that the liver is normal.

Community care
Prevention of the spread of infective hepatitis includes attention to general and personal hygiene. Special precautions must be taken for the safe disposal of urine and faeces from an infected patient. The virus is usually present in all the members of the patient's household and it is recommended that each person have a prophylactic intramuscular injection of gamma globulin. Such precautions may prevent or lessen the severity of an attack of infective hepatitis but are of little value in serum hepatitis.

Serum hepatitis

This is a less common but more severe form of viral hepatitis. The incubation period is about 3 months and the virus is transmitted by infected serum. Various body fluids such as saliva, vaginal discharge, seminal fluid and serous exudate have also been implicated. The condition can occur as the result of accidental innoculation during medical, surgical or dental procedures, blood transfusion, contaminated injection equipment, tattooing or laboratory accidents. It has been found that patients with serum hepatitis display specific antigens in their plasma. These antigens are highly infective protein particles. Initial infection may be followed by a persistent carrier state, so special care must be taken when nursing those who have positive serum. Patients who present with acute symptoms of serum hepatitis must be nursed in an isolation unit. The outcome of acute serum hepatitis may be either complete resolution, massive liver necrosis, chronic hepatitis, or resolution with scarring.

DISORDERS OF THE BILIARY TRACT
Gall-stones

Gall-stone formation is known as **cholelithiasis** and is thought to be a condition related to the Western pattern of living. It has become a common disease, with increasing incidence over the past 25 years. The stones may consist of pure bilirubin, cholesterol or a combination of both with some calcium deposits. While they are in the gall-bladder they may be entirely asymptomatic; problems arise when the stones move out into the cystic duct, where they tend to become impacted and cause inflammation of the gall-bladder or **cholecystitis**. A stone which has reached the bile duct and become impacted will obstruct biliary drainage (Fig. 5.20). This results in biliary colic and jaundice.

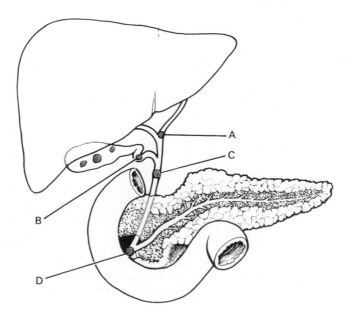

Figure 5.20
Sites of biliary tract obstruction due to gall-stones A. Hepatic duct B. Cystic duct C. Bile duct C. Sphincter of Oddi

Trauma from stones in the biliary tract causes stricture formation. Impaction of a stone or stricture at the sphincter of Oddi will prevent bile and pancreatic secretion from entering the duodenum.

The formation of gall-stones is thought to occur more frequently in women of child-bearing age.

Clinical features

The patient may have a history of dyspepsia and a special aversion to fatty foods. Pain occurs in the right epigastrium and radiates to the subscapular area. Typically, it is of sudden onset, colicky and very severe. Obstruction of the bile duct or the sphincter of Oddi results in high levels of bilirubin circulating in the blood. This produces a yellow tinge of the skin called jaundice, very dark coloured urine and pale, fatty stools.

The patient who is suffering from an acute attack of biliary tract disorder appears restless, in pain, nauseated and dehydrated. The jaundiced patient may have coagulation defects caused by inability to absorb fat and fat-soluble vitamins, including vitamin K.

Investigations

History and clinical examination.

X-ray of abdomen.

Examination of blood, urine and stools.

Cholecystogram to demonstrate gall-bladder appearance and function.

Cholangiogram to estimate biliary duct function and to show the presence of stones or stricture.

Ultrasound.

Nursing observations and records

Temperature, pulse, respiration and fluid balance.

Colour of stools, urine and skin.

Course and complications

Most patients with acute cholecystitis recover within a few days with conservative treatment. Recurrent episodes may occur and some have serious complications. Ascending infection in the hepatic ducts will cause cholangitis which will obstruct the flow of bile from the liver. Impaction of a stone in the gall-bladder neck or cystic duct will result in stasis of bile, infection and the possibility of pus formation in the gall-bladder which will distend and may eventually rupture resulting in peritonitis. Obstruction of the bile duct or the sphincter of Oddi prevents the flow of bile and pancreatic secretions into the duodenum. This will cause pancreatitis and inability to absorb protein, carbohydrates and fat.

Treatment and nursing care

During the acute inflammatory stage the patient is confined to bed and is more comfortable when nursed in a well-supported, upright position (Fig. 6.11, p. 198).

Medical treatment

Specific care of these patients includes the relief of pain using drugs to relieve spasm; this may allow the obstructing stone to be passed into the duodenum. The patient has nothing orally, thus avoiding the normal stimulus to the gall-bladder to contract. Hydration is maintained by intravenous infusion.

Surgical treatment

When the patient has recovered and the signs and symptoms of inflammation have disappeared, surgery may be advocated to prevent the serious complication of biliary tract obstruction. The diagnostic procedures cholangiogram and cholecystogram are performed and the gall-bladder, which is the source of gall-stones, is removed. The operation is fairly common and is known as **cholecystectomy**.

The patient has routine preparation for theatre. Special preparation includes estimation of the prothrombin index, particularly if the patient has had biliary obstruction which has prevented the absorption of vitamin K. A nasogastric tube is passed before surgery as the procedure is less distressing to the patient at this stage. During the operation a cholangiogram is performed following the removal of the gall-bladder. This is to ensure that the bile duct is patent. Any exploration of the bile duct, which may be necessary as a result of the cholangiogram, will cause oedema and it therefore becomes necessary to insert a T tube drain to allow free flow of bile from the liver. At the end of the operation the patient will have a drain at the site of the gall-bladder to prevent the formation of haematoma and also a T tube drain in the bile duct if it has been explored (Fig. 5.21). General postoperative care is described on page 000.

Management of T-tube drainage following exploration of bile duct. Initially there will be free drainage of bile into the collecting bag attached to the drain. After a period of 48 hours the drain is clamped off for short periods and the patient is observed for signs of increasing pain, which indicates obstruction. If this occurs free drainage must be resumed immediately. When there is no adverse reaction to the drain being clamped off then this should be continued for longer periods each day until there is very little or no bile draining into the collecting bag.

Observation of stools and urine will also indicate whether or not proper flow of bile has been re-established. Usually after 10 days a postoperative cholangiogram is performed to confirm patency of the duct and then the T tube may be removed.

Follow-up. The patient who has a straightforward cholecystectomy will probably leave hospital after 10 days. At this stage he should be having a normal diet. One month after the operation he is reviewed at a follow-up clinic and should be ready to resume normal activity.

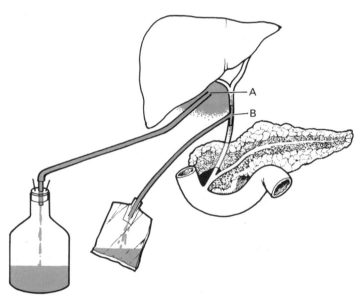

Figure 5.21
A. Drainage tube in gall-bladder bed following cholecystectomy
B. Site of T tube drain following exploration of the bile duct

DISORDERS OF THE PANCREAS

Diabetes, a disease of the pancreas related to its endocrine function, is described in Chapter 11.

When malignant tumours arise in the pancreas they are usually rapidly fatal; involvement of the head of the organ causes obstructive jaundice. Other important and serious conditions of the pancreas are the result of inflammatory processes.

Pancreatitis

This inflammatory disease of the pancreas may affect either sex, usually between the ages of 40 and 70; it can be either actue or chronic.

Acute pancreatitis
In the acute form the inflammatory changes cause oedema and haemorrhage into the gland; however, the pancreas can recover normal function when the precipitating factors have been removed.

Chronic pancreatitis

In chronic pancreatitis the eventual calcification and necrosis of exocrine cells and islets of Langerhans reduce normal function. The predisposing causes are obstruction of the flow of pancreatic secretions and excessive stimulus of pancreatic secretions. Obstruction of the pancreatic duct or the sphincter of Oddi may be caused by impacted gall-stones, tumour or inflammatory changes caused by regurgitation from a chronically infected biliary tract. The damming-back of pancreatic enzymes within the gland results in autodigestion and the possible erosion of blood vessels. Alcohol in excess is thought to produce spasm of the sphincter of Oddi and to stimulate pancreatic cells to produce excessive amounts of their secretions.

Clinical features

There may be a history of dyspepsia, biliary colic or alcoholism. In the acute form the patient appears ill and is in acute pain. The onset of the pain is sudden, starting in the epigastrium and later penetrating to the back. It is usually constant. Nausea and vomiting are common. The patient has tachycardia and a mild fever and is hypotensive.

Investigations

Pancreatic function tests

1. The degree of duct obstruction and the excretory ability of the gland can be estimated by the levels of serum amylase and lipase. In acute pancreatitis the levels will be high in blood and urine.

2. Pancreatic function can be measured by taking specimens of duodenal aspirate and blood samples before and after giving intravenous injections of secretin and pancreozymin.

Radiology

Plain X-ray of abdomen may show pancreatic calcification or the presence of stones in the biliary tract.

Surgery

Laparotomy may be necessary to confirm the diagnosis because the clinical features are very similar to those of a perforated ulcer.

Nursing observations and records

Accurate records of fluid intake and output.

Observation of signs of adynamic ileus, a possible result of constant acute abdominal pain.

Observation of stools — steatorrhoea will occur because absence of lipase causes malabsorption of fat.

Observation of urine — glycosuria may be present due to a temporary diabetic state.

Course and complications

When the acute phase subsides and the cause of inflammation has been diagnosed, the patient may require surgery to remove the obstruction or may need treatment for alcoholism if this was a predisposing factor. Recurrent acute inflammatory changes may result in the formation of fibrosis and the destruction of acinar and islet tissue. This state of chronic pancreatitis will eventually produce symptoms of malabsorption and diabetes due to the reduction of exocrine and endocrine function of the pancreas.

Treatment and nursing care

Medical treatment

Conservative treatment in the acute stage is aimed at:

1. **Treatment of shock**. Bed rest and total nursing care. In severe shock plasma transfusion may be necessary to correct dehydration and electrolyte imbalance.

2. **Relief of pain**. Adequate control of pain may be difficult; morphine is seldom used as it causes spasm of the sphincter of Oddi and there is the risk of the patient becoming addicted since only opiates give relief.

3. **Inhibition of pancreatic secretion**. This can be achieved by continuous gastric suction to prevent gastric acid entering the duodenum, so stopping the production of secretin. Pancreatic and gastric acid secretion can also be reduced by drugs which prevent stimulus through the vagus nerve, for instance probantheline bromide.

4. **Prevention of infection**. Antibiotics may be given intramuscularly to prevent secondary infection of damaged tissue.

Surgical treatment
This is aimed at the relief of obstruction and at increasing drainage. Obstruction due to impacted gall-stones or from inflammation due to regurgitated bile from a chronically infected biliary tract can be relieved by removal of stones and the gall-bladder.

Increased drainage can be effected by first demonstrating the stricture of the pancreatic duct by an operative pancreatogram, then subsequently by reconstructing drainage. The pancreatic duct can be anastomosed to the duodenum, by-passing the sphincter of Oddi. If the duct has become narrowed, a polythene tube can be inserted to increase drainage.

Total pancreatectomy may be necessary for the relief of intractable pain of acute recurrent pancreatitis. This radical operation requires immediate insulin replacement and oral pancreatic supplements at meal-times.

DISORDERS OF THE PERITONEUM

Ascites

The fluid of the peritoneal cavity acts as a lubricant and allows the abdominal organs to glide smoothly over one another. Excess fluid in the cavity is termed ascites. Most commonly, ascites complicates conditions which increase venous pressure in the abdomen, such as congestive cardiac failure (Ch. 7), liver cirrhosis or portal vein thrombosis. Because of the high venous pressure, fluids leave the capillaries and enter the peritoneal cavity. Although rare, tuberculosis and malignancy of the peritoneum may also cause ascites.

Clinical features
Symptoms of the underlying condition are accompanied by a progressive and regular distension of the abdomen. Pressure symptoms such as dyspnoea are troublesome.

Treatment and nursing care
The underlying cause must be treated first. To relieve the distressing pressure symptoms abdominal paracentesis is carried out. Following local anaesthesia with lignocaine 2 per cent, a small trochar and cannula are inserted through the abdominal wall into the peritoneal cavity. Maintaining strict asepsis fluid is withdrawn and a specimen is sent for pathological examination. Since there is risk of the patient collapsing when a large quantity of fluid is withdrawn from the body, careful check is made of his pulse and general condition during the procedure.

Peritonitis

This is an inflammation of the peritoneum which is usually due to invasion by micro-organisms. Infection may be blood-borne as part of a generalized septicaemia. More commonly, however, rupture or perforation of some diseased abdominal organ causes a breach in the visceral peritoneum and allows infected material to spill into the cavity. The local infection may spread rapidly causing generalized peritonitis. A similar result may follow the use of corticosteroid drugs when the normal reaction to inflammation is inhibited. Any abdominal organ is then susceptible to inflammation, perforation and contamination of the peritoneal cavity by bacteria.

Clinical features
The onset of peritonitis may either supervene on the symptoms of an existing disease or occur dramatically, as in the case of perforated peptic ulcer. Less frequently it results postoperatively from breakdown of an anastomosis. Pain is acute, severe and

continuous, rapidly spreading over the whole abdomen which becomes tender and rigid. Peristalsis is inhibited. The vomiting that occurs initially becomes more frequent and ultimately contains faecal material. As the state of collapse becomes more severe, the abdominal rigidity gives way to a less painful distension. The patient lies motionless, eyes sunken, face pale and anxious looking. The skin is cold and clammy, pulse rapid, blood pressure and temperature lower than normal. Urinary output is diminished.

Treatment and nursing care

Intravenous fluid replacement and antibiotic therapy are initiated immediately whilst continuous gastric suction, via a nasogastric tube, is established to relieve vomiting. The greater the amount recovered, the less the peritoneal contamination. No fluids are allowed orally.

A nurse in constant attendance can do much to allay anxiety and make such observations of the patient as will indicate any change in the course of the condition. Blood-borne peritonitis is treated medically and should respond well to intensive antibiotic therapy. Peritonitis due to perforation of some abdominal organ is more complicated and requires surgical treatment. A rising pulse, hypothermia, increasing pallor and collapse indicate that medical therapy is ineffective and surgical repair must be carried out immediately. If the peritonitis is localized, prognosis is much more favourable. However, in a generalized peritonitis, the condition is usually so severe and acute that the outcome is often fatal.

Such catastrophies can be avoided if threatening abdominal conditions are resolved before peritonitis is established.

DEFECTS OF THE ABDOMINAL WALL

Hernia

A hernia is the protrusion of an organ from its own cavity. A hernia of the anterior abdominal wall can be caused by congenital weakness of the supporting muscles. Alternatively it can be due to physical strain at work or strain produced by some disease such as chronic bronchitis, enlarged prostate gland or chronic constipation. Inadequate wound healing because of infection or poor physical condition may also result in the development of a hernia. If the organ can be returned to its cavity the hernia is termed **reducible**; if the size of the defect in the muscle does not allow the organ to be returned it is said to be **irreducible**.

Clinical features

The patient or the mother of a small child may notice a swelling at the site of the hernia (Fig. 5.22). This swelling or lump may enlarge when the patient coughs, strains or lifts heavy objects. There may also be some local discomfort which disappears when the patient lies down.

Course and complications

Initially, a sac of peritoneum protrudes through the weakened area and a loop of intestine may follow as the area enlarges. The hernia may become irreducible as a result of inflammatory adhesions or because of constriction of the protruding organ by the narrow opening into the hernial sac. If the blood supply to the organ becomes impaired the hernia is said to be strangulated (Fig. 5.23). This causes severe pain, nausea, vomiting and abdominal distension. The damaged part of the intestine becomes necrotic and intestinal obstruction ensues.

Treatment and nursing care

Surgical repair of the hernia, while the patient is in reasonably good physical condition, will prevent serious complications. The operation is called herniorrhaphy. During the preoperative period, any physical condition which will cause extra strain on the newly repaired tissue should be corrected. The herniating structure is returned to its cavity and the defect in the supporting muscle is sutured. A patch may be used to strengthen the muscle wall and prevent recurrence of the hernia. During the postoperative period,

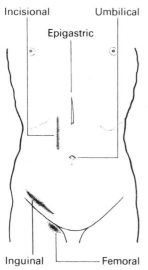

Figure 5.22
Common sites of hernia of the anterior abdominal wall

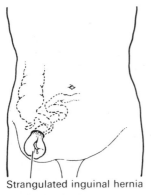

Figure 5.23
Strangulated hernia

early recognition of symptoms which may cause greatly increased intra-abdominal pressure will prevent disruption of the repaired tissue. The nurse can help the patient to support his wound during sneezing, coughing or postoperative vomiting. Signs of bladder or abdominal distension should be reported immediately. The patient may be in hospital for 7 days, but if home and community care are adequate, he may be discharged within 2 to 3 days of the operation.

Community care
On discharge from hospital, the patient is advised to refrain from strenuous exercise for at least 3 weeks.

NURSING CARE OF THE PATIENT WITH A GASTRO-INTESTINAL DISORDER

When planning nursing care for the maintenance or restoration of health, it is important to consider the self-esteem of the patient. Disorders of the gastrointestinal tract often produce symptoms which intensify the physical and emotional distress caused by illness. For example, the apprehension and embarrassment experienced by the patient with diarrhoea and vomiting must be recognized. Observant, sympathetic nursing care can lessen the discomfort of the patient and those around him by ensuring privacy and proper ventilation and by preventing or dispelling offensive odour.

Psychological care

Anxiety may be allayed by giving the patient a simple explanation of nursing procedures and the part he has to play, so gaining his confidence and co-operation. Explanation and support during diagnostic and therapeutic procedures will help the patient to cope with a situation which he may find unpleasant and exhausting.

Since emotional disturbances also predispose to some gastrointestinal tract disorders, it is important that nurses in the course of their duties approach patients with a reassuring and optimistic attitude. They should be encouraged to express and share their stressful problems.

Physical care

The physical care of the patient includes the maintenance of respiratory and circulatory functions and the provision of an adequate fluid and nutritional intake.

Nutrition
The normal way to take nourishment is by oral ingestion. Some patients may be prevented from eating and drinking because of symptoms such as pain, nausea and vomiting. At this time intravenous infusion may be given to prevent dehydration and electrolyte imbalance. Satisfactory nutrition can be achieved by feeding via a nasogastric tube or by a tube opening into the jejunum, a jejunostomy. Others may have disorders which cause inflammatory changes, preventing digestion and absorption of nutrients. The only alternative for these patients is to be fed via the circulatory system, **parenteral nutrition**. In this situation the nutritional and biochemical requirements of the patient are estimated on a daily basis. The physician, with the aid of the biochemist, prescribes the nutrient solution for the individual's needs over 24 hours. Administration is achieved by cannulation of a large central vein. The doctor passes a catheter (most commonly via the subclavian vein) until the tip lies just above the right atrium of the heart. This procedure is carried out aseptically, preferably in the operating theatre. An X-ray is taken to check the position of the catheter.

Nursing care of the patient being fed parenterally requires skill and understanding. The patient's general condition and morale is likely to be low, therefore much encouragement will be necessary. There are several hazards associated with administration of nutrients parenterally, one of the most sinister being the risk of septicaemia. Great care must be taken by all involved to prevent the introduction of infection.

Many patients have been maintained solely on parenteral feeding for over a year, by which time the underlying condition has healed or corrective surgery has been possible. For the majority of patients parenteral nutrition is only required for a week or two. In either situation successful treatment may be life saving.

The mouth

Inspection of the mouth and pharynx reveals signs of systemic illness as well as local disease and must be carried out thoroughly as part of basic nursing observation. The appearance of the tongue in particular provides valuable information about the state of the gastrointestinal tract. The healthy tongue is pink and is kept moist by saliva which continually bathes the inside of the mouth.

A dry tongue is common in patients who mouth-breathe or who have lost excessive amounts of fluid and have become dehydrated. In dehydration, salivary secretion is diminished as body fluids are concentrated in vital areas and the patient experiences thirst. Often, for medical or surgical reasons, oral fluids are forbidden; therefore, thorough, regular mouth care must be provided in an effort to keep the mouth clean and comfortable.

A brown, furred tongue may indicate irregular oral toilet or inadequate elimination of waste — for example, renal insufficiency — but it usually accompanies underhydration. Frequent mouth care will help to cleanse and remove odour and unpleasant taste. Many patients during their treatment have a nasogastric tube inserted or are not permitted to eat or drink. If thirst is a problem, sucking small pieces of ice may afford relief, provided that too much fluid is not swallowed.

Observation of excreta

Vomitus

The volume and time in relation to food intake must be noted as well as the colour, presence of undigested food, frank or altered blood. In vomitus, blood changed by digestive juices has the appearance of coffee grounds.

Faeces

Stool consistency and regularity of bowel movement vary with the amount and type of food ingested. The faecal mass may be hard and dry when peristalsis is diminished, watery and offensive when the tract is inflamed and peristalsis is increased, or soft and ribbon-like in appearance when disease affects the lower bowel.

The faeces should not be unduly offensive and if they are bacteriological examination must be carried out to exclude the presence of pathogenic organisms. With this possibility in mind, specimens for observation and examination must be managed with care to prevent spread of infection (Ch. 1). Offensive stools are also likely in conditions of abnormal protein digestion when putrefaction occurs in the large intestine producing an unpleasant odour. Observation of the colour of stools is an extremely important aid to diagnosis. The normal brown stool becomes pale during a milk diet and dark when meat or iron containing preparations are ingested. When the biliary tract is obstructed the stool is clay-coloured due to the absence of bilirubin; excess of bilirubin produces dull green faeces. Bleeding within the tract may produce the typical black melaena stool. The presence of blood may be confirmed by using Occultest reagent tablets. Small quantities of blood may not be detected by the normal inspection, but this occult (hidden) blood will also react with Occultest reagents. In order to validate examination results three stool specimens are obtained on consecutive days. A melaena stool may, for example, be produced due to ingestion of blood following a tooth extraction thus giving a false sign of organic change.

The skin

The maintenance of an intact skin can prevent further discomfort and infection. This is of particular importance when the patient is confined to bed as the deprived tissues are at risk and easily damaged. By relieving pressure and keeping the skin clean and dry, damage may be avoided. When diarrhoea, faecal soiling or anal discharge exist, careful cleansing of the surrounding skin will prevent pruritis and excoriation. The use of a bidet or bath is the most efficient means of ensuring cleanliness and comfort.

Control of pain

Pain, in varying degrees of severity and character, is present at some time in most illnesses. Tolerance and reaction to pain vary from person to person and may be influenced by factors such as personality, cultural background or state of debility. The nurse's responsibility is to observe and make the patient as comfortable as possible. Reporting of observations can help the doctor prescribe appropriate treatment. Relief of pain permits diaphragmatic breathing, improves respiratory function and facilitates movement thus helping to prevent venous stasis and complications such as deep vein thrombosis.

Preoperative management

The nursing care of a patient having surgery should be directed towards meeting the varying physical, emotional and social needs of the individual. In this way each patient may be prepared to withstand the physiological and psychological stresses effected by anaesthesia and surgery.

The patient should be in the best possible physical condition before operation. For this reason examinations of the respiratory, circulatory and urinary systems are made to detect any coexisting disorder which may cause complications during or after surgery. The strange environment and procedures which are encountered when the patient comes into hospital may cause fear, depression or anxiety. Other stressful factors are pain, the uncertainty about survival, and doubts about retaining personal identity. In some patients this anxiety may reduce their understanding of the effects of surgery or of alternative treatment. The consequences of psychological stress result in physiological stress which may delay recovery. By giving the patient adequate information and allowing time to discuss socioeconomic problems, stress may be minimized. Indications are that patients who are carefully prepared in this way are more likely to make an uncomplicated recovery.

Postoperative management

In the immediate postoperative period when the patient has not yet fully recovered from the effects of anaesthesia an observant nurse can help to prevent the development of complications.

Frequent regular recording of blood pressure and pulse rate will indicate the state of the patient's circulatory system. Changes such as an increased pulse rate and a fall in blood pressure are signs of haemorrhage and must be reported immediately. The patient's colour and breathing pattern must be noted and attention drawn to deviations from normal. Shallow, inadequate ventilation may be due to the effects of drugs on the respiratory centre or the muscles of respiration and may result in respiratory failure. Noisy rapid breathing is usually caused by obstruction in the respiratory tract possibly by the tongue or a collection of secretions. Because of this possibility most patients are nursed on their side so that the tongue falls forward and secretions drain away.

Wounds and drains should be looked at as soon as possible so that the nurse can assess any further blood loss.

Any intravenous infusion should be inspected to ensure that the needle is in the vein and that the fluid is being administered at the correct rate.

As the patient regains consciousness he should be reassured and calmed. A restless patient can cause damage to his wound and may injure himself. Pain is another cause of apprehension and restlessness; therefore effective anagelsia is necessary to give the patient much needed rest, relaxation and sleep.

The body's natural reaction to injury of any sort is to rest. This loss of function is apparent following surgery of the gastrointestinal tract and results not only from the surgical procedure itself but also from trauma associated with disturbance of the abdominal organs. Peristaltic action is lost because of post-traumatic paralysis or adynamic ileus.

Adynamic ileus
This loss of function may be:

1. Transient following for example, a simple appendicectomy.
2. Persistent following major surgery.
3. Present later if the repaired intestinal tract again becomes disordered.

Clinical features. There is absence of bowel sounds, faeces and flatus. Abdominal distension ensues due to the accumulation of intestinal gas and secretions. This causes discomfort and pain.

Vomiting will result when the stomach becomes dilated with an accumulation of gastric and intestinal secretions and gases.

Treatment includes intravenous replacement of fluids, nutrients and electrolytes; decompression of the intestinal tract by intermittent aspiration via a nasogastric tube. Decreasing amounts of aspirate suggest that normal function is returning.

Accurate records of fluid intake and output are necessary for the assessment of fluid replacement. Nothing is given by mouth until peristalsis is resumed. Restricted fluids are then allowed and the amount gradually increased as normal function returns.

Healing of abdominal wounds
This is normally straightforward provided that the wound is not contaminated or subjected to undue tension. Most uncomplicated wounds are exposed after 3 days and the patient is encouraged to bath or shower daily. Healing is fairly well established in 10 days and sutures can be removed.

Wound infection. A tense, painful and inflamed wound suggests that infection is present in the deeper tissues. In most cases, bacteriological examination of any discharge reveals the offending organism and a course of an appropriate antibiotic accompanied by aseptic wound care should effect speedy healing. Sometimes wound probing is required to open pockets of pus which should then be allowed to drain freely.

Regional abscesses may form in the pelvis or, less frequently, in spaces under the diaphragm (subphremic abscess). Signs of infection persist long after surgery and necessitate drainage of the abscess.

Wound dehiscence (burst abdomen). This is a very alarming complication of abdominal wound healing which may occur about 10 days after surgery. The wound suddenly leaks serosanguineous fluid and subcutaneous and deeper layers of the wound edges separate allowing loops of intestine to appear on the surface of the abdomen. It is due to poor healing of the tissue which may be the result of:

1. Poor general health, anaemia, malnutrition and vitamin C deficiency.
2. Stress and strain during the postoperative period, for example from coughing or vomiting.
3. Wound infection and poor drainage procedures or the premature removal of sutures.

Treatment. As soon as possible the prolapsed intestines are wrapped in sterile towels soaked in warm saline. Meanwhile the operating theatre is alerted. A nurse in constant attendance can help to allay the anxiety produced by this dramatic event. The patient is prepared for theatre and the wound resutured under general anaesthesia. The degree of fluid loss and circulatory collapse is minimized if prompt treatment is provided.

Surgery is a traumatic experience for any patient but a confident, optimistic nurse can do much to avert anxieties, depression and apathy.

Early ambulation gives encouragement to most patients, but for those whose progress is hindered some light occupational or recreational therapy may be required.

SUGGESTED ASSIGNMENTS

Projects
1. Select a unit where there is a planned early discharge scheme for surgical patients. Find out how continuity of care is ensured and how the interests of the patient are safeguarded. If possible follow up one or two patients whom you know in consultation with the community nurse.

2. Where is the nearest stoma clinic for your area? What are its functions? If there is a stoma nurse what are her duties?

3. Choose two (or three) patients with a similar common disorder, for example peptic ulceration, on whom you could carry out a small comparative study. Headings under which you make your observations should be your own but could include previous history and circumstances which aggravated symptoms, reactions to admission to hospital, response to nursing care and treatment, length of stay, your own conclusions.

Discussion topic
Consider the hazards of living in an overcrowded environment with poor sanitation and its relevance to disorder of the gastrointestinal tract.

FURTHER READING

Bouchier I A D 1977 Gastroenterology, 2nd edn. Bailliere Tindall, London
Capia L G 1972 The care of the cancer patient. Heinemann, London
Chamberlain E N, Ogilvie C M 1974 Symptoms and signs in clinical medicine, 9th edn. Wright, Bristol
Naish J M, Read A E 1974 Basic gastroenterology including diseases of the liver, 2nd edn. Wright, Bristol
Ryall R J 1973 The digestive system. Penguin Library of Nursing Series. Churchill Livingstone, Edinburgh

6. *The Respiratory System*

The many diseases that may affect the respiratory system can cause both acute and chronic illness. Often the early symptoms of illness are unobserved or ignored. The disease may then slowly progress to become a chronic condition. The high incidence of disability caused by chronic respiratory illnesses indicates that they are a major health problem. Health education can help by advocating means of prevention, early detection and treatment of disease.

ANATOMY AND PHYSIOLOGY

The respiratory system comprises passages and organs by means of which oxygen (O_2) is absorbed into the blood and carbon dioxide (CO_2) is excreted. The lungs are situated within the thoracic cavity (Fig. 6.1). Breathing is achieved by increasing and decreasing the size of the cavity. Enlargement of the thoracic cavity occurs as a result of nerve stimuli to the intercostal muscles and the diaphragm which cause them to contract, thus increasing the size of the cavity and drawing air into the lungs (inspiration) (Fig. 6.2). When the muscles relax the elastic recoil of the lungs expels the air (expiration). **Respiration** is the inspiration of air containing a relatively high proportion of O_2 and the expiration of air containing an increased amount of CO_2. The process of respiration is controlled by a group of nerve cells in the medulla oblongata known as the **respiratory centre**.

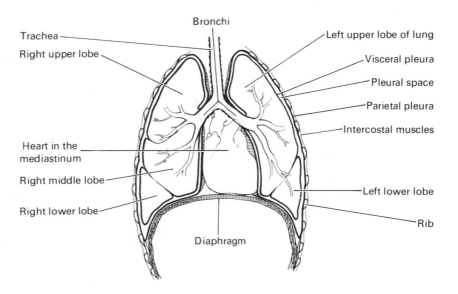

Figure 6.1
The lungs

The respiratory centre is influenced by the level of CO_2 and O_2 in the blood. High levels of CO_2 and low levels of O_2 stimulate the respiratory centre, causing an increase in the rate and depth of respiration in an attempt to 'wash out' or reduce the level of CO_2. Conversely, low levels of CO_2 diminish the stimulus to the respiratory centre, causing respiration to become slow and shallow. The maintenance of normal levels of oxygen and carbon dioxide in the blood depends on an adequate amount of oxygen in the inspired air and efficient respiratory and circulatory systems.

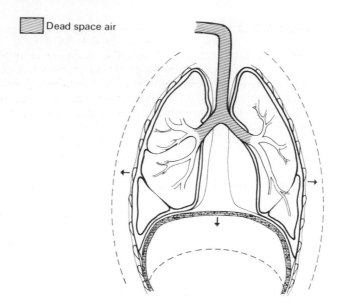

▨ Dead space air

Figure 6.2
Inspiration
The arrows indicate the direction
of chest expansion

CO_2 passes from the blood in the capillaries to the alveoli in the lungs and O_2 is passed from the alveoli to the capillary blood. This gaseous exchange is known as **diffusion**. The structures which enable it to take place are shown in Figure 6.3. The carriage of oxygen through the lung tissue is called **perfusion** and is dependent on an effective circulatory system. Lungs contain 3000 ml of air; this is the **vital capacity**. With each inspiration 400 ml of air enters the upper respiratory tract; of this amount, 150 ml (known as the **dead space air**) is held in the passages of the upper respiratory tract and the remaining 250 ml reaches the lungs for diffusion. This amount is known as the **tidal volume** and is necessary for normal metabolic function (Fig. 6.2). All tissues, including the medulla oblongata, require adequate oxygenation to maintain their normal function.

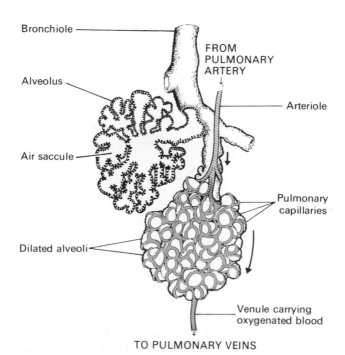

Figure 6.3
Structures enabling the diffusion
of O_2 and CO_2

Bronchiole

Alveolus

Air saccule

Dilated alveoli

FROM
PULMONARY
ARTERY

Arteriole

Pulmonary
capillaries

Venule carrying
oxygenated blood

TO PULMONARY VEINS

AETIOLOGY

The high incidence of respiratory disorder in temperate climates, especially in the United Kingdom, is associated with air pollution, cigarette smoking and cold, damp, foggy weather. These unfavourable conditions greatly aggravate any infective or allergic inflammatory changes present in the respiratory tract. The gravity of the situation in many countries has led to greater control of atmosphere pollution and of working conditions in occupations where dust and irritants are a problem.

Inflammation, increased secretion and infection prevent adequate alveolar ventilation and diffusion of gases. When these conditions become chronic there is a continuously lower percentage of O_2 in the blood (anoxaemia) and a higher percentage of CO_2 in the blood. Under these abnormal circumstances the respiratory centre is no longer influenced by the constant high percentage of CO_2 but by the low percentage of O_2 in the blood. In this situation great care must be taken to administer only the prescribed amount of O_2. Too high a percentage of O_2 in the blood will result in respiratory failure. If pulmonary oedema is present due to failure of the left side of the heart to transfer blood from the pulmonary veins, the diffusion of gases will also be inadequate (Ch. 7).

Trauma to the respiratory centre or to the muscles of respiration may prevent ventilation and necessitate the use of positive pressure ventilators. Failure of ventilation may also occur during the early postoperative period when obstruction of the airway or the effect of drugs on the respiratory centre may cause respiratory failure. Interruption of nerve pathways to the muscles of respiration in neurological diseases such as poliomyelitis and myasthenia gravis will also cause respiratory failure. Failure can also be of cardiac origin, for example following cardiac arrest when breathing usually stops within thirty seconds requiring immediate ventilation of the lungs by artificial means. Local spread of bronchial carcinoma embarrasses respiratory function by causing obstruction, collapse of a lobe or pleural effusion.

The accumulation of silica, asbestos fibre or coal dust results in **pneumoconiosis**. This is a collective term for a group of diseases caused by mineral dusts, which are progressive, and which produce fibrotic changes in the lungs; the pleura may also be involved. Recently there has been considerable concern regarding the role of blue asbestos in causing mesothelioma of the pleura; this is a malignant condition.

GENERAL FEATURES OF DISORDER
Cough

Cough is the most common symptom of respiratory disease and is a means of keeping the respiratory tract clear. The cough reflex is stimulated by any irritant touching the lining of the tract. The respiratory centre is the controlling factor in this reflex action, which causes forced expiration of mucus or foreign bodies. A cough may be dry or may produce sputum. Dry, unproductive coughing can be painful and exhausting to an ill patient and therefore a cough suppressant may be prescribed. A productive cough should not be suppressed but can be made less exhausting by giving an expectorant, a medication that loosens secretions.

Sputum

In health, sputum is not produced; it results from inflammation, infection or congestion, and may occur in varying amounts. Sputum produced by irritants is clear, white and mucoid; when infected sputum will be purulent (yellow or green) or mucopurulent; it may also contain blood.

Haemoptysis

The production of bright red, frothy blood from the lungs is usually associated with lung disease and vigorous coughing. The severity of the haemoptysis varies greatly from a few bloodstained streaks in the sputum to a very large haemorrhage that may be fatal.

Chest pain

Pain associated with respiratory disease may be

1. retrosternal pain made worse by coughing but not by deep breathing and most commonly caused by tracheitis.
2. lateral or posterior chest pain usually occurring on inspiration; it is sharp and stabbing, increasing on deep breathing and coughing.

Dyspnoea

Difficulty in breathing that produces obvious changes in the normal respiratory pattern is called dyspnoea. It results from any obstruction to air intake, such as excessive secretions, spasm of air passages or the presence of a foreign body or tumour. Any condition affecting either the respiratory centre or the thorax, such as trauma to the chest wall, will also cause dyspnoea.

Hypoxia

Hypoxia is shortage of oxygen. It may be due to shortage of oxygen in the inspired air or to lung diseases which prevent oxygen reaching the blood.

Finger clubbing

This is a characteristic feature of lung abscess, bronchiectasis and bronchial carcinoma; the cause is not known (Fig. 6.4).

Cyanosis

This is blue discolouration of the skin or of the mucous membranes. It results from an abnormally high proportion of haemoglobin which has not combined with oxygen in the circulation. It is associated with the conditions causing hypoxia.

Pleurisy

Pleurisy is the term used to describe inflammatory changes occurring in the pleura. It is one of the symptoms of pneumonia, tuberculosis, malignant invasion of the pleura and pulmonary infarction. There are two forms of pleurisy. **Dry pleurisy** is characterized by a sharp, stabbing pain on deep breathing and coughing which restricts respiration. **Pleurisy with effusion** is caused by changes in the pleura which prevent the normal secretion and reabsorption of pleural fluid. This causes fluid to collect in the pleural space and inhibits lung expansion, necessitating pleural aspiration (thoracentesis).

Empyema

Is a condition in which there is infection causing pus formation in the pleural space.

Pneumothorax

Pneumothorax is the condition in which air is present in the pleural space, thus preventing normal lung expansion. This may result from chest trauma or be spontaneous. **Spontaneous pneumothorax** occurs when the rupture of a small air sac or bulla beneath the surface of the visceral pleura allows air to enter the pleural space. The collapse of the affected lung can cause displacement of the heart towards the opposite side. The resulting pressure on the opposite lung inhibits its expansion. If, as a result of chest trauma, blood is also present in the space the condition is known as **haemopneumothorax**.

The patient who has a spontaneous pneumothorax presents with a sudden onset of breathlessness and tightness in the affected side of the chest. Moderate or severe dyspnoea will occur according to the degree of displacement of the heart. On physical examination there will be absence of breath sounds on the affected side of the chest. X-ray of the chest will demonstrate the edge of the collapsed area of lung and the degree of displacement.

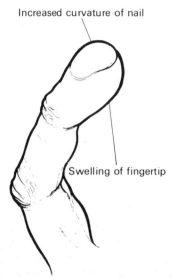

Increased curvature of nail

Swelling of fingertip

Figure 6.4
Finger clubbing

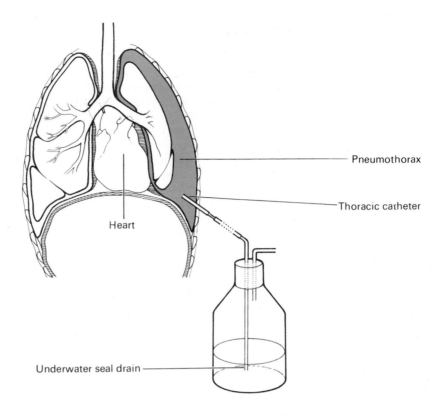

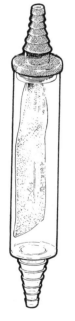

Figure 6.5
Underwater seal drainage

Figure 6.6
Heimlich valve

Figure 6.7
Heimlich valve in use

Treatment is aimed at the re-expansion of the lung by introducing a thoracic catheter and connecting it to an underwater seal drainage bottle. Air can be removed by placing the catheter in the upper intercostal region, but if it is placed lower, air and serosanguinous fluid can be drained from the pleural space (Fig. 6.5). When there is only air present in the pleural space a **Heimlich valve** (Figs 6.6 and 6.7) may be inserted.

These are aseptic procedures carried out under local anaesthesia.

INVESTIGATIONS
Clinical examination

During the clinical examination the comfort and safety of the patient is the nurse's main concern. The patient requires an explanation of the procedure, reassurance, warmth and privacy. He will also need help and support while moving into suitable positions for the clinical examination. When the patient has been settled comfortably and well supported with pillows, his temperature, pulse and respirations should be taken and recorded accurately.

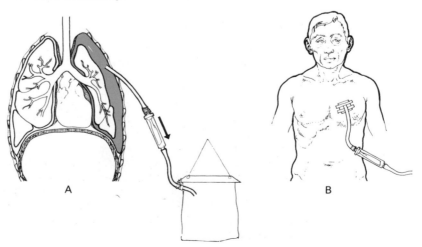

It is particularly important to observe the rate and depth of **respirations**. Any changes due to exertion, position or time of day should be noted and reported. When the airway is obstructed, noisy laboured breathing will result; this is called **stridor**. Pain or depression of the respiratory centre causes shallow inadequate breathing. The terminally ill or unconscious patient may develop periods of *apnoea* — that is an absence of breathing which is the result of a deficient blood supply to the respiratory centre.

While the doctor is taking the patient's medical and family history and details of occupation the nurse should collect instrumetnts for examination including sphygmomanometer, stethoscope, ophthalmoscope and syringes for venepuncture: she will then be free to assist and support the patient during palpation and auscultation.

Sputum

The investigation of sputum is important as treatment is based on the results of microbiological (Ch. 2) or cytological examination. It may be necessary to support and assist the patient during expectoration to ensure that an adequate sputum specimen is obtained. Once obtained the specimen must be clearly labelled and sent to the laboratory as soon as possible. When a specimen is being sent for microbiological examination it must be collected in a sterile container. A wax carton should always be available near the patient's bed. This will allow general observations to be made of amount, colour and consistency of the sputum.

X-ray

There are various types of X-ray procedures included in the investigations of chest diseases. Before any X-ray is taken a full explanation to the patient is necessary. The patient must be warmly clad while being transported to the X-ray department, he should have some form of identification and all his previous X-rays should be sent with him to allow comparison by the radiologist. Initially all patients have a straight X-ray of the chest which may be followed by more specialized techniques such as *tomography* or *bronchography*. During bronchography a special radio-opaque dye is used to outline bronchi and bronchioles. It is important that the bronchi are cleared of secretions before the procedure, and afterwards the physiotherapist should assist the patient to expel the radio-opaque dye from the bronchi.

Endoscopy

Examination under direct vision can be carried out during bronchoscopy, *thoracoscopy* or *mediastinoscopy* (Fig. 6.8). Preparation for these examinations includes explanation of the procedure and reassurance, as the patient may be very apprehensive. The

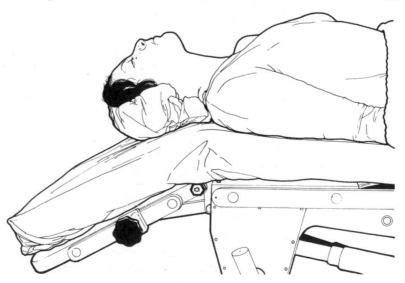

Figure 6.8
Position of the patient for bronchoscopy

examinations may be performed under either general or local anaesthesia, but the patient is usually required to fast to prevent regurgitation and inhalation of stomach content. The patient wears clothing which is warm and which can be easily removed. Identification bands are applied, premedication given, any prostheses and valuables are removed and stored in a safe place and he is allowed to rest. Notes and X-rays must accompany the patient to the diagnostic theatre. Following bronchoscopy under local anaesthesia the patient must not have anything by mouth until cough and swallow reflexes have returned. Mouth care should be carried out to make the patient more comfortable. Following thoracoscopy the patient may return to the ward with an **underwater seal drain** to facilitate the re-expansion of the lung (see p. 195 and Fig. 6.5).

Biopsy

Biopsies of pleural and lung tissue can be taken during thoracoscopy, of the respiratory tract during bronchoscopy and of the lymph nodes during mediastinoscopy. These biopsies are sent for pathological examination and great care should be taken when labelling; in particular, the **site** of the biopsy should always be noted.

Pleural aspiration

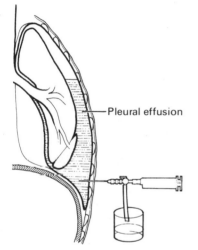

—Pleural effusion

Figure 6.9
Pleural aspiration

Specimens of pleural effusion can be obtained during therapeutic or diagnostic pleural aspiration. The specimen is sent for microbiological or *cytological* examination. In order to withdraw fluid from the pleural cavity the patient must sit in the upright position so that fluid in the pleural cavity will drain towards the base. The most recent X-rays, showing fluid levels in the chest, must be available to enable the doctor to decide where to introduce the aspiration needle (Fig. 6.9). The main concern of the nurse during pleural aspiration is to position, support and reassure the patient. Whenever possible the patient should be in the upright position, sitting either on the side of a bed or astride a chair with his feet supported and his arms and head resting on a bedtable or the back of the chair. In this position the shoulders and arms are raised, the rib-cage elevated, the intercostal spaces increased, thus facilitating the introduction of the aspirating needle into the pleural space. Observations of pulse, respirations, colour and pain are made during the procedure. To prevent the aspirating needle puncturing the visceral pleura the patient is asked to remain quite still and not to cough without warning, and if possible not to cough at all. At the end of the procedure an occlusion dressing is applied over the site of the aspiration and the amount of fluid is measured and recorded. Specimens of pleural fluid that have been collected in sterile containers must be labelled accurately before being sent to the microbiology laboratory.

Respiratory function tests

Lung function tests involve the use of a **spirometer** (Fig. 6.10) to measure the volume changes within the lungs during inspiration and expiration. A spirometer consists of a drum inverted inside another drum which contains water. A tube is passed through the drums and ends above the water level. The drum is balanced with a weight. As the patient breathes in and out a pen attached to the weight records volume changes on the calibrated spirograph paper.

One of the most commonly performed tests is that used to measure, in individuals, the volume of air that can be expired forcefully (FEV) at one, two or three second after full inspiration. Forced expiratory volume after one second following full inspiration is expressed as FEV.

Blood tests

Examination of arterial blood will demonstrate the amount of circulating haemoglobin and therefore its oxygen-carrying capacity. Samples will also be analysed to estimate the percentage of oxygen and that of carbon dioxide in the blood.

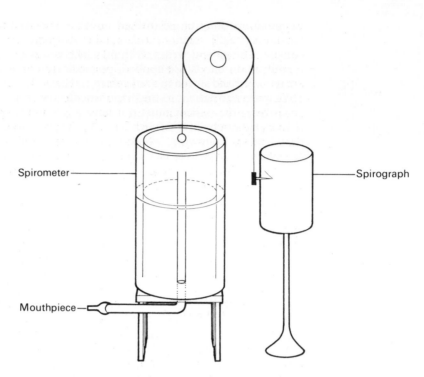

Figure 6.10
Spirometer

Spirometer

Spirograph

Mouthpiece

NURSING CARE OF THE PATIENT WITH RESPIRATORY DISEASE

The nursing care of the patient with a respiratory disorder must be directed to meeting his physical, psychological and social needs. One must consider the clinical features of the disease and in this way choose the most effective means of relieving the patient's discomfort. It must also be remembered that the patient's needs and dependence will relate directly to the severity of his illness.

The objective, when planning a patient's physical care, should be the maintenance of cell functions. The assistance of a physiotherapist is always desirable and may be life-saving. The aims when meeting this objective are:

1. To maintain the best possible ventilation.
2. To maintain circulation.
3. To maintain a balance of body fluids.

1. **The maintenance of the best possible ventilation** can be achieved by nursing the patient in a warm, well-ventilated environment. This will provide an adequate supply of

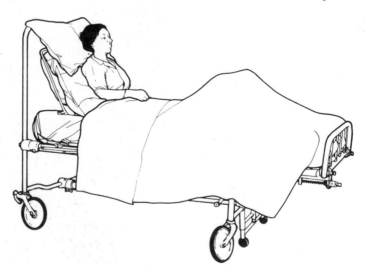

Figure 6.11
Upright position in bed

oxygen from the atmosphere and reduce the possibility of cross infection. Mechanical ventilation can be improved by nursing the patient in the upright position supported with a back-rest and pillows (Fig. 6.11). This position will ensure the best possible chest expansion unhampered by the pressure of abdominal organs under the diaphragm. The aid of a physiotherapist is essential to remove secretions which may be obstructing alveolar ventilation. The purpose of physiotherapy is to remove bronchial secretions, improve gaseous exchange and decrease sputum, so preventing further bronchopulmonary infection. The methods used by the physiotherapist to achieve this end will be breathing exercises, chest percussion, vibration and postural drainage. It is important that the patient himself is taught to breathe and expectorate effectively.

2. **The maintenance of an adequate circulation** will ensure an adequate flow of oxygenated blood to the tissues. This can be achieved by assisting venous return, which will prevent the formation of deep venous thrombosis and decubitus ulcers.

Venous return is promoted during physiotherapy to the chest and by leg exercises, which may be active or, if the patient cannot move without assistance, passive. The maintenance of circulation allowing adequate oxygenation to the body tissues will, in conjunction with turning the patient to relieve pressure on vulnerable areas, prevent the formation of decubitus ulcers.

3. **The maintenance of fluid balance** is necessary for the well-being of the body's internal environment. The balance will be disturbed if the intake of fluids does not replace that lost from the body by the kidneys, lungs and skin, especially if the loss of water by skin and lungs is increased because of pyrexia and increased respiration rate. Accurate records should be made of all fluids taken orally or parenterally and of those lost from urinary or alimentary tract, aspiration or drainage from wounds. An accurate record of fluid balance can be used to assess the amount of replacement fluids necessary to prevent dehydration. Normally fluid balance is maintained by diet and fluid intake. During illness the metabolic rate is increased and therefore the diet should contain increased kilojoules, protein and fluids (see Ch. 4).

Patients who have respiratory diseases may be admitted to hospital in a critical condition. They will require a great deal of reassurance and support initially while in this stressful situation and unusual environment. These diseases can be progressively incapacitating. The patient should be made aware of and helped to accept his limitations. Because his condition may alter his life pattern and those of his dependents considerably, he should know that support will be available. While in hospital medical and social service personnel can be alerted and can continue to provide help and support if necessary after discharge from hospital.

Care of the patient having oxygen therapy

Patients with a low oxygen concentration in their blood, that is **anoxia**, will have impaired metabolic function. An oxygen supplement will therefore be necessary and

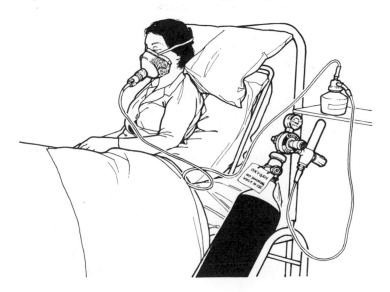

Figure 6.12
Administration of oxygen by Ventimask and oxygen cylinder

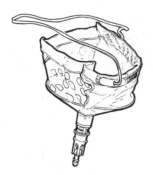

Figure 6.13
Ventimask

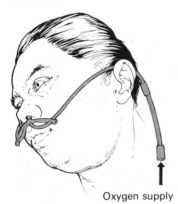

Oxygen supply

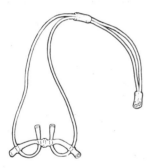

Figure 6.14
Nasal cannulae in use

can be administered by various types of equipment. When the anoxia is due to insufficient gaseous exchange oxygen can be administered by mask, nasal catheter or oxygen tent (Ch. 18). The oxygen can be obtained from an oxygen cylinder or from a system of pipes from a central supply. The administering apparatus is connected to the oxygen source by tubing which allows the oxygen to pass through a flow meter and a humidifier (Fig. 6.12). The nurse can then administer the prescribed amount of humidified oxygen. Most oxygen masks are disposable and can be adjusted to fit the patient comfortably. A high concentration of oxygen can be given by using a closed mask such as the Polymask. When an accurate percentage of oxygen supplement is required, as in some chronic respiratory conditions, a mask such as a Ventimask will be required (Fig. 6.13). This mask is available in three models which deliver 24 per cent, 28 per cent and 35 per cent O_2 respectively.

Nasal cannulae (Fig. 6.14) provide a rather unpredictable O_2 concentration but an O_2 flow rate of 2L/minute will usually provide an O_2 intake of about 30 per cent. The advantage of this method of O_2 therapy is that the patient can communicate and take food uninhibited by a face mask. Even though the oxygen is humidified the patient may feel dry; therefore oral and nasal hygiene are very important for his comfort. Since oxygen supports combustion, relatives and neighbouring patients must be warned of the hazard of fire and therefore the danger of smoking in the vicinity of any patient who is receiving O_2 therapy.

Care of the patient with underwater seal drainage

To allow re-expansion of the lung or lobe following chest surgery, trauma or spontaneous pneumothorax, a thoracic catheter is introduced into the pleural space and connected to an underwater seal drainage bottle.

Under local anaesthesia a trocar with a cannula attached to it is introduced through an intercostal space. The sterile catheter is then passed through the cannula into the chest and the cannula is withdrawn. The catheter is held in place by a stitch and attached to the drainage tube and bottle. This allows air to leave the pleural space, prevents its re-entry and permits the re-expansion of the lung or lobe (Fig. 6.5, p. 195).

The patient is nursed in the upright position and care is taken to prevent traction or compression of the drainage tubing. To prevent water entering the chest cavity the tubing **must** be clamped firmly before raising the bottle from floor level. The bottle stopper must be firmly in place to prevent ascending infection of the pleural cavity. During inspiration the pressure within the chest is reduced and the water level in the tube rises. On expiration the water level falls. This is often termed 'swinging' and demonstrates that the tube is patent. When no 'swinging' is observed this fact should be reported immediately. X-ray will demonstrate when lung re-expansion has been achieved and the catheter can be removed using aseptic technique; an occlusion dressing is then applied. When a more rapid removal of air from the pleural space is necessary a low pressure suction pump is used.

Care of the patient with a tracheostomy

A tracheostomy is an opening made into the trachea to facilitate breathing. The indications for tracheostomy are failure of respiratory function due to upper respiratory tract obstruction and conditions affecting the respiratory centre or muscles of respiration. Today it is more often an elective rather than an emergency procedure and is usually performed under general anaesthesia. The selection of the tracheostomy tube is very important as there are various types and sizes. Examples are:

1. Silver metal Jackson tube.
2. Red rubber James tube.
3. Portex disposable tube.

The Jackson tube is a double silver tube used when the patient does not need **assisted ventilation** but requires aspiration of secretions.

When assisted ventilation is necessary the James and Portex tubes which have a single or double cuff are used. These tubes have a fitting which can be attached to the ventilating machine. The cuff, when inflated, seals the area between the trachea and the

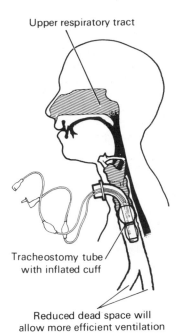

Upper respiratory tract

Tracheostomy tube
with inflated cuff

Reduced dead space will
allow more efficient ventilation

Figure 6.15
Tracheostomy tube *in situ*

tube (Fig. 6.15) and thus allows **positive pressure ventilation** and prevents aspiration from either the upper respiratory or the alimentary tract. For patients who need assisted ventilation for only a short time, an endotracheal tube may be passed, to avoid the hazards of a tracheostomy. In addition to the basic nursing care required for all patients, there are some specific nursing responsibilities for tracheostomy patients; these are: to maintain a clear airway, to prevent infection or trauma and to ensure adequate humidification of inspired air.

Maintaining a clear airway
This can be achieved by turning the patient from one side to the other (if this is possible), by physiotherapy to the chest and by aspiration of bronchotracheal secretion (see below).

Preventing infection
The aspiration of bronchotracheal secretion is an aseptic procedure performed to prevent descending infection. If the patient is conscious, he should be given a reassuring explanation to allay apprehension. Prior to aspiration, oral hygiene is carried out and oropharyngeal suction is used to remove secretions from the area above the tracheostomy tube. The deflated cuff of the tube is inflated and the other deflated. This is to prevent necrosis due to constant pressure on the wall of the trachea. The aseptic procedure of bronchotracheal suction is then begun, using a catheter which will not occlude the tracheostomy tube. The ventilator is disconnected during aspiration, therefore the procedure must be done deftly and quickly. Suction should only be applied when withdrawing the catheter (Fig. 6.16) and this can be controlled by a Y connection attached to the suction catheter to prevent trauma to the lining of the trachea and bronchi. Secretions from the other side can be removed by turning the patient and repeating the aseptic procedure. It is important to use an aseptic technique when changing tracheostomy tubes or dressings to prevent infection.

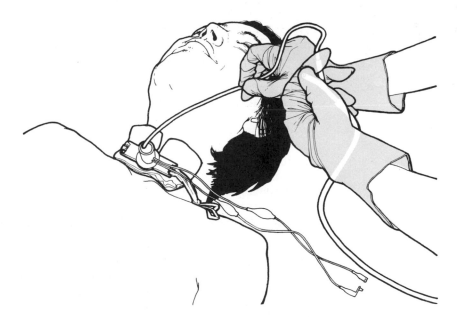

Figure 6.16
Aspiration via tracheostomy tube

Humidification of inspired air
Air entering the tracheostomy bypasses the humidifying area of the respiratory system. It is therefore necessary to provide an alternative source of moisture to avoid the drying of the secretions and mucosa. There are various methods of adding moisture; a common one is to bubble the oxygen through water.

Special aspects of nursing care
Patients with assisted ventilation may not necessarily be unconscious but they are totally dependent on nursing staff. The conscious patient may be apprehensive and

requires a great deal of psychological support. He will be unable to talk while the tracheostomy or endotracheal tube is in use and therefore should be given an alternative means of communication, such as a bell or a note book. He may also be anxious about eating and drinking and should be told how the nurse will care for his needs. If respiratory failure is due to chest trauma, for instance, the patient may be conscious but unable to tolerate or synchronize with the ventilator. In such circumstances heavy sedation may be necessary to allow effective ventilation.

While a patient is being cared for with a mechanical ventilator (Fig. 6.17) he must be under constant supervision. The patient's relatives will also need help and advice, particularly concerning his communication problems.

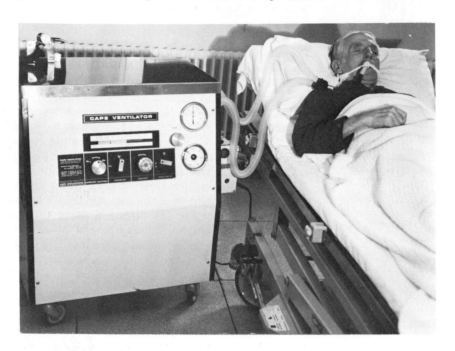

Figure 6.17
Patient on intermittent positive pressure (IPP) ventilator

COMMON DISORDERS OF THE RESPIRATORY SYSTEM
Coryza

Coryza, or the common cold, is a droplet infection caused by a virus; most people succumb to it at least once a year.

The symptoms of the common cold, which usually appear suddenly, are dry throat, nasal congestion causing thin, watery discharge and sneezing. There may be a moderate rise in temperature, the voice may become husky and the eyes watery, and the sense of taste or smell may be diminished. Often a cough develops, which may become productive.

The common cold usually lasts 7 to 10 days but may be complicated by sinusitis, otitis media, laryngitis, tracheitis or simple bronchitis.

Treatment is directed towards relief of symptoms and prevention of complications and of spread of infection to others. The patient requires a warm, well-ventilated environment, preferably not in close contact with others who may become infected. Nasal decongestants will reduce swelling and allow increased air flow. A dry mouth and throat will be soothed by hot drinks. To prevent excoriation of nasal skin, soothing cream can be applied with soft, easily disposed of tissues.

Influenza

This is an acute viral infection, affecting any age group, that occurs especially during the winter months. It is a febrile illness of sudden onset starting with general malaise, headache, backache and joint pain. There may be a painful, unproductive cough, conjunctivitis and enlarged lymph glands.

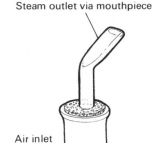

Figure 6.18
Nelson steam inhaler
The steam which is inhaled
through the mouth condenses on
the bronchotracheal mucosa and
stimulates the expectoration of
secretions.

The course of the disease is about 4 to 5 days but may be prolonged by secondary bacterial infection of the lower respiratory tract.

The patient should be isolated in a warm, well-ventilated environment. While he is febrile and suffering from anorexia, fluids must be encouraged. A linctus may be given to control a dry, unproductive cough. Steam inhalations will provide moisture to the upper respiratory tract (Fig. 6.18).

Bronchitis

Bronchitis is a general term describing an inflammatory condition of the bronchi. It may be acute or chronic.

Acute bronchitis

Inflammation of the bronchi may result as a complication of an upper respiratory infection such as coryza, influenza or measles.

Clinical features
There is mild elevation of temperature, a feeling of soreness behind the sternum, general malaise and an unproductive cough which may become productive due to secondary infection. The infection may spread downwards to the bronchioles.

Nursing observations
Four hourly recording of temperature, pulse and respirations.

Observation of amount and colour of sputum, which is usually abundant and purulent.

Investigations
A specimen of sputum — sent for culture and sensitivity of organisms.
Chest X-ray.

Course and complications
Gradual improvement in 4 to 8 days occurs in the majority of cases. However, those patients who smoke or live in areas of high atmospheric pollution may have a prolonged illness. Infection descending to fine bronchi and bronchioles becomes a serious complication in young children, debilitated patients and those suffering from chronic bronchitis.

Treatment and nursing care
Bed rest is necessary while the patient is pyrexial and having antibiotics. Pain caused by the inflammation can be relieved by medicated steam inhalations and an unproductive cough can be eased by the administration of a cough suppressant drug.

Rehabilitation and community care
Most patients only need advice about rest and diet during the convalescent period.

Chronic bronchitis

This is a progressive degenerative disease affecting the mucous membrane and cilia of the bronchi; it is caused by irritants associated with industrial pollution or the personal pollution of cigarette smoking. An acute exacerbation of the condition can be precipitated by viral or bacterial infection.

The changes which occur during the course of the disease greatly reduce the number of cilia and destroy normal function. The mucous glands enlarge and the increased amount of secretions block bronchioles and impair alveolar ventilation. As a result of infection fibrosis and stenosis of bronchioles occur (Fig. 6.19).

Clinical features
The patient will have a chronic cough, wheeze and tightness of the chest, especially in the morning before bronchial secretions have been expectorated. The sputum is usually

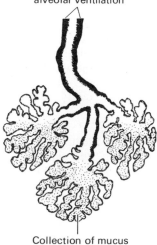

Narrowing of bronchiole
preventing adequate
alveolar ventilation

Collection of mucus
preventing adequate
gaseous exchange

Figure 6.19
Chronic bronchitis

thick, tenacious and mucoid, often copious, and may become purulent due to secondary infection. The patient may be cyanosed and dyspnoeic even at rest, cyanosis and dyspnoea becoming more evident on exertion. Chest expansion is poor and expiration is slow and difficult, leading to a higher level of carbon dioxide in the blood.

Nursing observations
Temperature, pulse and respiration.
Sputum, amount and colour.

Investigations
Chest X-ray.
Respiratory function tests.
Microbiological examination of sputum.

Course and complications
The symptoms slowly progress over the years and eventually lead to emphysema and right-sided cardiac failure (see Ch.7). Loss of elasticity of lung tissue prevents adequate expiration and may be the cause of the typical 'barrel chest' of the chronic bronchitic. The respiratory centre is no longer stimulated by high levels of CO_2 but by the lower than normal level of oxygen. This is very important to remember when administering oxygen because to overoxygenate the patient would result in a higher than normal level of oxygen in the blood. There would then be no stimulus to the respiratory centre and the patient would go into complete respiratory failure, requiring assisted ventilation with a positive pressure ventilator.

Treatment and nursing care
Bed rest is essential. Nursing care is as described on page 198. There should be careful administration of oxygen using a Ventimask which allows a regulated percentage of oxygen to supplement the atmospheric air. The percentage of oxygen and the length of time the patient requires oxygen therapy will be prescribed by the doctor following analysis of arterial blood samples. Antibiotic therapy will depend on the culture and sensitivity report on the sputum specimen.

Drugs which dilate the bronchi, especially salbutamol, are more effective when given by inhalation. In acute exacerbations they may be administered by an intermittent positive pressure ventilator with oxygen-enriched air over a period of 3 minutes four times daily.

Chest physiotherapy and the use of drugs to reduce the viscosity of mucus help to prevent the accumulation of excess mucus which would obstruct the airway.

Rehabilitation and community care
The patient must be well supported in the community as it may be necessary for him to change his whole life-style, housing and means of livelihood. Attendance at follow-up clinics to assess his condition should be encouraged. He should also continue physiotherapy and he and his family should be instructed in the use and dangers of oxygen therapy.

Pneumonia

Pneumonia is a general term describing an inflammatory condition of the lungs. There are two types: specific pneumonia, caused by a particular organism, and aspiration pneumonia, a secondary descending infection affecting lungs with an existing abnormality.

Specific pneumonia

Specific pneumonia can be caused by bacteria, viruses or mycoplasma (see Ch. 1) affecting one or more lobes. Young adults are more commonly affected by this type. The incidence is higher in winter and the spread is by droplet infection. The affected lobe becomes consolidated with exudate in the alveoli. When liquefaction of the exudate occurs, the infected material is either absorbed or expectorated.

Clinical features

The onset of the condition is sudden with the temperature rising to 40°C within a few hours; the patient may have rigors. General malaise, anorexia and headache accompany the pyrexia. The patient is dyspnoeic, he may have pleuritic pain and a painful, unproductive cough. The patient is made particularly uncomfortable by hot, dry skin and mouth. Herpes simplex may be present on or near the lips. The painful cough, caused by the inflamed pleura and consolidation, disappears when resolution occurs, allowing copious amounts of rusty-coloured sputum to be expectorated.

Nursing observations

Sputum, amount and colour.
Temperature, pulse and respirations.

Investigations

Chest X-ray.
Sputum for microbiological examination and sensitivity of any cultured pathogens.
Blood for culture and sensitivity.

Course and complications

There is usually a quick response to antibiotic therapy and a corresponding fall in temperature, pulse and respiration. With resolution other symptoms gradually abate, usually within 7 days. Complications which may occur are pleural effusion, emphysema and lung abscess.

Treatment and nursing care

The patient needs bed rest; nursing care is as described on page 198, with particular attention to oral hygiene and the care of herpes simplex. Pain can be relieved by local heat and analgesics, while antibiotics will reduce temperature and toxic symptoms. Oxygen therapy may be prescribed during the early stages of the disease and given via a Polymask. Fluids must be encouraged especially when there is pyrexia and the possibility of the patient becoming dehydrated. Efficient expectoration and chest expansion can be achieved with the aid of physiotherapy.

Rehabilitation

This is a debilitating disease requiring a fairly long convalescence to return the patient to health.

Aspiration pneumonia

Any abnormality in the respiratory system predisposes the lungs to invasion, even by organisms of low virulence. Generally, infections reach the alveoli by aspiration of infected material from the upper respiratory tract. An acute reaction may be the result of a breakdown in the normal defence mechanism of the respiratory tract due to unconsciousness or ineffective coughing, particularly following an operation. Bronchial obstruction by a foreign body or carcinoma will also prevent efficient drainage of secretions.

This condition can affect the young, the elderly and the debilitated and has a high morbidity rate.

Clinical features

There are signs of acute bronchitis with a gradual rise in temperature, pulse and respirations, dyspnoea and cyanosis. Cough is severe with purulent sputum. The course of the disease is longer than in specific pneumonia and the patient is often drowsy, lethargic and confused as a result of cerebral anoxia.

Nursing observations

Temperature, pulse and respiration.

Investigations
  Chest X-ray.
  Sputum for culture and sensitivity.
  Blood for culture and sensitivity.

Course and complications
The bronchi become inflamed and the alveoli collapse or become consolidated and
therefore gaseous exchange is greatly reduced. A bronchus may become obstructed by a
plug of mucus, causing *atelectasis* of the affected lobe. Bronchiectasis will occur if there
is incomplete resolution of the consolidation.

Treatment and nursing care
The treatment and nursing care is as previously described (p. 198), with special care
necessary during the period of confusion when the patient is unable to co-operate. It is
particularly difficult to ensure an adequate diet and fluid intake for this patient, who may
be both aggressive and resentful. Because the patient may be very young or elderly and
debilitated, particular attention must be given to skin care especially for those who are
incontinent. Oxygen can be administered to a baby in an incubator, to a young child in
an oxygen tent (Ch. 18) and to adults by an oxygen mask or nasal cannula.
Physiotherapy is essential in the management of this patient.

Rehabilitation and community care
Rehabilitation and community care depend upon the age of the patient and the
underlying cause of the aspiration pneumonia. If the cause is unknown, diagnostic
investigations will have been carried out in hospital and treatment instituted. Generally
the patient's return to health is prolonged and the elderly may require long-term
nursing care either in hospital or in the community if their home conditions are
suitable.

Bronchiectasis

In this disease the small bronchi become permanently dilated as a result of obstruction.
This can be caused by acute pulmonary infection or a bronchial tumour causing
collapse of a lobe. When the lobe collapses the alveoli and bronchi dilate to take up the
space. If infection occurs this dilatation is permanent due to loss of elasticity caused by
fibrotic changes. The condition may exist without symptoms until there is infection of
the dilated bronchi; then the symptoms vary according to the degree of infection
present.

Clinical features
Usually the patient presents with a history of recurrent cough and sputum which are
more troublesome in the morning. The reason for this symptom is that lower lobes are
more frequently affected and the change in position from arising stimulates the need to
cough up the copious secretions that have collected during the hours of sleep.
Haemoptysis can occur as a result of vigorous coughing which may rupture distorted
blood vessels. Typically the patient who has suffered from this condition for some years
has a decline in general health. A very common feature of this disease is finger clubbing.

Nursing observations
  Sputum, amount and colour.
  Temperature, pulse and respiration.

Investigations
  Bronchography, sputum culture.

Course and complications
Complications of the disease have been greatly reduced by the emergence of antibiotic
drugs. However, recurrent pulmonary infection such as pneumonia, emphysema and
haemoptysis may occur.

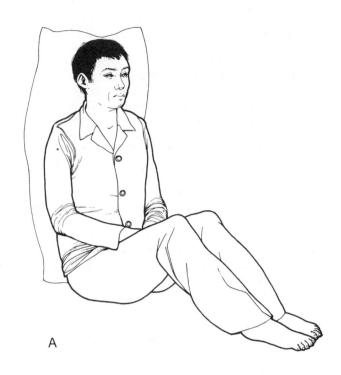

Figure 6.20A
Position used to facilitate the removal of secretions from right upper lobe and upper segment of left upper lobe

A

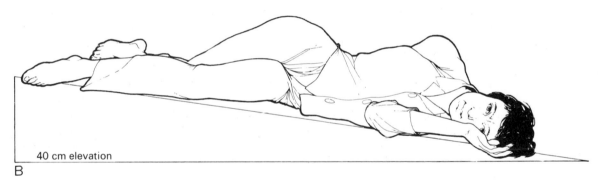

40 cm elevation

B

Figure 6.20B
Position used to facilitate removal of secretions from right middle lobe

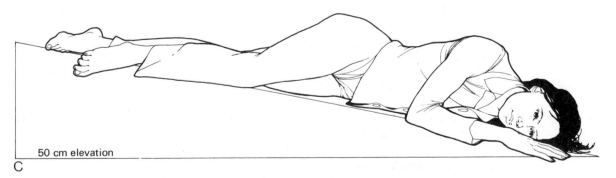

50 cm elevation

C

Figure 6.20C
Position used to facilitate removal of secretions from right lower lobe

Treatment and nursing care

When the bronchiectasis is confined to one lung surgery may be advocated and the affected lobe removed. However, if bronchography demonstrates extensive damage, surgery may not be possible. Medical treatment will be aimed at the control of infection and the drainage of sputum. The choice of antibiotic drugs will depend on the sensitivity of the cultured organism. During winter months it may be possible to prevent acute infection by giving the patient long-term antibiotic therapy. The method used to remove sputum efficiently is called **postural drainage.** It involves placing the patient in a position most suitable for drainage by gravity from the affected area (Fig. 6.20A, B, and C).

Rehabilitation and community care

The patient should be helped to understand the importance of a balanced diet with a high fluid intake. He should be advised to avoid chest infections and to continue breathing exercises, including postural drainage when necessary. These measures will help to prevent exacerbations of the condition. A light, outdoor occupation and leisure time spent in fresh air and sunshine will be beneficial to him.

Asthma

Asthma is a disease characterized by recurrent attacks of dyspnoea and wheezing. This is due to a temporary narrowing of the small bronchi caused by muscular spasm and oedema of the mucosa.

There are two clinical types of asthma: extrinsic and intrinsic.

Extrinsic asthma occurs in children who have a family history of allergic disease. Attacks of asthma may be precipitated by a hypersensitivity to certain *allergens* or as a result of psychological stress.

Intrinsic asthma occurs in later life in a person who has neither a personal nor a family history of disease caused by allergens. No obvious allergic factor is isolated when the disease does occur.

Clinical features

There is a history of periodic attacks of dyspnoea and of wheezing, especially on expiration. These episodes may be the result of inhaled or ingested allergens, or of emotional stress. The patient adopts the upright position and the accessory muscles of respiration are used in an attempt to increase expiration. The attacks may last several hours and leave the patient physically and emotionally exhausted.

Nursing observations

Signs of alterations in respiratory pattern and anxiety.

Investigations

Sensitivity tests to identify the allergen.
Identification of psychological factors.
Investigation of personal and family history — important in reaching a diagnosis.

Treatment of the acute attack

A vigilant nurse will notice at once when an attack is imminent, and, by initiating prompt treatment, will often avert the development of a severe attack. The patient is nursed in the upright position supported by pillows. A pillow on a bed table placed in front of the patient will support him in the optimum position during the acute episode. Psychological reassurance may be given by the presence of a calm nurse. When the attack has subsided, hot sweet drinks can be given to replace fluids lost due to increased metabolic rate during the attack. In a more prolonged, severe attack drugs may be necessary to relax the bronchial spasm.

A broncho-dilating drug such as salbutamol can be given by inhalation, and oxygen therapy may also be prescribed to raise the oxygen content of the blood. Oedema caused by inflammatory changes can be controlled by the anti-inflammatory effects of steroid therapy.

Course and complications

When asthmatic attacks do not respond to treatment with drugs, status asthmaticus exists and may last for many hours. This is a medical emergency requiring intensive steroid therapy which will be prescribed immediately. Salbutamol will be given via an intermittent positive pressure ventilator so that the drugs will reach the bronchi and be effective as quickly as possible. Oxygen therapy will be prescribed by the doctor and the amount to be given is estimated after examination of oxygen levels in the arterial blood. Reassurance is essential for the patient in this stressful situation to allow effective treatment.

Rehabilitation and community care

The asthmatic child and his parents must be educated in how to avoid those things which trigger off attacks—causative allergens, emotional stress and respiratory infection. To do so is important, because it allows the child's educational and physical development to progress as normally as possible. Sometimes parents become overprotective and it is then necessary to place the child in a special school or in residential care.

Carcinoma of the bronchus

The term lung cancer is often used to describe carcinoma of the bronchus. There is a higher incidence of the disease in men than in women, the age group being 40 to 70 years. The incidence is also higher in cigarette smokers and in those whose occupation exposes them to the inhalation of carcinogens such as asbestos and nickel.

Clinical features

The patient may present in the early stages with a history of weight loss, lassitude, cough and dyspnoea. Sputum can be bloodstained or there may be episodes of haemoptysis. In some instances the reason the patient seeks medical advice is due to symptoms arising from metastases.

Investigations

Chest X-ray normally includes posteroanterior and lateral views so that the whole lung area is examined. These areas can be examined in depth by tomography. Bronchoscopy will demonstrate vocal cords, trachea, main *carina* and bronchi. The surgeon may, by direct vision, assess the possibility of surgery and obtain a biopsy of any obvious tumour for histological examination.

Mediastinoscopy allows the surgeon to examine an area on both sides of the tracheal bifurcation and to obtain a biopsy from the lymph nodes situated there. These lymph nodes are frequently invaded by tumour cells and may be excised for histological confirmation of diagnosis.

A sputum specimen is sent for microbiological and cytological examination. Tests are carried out with the spirometer to estimate lung function and assess whether this will be adequate following surgery. Thoracotomy, an exploratory operation through the chest wall, may be necessary to assess the possibility of removing the tumour.

Treatment and nursing care

Adequate lung function and the localization of the disease should enable surgery to be considered, as excision of the affected lobe or lobes is the treatment of choice.

During the preoperative period smoking must be discouraged; intensive chest physiotherapy will help to prevent sputum retention and will encourage full lung expansion. It is also important to instruct the patient in effective breathing and coughing exercises, which will be necessary in the postoperative period. The operations which may be performed are **lobectomy**, the removal of a lobe or **pneumonectomy**, the removal of a whole lung. Postoperatively the usual care of a patient following major surgery will be carried out.

Following a lobectomy the patient will return to the ward with one or two chest drains, an upper one to remove air and a lower one to remove serous fluid, to prevent infection and promote lung expansion (Fig. 6.21). Care of the patient with underwater seal drainage is as discussed on page 200.

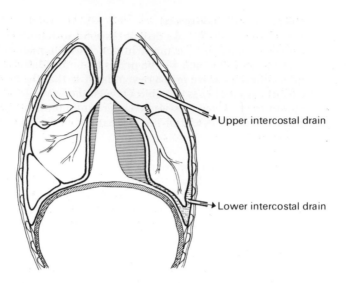

Figure 6.21
Lobectomy

Upper intercostal drain

Lower intercostal drain

Following a pneumonectomy there will be no need for drainage tubes because there is no raw lung tissue remaining on that side to cause air leakage or serous oozing. Before leaving the operating theatre a negative pressure is introduced on the side of the pneumonectomy to draw the mediastinal contents slightly towards the space and allow full expansion of the remaining lung.

In the early postoperative period the patient may be sat up if his blood pressure is satisfactory. This will facilitate chest movement and pleural drainage. Observation and control of pain by the administration of analgesics will allow physiotherapy to be recommenced as soon as possible to prevent mucus remaining in the bronchi, which may cause atelectasis and require emergency bronchoscopy to remove the obstruction.

Radiotherapy may be used as primary treatment if the site of the tumour makes surgery impossible. It can be of palliative value in some recurrent or advanced cases of the disease or in the treatment of metastases.

Course and complications
The complications are bronchial obstruction, causing atelectasis and leading to pneumonia and lung abscess. If there is pleural involvement the normal secretion and absorption of pleural fluid will be impaired, causing pleural effusion. Involvement of lymph nodes will cause venous congestion of the superior vena cava. A primary tumour in a bronchus may produce metastases in the brain, bone or liver. These deposits cause pain and debilitation and a variety of symptoms each requiring specific treatment.

Community care follow-up
The prognosis is generally poor, but following successful surgery 25 per cent of patients survive for an average of 5 years. These patients and their families face a difficult future in which much support can be given by their general practitioner, nurse and medical social worker.

Cancer research has not yet discovered how carcinogens act nor has it produced any dramatic breakthrough in treatment. Therefore, prevention cannot be stressed enough. It is known, for example that cigarette smoking produces a high incidence of the disease, although this does not seem to have changed attitudes towards the habit.

Pulmonary tuberculosis

Pulmonary tuberculosis is caused by the micro-organism *Mycobacterium tuberculosis*. The route of infection is by inhalation of air containing tubercle bacilli which have been coughed and sneezed into the atmosphere by an infectious patient. When a large number of tubercle bacilli have entered the lung tissue the white blood cells surround the bacilli and invade the alveoli. This can result in a pneumonia-type condition, which may resolve after a period of time, or caseation may occur. Caseation means that the infected area has a cheesy consistency, which later becomes fibrosed, then calcified, with the formation of lung cavities. There will be extensive cavities in a severely affected lung and sputum culture will be strongly positive. Minimal or no cavities will be present in a mildly affected lung and the sputum may or may not produce a positive culture.

When infected with tubercle bacilli for the first time the lesion is known as primary and may heal spontaneously, providing the patient with an acquired immunity. A healed primary lesion may be reactivated in later life if the patient's general health deteriorates. Those susceptible to the disease are people who are in close contact with an infectious patient, those in poor general health or those whose social conditions are unfavourable and immigrants who have a low racial resistance to the disease.

Clinical features
Usually the onset is insidious, with tiredness, anorexia, loss of weight and a dry, irritating cough. If undiagnosed or untreated at this stage the patient will later present with dyspnoea, productive cough and elevation of temperature in the evening. The patient may also have enlarged glands in the axillae, neck or groin.

Nursing observations
Recording of temperature, pulse and respiration particularly in the evening.

Observation of sputum amount and colour, and whether it is bloodstained.

Side-effects of drug therapy are fairly common and may include gastrointestinal disturbance, skin rash, tinnitus and eye focusing problems. Any of these manifestations should be noted and reported.

Investigations
When a patient has been to a mass X-ray unit and the results suggest infection by tubercle bacilli, he will be asked to undergo further investigations. These include chest X-ray and tomography to demonstrate cavitation and the presence of enlarged lymph nodes. Because bacilli may be scanty, sputum specimens are taken on 3 consecutive days to see if they are present. The tubercle bacilli are described as 'acid fast' because of the method used in the laboratory to demonstrate them. Sputum specimens will also be sent for concentration tests which demonstrate the virulence of the infection. Skin tests using purified tubercle protein are used to assess hypersensitivity to tubercle bacilli. This sensitivity is associated with previous infection that has resulted in an acquired immunity, or with effective artificial immunization against infection. Redness and swelling at the site of the skin test denote a positive reaction and show that the patient is immune to the disease.

Blood specimens will be taken to estimate the blood sedimentation rate, which is raised during infection (see Ch. 12). Once diagnosed the health authorities are notified and, through consultation with the patient, an attempt is made to trace the source of the infection and to follow up contacts. The contacts will then attend a clinic for X-ray and investigation.

Course and complications
The disease will progress and cause increasing debility, haemoptysis and spontaneous pneumothorax. Pleurisy may develop with or without pleural effusion. An undiagnosed and untreated infectious patient becomes a risk to the community in which he lives and works.

Treatment and nursing care
The objectives of treatment are to return the patient well and safe to his or her family, to solve immediate medical, physical and social problems and to prevent the spread of infection to the community. Treatment depends on whether the patient is only infected or is both infected and infectious. An infected patient can be cared for in the community under the supervision of the health authorities, but if the patient is also infectious as shown by acid fast bacilli in his sputum he must be nursed in isolation until his sputum culture and concentration tests are negative. Initially the treatment is bed rest because of the patient's general debility and he will need a high protein diet with milk supplements. Drug therapy will be in triplicate — that is, three drugs will be given at once — because the bacilli can become resistant very quickly to a drug and there is a limited number of suitable drugs available. Examples of triplicate drug therapy are

streptomycin daily for three months, isoniazid and sodium aminosalicylate (para-aminosalicylic acid — PAS) given over a period of 18 months to 2 years or Rifampicin, Isoniazid orally once daily for a year and Ethambutol orally for at least a year.

While nursing patients in isolation wards of hospitals, it is important to conform to the specific regulations regarding the disposal of sputum and infected material. Although there is no need to have separate crockery or special laundering arrangements, it is important to remember that the rules regarding the prevention of cross infection must be adhered to. The nurse must also be aware of the need to maintain her own general health and to protect her hands when administering injections of streptomycin, a drug which is known to produce skin rashes. When the infectious patient has a negative sputum concentration and culture he can be discharged from hospital and continue his drug therapy at home.

Community care
In the community the patient should be advised by the health authorities on drug therapy, diet, and rest for approximately 2 years or until the patient no longer requires treatment. It is important to stress the role that a nurse may assume in helping the patient to lead a healthy life.

SUGGESTED ASSIGNMENTS

1. Consider the measures which may be taken to detect, diagnose and control spread of pulmonary tuberculosis among and from:
   a. Vagrants.
   b. Immigrants.

2. The direct relationship between respiratory disease and air pollution from smoke and chemical agencies is undeniable. Discuss the means whereby prevention of disease and promotion of health can be achieved.

3. Discuss the problems which may confront both patient and family with regard to drug administration in the following circumstances:
   a. A man with chronic bronchitis going on holiday.
   b. A school-age girl with asthma.

4. Recognizing the psychological and physical problems of a person suffering from carcinoma of the bronchus, consider the role of the nurse when assisting the patient during complicated diagnostic tests and treatment.

FURTHER READING

Capra L G 1972 The care of the cancer patient. Heinemann, London
Goldman K P 1970 The chest in health and disease. Health Horizon, London
Grenville-Mathers R 1973 The respiratory system. Penguin Library of Nursing Series. Churchill Livingstone, Edinburgh
Grenville-Mathers R 1973 Thoracic medicine and surgery for nurses, 3rd edn. Sylviro Publications, London
Hume K M 1970 Asthma A guide for patients. Health Horizon, London
Mcleod J (ed) 1977 Davidson's principles and practice of medicine, 12th edn. Churchill Livingstone, Edinburgh
Sykes M K, McNichol M W A, Campbell E J M 1976 Respiratory failure, 2nd edn. Blackwell Scientific, Oxford

7. The Cardiovascular System

Caring for patients with cardiovascular disease presents a challenge to the nurse's skills of observation and communication. The presentation of cardiac disease is extremely variable, and appearances are often deceptive. Many patients with severe heart disease seem healthy and robust, but on clinical examination and questioning they are found to be badly disabled by dyspnoea or pain on even slight exertion, and are therefore unable to cope with normal daily activities, household duties or employment. The patient with disturbance of heart rhythm and conduction may have few symptoms, yet he is at risk of unexpected collapse from a sudden fall in cardiac output at home, at work, or even crossing the road. On the other hand, those with acute myocardial infarction may be in severe pain, pale and sweating, and the patient with infective endocarditis may be ill with fever and general malaise.

Time and patience are necessary to reassure patients that a normal, active life is possible despite cardiac disease. Yet there are many who do not understand clearly or who are not realistic about their disease. They need careful explanation and persuasion to encourage them to alter their life-styles so that they can live happily and safely within the limits of their disability. The possibility of cardiovascular disease, its investigations, final confirmation and treatment, will mean a time of anxiety for a patient and his family. To help him overcome it, the nurse must try to see her patient not only in the hospital setting but in his home and with his family, at work and in the community.

ANATOMY AND PHYSIOLOGY OF THE HEART

The heart has three layers:

The pericardium — a smooth membranous sac surrounding the heart, consisting of an outer fibrous and inner serous coat.
The myocardium — specialized muscle tissue.
The endocardium — an inner layer of endothelium which lines the chambers of the heart and the valve surfaces.

The heart is divided by a muscular septum into left and right sides which do not communicate with each other (Fig. 7.1). Each side is subdivided into upper and lower chambers, the **atria** and the **ventricles.** Thus there is a right and left atrium and a right and left ventricle. Separating the atria from the ventricles are one-way valves, the **tricuspid** and **mitral valves.** At the outlet of the ventricles to the major vessels are the **pulmonary** and **aortic valves** which prevent backflow into the ventricles.

Pulmonary and systemic circulation (Fig. 7.2)
The heart pumps **venous blood** to the lungs, where carbon dioxide, a waste product of metabolism, is given off and oxygen is received, and **arterial blood,** carrying oxygen and nutrient materials to all body tissues.

Venous blood from the superior and inferior venae cavae passes into the right atrium, and then through the tricuspid valve to the right ventricle. As the right ventricle contracts, blood is pumped through the pulmonary valve to the pulmonary artery and lungs **(pulmonary circulation)**. Arterialized blood from the four pulmonary veins passes into the left atrium and through the mitral valve to the left ventricle. As the left ventricle contracts, blood is pumped through the aortic valve to the aorta and the **systemic circulation**.

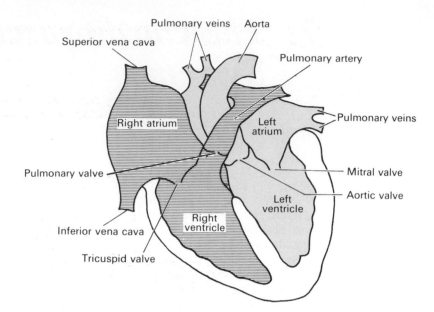

Figure 7.1
The anatomy of the heart

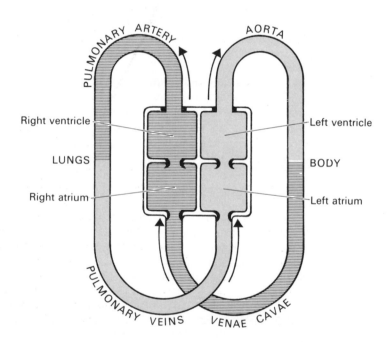

Figure 7.2
Pulmonary and systemic
circulations

Blood supply
The myocardium itself requires a blood supply. Arterialized blood is passed to the heart muscle by the right and left coronary arteries (Fig. 7.21). Coronary venous blood is returned to the right atrium together with the venous return from the rest of the body.

Nerve control
Both sympathetic and parasympathetic nerves play a part in regulating heart action. **Parasympathetic nerves**, the vagi, decrease the rate and force of contraction and decrease blood flow through the coronary arteries supplying the myocardium. **Sympathetic nerves** have the opposite effect, increasing the heart rate and force of contraction and increasing blood flow to the myocardium, thus improving the oxygenation and nutrition of the myocardium. When a person is subjected to stress, sympathetic nerve stimulation allows the heart to cope by making it a more effective

pump and improving blood flow through the circulatory system. While the body is resting, parasympathetic stimulation allows the heart to rest, thus preserving the heart's strength.

Conducting pathways
These are shown in Figure 7.3. Every heartbeat is initiated by an electrical impulse which passes along conducting pathways of specialised cells, some of which are grouped to form nodes.

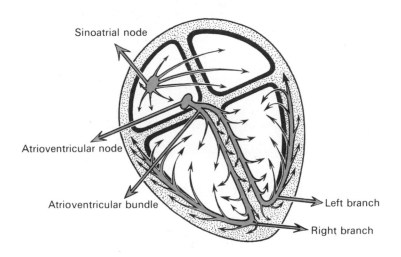

Figure 7.3
Conducting pathways

Sinoatrial (SA) node or 'pacemaker'. The electrical impulse arises in this node and spreads in all directions across the walls of both atria causing them to contract **(atrial systole)**.

Atrioventricular (AV) node and atrioventricular bundle. The impulse from the atria is conducted to the AV node situated in the right atrium close to the tricuspid valve. The AV node passes impulses to the specialised conducting muscle fibres of the AV bundle, which divides into right and left branches. The impulse, spreading rapidly through these branches, causes the ventricles to contract **(ventricular systole)**. After contraction, the atria and ventricles relax **(cardiac diastole)**.

A block in the conducting pathways may occur, preventing the passage of impulses from atria and ventricles. This may follow acute myocardial infarction and can be corrected by the use of a temporary or permanent **artificial pacemaker**. An electrode is introduced through a peripheral vein and its tip is positioned in the apex of the right ventricle. The other end is attached either to a portable, battery-operated pacemaker for temporary pacing, or to a pacemaker box buried under the skin of the axillary area or the anterior chest. In this way the ventricles are artificially stimulated to contract, should normal conduction of the impulse be blocked.

AETIOLOGY

The causes of cardiac disease are many and complex; also, cardiac diseases may occur singly or in association. The heart may be affected directly by **congenital defects** and **structural abnormalities**, such as atrial septal defect or pulmonary stenosis, or by **impaired blood supply** to its structure for example from diseased coronary arteries causing angina and myocardial infarction.

The heart may also be affected by **infection** both directly, as in diphtheria, syphilis, and a variety of bacterial and viral infections and indirectly, as in rheumatic fever.

Changes in cardiac function are associated with many other diseases, such as hypertension, thyrotoxicosis, myxoedema and anaemia, and the cardiovascular changes of pregnancy and childbirth may place such a circulatory strain on an already diseased heart that both the pregnancy and the mother's life may be in danger. Whether the structure and function of the heart are affected directly or indirectly, in time the heart muscle itself fails and cardiac failure results, precipitated by one or a combination of several of the factors mentioned above.

The diseases to be discussed in this chapter are those commonly seen in clinical practice (Table 7.1).

Table 7.1
Classification and incidence of cardiac disease

Type	Incidence (%)	Age group
Coronary heart disease Hypertensive heart disease }	60% (increasing)	Middle and old age
Rheumatic heart disease	20% (decreasing)	Childhood and adolescence (acute) Middle and old age (chronic)
Pulmonary heart disease	10%	Middle and old age
Congenital heart disease	1–3%	Infancy
Others	7%	

GENERAL FEATURES OF DISORDER

Dyspnoea

Difficult or laboured breathing, though not peculiar to heart disease, is the most common and often the earliest symptom; when severe it can cause great distress and anxiety. In cardiac disease dyspnoea is usually progressive.

1. Dyspnoea on exertion
This first appears when climbing hills or stairs or when doing heavy household work. Gradually, even less strenuous exercise will cause shortness of breath, for example walking slowly on level ground (Fig. 7.4).

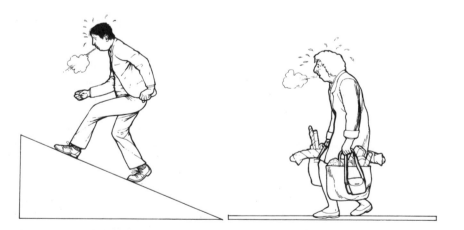

Figure 7.4
Dyspnoea on exertion

2. Dyspnoea at rest
Eventually breathlessness is present even when the patient is at rest, and finally **orthopnoea** occurs, that is the need to sit upright in order to breathe more easily. Many patients prefer to sleep using three or four pillows. Cardiac dyspnoea is usually due to pulmonary venous congestion. As left heart failure develops, back pressure of blood is transmitted to the pulmonary veins and capillaries. As the pressure rises, fluid exudes into the alveoli making the lungs less compliant and reducing the volume of air passing into and out of the lungs. Because the lungs are stiffer, the work of breathing becomes more difficult (Fig. 7.5).

3. Paroxysmal nocturnal dyspnoea (cardiac asthma)

Attacks of dyspnoea often occur during sleep in patients with left heart failure. The patient wakens gasping for breath and intensely anxious, and will sit on the edge of the bed or often walk to an open window for fresh air to ease the distress. When lying flat or having slipped down in bed, venous return to the heart is increased and pulmonary venous congestion increases. In addition, the diaphragm is elevated when lying, thus reducing the vital capacity of the lungs (Fig. 7.5).

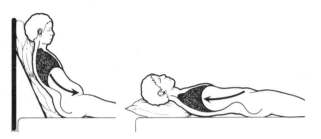

Figure 7.5
Reduced vital capacity of the lungs
—the effect of posture

Pain

Cardiac pain is experienced in myocardial ischaemia, myocardial infarction and pericarditis.

1. Myocardial ischaemia

This is a reduction in oxygenated blood supply to the myocardium due to atherosclerosis and narrowing of the coronary arteries. It may cause a pain known as **angina pectoris**, a central chest pain which may radiate to the neck, jaw and arms, more often the left arm. Angina is described variously as a tightness in the chest, a numbness or heaviness in the arms, a choking in the throat or an ache in the jaw. It is associated with exertion, such as walking up stairs, and with emotion, cold weather or eating a heavy meal. It is relieved by rest and by sucking a glyceryl trinitrate tablet. Episodes of angina are brief, seldom lasting more than 15 minutes.

2. Myocardial infarction

Inadequate blood supply to the myocardium due to blocking of a coronary artery by thrombus and atheroma may cause pain as the part of the myocardium supplied by that artery becomes irreversibly damaged. Distribution of the pain is similar to that of angina, that is central chest with radiation, but the pain is much more severe and is described as a crushing or constricting pain. Unlike angina, the pain generally comes on at rest and is unrelieved by rest; it is also prolonged, usually lasting more than 30 minutes.

3. Pericarditis

Inflammation of the pericardium may complicate rheumatic fever and acute myocardial infarction, often producing pain similar in distribution to the pain of myocardial infarction. It may be worsened by inspiration, swallowing and movement. Diagnosis is confirmed by the presence of a pericardial friction rub, which is heard as a scratching noise over the heart on auscultation. A chest radiograph may show a pericardial effusion — a collection of fluid in the pericardial sac — which is often serous but may be purulent in pyogenic pericarditis or bloodstained in malignant pericarditis. The effusion can cause compression of the heart and impair its action.

Palpitations

Cardiac disease and arrhythmias may produce an awareness of the heart's action as a thumping or as a very fast or irregular beating. In the healthy person, anxiety may lead to palpitations as a result of sympathetic nervous stimulation.

Oedema

Accumulation of excess fluid in the tissues is often a feature of cardiovascular and other diseases. There are three types of mechanism which may be involved in the formation of oedema:

Physiological mechanisms.
Physical obstruction to circulation.
Impaired muscle action.

Physiological mechanisms

1. Retention of salt (sodium chloride) and water. In cardiac failure the retention of water follows retention of sodium ions in the kidneys. The filtration of sodium ions by the glomeruli is reduced and the reabsorption of sodium ions from the tubules is increased.

2. Raised blood pressure in capillaries. Tissue fluid is formed at the arterial end and reabsorbed at the venous end of the capillary (Fig. 7.6). Normally balance is maintained by the following two pressures: first, blood pressure or hydrostatic pressure which forces fluid out through the capillary walls to the tissue spaces; second, osmotic pressure exerted by the plasma proteins, which draws fluid back into the capillary. At the arterial end, the blood pressure is greater and fluid exudes into the tissues. At the venous end the osmotic pressure is greater and fluid is reabsorbed from the tissues. When back pressure develops in veins and venous return is impaired, as in right heart failure (p. 241), engorgement at the venous end of the capillary will increase the blood pressure, and fluid will exude into the tissues and will not be adequately reabsorbed, that is, oedema develops.

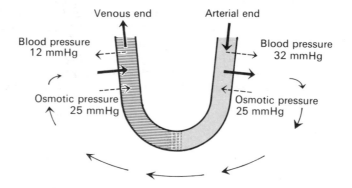

Figure 7.6
The formation of tissue fluid

Physical obstruction to circulation
Back pressure on capillaries can also accompany localised blockage of veins, for example, when stockings, garters or constrictive clothing are worn. Venous return may also be impeded by pressure on the popliteal area, for example, when sitting with the legs crossed at the knee or with the bend of the knee at the edge of a chair. Below the point of pressure, venous capillary hydrostatic pressure will increase due to venous stasis, causing movement of fluid into the tissues.

Impaired muscle action
When there is little or no muscular activity in a limb, as occurs during prolonged sitting, or lying in bed, then venous return will not be assisted by the action of the 'muscle pump'. Lack of muscle contraction leads to pooling of blood in veins; venous stasis and oedema follow. Impaired lymphatic drainage also plays a part in oedema formation. Minute lymphatic capillaries in tissue spaces act as an extra system for the flow of fluid from tissues into the circulation. The oedema seen in a weak or paralysed limb following a cerebral vascular accident may be due to a combination of impaired lymphatic and impaired venous return. This occurs when the 'muscle pump', which acts on both lymphatic vessels and veins, fails to work effectively in the weak or paralysed muscles (p. 248).

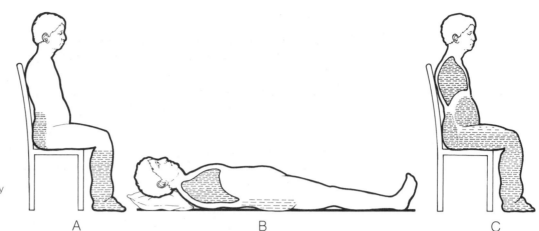

Figure 7.7
Sites of oedema
A. Dependent parts
B. The effect of recumbency
C. Total body oedema

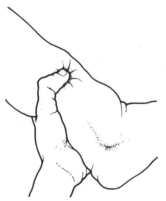

Figure 7.8
Pitting oedema

Sites of oedema

Oedema accumulates first in the lowest parts of the body, that is, the site depends mainly on gravity (Fig. 7.7). Oedema which occurs in any part of the body lower than the heart is known as dependent oedema. The severity of the oedema will depend on the length of time the part remains dependent, on the degree of slowing of venous return and on the extent of the loss of 'muscle pump' action. In the ambulant patient, or when sitting, oedema occurs first in the feet and ankles, then in the legs. When the patient is in bed, oedema gathers in the sacral areas and thighs. In left heart failure (p. 240), fluid accumulates in the lungs (**pulmonary oedema**). In right heart failure, oedema shows first in the lowest dependent parts. As the heart failure progresses and venous stasis increases, oedema increases. Fluid may accumulate in the peritoneal cavity (**ascites**) or in the pleural cavity (**hydrothorax**). In very advanced heart disease total body oedema may develop.

Cardiac oedema is said to 'pit' on pressure. This means that if an oedematous area is pressed by the finger, an indentation remains when the finger is removed (Fig. 7.8).

Changes in the amount of fluid retention can best be assessed by daily weighing of the patient.

Effects of oedema

Oedema creates many problems. For example, it can cause varying degrees of distress and discomfort; it impairs the function of vital organs; and it impairs cell function.

A gradual onset of swelling of feet and ankles may be no more than an unsightly irritation to some. Grossly oedematous feet and ankles might prevent the wearing of shoes and could lead to an elderly person becoming housebound. The sudden onset of acute pulmonary oedema may produce major discomfort and distress from severe shortness of breath. In this instance, oedema severely impairs the function of vital organs, the lungs.

Oedema also impairs cell function and increases the possibility of cell death. In oedematous areas the distance between the cells and nutrient bearing materials is increased. This has important implications for skin care and for potential to absorb medications. Pressure sores develop readily due to impaired cell nutrition and oedematous tissue is especially vulnerable if damaged or subjected to pressure; for example, the dependent areas of sacrum and heels in a bedfast patient. All such areas must be routinely inspected and protected (p. 448). Where there is increased tissue fluid and reduced capacity of cells to absorb, it should be obvious that an oedematous site must not be used for intramuscular injections.

Cyanosis

Cyanosis is indicated by a blue discoloration of the skin or mucous membranes (Ch. 6). Distinction should be made between peripheral cyanosis and central cyanosis.

Peripheral cyanosis

This is due to high oxygen extraction from the blood in the peripheral tissues, as in patients with a low cardiac output or with circulation impaired by vasoconstriction. A blue tinge appears in the lips and nails, and in the skin of the hands, feet, ears or cheeks. Peripheral cyanosis also develops in normal people when they are cold due to low blood flow through the skin, but it disappears when the skin is warmed.

Central cyanosis

This is due to inadequate oxygenation of the blood resulting from impaired gas exchange in the lungs, for example in pulmonary oedema or an intracardiac shunt in congenital heart disease. Unlike peripheral cyanosis, central cyanosis affects the warm mucous membranes such as the tongue.

INVESTIGATIONS

Clinical examination

Every patient admitted to hospital requires a full clinical examination, which includes a history of the current illness, previous state of health, family and social history and a physical examination. Routinely, the admitting physician will check all body systems but often one system requires special attention. In the diagnosis of cardiac disorders, **auscultation** plays an important part, that is, listening to heart sounds with the aid of a stethoscope. Altered heart sounds and the presence of murmurs caused by abnormally turbulent blood flow can be assessed accurately in this way by an experienced physician.

During clinical examination, the nurse should remain with the patient whenever possible. Both doctor and nurse should ensure that the patient has warmth and privacy throughout. The nurse should also remember that the doctor will appreciate quiet in the room during auscultation.

Temperature

Body temperature is controlled by the heat-regulating centre in the hypothalamus. When the centre is affected by pyrogens from micro-organisms or broken-down tissue cells, pyrexia occurs. In cardiac disease, micro-organisms produce bacterial endocarditis and purulent pericarditis; rheumatic fever is also related to infection. Following myocardial infarction, a low grade fever begins within 24 to 48 hours and gradually subsides during the first week. This pyrexia is thought to be a reaction to myocardial necrosis. Nursing responsibility lies in the accurate recording and reporting of changes in temperature. A neat graph is vital for correct assessment of the patient's progress, and in particular his response to treatment.

Pulse

A pulse is the wave of expansion felt in an arterial wall when a superficial artery is compressed by the finger. As the left ventricle contracts, the blood ejected distends the aorta and the arteries, which contain elastic tissue in their walls. Some sites of the pulse are illustrated in Figures 7.9 and 7.10.

Attainment of skill in feeling the pulse requires practice. The rate, rhythm and volume of the arterial pulse are all assessed. Accurate observation, recording and reporting of the features of the pulse of cardiac patients are essential. Accuracy requires concentration and the consistent assessment of every pulse feature, not merely the rate.

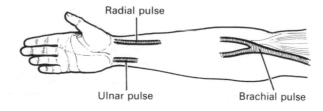

Figure 7.9
Arterial pulses in upper limb

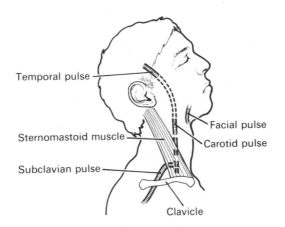

Figure 7.10
Arterial pulses in head and neck

Temporal pulse

Facial pulse

Sternomastoid muscle

Carotid pulse

Subclavian pulse

Clavicle

Rate

Pulse rate normally reflects heart rate. In a resting adult, the normal range is 60 to 100 beats per minute.

Bradycardia

This is the term for a slow pulse — that is less than 60. This is a normal rate in athletes but is also associated with excess vagal stimulation, for example due to raised intracranial pressure; with myxoedema when metabolic rate is decreased; with digitalis excess; and with 'heart block' where disease of the conducting system of the heart prevents normal conduction from atria to ventricles, thus allowing the ventricles to contract at their own intrinsic rate of 20 to 40 beats per minute.

Tachycardia

This denotes a rapid heart rate — that is greater than 100 beats per minute. It is normal in infants and young children, and in adults it is usual with exercise and anxiety. It also accompanies fever, shock, haemorrhage, thyrotoxicosis and cardiac failure.

Having recorded the patient's pulse rate on a graph the nurse should look at the trend of the recordings on the graph — steady, gradual increase or decrease, sudden increase or decrease. Any change over time should be reported, but sudden change should always be reported at once; failure to do so may endanger the patient.

Rhythm

The normal heart rhythm is regular, but **sinus arrhythmia**, where the heart rate increases on inspiration and decreases on expiration, is common to children and young adults and is considered normal.

Extrasystoles or ectopic beats may appear as isolated irregularities in an otherwise regular pulse. These extra beats of the ventricles follow quickly upon the previous beat and are followed by a compensatory pause.

Pulsus bigeminus or bigeminy takes the form of coupled beats when normal and ectopic beats alternate. Extrasystoles and coupling may indicate digoxin toxicity.

Atrial fibrillation (p. 229) produces a totally irregular pulse and is often associated with thyrotoxicosis, coronary artery disease and mitral stenosis. In atrial fibrillation, if the heart rate is rapid, the number of pulsations felt in the peripheral artery will be fewer than the number of beats (ventricular contractions) heard at the apex, that is the pulse rate may not reflect the heart rate. The discrepancy between apical and radial recordings is called the **pulse deficit**. The pulse deficit is estimated by simultaneous recording by two people of heart rate and pulse rate. The rate of an irregular pulse must be counted for not less than a minute. The finding of an irregular pulse must always be reported; failure to do so may have serious consequences for the patient.

Volume

Pulse volume is reflected in the amount of movement of the finger caused by the pulse wave. Volume is related to the cardiac output.

Cardiac failure, shock and acute myocardial infarction are associated with low cardiac output and small volume pulse. In the elderly, calcification of the arterial wall reduces pulse volume. An incompetent aortic valve, severe anaemia and thyrotoxicosis are associated with high cardiac output and large volume pulse, but physiological factors such as emotion, exercise, heat and pregnancy will also increase pulse volume.

Respiration

Dyspnoea, or difficulty in breathing, is the commonest symptom of heart failure (p. 240). The normal respiratory rate for adults is 16 to 20 per minute, and for a child 20 to 40. Rate is assessed by observing chest wall expansions, or by touch, laying the hand gently on the patient's chest wall. Breathlessness of cardiac origin which indicates pulmonary venous congestion or pulmonary oedema may be observed both on exercise and at rest and especially when the patient lies flat. The nurse should use her eyes and her ears to be on the alert for changes in respiratory rate. Changes must be reported quickly, since acute pulmonary oedema may develop rapidly with a rate of 40 to 50 or more per minute, causing great distress and anxiety to the patient. **Cheyne-Stokes respiration** may indicate advanced left heart failure and is often a preterminal sign. The characteristic waxing and waning phases occur when the respiratory centre is affected by lack of oxygen from decreased cerebral blood flow.

Blood pressure

Blood pressure is the pressure exerted by the blood upon the walls of the blood vessels. It depends mainly on the cardiac output and the peripheral resistance in the arterioles. The normal blood pressure of a young adult is around 120 systolic and 80 diastolic, measured in millimetres of mercury (mmHg). Blood pressure rises with age, and also with anxiety and on exercise. It should be recorded when the patient is resting and relaxed.

Hypertension indicates high blood pressure with levels above 150 mmHg systolic and 90 mmHg diastolic (p. 237).

Hypotension indicates low blood pressure with levels below 100 mmHg systolic and 60 mmHg diastolic.

Blood pressure is assessed using a sphygmomanometer at the brachial artery. The inflatable cuff, acting as a tourniquet, compresses the artery until no pulse is discernible. The returning pulse can be heard with the aid of a stethoscope on gradual deflation of the cuff. The sounds at first are faint and tapping, gradually becoming more intense, and then changing to an abrupt muffling before their final disappearance. **Systolic pressure** is that at which the sounds are first heard. **Diastolic pressure** may be taken either as the muffling or the disappearance of sounds, but it is important that one level be decided upon when a patient is being treated for hypertension, since consistency is needed to assess progress accurately.

Electrocardiography

The electrocardiogram (ECG) is a means of demonstrating on paper the electrical changes which initiate contraction of heart muscle (Fig. 7.11). Cardiac cells are electrically charged. The discharge and recharging of these cells during each cardiac cycle is detected at the body surface when electrodes are attached to the body at conventionally determined sites.

The ECG is important for the diagnosis and treatment of cardiac disease. It is used for the detection of arrhythmias and hypertrophy of the chambers of the heart, for the diagnosis of injury to heart muscle from ischaemia and to confirm the exact site and extent of a myocardial infarction.

While the ECG is being recorded, the patient must be at rest, and is asked to keep quite still and relaxed, to avoid distortion of the tracing by muscle activity. An ECG may be recorded at home, in the doctor's surgery or in an out-patient department to which the patient is referred for specialist opinion before hospital admission. Each patient's ECGs are kept on file, to allow assessment of any change in heart muscle activity over a period.

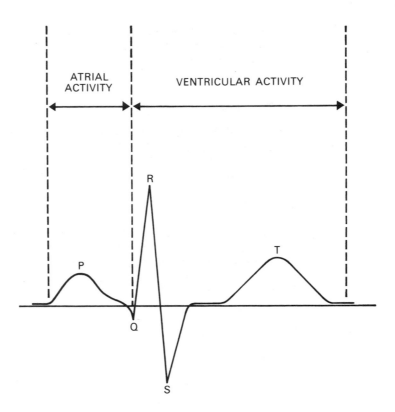

Figure 7.11
Normal ECG deflections

Cardiac monitoring

Cardiac monitoring is a means of demonstrating continuously on a small screen the electrical activity of the heart. Monitoring is especially valuable when serious disturbance of heart rate and rhythm is present or suspected, for instance, following myocardial infarction or cardiac surgery. Serious arrhythmias may endanger life. Prompt observation, reporting and treatment of changes on the oscilloscope may prevent sudden death.

Valuable as monitoring is, the nurse must remember that it is merely an aid to, not a substitute for, skilled observation of the patient.

Chest X-ray

X-ray is essential for full cardiac assessment of the patient. It shows an outline of the heart and lungs indicating enlargement of the chambers of the heart, displacement of the vessels, calcification of the valves and the diffuse congestion of lung fields in pulmonary oedema.

Anteroposterior and oblique films are taken either in a radiography department or by a portable machine at the patient's bedside. A nurse should remember the need for warmth, privacy, explanation and reassurance during the procedure, and should ensure that it is carried out with minimal strain to the patient.

Cardiac catheterization

The passing of a small flexible tube into either side of the heart and the coronary arteries is now a widely practised technique to establish the exact cardiac diagnosis and to measure the severity of abnormalities, generally prior to surgical correction (Fig. 7.12).

Right heart catheterization
A radio-opaque catheter is passed into an arm or leg vein and advanced to the chambers of the right side of the heart, entering the right atrium and passing on as far as the pulmonary artery (Fig. 7.13).

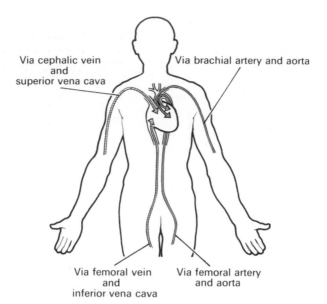

Figure 7.12
Cardiac catheterization routes

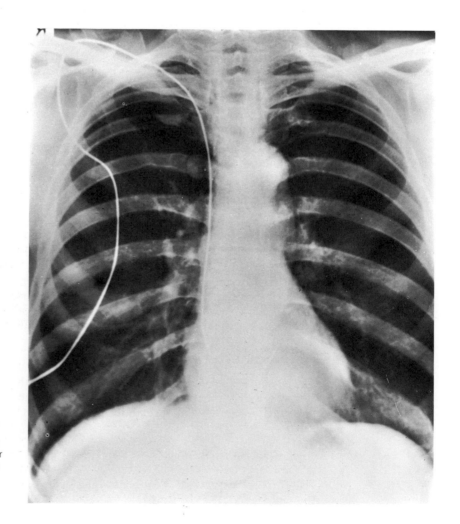

Figure 7.13
Right heart catheterization
The catheter has been passed via
the right subclavian vein, superior
vena cava and right atrium to the
right ventricle

Left heart catheterization

The catheter is introduced into the femoral artery in the groin or the brachial artery in the arm and is passed back to the left side of the heart, entering by the aorta. This route is also used to examine the coronary arteries which arise from the aorta.

Angiography

A radio-opaque dye can be injected via the catheters and simultaneous, high-speed cine-radiography carried out. This will demonstrate the anatomy of the heart, any abnormalities of the blood flow, or of the chambers, great arteries and coronary arteries.

The uses of cardiac catheterization are:

1. To measure pressure within the chambers and vessels of the heart. When the mitral valve is stenosed or narrowed, for example, pressure will be abnormally high in the left atrium.

2. To obtain blood samples from the chambers and vessels. In atrial septal defect, for instance, oxygenated blood from the left atrium may shunt to the right atrium, producing abnormally high oxygenation of the venous blood in the right atrium.

3. To outline abnormal anatomy or function by the injection of dye — angiography. This will show, for example, narrowed or blocked coronary arteries, abnormal blood flow through septal defects and backflow of blood through incompetent valves.

These procedures require great skill and involve risks to the patient of haemorrhage, arrhythmias and infection. Explanation of the procedure should only be given by a person thoroughly familiar with it. The amount of detail provided will depend on the intelligence and knowledge of the patient, the extent of his almost certain anxiety or fear and his desire or demand to know about the procedure. The test may involve several hours lying on an X-ray table surrounded by seemingly threatening equipment and machinery. Administration of a mild sedative before the procedure, plus careful explanation and reassurance during it, is necessary.

Precatheter preparation

A light meal may be given before the test. Local anaesthetic is injected at the site of introduction of the catheter.

Postcatheter care and observations

The nurse's main responsibilities are:

1. *The site.* Quarter hourly observations for haemorrhage must be made for the first few hours. This is especially important after arterial puncture, since arterial bleeding may be brisk and heavy. Bruising or swelling around the pressure bandage may indicate formation of a haematoma (collection of blood). If bleeding occurs, firm pressure must be applied and help called immediately. The patient must have access to a bed-side bell to call a nurse if bleeding occurs.

2. *Pulse.* Quarter hourly observation for the first 2 hours, or longer if necessary noting rate, rhythm and volume. Rising rate and weak volume may indicate haemorrhage. Irregularity of rhythm may indicate the onset of an arrhythmia. Changes should be reported immediately.

3. *Temperature.* Pyrexia may indicate infection.

4. *Pain.* Any complaint of pain whether at puncture site, limb, chest or abdomen should be considered abnormal and reported at once to the doctor.

CONGENITAL HEART DISEASE

Congenital abnormalities may be mild or severe, single or multiple; the clinical manifestations are therefore variable. The owner of a minimally malformed heart may go through life symptomless and completely unaware of the defect. Severe or multiple defects, on the other hand, will cause serious incapacity and may be incompatible with life, the child being born dead or dying soon after birth.

The cause may be genetic, or it may be an environmental factor affecting the mother during early pregnancy. German measles occurring during the first 3 months of pregnancy may give rise to heart lesions through arrested or faulty development of the fetus. There may be other causes as yet unknown.

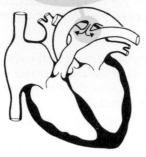

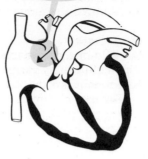

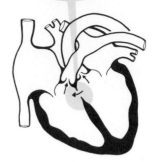

Figure 7.14
Example of congenital defect: Patent ductus arteriosus (PDA)

Figure 7.15
Example of congenital defect: atrial septal defect (ASD)

Figure 7.16
Example of congenital defect: ventricular septal defect (VSD)

Examples of some clinical conditions are shown in Figures 7.14 to 7.16.

Clinical features

In general, the larger the defect the earlier its presence becomes apparent, and if it permits the mixing of arterial and venous blood, as in ventricular septal defect, the child will be cyanosed. Cyanosis, dyspnoea, failure to thrive, clubbing of the fingers and heart murmurs are features common to many congenital heart diseases. A small defect may go unnoticed until the child or adult is much older and perhaps being examined at school, for employment or for insurance.

Investigations

Full clinical examination.
Chest X-ray.
ECG.
Cardiac catheterization.

Complications

Bacterial endocarditis.
Chest infection.
Cardiac failure.

Treatment and nursing care

Many congenital abnormalities are corrected by surgery. The prognosis depends largely upon the severity of the defect, the success of surgery, the patient's resilience to surgery and its possible complications.

Preferably a patient undergoing cardiac surgery is nursed at first in an intensive care unit by specially trained staff, and convalescence is continued in a general ward until he is ready to go home. Since important complications include haemorrhage, arrhythmias and infection, it is essential that the nursing staff observe him closely during this period. Supervision will continue at home and progress will be assessed carefully at hospital out-patient clinics for at least a year.

RHEUMATIC HEART DISEASE

Rheumatic fever is a chronic, inflammatory disease commonest between the ages of 5 and 15 years. The course of the disease is generally punctuated by recurrent, acute attacks.

Acute rheumatic fever

Acute rheumatic fever is still the principal cause of cardiac death and disability in the young adult. It follows infection with, and abnormal immunological response to, the

Group A haemolytic streptococcus. Between the streptococcal infection, usually as a sore throat, and the onset of rheumatic fever there is a latent period of 1 to 3 weeks. The effect of the disease may be widespread throughout the body, but especially involved are connective tissues, such as heart valves, heart muscle, joints and tendons.

Clinical features
Onset. Acute pharyngitis is followed after a few weeks by either a gradual onset of malaise, anorexia, low grade fever and weight loss, or a sudden onset of joint pain with high fever, sweating and tachycardia.

Polyarthritis. This is characterized by pain in joints. The joints most often affected are knees, ankles, elbows and wrists. They become swollen, painful, hot and tender, and the pain tends to be 'flitting' in nature, moving from one joint to another.

Rheumatic nodules. Painless, subcutaneous nodules appear, attached to tendons or over bony prominences such as the elbows, knees or back of the head.

Erythema marginatum. Reddish, crescent-shaped patches appear on the trunk.

Carditis. Heart involvement is the most serious feature of acute rheumatic fever. It takes three forms: endocarditis, myocarditis and pericarditis.

1. *Endocarditis.* Inflammation of the endocardium affects the valves. Characteristic minute warty vegetations form along the valve margins. Dilatation of the valve ring may result in the valve leaking, and when the doctor listens to the heart there may be abnormal murmurs.

2. *Myocarditis.* Inflammation of the myocardium is suggested by a rapid pulse rate. Often the pulse is faster than one would expect for the degree of fever present, and it may persist when the fever subsides. Irregularity of heart rhythm and pulse may occur. Cardiac failure may develop, and the heart may enlarge. Such an enlargement can be seen on X-ray and may be accompanied by changes in ECG.

3. *Pericarditis.* Inflammation of the pericardium usually indicates severe infection. Chest pain may result and is often aggravated by movement, breathing or coughing. An effusion of serous fluid may accumulate in the pericardial sac.

Investigations
Full history of past and present illness is taken, noting particularly any episodes of sore throat. Full physical examination and auscultation of the heart are carried out. ECG and chest X-ray are necessary. Common findings in the blood are a raised white cell count, anaemia, a raised erythrocyte sedimentation rate and a high ASO (antistreptolysin 'O') titre giving evidence of a recent streptococcal infection. A throat swab is sent for bacteriological investigation; it may show haemolytic streptococcus.

Nursing observations
Temperature. Fever is common and is reduced by the administration of salicylates. The fever is associated with profuse sweating, which is increased by the salicylates.

Pulse. A rapid pulse is associated with fever but the tachycardia of rheumatic fever is often unusually persistent and disproportionately severe and it may indicate damage to the heart muscle. To assess the rate more accurately, sleeping pulse rates are recorded; this eliminates increase caused by anxiety, activity or excitement. Any irregularity of rhythm must be reported immediately as it may give early indication of myocardial damage.

Blood pressure and respiratory rate. Both are important when there is risk of cardiac failure with associated dyspnoea and fall in cardiac output.

Fluid balance. While fever, sweating and anorexia persist, careful assessment of fluid and dietary intake and of urinary output is essential.

Course and complications
The course of rheumatic fever may be short and acute or it may be prolonged for many months. Recurrent attacks are common with the risk of increasing cardiac damage and heart failure with each attack. The very young child rarely escapes cardiac damage, but risk diminishes with age. Most people affected live relatively normal lives until 40 or 50 years of age when the complications of chronic rheumatic heart disease become evident. The incidence and severity of rheumatic fever and of its sequel, chronic rheumatic heart disease, has declined in the last 50 years in the Western world due to better social

conditions, less overcrowding and risk of cross infection, the use of antibiotics and change in the virulence of streptococci.

Treatment and nursing care

Until the active stage of the disease is over, complete rest is essential until joint pain eases, fever and pulse rate subside and white cell count and ESR are normal. This may take several weeks. During the acute stage, help with washing and personal hygiene and with meals will be wanted and needed, but it is important that independence should be restored as quickly as possible, especially with children and adolescents who may easily become restless and bored. Continuous bed rest, profuse sweating, and inadequate nutrition increase the risk of pressure sores. Frequent washing and drying of the skin and observation of all pressure areas, relief of pressure, dry, crease-free bed linen and a daily bed-bath are necessary. Tepid sponging and the use of a bed-side fan and salicylates will reduce pyrexia.

Painful joints should be handled gently and warm cotton wool wrappings may ease discomfort. Passive limb physiotherapy is given to promote adequate circulation and venous return, and a bed cradle is used to protect joints from the weight of the bed clothes. During the acute illness when there is fever, malaise and poor appetite, weight will be lost and dehydration will be a danger. A light diet is given with additional nourishing fluids until appetite and temperature return to normal. No dietary restrictions are necessary except salt restriction if cardiac failure develops (p. 240).

A dry, furred tongue is associated with fever. The mouth should be examined regularly for cleanliness and rinsed frequently. It is important to observe the teeth for dental caries and the gums for infection, since such an infection may be associated with subacute bacterial endocarditis (p. 231).

Urinary output must be observed, especially while fever and sweating persist. Constipation is common during fever and a mild oral aperient may be given. If the patient is allowed to use a bed-side commode or is wheeled to the toilet on a sani-chair, some of the anxiety and stress of having to use bedpans will be avoided.

Sound, pain-free rest is essential, and the nurse should report episodes of restlessness or wakefulness.

Penicillin is given to combat the streptococcal infection in the nose or throat. A course of intramuscular injections is followed by prophylactic oral therapy, lasting possibly for many years into adult life, to prevent further attacks of the disease. It is vital that any recurrence of symptoms be reported immediately to the family doctor.

Salicylates are given in large doses to reduce fever and pain. Calcium aspirin is preferred to sodium salicylate, since the former is more soluble and less likely to cause gastric irritation or to precipitate cardiac failure. Steroids are given because of their anti-inflammatory properties. They are most effective in severe cases where there is evidence of cardiac involvement, for instance carditis.

Digitalis, diuretic therapy and salt restriction will be started if cardiac failure develops (p. 240). A tranquilliser to ease anxiety and a sedative to promote rest and sleep may be given.

Support, encouragement and reassurance must be given not only to the patient but also to his parents and family, who may be frightened by the prospect or presence of heart damage. The family must be helped to understand the illness and the reasons for the care given, and their assistance must be obtained in planning activities for convalescence in hospital or at home. Parents are encouraged to visit young children frequently, and schooling may be continued in hospital. Whenever possible, convalescence continues at home under the supervision of the family doctor and community nurses, provided that the parents, family and the patient are able to cope reliably with continuing drug therapy and with regulating a gradual increase in activity.

Chronic rheumatic heart disease

Following acute rheumatic fever and recurrences of the disease, rheumatic endocarditis may smoulder on for many years producing chronic rheumatic heart disease. This takes the form of valvular heart disease and presents sometimes in early adult life, but more often many years later, in middle or old age. Rheumatic endocarditis causes

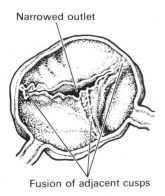

Narrowed outlet

Fusion of adjacent cusps

Figure 7.17
Valve stenosis

inflammation and distortion of the valve cusps and eventually fibrosis and calcification of the valve ring. This leads to different degrees of:

Stenosis or narrowing of the valves, causing obstruction to blood flow.
Incompetence or imperfect closure of the valve, resulting in leakage and backflow of blood (regurgitation).

A valve may be stenosed or incompetent, or both (Fig. 7.17). Patients may have disease of more than one valve.

Mitral valve disease

Mitral stenosis is more common than incompetence, but combined stenosis and incompetence often occur. As the mitral valve narrows, pressure in the left atrium rises and is transmitted back to the pulmonary veins and capillaries (p. 214). Lung congestion follows, making breathing more difficult, and the patient complains of progressive shortness of breath and tiredness. Dyspnoea appears first on exercise, but eventually less and less exercise is required to produce it. Orthopnoea, paroxysmal nocturnal dyspnoea and acute pulmonary oedema may result — that is the features of left heart failure occur, followed eventually, perhaps after many years, by right heart failure (p. 241).

Atrial fibrillation

This is commonly associated with mitral stenosis. Atrial fibrillation is an arrhythmia of the heart in which the atria fail to contract regularly but rather 'twitch' feebly and rapidly. Normally each atrial contraction is followed by ventricular contraction as the nervous impulse is passed through the heart's conducting system (p. 215). When the atria fibrillate, the ventricles respond erratically and inefficiently.

The pulse is the wave of distension felt in the arteries in response to each contraction of the left ventricle. Therefore, if the ventricles contract irregularly and with variable force, not every contraction will be strong enough to open the aortic valve and produce a palpable pulse wave of distension, and the pulse will be irregular in both time and force (rhythm and volume). This will produce what is known as a **pulse deficit**, where the heart rate is greater than the pulse rate. The pulse deficit is estimated by simultaneous recordings of heart rate, by auscultation at the apex, and of pulse rate, by taking the radial pulse at the wrist. It is vital that the nurse reports immediately an irregularity of the pulse because it might indicate the onset of atrial fibrillation.

Atrial fibrillation is an important complication; weak and erratic contraction of the atria and the ventricles, altered blood flow and poor emptying of the chambers will result in stasis of blood, which in turn will allow thrombi to form. When dislodged from the left side of the heart, systemic embolism occurs, which may block cerebral, limb, renal or mesenteric arteries (Fig. 7.37).

Mitral valve disease is also assessed on auscultation by the presence of altered heart sounds and murmurs. X-ray will show an enlarged left atrium; this is best seen when the patient has a barium swallow, in which the barium-filled oesophagus is displaced backwards by a bulging left atrium. Cardiac catheterization may be carried out to measure the pressures in the chambers of the left side of the heart, or dye may be injected to assess whether backflow of blood is present, indicating mitral incompetence. The course of mitral valve disease is one of gradual deterioration, and complications are common.

Mitral valve disease also increases the risk of chest infection and chronic bronchitis, since either is more likely to develop when there is pulmonary congestion. Following left-sided heart failure and pulmonary congestion right heart failure gradually appears.

Aortic valve disease

Disease of the aortic valve is often due to rheumatic endocarditis, but it may also be caused by congenital malformation or syphilis. Stenosis and incompetence may occur singly or together.

Aortic stenosis

Stenosis causes an increased work load for the left ventricle, as it tries to overcome the obstruction of the narrowed valve. The left ventricle compensates by enlargement of individual muscle fibres (hypertrophy). Left ventricular hypertrophy increases as stenosis increases. Gradually, the coronary arteries become unable to meet the demands of the hypertrophied muscle for blood and angina is felt. While the heart compensates in this way fairly normal activities are possible, but eventually the heart fails. Left heart failure is followed by right heart failure; the earliest symptoms of the former are breathlessness and fatigue. Angina and syncope on exertion, for example fainting on climbing a hill, are both important features. Sudden death may occur.

On auscultation, heart murmurs and altered heart sounds are heard, and ECG and X-ray will show evidence of left ventricular enlargement. Cardiac catheterization will give detailed information about the severity of the valve lesion. Heart failure is the most frequent complication requiring treatment (p. 240). Cardiac surgery is carried out in severe cases where there is great risk of sudden death. Because of this risk, skill and patience are required from doctors and nurses to explain to the patient the need for major cardiac surgery, especially when the signs of the disease outweigh the symptoms and the patient does not perceive himself as being either severely disabled or at risk.

Aortic incompetence
Incompetence of the valve allows backflow of blood into the left ventricle during diastole. By increasing the volume of blood to be expelled, the work load of the left ventricle is increased, leading to left ventricular hypertrophy and eventual left heart failure.

Pulmonary and tricuspid valve disease
Pulmonary valve disease is uncommon; it is usually congenital in origin, and may be associated with a ventricular septal defect or Fallot's tetralogy.

Most patients with tricuspid disease will also have mitral and aortic disease, rheumatic in origin. Stenosis and incompetence give rise to right heart failure. Obstructed blood flow through the narrowed valve and backflow through the incompetent valve will cause, in the right atrium, a rise in pressure, which will be transmitted back to the venae cavae and systemic venous return.

Since chronic rheumatic heart disease is progressively disabling, careful follow-up is necessary at intervals dictated by the rate of progression of the disease, by the development of complications and by the degree of cardiac failure present. Cardiac failure must be treated and controlled (p. 240), but eventually cardiac surgery will be advised, usually following a very careful assessment of the nature and extent of the valve disease.

Treatment of valvular heart disease
Cardiac surgery may greatly improve a patient's condition and increase life expectancy. The risks of surgery itself and of subsequent complications are nevertheless considerable. Physicians and surgeons will make careful assessment of a patient's condition and discuss their clinical findings in detail before a decision is made. Surgery may be 'closed' or 'open'.

Closed heart surgery
In closed heart surgery, the circulation continues to flow through the heart. To relieve stenosis of the mitral valve, for example, a dilator is positioned in the valve to stretch it and thus relieve obstruction. This procedure is known as **mitral valvotomy**. Restenosis may occur several years after surgery and valvotomy may be repeated two or three times. As the valve becomes more rigid and calcified, replacement using artificial valves becomes necessary.

Open heart surgery
In open heart surgery or **cardiopulmonary bypass**, the heart and lungs are emptied of blood. Venous blood is drained from the superior and inferior venae cavae into an oxygenator. A pump recirculates the blood and returns it via the femoral artery or the aorta (Fig. 7.18). This technique is used for **replacement of valves**. There are several types of valve in use:

1. *Mechanical valves.* (a) Ball and socket type — Starr-Edwards valve (Fig. 7.19). (b) Disc type — Bjork Shiley valve. Because of the risk of thrombus formation on the

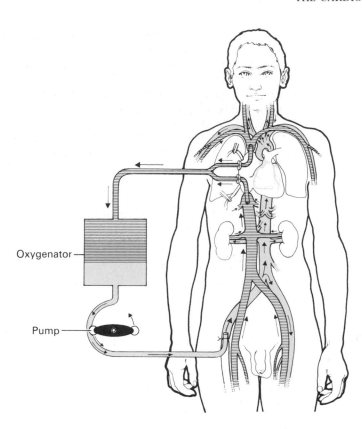

Figure 7.18
Cardiopulmonary bypass

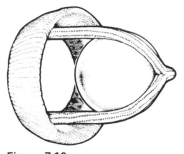

Figure 7.19
Starr-Edwards aortic valve
prosthesis

valves, patients require anticoagulant therapy, sometimes for life; although this may successfully prevent embolism, it will add to the risk of haemorrhage.

2. *Biological valves.* (a) Homografts — these are of human tissue and include valves which are obtained within 12 hours of death but which may be stored for a limited period only, and valves fashioned from tissue taken from the patient himself, such as the fascia lata valve. (b) Heterografts — non-human tissue is used, for instance pig valves. Anticoagulant therapy is not necessary with homograft and heterograft valves, but infection is a risk with all three types, and the Starr-Edwards valve may cause anaemia, since the action of the valve causes destruction of blood cells (haemolysis). Patients who are about to undergo surgery may appreciate the chance to talk to someone who has already successfully undergone the same operation. Many such patients are members of special clubs or associations. However, some postoperative patients take delight in giving detailed accounts of their own experiences which, to the anxious pre-operative patient, are very frightening. Nurses should be alert to this danger and should refer the patient to a senior member of staff who will be able to give the necessary information clearly and with reassurance.

Subacute bacterial endocarditis

Subacute bacterial endocarditis is most often caused by the micro-organism *Streptococcus viridans*. The disease usually affects hearts already damaged by rheumatic valve disease or by congenital defects, or it may infect prosthetic valves. Because *Strep. viridans* is often found in infected gums, teeth, or tonsils, bacterial endocarditis may occur after dental treatment or extraction when the bacteria are released into the bloodstream. The infection in the bloodstream causes large, loosely adherent vegetations to form on the valves (Fig. 7.20). The vegetations of rheumatic endocarditis are smaller and more adherent.

Clinical features

The patient complains of malaise, anorexia and tiredness. A prolonged, unexplained fever is often present. Many patients are anaemic, and the white cell count (Ch. 8) and the ESR are raised. Petechial haemorrhages into the skin (Ch. 8) and splinter

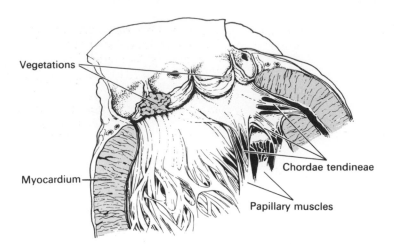

Figure 7.20
Vegetations of bacterial
endocarditis on valve

haemorrhages under the nails may develop. Osler's nodes, appear—raised, tender nodes on the fingers or toes. Heart murmurs develop, due to the inflammation of the valves. The spleen is often enlarged and haematuria may be present.

Investigations

The findings of unexplained pyrexia in patients with valvular or congenital heart disease, or in those who have undergone cardiac surgery, is significant. There may be a history of dental treatment or infection. The diagnosis is confirmed on obtaining a positive blood culture. Many specimens of blood are carefully taken under strict asepsis to eliminate the possibility of a false positive through contamination of the specimen. By examining the culture medium under the microscope, the infecting organism will be identified.

Nursing observations

Accurate recordings of temperature and of pulse rate and rhythm are vital to assess the course of fever and as an indication of effectiveness or abnormality of heart action. Weight gain or loss is assessed daily if cardiac failure is present, and observation of general appearance, appetite, vitality and mental state is important, particularly when the course of the disease is long and wearying.

Course and complications

The course of the disease may be long, and the length of treatment depends on the patient's response to antibiotics. Before antibiotic therapy was introduced, almost all patients died, and even to-day the disease is serious, especially if there is delay in starting antibiotics. The main danger is embolism from the vegetations on the endocardium of the valves. Emboli may lodge in the brain causing hemiplegia, in the kidneys causing renal damage, in the skin causing haemorrhages, in the retinae causing loss of vision, or in the spleen, limb or mesenteric vessels (Fig. 7.37). Because of severe valve disease, heart failure develops.

Treatment and nursing care

The selection of antibiotic depends on sensitivity tests. Benzylpenicillin is often used, large doses being given intramuscularly. Over many days and possibly weeks, this may cause severe discomfort to the patient, and careful observation of injection sites for local reaction is required, together with strict aseptic technique in the preparation and administration of injections. Continuous intravenous infusion of antibiotics may be necessary. Several antibiotics may be used where fever and infection persist or resistance develops. Oral antibiotics will be given when the temperature falls, indicating a response to treatment.

As in rheumatic fever itself, while endocarditis persists bed rest may be prolonged. During the period of bed rest and fever, the same meticulous care of the skin, pressure areas and mouth, and the same observation of bladder and bowel function and sleep pattern will be necessary. Mobilization begins when signs of a response to drug therapy appear. When the patient is discharged from hospital, the following are essential:

1. To take all drugs as prescribed to maintain therapeutic blood levels.
2. To attend follow-up clinics regularly.
3. To treat promptly any upper respiratory tract infection.
4. To undergo prophylactic penicillin therapy before and after dental extraction or treatment.

CORONARY HEART DISEASE

Coronary arteries (Fig. 7.21) are commonly affected by the degenerative disease atherosclerosis. **Atherosclerosis** is the condition in which fatty substances such as cholesterol are deposited in the lining of arteries in the form of atheromatous plaques. These plaques narrow the lumen of the artery causing reduction in the blood supply to the myocardium: **myocardial ischaemia**. This may result in the pain of **angina**. Thrombus may form on the surface of the plaque eventually blocking the artery: **coronary thrombosis**. Blockage of blood supply to the myocardium causes necrosis or death of the area of muscle served by that artery: **myocardial infarction**.

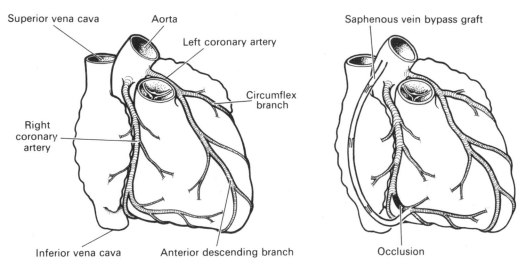

Figure 7.21
Normal coronary arteries

Figure 7.22
Coronary arteries showing blocked artery and bypass graft

Coronary artery disease is the most common type of heart disease and the most frequent cause of death in middle and old age in developed countries. It has been shown that certain risk factors are significant in the development of coronary artery disease. The incidence of the disease is rising and some risk factors may reflect the changing pressures and way of life in the Western world today. In the last 40 years there has been a steady increase in incidence in all classes, especially in men under 45 years and to a lesser extent in women over 50 years. The risk factors are:

1. **Diet.** A diet high in saturated (animal) fats (Ch. 4) is related to high blood cholesterol levels. The higher the blood cholesterol level, the greater the risk of developing atheroma.
2. **Hypertension.** Hypertension accelerates the development of atherosclerosis. The higher the blood pressure the greater the risk of developing coronary artery disease.
3. **Smoking.** Atherosclerosis, myocardial infarction and sudden death are far more prevalent in smokers than non-smokers.
4. **Heredity.** Atherosclerosis tends to run in families.
5. **Exercise.** Atheroma occurs more often in people with sedentary jobs than in those who do manual work. Lack of regular physical exercise is more common in this age of car transport, and it has been shown that exercise lowers plasma cholesterol levels.
6. **Obesity.** Through the association with hypertension, high dietary intake of animal fat and lack of exercise, obese people are more often at risk.

7. **Tension and anxiety.** People who show marked drive, who have a competitive nature and who experience emotional tension and stress, are claimed to have a higher incidence of coronary artery disease.

Angina pectoris

The pain of angina is caused by inadequate blood supply to and oxygenation of the myocardium (myocardial ischaemia) generally as a result of coronary atherosclerosis. Angina is also felt if the myocardial oxygen need is increased, for example in hypertension or aortic stenosis, which cause left ventricular hypertrophy (p. 238), or if the blood carries less oxygen, as in anaemia.

Clinical features
The characteristics of anginal pain are described on page 217. Anxiety and a rapid pulse rate often accompany pain.

Investigations
1. History. Diagnosis can usually be made from the history of pain. Often all the major characteristics are present.
2. ECG. During an attack of angina, ECG changes occur and these can be provoked by an exercise test. The patient is attached to ECG electrodes and exercises on steps or a treadmill. ECG changes often occur when the coronary arteries fail to supply the myocardium with enough oxygen to meet the extra demands made on it by exercise.
3. Cardiac catheterization — coronary angiography. The injection of dye outlines the vessels and shows the extent and severity of atheroma (p. 225).

Nursing observations
A nurse must observe a patient for any sign of restlessness or anxiety which might indicate the onset of angina and must train herself to assess and report an episode in terms of the major characteristics of pain already mentioned.

Course and complications
Patients with angina generally survive 5 to 10 years. Many live 20 years or more, but there is always risk of acute myocardial infarction or sudden death.

Treatment and nursing care
Rest is encouraged, but unnecessary restrictions can make the person consider himself an invalid, and an optimistic attitude will help him to overcome or adjust to his disability. Generally it is enough to use common sense to modify activity, avoid overwork, worry or anxiety and live within the limits of the pain.

Obesity should be corrected, large meals avoided and a diet low in saturated fat may be recommended. Cigarette smoking should be stopped. Exercise is encouraged provided it does not provoke pain.

Drugs
1. Glyceryl trinitrate. Angina may be prevented and relieved by taking a tablet of glyceryl trinitrate sublingually. The drug is not addictive and as many tablets as are necessary to relieve the pain may be taken; patients should always carry their tablets with them and should be taught to use them prophylactically before exertion. The drug causes lowering of blood pressure and hence a reduction in the work of the heart and, in some cases, dilatation of the coronary arteries.
2. Beta receptor blocking drugs, so-called 'beta blockers', propranolol, metoprolol, oxprenolol. These drugs block the stimulant effect of the sympathetic nervous system, which increases the rate and force of the heart beat. By reducing these, they reduce the oxygen demands of the myocardium. Angina is thus prevented by reduction of oxygen demand.

Surgery
In recent years, surgery has been used for severe angina. It is carried out by grafting blood vessels to bypass blocked arteries, for example by using a saphenous vein from

the patient to provide a bypass from aorta to peripheral coronary artery (Fig. 7.22), or by implantation of an internal mammary artery into the myocardium.

Myocardial infarction

Irreversible damage to an area of myocardium occurs when the coronary artery serving that area is blocked by thrombus or atheroma (p. 233). The site of infarction depends on the vessel blocked; the size of infarction varies, and the area of muscle involved may be small or very extensive.

Clinical features

Pain is the major symptom. The nurse should note carefully its features and how it compares with anginal pain (p. 217). The sudden onset of severe, prolonged pain is associated with distress, sweating, pallor, nausea and vomiting. Many patients will describe having had a worsening of angina or a vague feeling of illhealth for some weeks before the acute attack.

Investigations

Diagnosis is established according to:

1. Clinical examination and history of the characteristic features of the pain.
2. ECG changes—daily recordings of ECG are taken, as infarction produces a recognizable series of changes over several days in most patients.
3. Levels of serum enzymes — when heart muscle is damaged, enzymes present in the muscle are released into the bloodstream and their levels are measured daily over several days. Serum glutamic oxaloacetic transaminase (SGOT)–peak level is reached quickly and returns to normal in 3 to 5 days. Lactic dehydrogenase (LDH)–peak level is reached more slowly and levels are elevated for up to 2 or 3 weeks.

Nursing observations

Relief of pain and anxiety is vital, and nurses must observe for and report any sign of pallor, sweating, anxiety or restlessness which might indicate returning pain.

Temperature. Fever occurs during the first few days. The temperature is usually recorded 4 hourly during this period.

Pulse. Recordings are made hourly at first, noting rate, rhythm and volume. When cardiac monitoring ends, usually after 48 hours, and there is no longer a visual image of the heart beat, it becomes all the more important to report any change in the pulse so that an ECG can be taken to establish the exact nature of the change.

Blood pressure. Hourly recordings are taken initially; changes will indicate altered cardiac output.

Respirations. Dyspnoea may indicate the onset of left heart failure.

Fluid balance. When cardiac output is impaired and renal blood flow is reduced, fluid intake and output must be accurately measured.

Complications

The risk of sudden death is great, and it occurs within minutes of onset in 25 per cent of cases. For this reason mobile coronary care units carrying equipment for immediate treatment or for resuscitation are being used in several centres. They enable help to reach the patient during the first critical hours by providing treatment in his home and by stabilizing his condition sufficiently and keeping him under continuous cardiac monitoring before undertaking the journey to an intensive care unit. The overall risk will depend on the patient's age, the size of infarction and whether there has been previous infarction; after the first 48 hours, the risk quickly lessens.

There are several important complications following myocardial infarction.

Arrhythmias

Most patients have an alteration in heart rate, rhythm or conduction during the first 48 hours. Nursing and medical staff of coronary care units are specially trained in the use of cardiac monitors to observe, interpret and treat arrhythmias as they occur, thus preventing cardiac failure and cardiac arrest. Ventricular fibrillation (in which the ventricles do not contract but rather 'twitch' so that cardiac output ceases) is the most serious arrhythmia. Death results in the untreated case (p. 246).

Cardiogenic shock
In extensive infarction, the condition may deteriorate very quickly due to a fall in cardiac output and blood pressure. The patient will be cyanosed, pale, cold, sweating and often has mental confusion.

Other complications
These include:

Cardiac failure, both left-sided, with pulmonary oedema early, and right-sided later.
Systemic arterial embolism blocking cerebral, mesenteric, renal or peripheral arteries resulting from 'mural' thrombi on the infarcted wall of the left ventricle (Fig. 7.37).
Pulmonary embolism following deep venous thrombosis in the legs.
Ventricular aneurysm and rupture of the heart wall causing sudden death.

Treatment and nursing care

Relief of pain. This is urgent. An opiate, usually morphine, is given immediately intramuscularly, together with an antiemetic such as cyclizine, since morphine causes vomiting. This is repeated until the acute pain has eased. To relieve fear and anxiety, a tranquilliser, for example diazepam, is given for several days or longer if anxiety persists despite reassurance. Other drugs are started as necessary such as a night sedative to aid sleep, drugs to control arrhythmias or anticoagulants to reduce the risk of thromboembolism.

Rest. Complete bed rest is essential at first. If shocked and hypotensive, the patient lies flat in bed and everything is done for him. If the infarction is not severe, once pain is eased he is allowed to feed himself; is encouraged to exercise his legs in bed to improve venous return and to help prevent the formation of deep venous thrombosis; and is allowed to use a bed-side commode. The nurse must anticipate the patient's needs to avoid his straining. The bed-side locker must be within reach and anything he might need must be at hand. He must have some means, such as a bell, of summoning a nurse. All movement must be gentle and two nurses must 'double lift' the patient.

Personal hygiene. While bed rest continues the following are necessary: daily bed-bath, frequent observation and care of pressure areas and observation of the mouth. Oxygen is given while there is pain, dyspnoea or cardiac failure. Although humidified, oxygen therapy may dry the mouth, therefore frequent mouthwashes are usually necessary. After 2 or 3 days the patient is allowed to wash himself with help. Most patients worry about bowel function but find using a commode less stressful than using a bed-pan. Straining at stool must be avoided and constipation for 2 or 3 days is not harmful provided the patient is reassured that normal function can easily be restored by giving a mild oral aperient or suppositories. A sanichair is used to wheel the patient to the toilet until he is able to walk.

Diet. If the patient is obese, a low calorie diet is started. Restriction of animal fat may be advised. Meals should be light initially. Salt restriction is necessary only if severe cardiac failure develops (p. 240).

Mobilization. The pattern of mobilization has changed greatly in recent years and early ambulation is now encouraged. The patient may be allowed to sit out of bed from the second or third day and to walk from the sixth or seventh day. The length of time out of bed and the distance walked are gradually increased, but both are delayed or restricted if the patient becomes tired, if the infarction is extensive or if complications develop. After two or three weeks in hospital the patient is discharged home. The family doctor then supervises convalescence.

Rehabilitation

Following infarction both the patient and his family will be anxious about the future and the possible alteration of their lives. A nurse can help to relieve this anxiety by calmly explaining with reassurance and optimism what is meant by a heart attack and that normal life is possible despite it.

The team involved in helping the patient and his family includes not just hospital staff but also community colleagues. In many areas liaison schemes are being developed in which the community nurse visits the patient and his family while he is in hospital and continues to give support when he is discharged. Booklets have been compiled giving advice and answering some questions which often arise regarding, for instance, diet, how to lose weight or restrict animal fat, the need to stop smoking, the need to take exercise and how to gradually increase it, the need to avoid emotional stress. Car driving may not be advisable for 3 months. Sexual intercourse, which greatly increases heart rate, is not advisable during the first 2 months. Return to work is usually possible after 2 to 3 months but a change to a lighter job may be beneficial.

It is hoped that in years to come we may be able to reverse the present trend of rising incidence of coronary heart disease by preventive measures — such as preventing the development of atheroma. Health visitors, district nurses and general practitioners are assisting with prevention schemes. Patients who have had myocardial infarction, their families and selected groups of the population, are being screened about their health and way of life in terms of the risk factors previously mentioned (p. 233). Success may depend on each of us being prepared to alter in some way our present mode of living.

ABNORMALITIES OF BLOOD PRESSURE

Blood pressure varies widely from person to person and, within one individual, it varies throughout the day; therefore, it is difficult to define normality.

The cardiac output and the peripheral vascular resistance are the two main factors which determine arterial blood pressure. Peripheral resistance is determined by arteriolar tone. If the arterioles are narrowed by vasoconstriction the pressure in the arterioles rises and hypertension results.

Hypertension

Blood pressure is considered abnormally high if it consistently exceeds 150/90 mmHg in a person who is resting quietly.

When high blood pressure is secondary to a recognizable disease it is called **secondary hypertension**. In the younger patient, hypertension is more often 'secondary' and successful treatment is more likely through correction of the cause. The most important conditions to which hypertension can be secondary are:

1. Renal diseases, such as glomerulonephritis and chronic pyelonephritis.
2. Endocrine diseases, for example tumour of the adrenal gland.
3. Coarctation (narrowing) of the aorta.
4. Toxaemia of pregnancy.

In some forms of kidney disease the enzyme renin is liberated into the bloodstream from the damaged kidney. Renin acts on a substance in the blood to produce a vasoconstrictor agent, thus causing hypertension.

In most middle-aged persons no definite cause can be found; this type is called **essential hypertension**. It is the commonest form, affecting men and women equally, usually between the ages of 40 and 60 years.

Essential hypertension can be further divided into two groups, benign and malignant. Benign hypertension is mild and may even be symptomless. Malignant hypertension, on the other hand, is a severe form of the disease characterized by papilloedema (p. 238), a very high diastolic pressure and renal failure. Usually the onset is rapid and the course brief, although it is possible for a person known to have benign essential hypertension to move into the malignant phase after a number of years. Younger people are more often affected, typically between the ages of 30 to 40 years. The prognosis is poor and few patients survive more than a year without treatment.

Associated factors
In normal individuals, a transient increase in blood pressure occurs with anxiety, cold and exercise. Pressure also rises with age. Obesity and emotional stress are contributory factors and there is definite evidence of an hereditary factor and strong familial tendency to hypertension.

Clinical features

These are extremely variable and there may be no symptoms for many years. The disease affects coronary, renal and cerebral vessels and the myocardium; it should also be remembered that hypertension accelerates the development of atherosclerosis in coronary, renal and cerebral vessels (p. 251).

Level of blood pressure

Severity of hypertension is not judged by level of blood pressure alone. The course of the disease may vary in patients with similar heights of blood pressure. At first the blood pressure is 'labile', that is, it becomes abnormally high in response to emotion, anxiety or exercise. Eventually hypertension is found at rest, and in the later stages the clinical features indicate cardiac, renal and cerebral involvement.

Cerebral features

Headache is common but not always present, even in severe hypertension, and is thought to be due to vasodilatation of cerebral vessels and subsequent stimulation of pain-sensitive nerve endings in their walls. Dizziness, vertigo and memory impairment with cerebral deterioration may occur. Raised pressure and atherosclerotic changes in cerebral arteries may lead to cerebral haemorrhage or thrombosis (p. 105).

   Hypertensive encephalopathy is a rare but severe condition characterized by paroxysms of very high blood pressure and associated with disturbance of vision or speech, vomiting, paralysis, fits or loss of consciousness. It may occur in malignant hypertension and is due to acute localized cerebral ischaemia.

Renal features

Raised pressure and atherosclerotic changes in renal arteries cause thickening and narrowing of the vessels. Diminished renal blood flow causes impaired renal function and proteinuria appears. Eventually renal failure develops and in malignant hypertension death often occurs from uraemia (p. 290).

Cardiac features

High arterial pressure increases the work load of the myocardium, particularly that of the left ventricle. As a result, the left ventricle hypertrophies and eventually left heart failure develops (p. 240). Dyspnoea is the first symptom of left heart failure. As the disease progresses, the features of right heart failure appear.

   Hypertrophied myocardium demands increased coronary blood supply. If atherosclerotic coronary artery disease, which tends to be aggravated or accelerated by hypertension, is present, then angina and myocardial infarction may occur (p. 234).

Eye features

Changes in the eyes, particularly the retinae, are assessed using an ophthalmoscope. Such changes are significant and directly proportional to the severity of the disease. In severe hypertension — especially malignant hypertension — papilloedema, that is oedema of the optic disc, occurs.

Investigations

The priorities are to establish the cause and to assess the effect of raised blood pressure on the heart and the kidneys. The following are necessary:

   Detailed history and physical examination.
   Urinalysis for blood and protein.
   Serum urea levels.
   Creatinine clearance test and intravenous pyelogram (IVP) to assess renal function.
   A series of midstream specimens of urine to exclude urinary tract infection.
   Chest X-ray to show heart enlargement.
   ECG.

   Assessment of blood pressure must be accurate. The patient should be relaxed, with his arm bare to allow smooth application of the cuff and to prevent constriction from the sleeve. The nurse should know whether the doctor wishes diastolic pressure to be recorded as the muffling or as the disappearance of sounds. Recordings may be as frequent as quarter hourly if pressure is very high and treatment is being given to lower the pressure. Casual recordings may be preferred to regular 4-hourly recordings, but once daily is the minimum. Results must be charted neatly and any marked rise or fall in blood pressure must be reported at once and rechecked, since failure to do so may have serious consequences for the patient.

Course and complications

Hypertension is often present for many years and eventually found during a routine examination, such as for life insurance. Although many patients have no complications throughout the course of the disease, the possibility of cardiac, renal and cerebral complications means that the outcome of the disease may be serious.

People with high blood pressure levels generally have a shorter life expectancy than people with normal blood pressure levels, although many live to old age in good health or with few symptoms.

Treatment and nursing care

Mild hypertension may not require any treatment, and often to avoid unnecessary anxiety patients are not told that the blood pressure is raised or, if told, they are carefully reassured. There is increasing interest among doctors in the possibility of assessing hypertension outside a hospital ward or clinic. If the stress of hospital visits can be avoided then patient anxiety may be reduced and more reliable recordings of blood pressure obtained, for example by the general practitioner. Many other investigations can also be made by the general practitioner or at an out-patient clinic.

Rest and relaxation are advised. Rest in bed is not important in the early stages, although extra rest should be taken after meals or by going to bed earlier. As the condition becomes more severe rest is increased, and if serious complications develop, such as cardiac failure, then rest in bed is essential.

Diet. Restriction of animal fat may be advised, and if the patient is obese a low calorie diet is required. The hospital dietician should discuss diet content with the patient and his family if a restricted diet has to be continued at home.

Smoking must be stopped.

Drug therapy

Hypotensive drugs act by reducing cardiac output or by reducing peripheral vascular resistance. Beta receptor blockage, using propranolol, decreases heart rate and cardiac output. Sympathetic blocking drugs such as debrisoquine and methyldopa reduce vasoconstriction. Treatment is started by giving a small dose. Dosage is gradually increased until the blood pressure is controlled or side-effects appear, for instance **postural hypotension** due to pooling of blood in the lower body. This is assessed by taking lying and standing blood pressures; a marked fall in pressure on standing may occur, and nurses should report this or any complaint of dizziness on rising from bed to the doctor.

Oral diuretics which reduce blood volume and are mildly antihypertensive are often given with hypotensive agents.

Other drugs frequently used are tranquillisers and sedatives to ease anxiety, tension and insomnia; analgesics and antiemetics are given for symptomatic relief of headache or nausea.

Hypertensive patients may look well but are often at considerable risk and may be anxious, particularly if they have heard of the association of high blood pressure with stroke. The nurse's contribution toward their care is considerable. Careful recording of blood pressure, teaching the patient about the disease and the importance of drug therapy, reacting with understanding, and relieving anxiety through reassurance are all essential responsibilities which nurses share with other members of the health team.

Hypotension

Hypotension or low blood pressure may cause **syncope or fainting** — a transient loss of consciousness due to decreased cerebral blood flow.

Fainting may occur due to postural hypotension when there is some loss of vasomotor tone, for example during antihypertensive drug therapy or after a long illness requiring prolonged bed rest. If the patient stands up suddenly, poor vasomotor tone results in a rapid fall in blood pressure due to widening of the arterioles by peripheral vasodilatation. A faint or vasovagal attack may also be psychogenic, that is associated with emotional upset such as fear and sudden anxiety, or it may be caused by a stuffy atmosphere or pain.

Treatment
The recumbent position, keeping the head low, improves the venous return to the heart and consequently the cerebral blood flow. Fresh air and a cold drink will help the patient to recover quickly.

To distinguish between a syncopal attack and cardiac arrest, check the pulse of the patient. The syncopal patient has a palpable pulse, but following cardiac arrest the patient is pulseless.

CARDIAC FAILURE

Cardiac failure is present when the cardiac output is insufficient for the needs of the tissues. The heart fails for many reasons. Thyrotoxicosis increases the metabolic rate thus increasing tissue demands for blood and oxygen, while in anaemia the blood carries less oxygen. In both instances an extra load is put on the heart to supply sufficient blood to the tissues. A stenosed valve causes resistance to the outflow of blood. An incompetent valve increases the volume of blood to be expelled from a chamber of the heart, as regurgitated blood is added to the normal volume in the chamber. Disease of the myocardium makes the pump less effective, as in myocardial infarction or in the myocarditis of rheumatic fever. Several of these factors may be combined, one or both sides of the heart may be affected, and the degree of failure may be small or great. In effect, all the heart diseases mentioned may cause cardiac failure, but there are also other precipitating factors: pregnancy, which causes an increase in blood volume and cardiac output; excessive sodium intake, which causes water retention; infections and excessive exertion, which add to the myocardial work load.

Left heart failure

Its causes are associated with (1) **outflow obstruction** as in mitral stenosis and (2) **left ventricular failure** due to hypertension, aortic valve disease, mitral incompetence or myocardial infarction.

Clinical features
These are due to rising pressure in the lungs. The combination of back pressure from the left side of the heart and the normal pressure of forward flow from the right side causes pulmonary venous congestion. Dyspnoea on exertion, then dyspnoea at rest, orthopnoea, paroxysmal nocturnal dyspnoea (p. 217) and acute pulmonary oedema may develop. A chest X-ray will show congestion of the lungs and enlargement of the heart and its chambers.

Acute pulmonary oedema
The onset may be sudden, requiring immediate medical and nursing attention. Fluid accumulating in the alveoli of the lungs causes intense dyspnoea, which is extremely frightening for the patient. Breathing is noisy, cyanosis develops rapidly, the skin is moist and cold and a cough develops with copious, frothy, blood-tinged sputum. Secretions can often be heard rattling in the larynx and trachea, and on auscultation, crepitations are heard throughout the chest.

Treatment of acute attack
Relief is dramatic with the following treatment:

1. Morphine intravenously, to calm the patient and relieve anxiety; the nurse must not leave the patient until the acute dyspnoea and fear begin to ease.

2. A diuretic intravenously, such as frusemide, to act quickly to get rid of excess fluid.
3. Aminophylline intravenously, to ease bronchospasm.
4. Upright position in bed to increase the vital capacity of the lungs.
5. High concentration of oxygen to relieve cyanosis.

Right heart failure

This may be due to disease of the right side of the heart itself, but it is usually secondary to left heart failure. Eventually, back pressure is transmitted from the lungs to the pulmonary artery, right ventricle, right atrium and to the systemic venous return. The causes are therefore (1) those of left heart failure, (2) pulmonary disease such as chronic bronchitis and emphysema, (3) pulmonary and tricuspid valve disease and (4) septal defects.

Clinical features
These are due to rising pressure in the systemic veins. Oedema is the principal sign, varying in degree from mild ankle oedema to generalised oedema, including ascites and pleural effusion (p. 219).

Hepatic vein engorgement and liver congestion develop causing enlargement of the liver with mild jaundice.

Loss of appetite, nausea and vomiting appear, due to portal vein engorgement and congestion of the stomach and bowel.

Engorgement of the jugular veins (Fig. 7.23) can be seen by examining the sides of the neck when the patient is reclining. The height of the pulsation wave in the jugular veins is related to the degree of failure; when severe the pulsation may be seen at the level of the ear lobes.

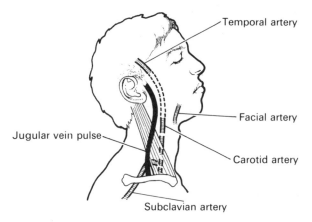

Figure 7.23
Jugular vein
Venous pulsation is seen but not felt; arterial pulsations are readily felt

Mental confusion occurs when the cardiac output is insufficient for cerebral tissue needs.

Kidney congestion causes a reduction in secretion of urine (oliguria).

When the right heart failure is secondary to left heart failure, dyspnoea is also present.

The course of the disease is variable; it is long if associated with chronic rheumatic heart disease, and short if associated with acute myocardial infarction.

Investigations
Clinical examination and history will reveal the underlying cause.

Nursing observations
The observations required will depend upon the precipitating cardiac disease, but those of temperature, pulse, respiratory rate and blood pressure will always be necessary. It is important that the nurse should observe, assess and report immediately any abnormality of pulse rate, rhythm or volume, or the development of shortness of breath. Accurate assessment of fluid balance is necessary because of the risk of impaired

renal function due to lowered cardiac output. Whenever possible, the patient is weighed daily to assess the development of fluid retention, or response to diuretic therapy. Nurses must look regularly for and assess changes in the amount of oedema present remembering to observe all possible sites.

Treatment and nursing care
The first principle of treatment is to correct the underlying cause whenever possible. When this has been done either medically or surgically and when a degree of failure persists, the following principles of treatment are applied.

Rest
Complete rest is essential at first to reduce the demands on the heart. The amount of restriction will depend on the severity of the failure. When the symptoms such as dyspnoea are relieved, and when the signs, say, of oedema diminish, the patient is allowed to increase activity very gradually. Impaired venous return greatly increases the risk of venous thrombosis, and lung hypostasis greatly increases the risk of pneumonia; therefore prolonged bed rest should be avoided.

Physiotherapy to improve both leg circulation and lung expansion is encouraged.
While the patient is acutely breathless, oxygen is given.
The upright position, well supported by pillows, and a bed table to lean on will improve the ability to breathe (Fig. 7.24). Sitting in an arm chair is sometimes more comfortable than lying in bed, and being out of bed even for a short time may improve the patient's morale.

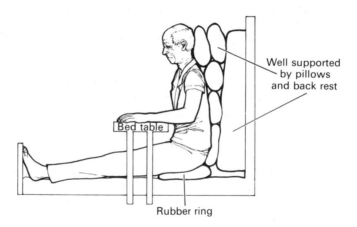

Figure 7.24
Upright position in bed

The pressure areas will be at risk and must be observed and treated regularly. Many patients find a rubber ring comfortable to sit on, and it may help to maintain position by preventing the patient from slipping down in bed, which would worsen dyspnoea. A bed cradle is used to take the weight of the bed clothes off the legs. Whenever possible, a bed-side commode or sanichair is used in preference to a bedpan.

If the patient becomes confused due to poor cerebral blood flow, he must be observed carefully for his own safety; for instance he may have to be prevented from lighting a cigarette beside an oxygen cylinder. Cot sides on the bed may also be required.

Diet
The diet must be light, easily eaten and easily digested, for the tired, dyspnoeic patient will have neither energy nor inclination to cut up or chew food or peel an orange. The appetite may be poor and nausea and vomiting are features of stomach congestion. For all these reasons, the nurse must ensure that the quantity of food is not too great, the food is appetizingly presented and the tray and utensils are easily reached.

Kilojoule restriction will be necessary if the patient is obese, as obesity increases the work load of the heart.

Salt restriction is effective in controlling the retention of fluid, but with the development of oral diuretics, severe restriction is now rarely necessary. Generally the patient is first advised not to add salt at table. This will reduce the daily intake of salt from 10 g to 5 g. Salt may also be withheld from the cooking, reducing intake to 3 g. When cooking for a family, this need not pose difficulties if the other members are prepared to add extra salt to their own food, but some patients prefer to prepare their own food separately. Salty foods such as bacon, meat extracts, sauces, salty fish, tinned food except fruit and baking powder should be avoided. Sodium-free salt can be bought. A 'salt-free diet' is very unpalatable and seldom recommended. It involves obtaining salt-free bread and butter and taking little milk, in addition to the other restrictions.

Drugs

Digitalis is most often used in the form of digoxin. Digoxin slows the heart by depression of the conducting pathways and by vagal stimulation. It improves the efficiency of the action of the myocardium by strengthening contraction, thus improving the cardiac output. Improved cardiac output will lead to improved renal blood flow and an increase in glomerular filtration; consequently digoxin has a diuretic action and will help to relieve oedema. Anorexia, nausea and vomiting are the most common side-effects. The pulse rate may become very slow, and the development of coupled beats (pulsus bigeminus) will indicate digoxin toxicity.

Diuretics. A diuretic is a substance which increases the excretion of sodium and water by the kidneys. The most commonly used diuretics are the thiazides, frusemide, and ethacrynic acid, all of which inhibit the reabsorption of sodium and water by the kidney, thus promoting a diuresis. Many diuretics act quickly, and nurses should know their speed of action in order to warn the patient what to expect after taking the drug. Frequent requests for bedpans may be embarrassing for the patient and inconvenient during tests or examinations or during visiting times. When at home, patients will decide the most suitable time to take a diuretic according to the daily pattern of activity. A long-acting diuretic may be more suitable for an elderly person.

Potassium. Potassium chloride supplements are given with most diuretics, since potassium is lost in large quantities in the urine. This is important when digitalis is being given, because potassium depletion causes increased sensitivity to digitalis and dangerous arrhythmias may develop.

Administration of diuretics, together with dietary salt restriction, is generally effective in relieving oedema.

Mechanical measures

Intractable oedema may be removed by mechanical means: pleural aspiration is carried out to drain a hydrothorax; abdominal paracentesis is performed to drain ascites. Southey's small silver tubes may be inserted into oedematous legs to drain fluid, but are seldom used now.

Pulmonary heart disease (cor pulmonale)

This is the name given to right heart failure secondary to disease of the lungs. Chronic bronchitis, emphysema or pneumoconiosis will increase the work load of the right heart, and cause chronic cor pulmonale. The incidence of this form of heart disease is greater in industrial areas. Acute cor pulmonale will follow massive pulmonary embolism (p. 256), since a major blockage of the pulmonary artery or one of its branches will put great strain on the right ventricle, causing right heart failure.

Cardiac arrest

Cardiac arrest is sudden failure of the heart to supply adequate circulation. The brain is the organ of the body most sensitive to lack of blood and oxygen, and effective circulation must be restored within 3 minutes to prevent irreversible brain damage. The commonest causes of cardiac arrest are myocardial infarction, anaesthesia, electrolyte imbalance, drowning and electrocution.

The nurse must know:

1. How to diagnose cardiac arrest quickly.
2. How to summon the emergency team promptly.

3. How to initiate resuscitation effectively.
4. Where to find the necessary equipment.

Cardiac arrest is diagnosed and treatment initiated on finding a patient **unconscious and pulseless** (absence of carotid or femoral pulse). Other signs include pallor, cyanosis, gasping, apnoea and, after a short interval, dilated pupils. The nurse must remember that the patient who has fainted has a palpable pulse.

The main objective of treatment is to restore an oxygenated blood supply to the brain by means of **cardiopulmonary resuscitation**.

Restarting the heart

The heart will sometimes be restarted by a sharp blow with a clenched fist (as one would thump a table) over the lower third of the sternum. External cardiac massage restores heart action and cardiac output by compression of the heart between the sternum and the spine. The compression, which empties the blood from the ventricles, is effective only when the patient is on a firm surface. For this reason, the patient should be lying flat and a cardiac arrest board should be placed under his chest. The heel of one hand is placed on the lower third of the sternum and the heel of the other hand is placed over the first (Fig. 7.25). The sternum is depressed forcefully and rhythmically by about 3 to 5 cm sixty times per minute in an adult. Rhythmic compression with the appropriate force will be easier to sustain if the arms are kept straight. It is important not to compress too quickly otherwise the ventricles will not have enough time to refill with blood. Some find it helpful to establish the rhythm by saying, 'one, one thousand: two, one thousand: three, one thousand'. The hands must be carefully positioned and should not lose contact with the point of compression in order to maintain the correct position. If too low, pressure on the xiphoid process may cause internal injury. The fingers should be raised: pressure by the fingers or the hand on the ribs may cause rib fractures.

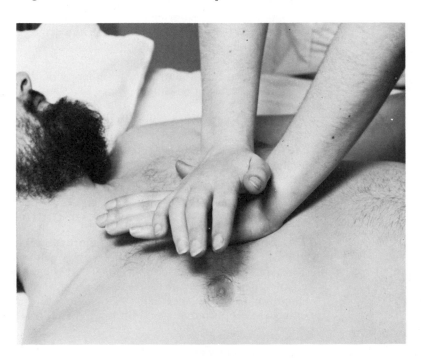

Figure 7.25
External cardiac massage
—position of hands

In infants the procedure is different. The hands encircle the chest. Much less pressure is applied by the thumbs, at mid-sternal level, at a rapid rate of 100 times per minute.

If external cardiac massage is effective, a carotid or femoral pulse will be felt.

Ventilating the lungs

To oxygenate the blood supply restored by external cardiac massage, lung ventilation must be started. First, the airway must be cleared. False teeth are removed and put in a safe place. Attention to this important detail only takes seconds and is vital, since dentures are easily lost or damaged during an emergency procedure. The neck is

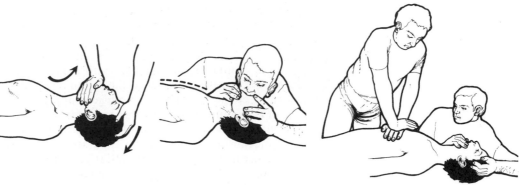

Figure 7.26A–C
Cardiopulmonary
resuscitation

A Head hyperextended
and chin raised to
clear airway

B Nose held. Mouth
to mouth breathing

C External cardiac massage
at lower end of sternum

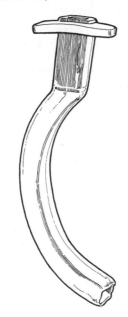

Figure 7.27A
Guedel airway

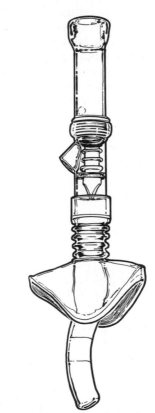

Figure 7.27B
Brook's airway

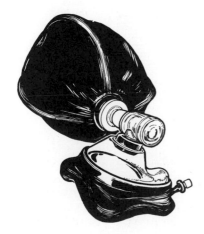

Figure 7.27C
Ambubag

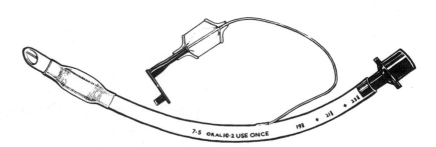

Figure 27.7D
Ventilation endotracheal tube

extended and the jaw pulled forward to stop the tongue falling back. A plastic oral airway is inserted. Direct mouth to mouth breathing at a rate of 12 respirations per minute will provide adequate ventilation (Fig. 7.26 A and B). The ratio should be one inflation of the lungs to 5 cardiac compressions.

The nurse should become familiar with aids to ventilation and their use — the Guedel airway, the Brook's airway, the Ambu bag and endotracheal tubes (Fig. 7.27) which can be connected directly to oxygen supply.

To be of maximum help to the emergency team, the nurse should also try to become familiar with the location and use of equipment and drugs on the emergency trolley, such as the defibrillator and suction apparatus. ECG electrodes will be required and applied at once to record heart rate and rhythm, and sodium bicarbonate will be used to correct the quickly developing, severe acidosis.

Cardiac arrest is due to **ventricular asystole** (a — without, systole — contraction of the heart), or **ventricular fibrillation**. In asystole, the heart muscle does not contract at all, there is no electrical activity, and the electrocardiogram shows a straight line (Fig. 7.28). In ventricular fibrillation, the ventricles 'twitch' or contract in an uncoordinated way due to chaotic electrical disturbance, and the electrocardiogram shows an irregular, bizarre pattern (Fig. 7.29). Cardiac output stops because the ventricles cannot fill or empty properly.

Ventricular fibrillation can be corrected by **electrical defibrillation**. The defibrillator machine delivers an electric shock to the heart muscle in order to stop the chaotic electrical activity, and to allow normal electrical conduction and normal heart rhythm

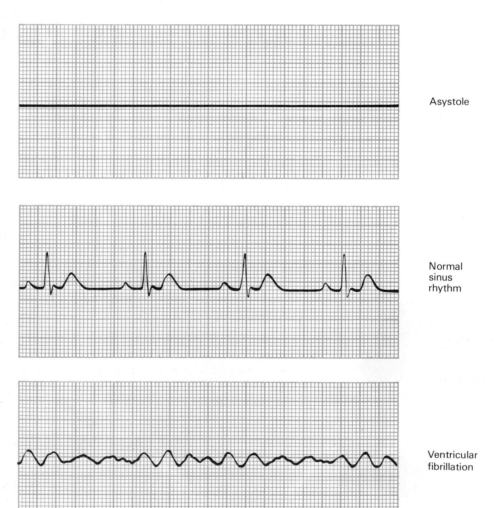

Figure 7.28
Asytole

Asystole

Normal sinus rhythm

Figure 7.29
Ventricular fibrillation
(compare with normal)

Ventricular fibrillation

to resume. The defibrillator paddles, covered with electrode jelly to prevent skin burns, are placed at the right upper chest and the left axilla so that the electric current will pass across the chest through the cardiac muscle (Fig. 7.30). To avoid getting an electric shock, everyone should stand well clear of the patient and the bed when the defibrillator is operated.

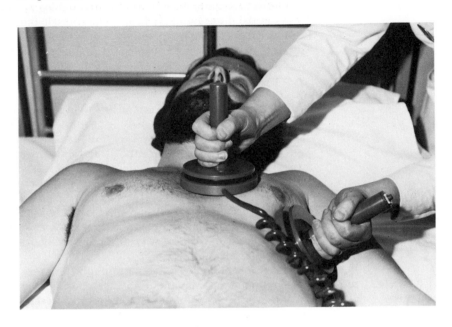

Figure 7.30
Defibrillation: position of paddles

ANATOMY AND PHYSIOLOGY OF THE BLOOD VESSELS

The **systemic** or **peripheral circulation** includes the whole vascular bed (Fig. 7.31) excluding the heart and pulmonary circulation. Arteries and veins have the same structure:

> Outer layer of fibrous tissue — **tunica adventitia**.
> Inner layer of muscle and elastic tissue — **tunica media**.
> Inner layer of endothelium — **tunica intima**.

Arteries differ from veins by having a smaller lumen, fewer muscle and more elastic fibres in the middle layer, and thicker walls. Most veins have valves, which consist of a fold of endothelium with the concave surface towards the heart, permitting flow only towards the heart (Fig. 7.32).

Arteries distribute the cardiac output, transporting oxygen and nutrient materials to the body tissues and cells according to their needs. Arteries also help maintain an adequate blood pressure by offering resistance to blood flow. The small vessels, arterioles, act as the main regulators of blood flow. By contraction and relaxation of their smooth muscle walls, the diameter of arterioles can change markedly, causing change in the resistance to blood flow through the vessels, that is change in **peripheral resistance**.

The vasomotor centre in the medulla is responsible for maintaining the arteriolar muscle in a partial state of contraction by continuous sympathetic action. Increased vasomotor centre activity causes **vasoconstriction** and increased peripheral resistance; decreased activity allows parasympathetic stimulation causing **vasodilatation** and decreased peripheral resistance.

The capillaries play an important part in cell respiration and nutrition by bringing blood into close relationship with all body cells. A capillary wall, composed of a single thin layer of cells, forms a semipermeable membrane. This allows the passage of water, oxygen and low molecular weight substances from the blood in the capillaries to the interstitial fluid, then to the cells, by the process of **diffusion**. At the arterial end of the capillary, oxygen diffuses through the capillary wall to the tissue fluid and cells; at the venous end, carbon dioxide diffuses from the cells to the tissue fluid and blood. By this

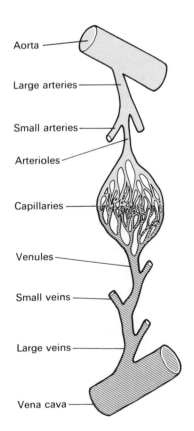

Aorta

Large arteries

Small arteries

Arterioles

Capillaries

Venules

Small veins

Large veins

Vena cava

Figure 7.31
Components of the vascular bed

TO HEART

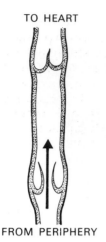

FROM PERIPHERY

Figure 7.32
Valves in vein

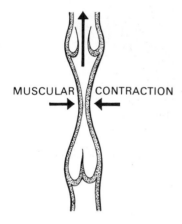

MUSCULAR   CONTRACTION

Figure 7.33
Action of the 'muscle pump'

same process of diffusion nutrient materials in solution in the blood pass through the semipermeable membrane to the cells.

Veins return deoxygenated blood from the body tissues to the heart. They act as a store of blood and return it at the rate required to maintain cardiac output. The action of the valves in the veins of the legs is of particular importance during exercise. When the veins are compressed by the contracted leg muscles the valves ensure that blood flows in the direction of the heart. This 'muscle pump' action is shown in Figure 7.33.

Valves which do not function properly subject the veins in the legs to high pressures, causing them to become tortuous and dilated (see varicose veins, p. 254).

AETIOLOGY

A blood vessel may be diseased in several ways, and causes of disease may occur singly or in association.

Arteries are affected by degenerative disease such as arteriosclerosis and atherosclerosis, and by thrombosis and embolism. Thrombosis is seen less often in arteries than veins, as arterial circulation is more rapid. Coronary artery thrombosis (p. 233) and cerebral artery thrombosis (p. 105) are considered elsewhere. Thrombosis and its association with degenerative disease in peripheral limb arteries will be considered here in more detail, as will the effect of embolism in limb arteries.

Arterial embolism is a complication of three cardiac diseases already discussed: mitral stenosis associated with atrial fibrillation, subacute bacterial endocarditis, and myocardial infarction.

Veins are affected by inflammation (phlebitis), by thrombosis (phlebothrombosis) or by combined inflammation and thrombosis (thrombophlebitis).

Varicosities are common. The term **varicose veins** describes the abnormal dilatation of leg veins caused by defective valve structure. Varicosities are also found as haemorrhoids (p. 175) and in the oesophagus as oesophageal varices due to obstructed portal venous return.

GENERAL FEATURES OF DISORDER

It is important to be able to differentiate between the effects of impaired arterial supply to, and impaired venous drainage from, a limb.

Arteries

Impaired arterial supply causes pain and cold extremities.

Intermittent claudication
This is the term which describes pain felt in a limb on exercise and relieved by rest. Usually the cramping pain is felt in the calf muscles or the foot when walking. As the arterial obstruction increases, the distance walked before claudication occurs shortens and the resting time required before the pain disappears lengthens. Eventually the degree of ischaemia is such that pain occurs at rest. These features can be compared with those of angina (p. 217). A similar pain can be reproduced if one raises an arm and rapidly clenches and unclenches the fist. Pain develops as the arterial supply fails to meet the exercised muscles' demands for oxygen and as waste products of muscle metabolism accumulate in the tissues.

Impaired arterial supply is associated with arteriosclerosis and atherosclerosis. In the early stages, symptoms may not appear if there is adequate **collateral circulation**, that is vessels arising behind and ahead of the affected vessel providing the necessary blood.

Distinction should be made between the features arising from impaired arterial supply and complete occlusion of an artery. When a limb artery is suddenly occluded by thrombosis or embolism there is not only pain and coldness but also pallor, numbness, absence of pulses distal to the block, and eventually tissue necrosis and gangrene. Alternative blood supply via collateral circulation may delay tissue death, but ultimately gangrene occurs.

Veins

Impaired venous flow is associated with inflammation and the formation of thrombus. These two processes cause local pain, tenderness, redness of the overlying skin if a superficial vessel is affected, dilated veins, increased warmth in the affected limb and oedema. When a vein is obstructed pressure in the vein distal to the obstruction is raised. This raises the blood pressure in the venous end of the capillaries causing oedema (p. 218). An adequate collateral circulation may prevent undue back pressure and oedema, but when a major vessel is blocked considerable swelling occurs.

INVESTIGATIONS

Pulse

Limb pulses are observed to assess the adequacy of blood supply when arterial vessel disease is present (Fig. 7.34 A-D).

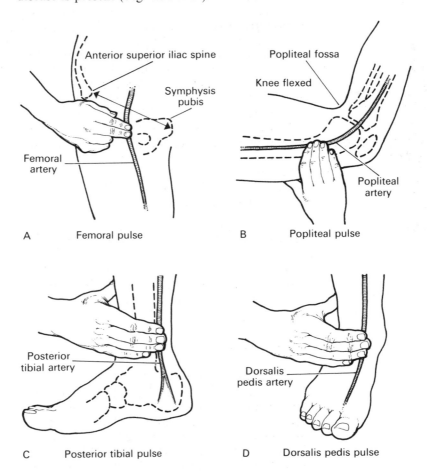

Figure 7.34
Arterial pulses in the lower limb

Arteriography

Femoral arteriography is performed under local anaesthesia to investigate lower limb arteries. Children or very anxious adults may require general anaesthesia. Following the injection of a radio-opaque contrast medium, a series of films is taken in quick succession down the length of the limb, demonstrating filling of the leg vessels and narrowing or obstruction of vessels.

Preparation

It is an essential courtesy to explain the procedure to the patient. Arteriography may not be pleasant. The procedure may be long and the injection of dye causes a feeling of heat. Detailed explanation is not necessary, but information about the length of the examination should be given together with warning about discomfort, since sudden pain or discomfort will alarm the patient and make him think that something has gone wrong.

The patient has nothing to eat or drink for 5 hours before the procedure. The groins are shaved and the bladder emptied before examination. A mild sedative may be given.

After care

A pad of gauze is firmly strapped over the puncture site to prevent arterial haemorrhage. Movement from trolley to bed may dislodge the pressure pad and a haematoma may form rapidly. The following routine is advisable: bed rest for 24 hours; quarter-hourly recording for 4 hours of pulse, blood pressure and of foot pulse for development of arterial occlusion; inspection of wound site for haemorrhage; then 4-hourly recordings including temperature and respiratory rate. After-effects should involve no more than local groin stiffness or bruising.

Venography

Peripheral venography or phlebography is the radiographic examination of the venous system of the limb following injection of a radio-opaque contrast medium. The procedure is carried out under local anaesthesia, usually on a lower limb. It demonstrates the patency of deep veins, areas of non-filling or irregular filling indicating past or present thrombosis and the competence of valves. It is also used to investigate cases of acute or recurrent pulmonary embolism where venous thrombosis is likely and venous ligation necessary.

Preparation

The examination may be carried out on an out-patient basis. Preparation is as for arteriography with the exception of the groin shave. In this case, the contrast medium is injected either directly into a vein on the dorsum of the foot or via a small cannula after venous cut-down under local anaesthetic. The flow of the contrast is watched and a series of films taken as it enters and fills the venous system.

After care

The patient may walk about at once or as soon as the effects of sedation have worn off. Cut-down sutures are removed after 5 days.

Ultrasonography

Ultrasonography is a diagnostic procedure employing high frequency sound waves. The ultrasound waves pass as a beam through body tissues and are partially reflected at junctions between various structures in the path of the beam. The Döppler effect, which depends on the echo from a moving surface, is used to demonstrate the presence or absence of pulsation in peripheral vessels. The sound reflected from a moving column of blood alters in frequency and the audible signal is monitored.

Apart from explanation of the procedure to the patient, no special preparation or after care is necessary.

DISORDERS OF THE ARTERIES
Arteriosclerosis

This disease, which may affect any artery, causes shrinking of the intima, loss of elasticity and atrophy of the muscle fibres of the media, as a result of which the lumen of the vessel gradually narrows. This is often called 'hardening' of the arteries.

Many middle-aged and elderly people are unaware of the presence of arteriosclerosis until vessel narrowing causes symptoms due to ischaemia (impaired blood supply to the tissues supplied by those vessels).

Atherosclerosis

Atherosclerosis affects mainly the aorta, large arteries, coronary and cerebral arteries. Although it becomes more common with age, it can develop at any age and may be present in seemingly healthy people.

As noted earlier atherosclerosis results from the deposition of fatty plaques in the intima causing reduced blood flow to tissues or a blockage to blood flow following associated formation of thrombus (p. 254). In coronary arteries this process causes angina and myocardial infarction (p. 233). Atherosclerosis in leg vessels causes intermittent claudication; in cerebral vessels mental changes may result from an impaired blood supply. When thrombosis follows in leg or cerebral vessels, gangrene of the limb or hemiplegia may occur (Fig. 7.35).

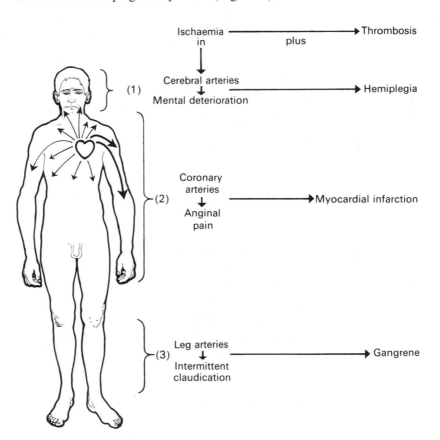

Figure 7.35
Some effects of impaired blood supply

Arterial degenerative disease may result in intracerebral haemorrhage when it occurs in hypertensive patients due to the high pressure of blood in diseased, weakened vessels.

The management of these two degenerative diseases is considered below, under peripheral vascular disease.

Peripheral vascular disease

This term describes the condition in which there is impaired blood supply to the limbs resulting in lack of oxygen and nutrients for the tissues. The main cause is degenerative disease, principally atherosclerosis. The disease is more common after the age of 50, and as the proportion of elderly people in the population increases, the incidence of these degenerative diseases rises. It affects men more often than women. It rarely affects upper limbs, and is associated with diabetes.

Clinical features

Early symptoms are pain on exercise, relieved by rest (intermittent claudication) and cold extremities. The course is usually progressive with the development of severe ischaemia and pain at rest. Eventually ulceration and gangrene may occur.

Investigations

Full clinical examination and medical history are taken, noting particularly the presence of risk factors of atherosclerosis. It is important to note whether limb pulses are absent or present. Arteriography will show the extent and severity of vessel occulsion and impaired blood supply, and it is necessary for determining whether reconstructive surgery is possible.

Nursing observations

Unless the nurse examines the state of the limbs and compares them in detail initially subsequent changes will not be noticed or will not be assessed accurately.

The nature of pain in the limb, its position and intensity and its relationship to exercise and rest are noted. Meticulous observation of the state of the skin for dryness and for any damage or ulceration is necessary. The first sign of any break in the skin should be reported at once. Colour and warmth of the limbs should be compared, and dorsalis pedis and posterior tibial pulses checked.

Treatment and nursing care

In the absence of a specific cure, management of peripheral vascular disease includes control of risk factors, education of the patient in the care of the limbs and measures to improve blood supply.

Control of risk factors

Obesity should be controlled, since weight reduction will ease the work load on the lower limbs. A reduction in dietary animal fat intake may be advised if blood cholesterol levels are high. Diabetes must be treated and stabilized. Diabetic patients are more susceptible to infection of limb tissue and to gangrene, and the presence of diabetic peripheral neuropathy increases the likelihood of ulceration and gangrene following injury.

Smoking must be stopped. Nicotine has three harmful effects: reduction of blood to the tissues through vasoconstriction of blood vessels, reduction of oxygen-carrying capacity in an already reduced blood flow and an increase in stickiness of blood platelets predisposing to thrombus formation.

Education of the patient

The nurse plays an important role in the education of the patient with peripheral vascular disease, and this teaching should extend to his family, particularly when the patient is unable to cope safely with his own limb care, for instance when generalized degenerative disease results in mental change and impaired cerebral function.

Since minor injury may precipitate gangrene, great care should be taken of the skin of the limb. Poorly nourished tissue heals badly, therefore all trauma, even minor trauma such as cut skin when trimming toenails or corns should be avoided. Regular attention to feet by a chiropodist is essential. Pressure from badly fitting shoes or stockings, or prolonged pressure of heels on a mattress can also lead to skin damage. Shoes should be checked for protruding nails and seams, lumps or torn linings, and new shoes should be broken in gradually by alternating their use with an old pair. Stockings, preferably seamless, must fit correctly. Pressure areas should be carefully inspected and treated. Patients with peripheral vascular disease should also be advised never to walk barefoot, and to avoid crowded areas where foot injuries are likely, such as supermarkets or football matches. A doctor should be told of any injury or infection. Fungal infection of the feet must be treated and the skin kept clean and dry.

Limb temperature is important. Direct heat increases tissue demands for oxygen and nutrients. In ischaemic areas these needs may not be met adequately by impaired blood supply. Therefore patients should be taught how to avoid increasing local tissue metabolism in their limbs. The limbs should be kept warm, but extremes of heat and cold must be avoided, for example, from fires or radiators, hot water bottles, sun-bathing, or wading in cold water.

Analgesia and sedation may be required, especially when continuous rest pain occurs.

Measures to improve blood supply

Blood supply to the limb may be improved by **reflex dilatation**. An electric heat pad is placed on the body trunk. Warmed blood stimulates the vasomotor centre in the brain causing vasodilatation of the vessels in the affected limb.

A physiotherapist may teach the patient **Buerger-Allen exercises** (Fig. 7.36). Several times in succession, the legs are alternately raised 45 degrees above the level of the bed for 1 minute then lowered for one minute and the feet exercised.

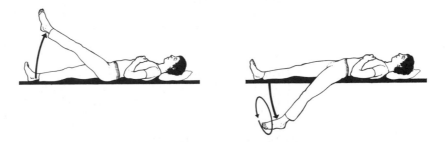

Figure 7.36
Buerger-Allen exercises

Several surgical measures are possible. In milder cases, lumbar **sympathectomy** is performed. Revascularization techniques are used for severe ischaemia with rest pain and early gangrene. There are two commonly used methods of direct reconstructive surgery: **endarterectomy**, in which the thickened, diseased, inner layer of the artery is cored out, and **bypass grafting**, in which synthetic material such as Dacron or the patient's own long saphenous vein is used. Because of the presence of valves, the length of vein is reversed before insertion to prevent blood flow being impeded. Such techniques often prevent the need for amputation and allow many elderly people to retain their independence; but despite success in retaining limb function, it must be remembered that many such patients will also suffer from generalized degenerative disease.

In addition to progressive atherosclerotic narrowing of vessels, thrombosis and embolism may occur in a limb artery causing complete occlusion of the vessel. Sudden occlusion will require prompt action and possible emergency surgery to save a limb, especially if a major artery is affected.

A nurse must report immediately to the doctor the occurrence of the following limb features: rapid onset of pain, coldness, numbness, pallor and absence of pulses distal to the block.

The limb should be rested and overheating avoided by keeping the limb at room temperature; a bed cradle is used to permit air to circulate freely. This also allows the limb to be observed easily, but overexposure of the patient must be avoided. Reflex dilatation is used, analgesia given and anticoagulation started. If surgery is required (embolectomy) it should be remembered that the combination of pain and haste in preparing for surgery will be alarming for the patient. The need for surgery must be calmly but carefully explained with reassurance to both the patient and his family.

Rehabilitation

The community health team is vital for the continued and successful care at home of patients with peripheral vascular disease, many of whom are elderly and without family help. As the disease progresses and exercise tolerance lessens, many patients must change to lighter, more sedentary work. Social service workers will help the patient find new employment. For the house-bound, the general practitioner, community nurse and chiropodist may all give support, and visits to a day centre are valuable in providing the stimulation of change of environment, interest and friendship.

DISORDERS OF THE VEINS

Superficial phlebitis

Superficial phlebitis, or inflammation of superficial veins, is a common condition caused usually by injury to vessels following surgery, childbirth or intravenous infusion. As veins have thinner walls than arteries they are more subject to endothelial damage. The intima thickens and narrows, and thrombus may form causing superficial thrombophlebitis — a condition often seen after prolonged infusion of intravenous fluids. Phlebitis of leg veins is frequently associated with varicosities.

The affected area becomes swollen, red and tender. Such inflammation may be seen tracking along a length of affected vein from the site of intravenous infusion. Pain is relieved by giving analgesia, and the application of local heat in the form of a kaolin poultice may be soothing. Careful observation of infusion sites is important and early signs or symptoms must be reported promptly, especially when life is being maintained by intravenous infusion and when progressive occlusion of veins from frequent change of site has occurred.

Varicose veins

Varicosities are the commonest vein lesions. The presence of valves in veins and the action of the muscle pump are responsible for maintaining venous return from the legs. When the valves are defective or incompetent, the veins dilate causing back pressure and stasis of blood which further dilates the veins. Superficial phlebitis often occurs, and stasis of blood predisposes to thrombus formation and oedema. Varicose eczema is common and a break in the skin may lead to varicose ulceration (p. 450).

The long and short saphenous veins are most often affected, and early symptoms are pain and fatigue in the leg on standing. Nurses will often care for patients who have varicose veins in addition to other diseases, and varicosities must not be overlooked, particularly as there is always the additional risk of the development of deep venous thrombosis. The legs must be observed carefully and handled gently to avoid trauma or rupturing a vein. A bed cradle should be provided and any abrasion or skin break reported. When out of bed, prolonged standing should be avoided and support elastic bandages or stockings should be worn.

Surgical treatment includes injection, ligation or stripping of the vessels.

Venous thrombosis

Thrombosis is the process of coagulation of circulating blood in the vessels.

Thrombus is the solid substance formed from blood constituents. A thrombus which becomes detached is termed an **embolus**. Atheromatous plaque, micro-organisms, fat cells or air may also be carried in the bloodstream as emboli and may become lodged in a blood vessel some distance from their original site.

Several factors may precipitate venous thrombosis:

1. Injury to endothelial lining. Intravenous infusion or injections, accidents, operations and inflammation may damage the inner lining to which platelets then adhere.

2. Increased blood coagulation. Dehydration causes the blood to become more viscous, as does polycythaemia where there is an excess of red blood cells. Blood clotting is also affected by tissue damage for example after operations, myocardial infarction or childbirth. There is also a small but significant increase in risk in women using oral contraceptives.

3. Slowing of venous circulation. This is the most important factor in the formation of venous thrombosis and any condition which produces slowing of venous circulation will predispose to thrombus formation in veins. Rest in bed, especially prolonged rest and immobility after an operation and the reluctance to move in bed which is characteristic of some elderly people, causes circulatory stasis. A pillow under the knees will compress the calves and slow the circulation, as will cardiac failure which causes impaired venous return.

Deep venous thrombosis

Deep venous thrombosis or phlebothrombosis is mainly a hazard of immobilization, with slowing of the rate of blood flow being the principal factor. Risk is particularly high after prolonged rest, limb paralysis or major surgery. Following surgery, the plasma becomes more viscous and there is an increase in the number and stickiness of platelets, which tend to adhere. Around the tenth postoperative day this aggregation of platelets is at its maximum, making this the most crucial period for the occurrence of the dangerous and often fatal complication, pulmonary embolus (Fig. 7.37).

Thrombosis often starts in the deep veins of the gastrocnemius muscles.

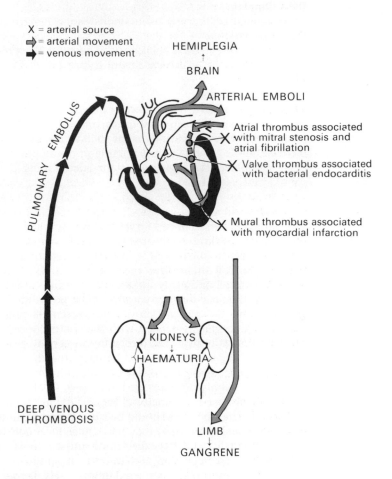

Figure 7.37
Sources and movement of emboli

Clinical features

The following may be present: slight calf pain or heaviness; limb oedema which may be gross if a large vessel is blocked and collateral drainage is poor; increased warmth in the affected limb; dilatation of veins; low grade fever.

Often the diagnosis is missed, either because there are no signs, as in about 50 per cent of cases, or because the signs, though present, are overlooked. When the thrombus is only loosely adherent to the vessel wall, the first indication may be sudden collapse or the onset of the clinical features of pulmonary embolus, the thrombus having loosened from the vessel wall and travelled in the venous return flow to lodge in the pulmonary artery or one of its branches (p. 254).

Prevention

Active measures can be taken to prevent deep venous thrombosis. To avoid slowing of venous return, prolonged bed rest should be avoided and early ambulation encouraged with active walking rather than just sitting in a chair. If bed rest is necessary, immobilization of the body or limbs must be prevented and the patient should not lie in one position for any length of time. Leg exercises, either active or passive, must be carried out to include both ankle and knee joints. The patient should dorsiflex and plantarflex the foot against resistance, or the nurse should put the patient's ankle and knee joints through their full range of movement.

Deep breathing exercises, which promote venous return, should be taught and encouraged.

Leg vein compression or injury are avoided by careful handling and positioning of the limbs during and after surgery. Any position in which pressure is exerted on veins should be avoided. For example, sitting or lying with pillows under the knee or calf, crossing the legs at the knee, or sitting in chairs which compress the popliteal space. Many patients are accustomed to these practices at home and should be advised about their dangers.

Anticoagulant therapy, using small doses of heparin, may be given subcutaneously to high risk patients.

Whether the patient is at home or in hospital, the nurse must share the responsibility with others in the health care team to prevent deep venous thrombosis.

Nursing observations

The nurse also has a major part to play in the prevention of pulmonary embolus by early detection of deep venous thrombosis through meticulous observation and prompt reporting of warning signs such as a slight temperature rise, slight pulse rate increase, ankle oedema or any complaint of calf pain or tenderness. While the legs are being examined, the opportunity for encouraging the patient to exercise the limbs should always be taken.

Treatment and nursing care

The patient is nursed in bed for a few days, by which time the pain and swelling should be resolved. The limb is elevated to promote venous drainage by raising the foot of the bed, and a bed cradle is used to keep the weight of the bed clothes off the limb. During this time, careful attention to the care of the patient's skin, pressure areas and mouth, and observation of dietary intake, bladder and bowel function and sleep pattern are necessary. In particular, dehydration must be avoided to prevent an increase in blood viscosity and the patient should be prevented from becoming constipated, since straining at stool is associated with the complication of sudden pulmonary embolus. The addition of bran to the diet, a mild aperient or suppositories may be necessary. Deep breathing exercises should be encouraged.

When the patient is allowed up, the full length of the affected limb should be supported by applying an elastic bandage or stocking before getting out of bed. Elastic stockings increase the velocity of blood flow in veins, but the fit and application are important. The stockings should be smooth and wrinkle-free. If too slack they will not be effective and if too tight they may cause local constriction and impair blood flow. High risk patients may have full length anti-embolism stockings applied to the legs as soon as bed rest begins on admission to hospital.

Anticoagulant therapy is started immediately. Intravenous heparin is given initially. Heparin is a powerful anticoagulant which works by preventing the conversion of prothrombin to thrombin. It has a rapid action but is short lasting; therefore oral anticoagulation using warfarin is started 24 to 48 hours before heparin is stopped to allow uninterrupted therapeutic action, since warfarin is not fully effective for 24 hours. Warfarin has no direct effect on the blood but works on the liver by reducing the formation of prothrombin. The nurse must remember that anticoagulant therapy involves the danger of haemorrhage. Any sign of bleeding must be reported. Analgesia and night sedation may be necessary and congestive cardiac failure will be carefully controlled.

Venography may be carried out, and if there is major risk, for instance when thrombus is known to be present and when several minor embolic episodes have occurred, it may be necessary to ligate or partially constrict the inferior vena cava to prevent further emboli passing to the pulmonary circulation.

SUGGESTED ASSIGNMENTS

1. How would you explain to a patient or relative of a patient in your ward the meaning of the terms 'pacemaker' and 'heart attack'?

2. Consider the anxieties a patient might experience following a coronary thrombosis. How can the hospital nurse and the community nurse help to relieve these anxieties?

3. If you were working in the community what dietary advice would you give to:

a. A family with a history of atherosclerosis?

b. A mother with cardiac failure?

How would you explain the reasons for the advice you offer, and how would you try to make your suggestions acceptable?

4. How well do you observe your patients? Much nursing care is planned on the basis of skilled observation of patients using all the senses. Your eyes, ears, nose and hands can tell you that a patient has suffered an acute myocardial infarction. Describe what you see, hear, smell and feel on admitting such a patient.

5. Many people in hospital and at home have a degree of cardiac failure. Select a number of such patients in your care and make your own estimation of the severity of their disease and of its effect upon their lives by:

a. observing, describing and comparing the signs of failure, and

b. interviewing each patient about his symptoms.

FURTHER READING

Aspinall M J 1973 Nursing the open heart surgery patient. McGraw Hill, New York

Conway N 1974 A pocket atlas of arrhythmias. Wolfe, London

Guyton A C 1974 Function of the human body, 4th edn. Saunders, Philadelphia

Hubner P 1975 Nurse's guide to cardiac monitoring, 2nd edn. Bailliere Tindall, London

Julian D G 1978 Cardiology, 3rd edn. Bailliere Tindall, London

Macleod J (ed) 1977 Davidson's principles and practice of medicine, 12th edn. Churchill Livingstone, Edinburgh

Meltzer L E 1978 Intensive coronary care. A manual for nurses, 3rd edn. Charles Press, London

Turner P P 1976 The cardiovascular system. Penguin Library of Nursing Series. Churchill Livingstone, Edinburgh

Report of a Joint Working Party of the Royal College of Physicians of London and the British Cardiac Society 1976 Prevention of coronary heart disease. Journal of the Royal College of Physicians vol 10 no 3 (April)

8. The Blood

Blood disorders are diverse; they may affect any age group and their treatments demand a wide variety of skills from doctors and nurses. Some conditions are common in all parts of the world, while others are extremely rare. A few serious blood diseases, notably some types of anaemia, respond very quickly to treatment, and although this is rewarding it may not present a particular nursing challenge. On the other hand, highly skilled nursing care is vital for a child with acute leukaemia, for example, and thoughtful support from all members of the health team is necessary for the child's parents.

ANATOMY AND PHYSIOLOGY

Blood is red in colour, sticky to the touch and salty to the taste. In health it is slightly alkaline (ph 7·4) and the normal volume is 3·5 to 6 litres. The main constituents are plasma, an aqueous solution of proteins, and, suspended in it, blood cells.

Plasma

Plasma is a yellowish fluid containing 91 per cent water. Of the remaining 9 per cent, approximately 7 per cent are the plasma proteins — albumin, fibrinogen and the globulins, which include prothrombin.

Many other substances, including electrolytes (notably sodium chloride, potassium and calcium), hormones, enzymes, nutrients and waste products are to be found in small amounts in plasma. Collectively these substances make up the remaining 2 per cent.

The cellular components

At birth blood cell formation (haemopoiesis) takes place in the marrow of all bones. As the child grows, his red haemopoietic marrow gradually becomes restricted to flat bones such as the ribs, sternum and skull bones, irregular bones, for example the vertebrae and pelvis, and the ends of the long bones.

Red blood cells (erythrocytes)
Red cells are small, biconcave, non-nucleated discs (Fig. 8.2). As there is no nucleus each cell has a short life span of about 120 days. In consequence constant replacement of red cells is necessary: normally the red bone marrow makes about 3 million every second. The normal red cell count is 5 000 000 per cubic millimetre (mm^3).

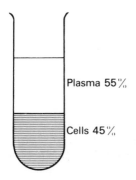

Figure 8.1
Blood proportions

Plasma 55%

Cells 45%

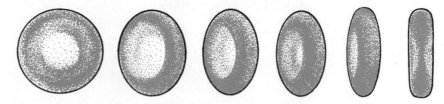

Figure 8.2
Red blood cells

Red blood cells contain a high concentration of **haemoglobin**, a compound composed of a protein, a pigment and iron. It enables oxygen (O_2) to be carried from the lungs to the tissues and carbon dioxide (CO_2) to be transported back from the tissues to the lungs. For the proper development of red cells (erythropoiesis, Fig. 8.3) various nutrients are essential; these include iron, vitamin B complex (in particular vitamin B_{12} and folic acid), vitamin C and protein. The formation of haemoglobin is shown in Figure 4.5, page 138.

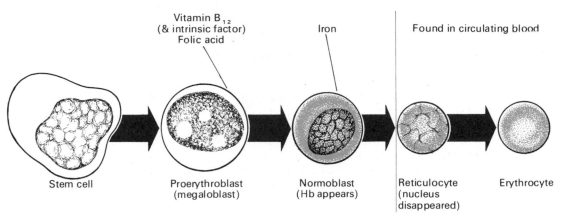

Figure 8.3
Erythropoiesis

The reticulocytes normally make up less than 1 per cent of the circulating red cells. An increase in this percentage indicates that the bone marrow is producing more red cells than normal.

Platelets (thrombocytes)

Platelets, also non-nucleated and formed in the red bone marrow, are much smaller than red blood cells. The life span of platelets is 9 to 11 days. The normal platelet count is 250 000 per mm^3 blood. Platelets play a vital role in the clotting of blood.

White blood cells (leucocytes)

White cells are larger than red cells; they are nucleated and there are two main types (Fig. 8.4):

1. **Granulocytes** (polymorphonuclear leucocytes), which are the most numerous type of cell, form up to 75 per cent of the total white count. There are three subgroups of granulocytes (Fig. 8.4).

2. **Lymphocytes**, which are found in the lymph nodes and spleen as well as in the red bone marrow.

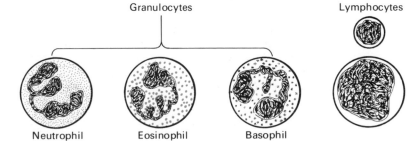

Figure 8.4
White blood cells found in circulating blood

The life span of white cells is variable. The normal count is also variable and ranges between 5000 and 8000 per mm^3 of blood. Figure 8.5 shows the normal development of white cells (leucopoiesis). Collectively the white cells form an important part of the body's defence system. Most granulocytes have the power to engulf micro-organisms and dead tissues: this process is known as **phagocytosis**. Lymphocytes multiply in response to virus infections and produce antibodies. Leucocytes are the only cells which can leave the circulation and return to it.

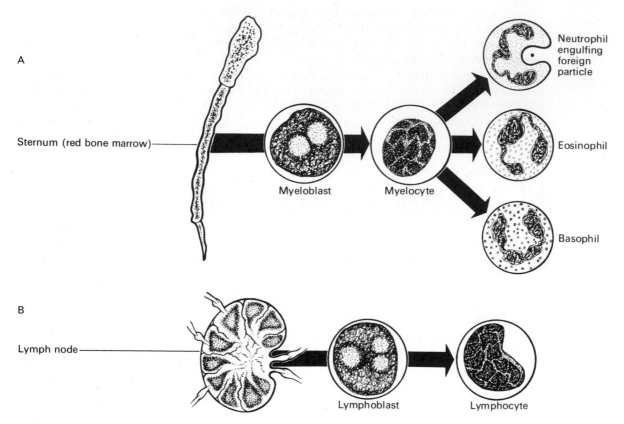

A

Sternum (red bone marrow)

Myeloblast

Myelocyte

Neutrophil engulfing foreign particle

Eosinophil

Basophil

B

Lymph node

Lymphoblast

Lymphocyte

Figure 8.5
Leucopoiesis
A. Myeloid
B. Lymphoid

Physiological arrest of haemorrhage (physiological haemostasis)

The phenomenon of natural haemostasis which includes clotting or coagulation of blood is important because without it even slight injury could result in a person bleeding to death. In health blood within the vessels remains fluid. This is partly because of the smooth lining of the vessels but also because platelets remain inactive until damaged and there is a small amount of anticoagulant present in the plasma.

When blood is shed a series of events takes place:

1. The severed artery or vein contracts.
2. Platelets adhere to the broken endothelium of the vessel, forming a plug. This alone is sufficient to stop bleeding from a very small vessel or capillary.
3. Coagulation occurs (Fig. 8.6).

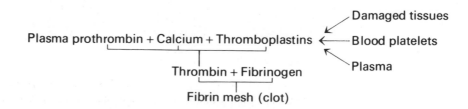

Figure 8.6
Coagluation of blood

(a) Thromboplastins liberated from the damaged tissue, disintegrated platelets and plasma activate the plasma prothrombin to form thrombin, provided calcium salts are present.
(b) Thrombin then acts on the soluble plasma fibrinogen, changing it into insoluble fibrin. Fibrin is precipitated in the form of a fine meshwork which

adheres to the platelet plug and traps red blood cells, forming a clot. In normal individuals this takes from 3 to 10 minutes.

4. The clot then retracts. As the mesh of fibrin contracts, serum (plasma minus fibrinogen) oozes out and the clot gradually hardens and dries.

Clotting may be accelerated by warmth which speeds up the chemical changes. Conversely, the process of clotting in shed blood may be slowed down by cooling. It is possible to prevent clotting altogether by removing or rendering inactive any of the factors necessary for clot formation, the easiest being calcium. Use is made of this knowledge in clinical practice when blood is to be collected and stored for various purposes such as:

1. Transfusion. The addition of sodium citrate to blood as it is shed by the donor causes the formation of calcium citrate. Since ionizable calcium in the plasma is now bound with citrate it is no longer available for coagulation. A 3.8 per cent solution of sodium citrate will ensure that blood remains fluid.

2. Examination of samples of peripheral blood. Various specimen bottles are issued by the haematology laboratory containing different types of anticoagulant, for example potassium oxalate (which gives rise to a precipitate of calcium oxalate, thus rendering the calcium inactive). The nurse should be familiar with the types of bottles and anticoagulants used in her own hospital so that she may select the appropriate ones when needed by the doctor.

Blood groups

It is always essential that the blood of a patient requiring a transfusion is cross-matched with the donor blood he is about to receive. The reason for this precaution is that individuals differ in the blood groups to which they belong. A person's blood group is identified by his red blood cells and his plasma. There are several grouping systems, although only the two most important in medical practice will be considered here. Other systems are of interest mainly in criminology and in paternity disputes.

A B O blood groups

An individual's blood is classified A, B, AB or O according to the chemical substances called agglutinogens carried by his red blood cells. The agglutinogens can be identified according to the way in which they react with antibodies or agglutinins, designated anti-A and anti-B, found in the plasma (Table 8.1).

Table 8.1
Blood groups and their distribution in Western Europeans

Blood group	Antibodies in plasma	Population (%)
A	anti-B only	42 %
B	anti-A only	9 %
AB	no antibodies	3 %
O	anti-A and anti-B	46 %

For transfusion purposes it is **the effect that the plasma of the recipient will have on the red cells of the donor blood that must be considered**. If, for example, a patient of Group A was to be transfused with Group B blood the relatively large volume of the patient's plasma containing anti-B agglutinins would cause the transfused Group B red cells to come together in clumps, that is to agglutinate. In some instances the red cells would break down (haemolyse, p. 265). Table 8.2 shows the blood groups which, in theory, safely 'mix', but since there are subgroups, direct cross-matching is the only means by which compatibility of blood groups can be ensured.

Table 8.2
Compatible blood groups

Red cells of donor	Blood group of recipient			
	A (anti-B)	B (anti-A)	AB (neither anti-B nor anti-A)	O (anti-A & anti-B)
A	compatible		compatible	
B		compatible	compatible	
AB			compatible	
O	compatible	compatible	compatible	compatible

The Rhesus factor

About 75 per cent of the people in Western populations carry a Rhesus factor in their red blood cells and are therefore classified as being Rhesus positive (Rh +ve). Those who lack this factor are called Rhesus negative (Rh −ve).

Although there is no naturally occurring Rhesus antibody, if a Rh −ve person is exposed to Rh +ve red cells, then antibodies may be formed, and once formed they stay in the blood. Exposure may occur through:

1. Transfusion of Rh +ve blood.
2. Pregnancy (Fig. 8.7), when the mother is Rh −ve and the fetus is Rh +ve. In this situation the mother may form Rhesus antibodies in her blood which then pass back via the placenta to the fetus. This results in breakdown of the baby's red blood cells (haemolysis) giving rise to haemolytic disease of the new born. If very seriously affected, the baby may be born dead; he may survive if given an immediate exchange transfusion of Rh −ve blood at birth. Subsequent pregnancies are always at greater risk because there is a progressive build-up of antibodies.

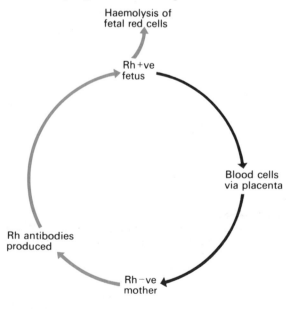

Figure 8.7
Rhesus antibody production in pregnancy

INVESTIGATIONS

History

From an accurate history, the doctor may find the cause and elicit the symptoms of a blood disorder, for example, frequent use of aspirin by the patient causing gastric irritation and blood loss.

General physical examination

This will indicate general level of health, features related to underlying conditions that cause blood disorders and features specific to the blood disorders themselves.

Examination of circulating blood

Venepuncture is the withdrawal of venous blood in small amounts (2 to 10 ml) for diagnostic purposes. Samples of venous blood are taken by a doctor from a peripheral vein, usually the cephalic vein. Laboratory findings often enable an accurate diagnosis to be made of comparatively simple blood disorders such as iron deficiency anaemia.

The correct bottles containing the appropriate anticoagulant should be available. Whenever possible, a nurse should be with a child and with an apprehensive adult during venepuncture. No special preparation is necessary. A haematoma may form at the puncture site, but this can be avoided by the application of digital pressure to the site.

The most common tests include cell count, haemoglobin estimation, and clotting and bleeding times.

Cell count
The number of circulating blood cells of each type is determined (Table 8.3) and their size, shape and maturity is noted.

Table 8.3
Normal range of blood cell values

Type of cell		Number of cells per cubic millimetre
Red blood cells	men	4 500 000–6 500 000
	women	3 900 000–5 600 000
White blood cells		
neutrophils		2500–7500
lymphocytes		1500–3500
monocytes		200–800
eosinophils		40–440
basophils		0–100
Platelets		100 000–350 000

Haemoglobin
To estimate haemoglobin level, a small quantity of blood is obtained in a tube containing an anticoagulant called sequestrene. Normal levels are:

Men: 13.5–18.0 g per 100 ml
Women: 11.5–16.5 g per 100 ml
14·6 g per 100 ml = 100 per cent

Clotting and bleeding times
The clotting time is a test of the clotting mechanism. The normal rate is 4–10 minutes. The bleeding time is the time taken for bleeding to cease. Normal is 2–5 minutes.

Investigations appropriate to the underlying conditions

Chronic blood loss, which is an important cause of iron deficiency anaemia, is commonly due to a gastrointestinal lesion (Ch. 5).

Barium studies
Barium studies are carried out when such lesions are suspected — hiatus hernia, peptic ulcer, carcinoma or diverticulitis.

Examination of faeces for occult blood
Occult bleeding occurs with gastrointestinal lesions such as those mentioned above.

Gastric analysis
In pernicious anaemia there is no hydrochloric acid in the gastric juice even after the injection of histamine or pentagastrine (Ch. 5) which will stimulate its secretion.

Examination of bone marrow

The procedure known as marrow puncture involves the removal of a specimen of red bone marrow by aspiration using a stout needle with an adjustable guard such as the Salah needle (Fig. 8.8). In adults, the sternum and the iliac crest are the most accessible sites. The tibia is preferred for very young children and on rare occasions the vertebral spines are used for the obese patient.

Figure 8.8
Salah needle

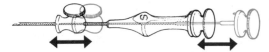

Laboratory examination of red bone marrow provides a useful aid to diagnosis in blood disorders such as pernicious anaemia and the leukaemias. It is also important when the diagnosis of a blood disorder is not clear following examination of the peripheral blood. During the course of the disease, repeated examination of bone marrow may be required to assess the effect of treatment.

The procedure is performed under local anaesthesia by a doctor using an aseptic technique. Nursing responsibilities are to ensure patient comfort before and after the procedure and to prepare the equipment. Adults will require careful explanation of the procedure, and light sedation may be given. Children are generally sedated beforehand, both to allay fear and to prevent excessive movement during the procedure. In this case two nurses will be required, one to assist the doctor and one to hold and comfort the child. In some instances it may be preferable for a parent to do this.

The actual removal of bone marrow is painful. Following the procedure, some patients may require mild analgesia as the effect of the local anaesthetic wears off. Patients who have been sedated should not be allowed up for 2 to 3 hours. Complications are rare, but infection could result from poor aseptic technique. When using the sternal site, especially in young children, the possibility of inadvertently inserting the puncture needle right through the sternum causing damage to the organs in the mediastinum is always present. For this reason, the iliac crest is the preferred site for children.

Schilling test

This is a method of assessing the body's ability to absorb vitamin B_{12} which is essential for formation of red blood cells

Following a fasting period of not less than 6 hours, an oral dose of vitamin B_{12} 'labelled' with radioactive cobalt is given. An intramuscular dose of vitamin B_{12} is also given, in the form of 1000 micrograms of cyanocobalamin. A 24-hour urine collection is then started, from which laboratory staff can estimate the amount of radioactive vitamin excreted.

A healthy person stores and requires a comparatively small amount of vitamin B_{12} and would therefore excrete most of a given dose. However, people with disorders of intestinal absorption and those in whom a compound of gastric secretion known as the intrinsic factor is absent cannot absorb vitamin B_{12} and the oral radioactive dose given would not therefore be excreted by the kidneys, while the intramuscular dose would be taken up by the bloodstream and used by the body deficient in vitamin B_{12}. In these instances, the amount of vitamin B_{12} found in the urine would be negligible, thus proving a deficiency in absorption. If disorders of the intestinal tract have been ruled out, it can be assumed that the intrinsic factor is absent, producing a condition known as pernicious anaemia (p. 267). The nurse must ensure that the patient fasts, that the correct dose of vitamin B_{12} is given at the appropriate time and that all urine is collected over an exact 24-hour period.

DISORDERS OF THE RED CELLS

Diseases affecting the red blood cells are common in all parts of the world. There may be overproduction or underproduction of cells or abnormality of the cells themselves.

An increase in the number of circulating red cells is called **erythrocytosis**. This will occur in response to anoxaemia (p. 193) and can be found among people living at high altitudes. The same compensatory mechanism operates in some disorders, for example congenital heart conditions and chronic pulmonary disease. No treatment is necessary because in these circumstances the erythrocytosis is beneficial to the individual as it increases the oxygen-carrying power of the blood. Treatment will of course be needed for the underlying condition.

Erythrocytosis also characterizes a rare condition of unknown origin called **polycythaemia vera**. In this disease of adults there is an extension of red marrow throughout the long bones. Treatment is usually by irradiation, but venesection, whereby a litre of blood or more is removed rapidly from the patient, may also be necessary.

The most common and the most important group of diseases affecting the red cells is the anaemias.

Anaemia

Anaemia may be defined as a level of circulating haemoglobin which is below normal for the person's age and sex. A reduction for any reason in the number of red cells or their haemoglobin content or both will cause anaemia.

Causes of anaemia

Blood loss (*posthaemorrhagic anaemia*)
The seriousness of haemorrhage depends on both the amount and the speed with which blood is lost; for example, a sudden rapid loss of 1·5 litres or more in an adult will result in collapse and shock. The same amount lost over a period of several days would be less harmful, although the reduction in haemoglobin will be similar.

Acute blood loss. Haemodilution, whereby fluid is drawn from the tissues into the circulation, follows rapid haemorrhage. The degree of anaemia which results is not measurable until the circulating volume is fully restored, and this takes several hours.

Chronic blood loss (Fig. 8.9). Repeated small losses of blood usually occurring internally, for example from a peptic ulcer or haemorrhoids, cause a progressive fall in haemoglobin and a gradual onset of symptoms.

Excessive destruction of red cells (*haemolytic anaemia*)
Whenever red cells are destroyed more rapidly than they are being formed anaemia will result. This may occur in one of two ways:

1. The red blood cells are abnormal and therefore break down more easily, as in pernicious anaemia and some rare hereditary diseases.
2. The red cells are normal but the presence of infection, such as malaria, toxins or the undesirable side-effects of certain drugs, causes them to break down. Antibodies to the Rhesus factor (p. 262) also cause haemolysis of red cells.

Failure to produce red cells (*aplastic or hypoplastic anaemia*)
Aplastic anaemia, in which no red cells are produced, is fatal and fortunately rare. Hypoplastic anaemia, in which blood formation is inadequate, is more common. Either condition may arise: (a) as an idiopathic disease or (b) secondary to a known cause, for example deficiency of important nutrients such as iron or vitamin B_{12} and factors such

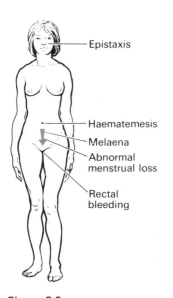

Epistaxis

Haematemesis

Melaena

Abnormal menstrual loss

Rectal bleeding

Figure 8.9
Types of chronic bleeding causing iron deficiency anaemia

as the intrinsic factor all of which are necessary to make blood. Exposure to radiation or idiosyncrasy to drugs may affect red bone marrow and are occasional causes, as are toxins resulting from kidney or liver failure.

Regardless of the cause all anaemias have certain clinical features in common.

Clinical features of anaemia

General symptoms and signs of anaemia whatever its origin are due to a lowered haemoglobin which results in a decreased supply of oxygen to the body tissues. According to the severity of the anaemia the patient will suffer to a greater or lesser degree from the following:

1. Increasing tiredness and lassitude, particularly at the end of the day when the body is finding progressive difficulty in coping with a poor oxygen supply.

2. Pallor of the skin and mucous membranes: a reduced pigmentation of the blood results from a lowered haemoglobin level, and blood supply to the periphery is cut down in favour of vital organs such as the heart and brain, hence the pale appearance.

3. Anorexia and dyspepsia which are often accompanied by some weight loss.

4. Breathlessness on exertion which occurs as the respiratory system tries to compensate for the reduced oxygen supply (Ch. 6). The oxygen-carrying power of the blood cannot, however, be improved until the anaemia is corrected and there is enough haemoglobin to carry the oxygen to meet the body's needs.

5. Tachycardia and possibly heart failure. As with breathlessness, the increase in heart rate is a direct result of the body trying to compensate for the reduced amount of oxygen available. In addition, since anaemia makes the blood less viscous or sticky, it flows much more rapidly than normal through the peripheral circulation. These two factors increase the workload of the heart and the heart may then fail, particularly if the patient is elderly or weak.

Iron deficiency anaemia

This is the most common type of anaemia in every country in the world. Women of child-bearing age are the most susceptible because of the increased demand for iron during pregnancy and following each menstrual loss. Insufficient dietary intake of iron and lack of hydrochloric acid necessary for the absorption of iron are other important factors. Haemorrhage as referred to previously results in an iron deficiency type of anaemia.

Clinical features

The condition has a gradual onset and the level of haemoglobin may be very low (7 g per 100 ml) before the patient seeks medical advice. Typically, the patient waits until he has become incapacitated before consulting his doctor. By this time he may have developed all the general symptoms and signs of anaemia due to diminished oxygen supply. In addition he may display those features specific to the nutritional deficiency of iron. These are:

1. Glossitis: an unusually smooth, shiny, sore tongue due to atrophy of the papillae.
2. Angular stomatitis: inflammation at the corners of the mouth.
3. Koilonychia: thin, brittle, dry nails which characteristically become concave and are therefore described as spoon-shaped (Fig. 8.10). The blood examination shows a hypochromic, microcytic anaemia.

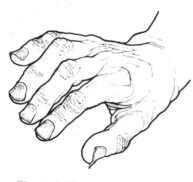

Figure 8.10
Koilonychia

Investigations

Examination of peripheral blood samples for haemoglobin estimation and a cell count is carried out. A variety of investigations may be necessary to elicit the cause; for example, a suspected carcinoma of stomach will call for a barium meal and tests of gastric acid secretion.

Treatment and nursing care

Treatment depends on the severity of the patient's clinical condition.

Rest. If the haemoglobin is below 5 g per 100 ml it is usual to confine the patient to bed and he must have complete bed rest if there is cardiac failure. In less severe cases the patient should be encouraged to rest for a few days but allowed up for toilet purposes.

Correction of anaemia. Blood transfusion is reserved as initial treatment for the severely ill patient. Oral preparations of iron, for example ferrous sulphate (200 mg) given three times daily after meals, is effective for the majority of patients. Gastrointestinal upsets may occur if the iron is not given after main meals. Occasionally a patient will have difficulty in swallowing pills, in which case a liquid preparation, usually in the form of a syrup such as Fersamal, will be prescribed.

If none of the oral preparations can be tolerated or if the anaemia is not responding, then intramuscular iron, for example Imferon or Jectofer, may be ordered by the doctor, the dosage being calculated according to the patient's body weight. Unless these preparations are injected very carefully and deeply into the muscle they will cause irritation and staining of the tissues. Some physicians prefer to give Imferon intravenously.

Mouth care. Oral hygiene is very important and mouth care is often necessary 4-hourly. Gentle swabbing and frequent rinsing are usually effective.

Treatment of underlying and associated conditions. Cardiac symptoms should improve with iron therapy but the physician may prescribe digoxin to control tachycardia.

When the anaemia is due to haemorrhage the cause must be found and treated.

Dietary deficiency must be corrected by encouraging the patient to eat iron-rich foods (Ch. 4).

If adequately treated, the patient's haemoglobin will rise by 1 per cent per day, which means that the normal level will be reached in 4 to 8 weeks.

Community care

Preventive care

Health education is important and the community nurse should advise on suitable diet, giving special attention to those whose sex or age group places them at particular risk. Medicinal iron should be administered to women during pregnancy and lactation and if menstruation is heavy. Infants, particularly if of low birth weight, should have iron-containing foods introduced into their diet by the age of 3 months. Elderly patients (Ch. 20) living alone often need a good deal of persuasion to eat suitable meals that contain adequate amounts of iron.

Follow-up

After immediate treatment for iron deficiency anaemia, continued iron therapy is necessary for a further 2 months. This is to ensure that the patient's depleted body stores of iron are replenished. Regular check-ups will also be necessary and iron will be administered as required.

Pernicious anaemia (Addisonian anaemia)

This condition is much less common than iron deficiency anaemia, but when it does occur it is most prevalent in the middle-aged group and affects women more often than men. It is very rare in younger people. The condition is the result of the inability of the stomach to produce the intrinsic factor which in health ensures the absorption of vitamin B_{12} from the alimentary tract.

The effects of the disease are particularly destructive and, if untreated, the patient will die — hence the adjective 'pernicious'.

Clinical features

The disease has a gradual onset and early symptoms are often unnoticed or ignored by the patient so that the anaemia may be well advanced by the time he visits his doctor.

The general symptoms and signs of anaemia will be present, and in addition the following features, which are specific to the lack of vitamin B_{12} will occur:

1. Achlorhydria, absence of hydrochloric acid in the stomach.
2. The skin, as well as being pale, has a slight lemon tint. This is due to the presence of bilirubin resulting from the excessive breakdown of red cells. Urobilinogen will then be found in the urine (Ch. 5).

3. The tongue is sore and sometimes ulcerated.

4. Intermittent diarrhoea may occur.

5. A feeling of numbness and 'pins and needles' (paraesthesiae) in the fingers and toes is present in advanced cases, particularly if a relapse occurs in the disease. It indicates involvement of the nervous system.

Blood examination shows a *macrocytic anaemia*.

Course and complications

Degenerative changes appear in the spinal cord if treatment is delayed or inadequate. Because both the ascending and the descending tracts are involved, the term subacute combined degeneration of the cord is used.

The disease will run a progressive course with increasing anaemia and further damage to the nervous system if it is untreated. The patient may die either from anaemia or from infection, to which he becomes increasingly susceptible.

Investigations

Examinations of samples of peripheral blood to estimate haemoglobin and number and abnormality of red cells.

Schilling test (p. 264).

Marrow puncture to reveal the presence of megaloblasts.

Treatment and nursing care

As with other types of anaemia this varies according to the severity of the disease.

Rest. The patient is confined to bed generally until his haemoglobin is up to 7 g per 100 ml. During this time he must be encouraged to move his legs to prevent venous stasis and to minimize the risk of deep venous thrombosis. Unless there is cardiac involvement he will be allowed up for toilet purposes and then gradually encouraged to become more ambulant as he feels able.

The nurse must be understanding in her approach, as the patient may feel irritable and depressed. He may have difficulty in sleeping at night, in which case simple nursing measures such as rearranging the bed clothes, making sure the bladder is empty and giving a hot drink should be tried before giving sedation.

Correction of anaemia. A blood transfusion of packed cells will be given if the haemoglobin is dangerously low (below 4 g per 100 ml). Replacement of vitamin B_{12} (cobalamin) must be by intramuscular injection for all patients since they are unable to absorb the vitamin if it is given by mouth. The preparation of cobalamin most commonly prescribed is hydroxocobalamin. The dosage is 1000 micrograms given twice in the first week and then 1000 micrograms once a week until the blood is normal. The nurse will find it very rewarding to see that after the first injection the patient begins to feel and look much better. As the bone marrow responds by producing normal red cells very rapidly, there is a much greater need for iron. For this reason ferrous sulphate may also be prescribed.

A light nourishing diet, rich in iron, protein and vitamin C, will also aid the production of normal cells.

Mouth care. This is similar to that outlined for iron deficiency anaemia.

Community care

The patient will need a maintenance dose of hydroxocobalamin for life. Dosage is regulated so that haemoglobin and blood count are kept within normal limits. Most patients require 1000 micrograms once every 4 to 6 weeks but some may remain healthy with even less frequent injections.

If the patient is elderly and living alone the community nurse may be asked to give the injections. At this time she will advise the patient about diet.

Anaemia secondary to other conditions

The treatment must first be directed at the underlying cause. If, for example, there is a hypoplastic type of anaemia in which the bone marrow is failing to produce blood cells due to some toxic factor, then the toxic factor must be removed if possible. This may mean treating an infection or discontinuing administration of a drug. When the toxins result from liver failure or from cancer then blood transfusion may be the only means of supporting life. Sometimes corticosteroids, such as prednisolone, are prescribed in order to stimulate the bone marrow to produce more blood cells.

DISORDERS OF THE PLATELETS AND HAEMOSTASIS

Absence of one of the substances in the blood necessary for clotting or disorder of the normal physiological process whereby haemorrhage is arrested (p. 260) will result in an abnormal tendency to bleed. Conditions in which this occurs are known collectively as the haemorrhagic disorders.

Bleeding due to defects in the clotting mechanism

Absence of one of the clotting factors (thromboplastins) in the blood plasma will, according to which particular factor is missing, give rise to either haemophilia or Christmas disease. In both conditions the patient suffers from a life-long tendency to spontaneous haemorrhages, often into joints (haemarthrosis) or into soft tissues, the nose being one of the commonest sites. These patients are at great risk if injured because haemorrhage after trauma is very slow to stop and prolonged bleeding will follow even the most trivial injury.

Treatment is symptomatic and infusion of fresh blood will be needed whenever there is an appreciable amount of bleeding. Children may need to attend special schools for the physically handicapped (Ch. 18). Since the diseases are hereditary genetic counselling should be given prior to marriage.

Bleeding due to defects of the capillary walls or a diminished number of platelets

Defects in the capillary walls may occur as a manifestation of some other (usually serious) disease or infection during the course of which the endothelium becomes damaged thus allowing blood to escape. Meningococcal meningitis, septicaemia, malignant disease and scurvy are a few examples of conditions which will cause this to happen. Occasionally some drugs have toxic side-effects with the same result, aspirin, phenobarbitone, phenytoin and phenylbutazone being among the culprits.

A diminished number of platelets (thrombocytopaenia) may accompany other conditions, for example leukaemia, or may arise spontaneously.

In all these conditions there is bleeding in small amounts into the skin or mucous membranes appearing as haemorrhagic spots called **purpura**. If the haemorrhages are only small they are termed **petechiae** (Fig. 8.11); larger purpuric spots are called **ecchymoses** or bruises.

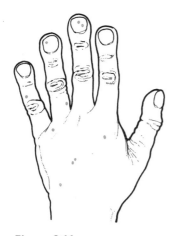

Figure 8.11
Petechiae

DISORDERS OF THE WHITE CELLS

An increase in the number of circulating white blood cells is called **leucocytosis**. This is the normal body response to bacterial invasion and will resolve when the infection has subsided.

Too few white cells is termed **leucopaenia**; this may occur in response to certain specific infections such as tuberculosis and enteric fever, or it can be the result of a very severe infection to which the body has no resistance.

Agranulocytosis
This is a rare, but very serious illness, where few or no granulocytes are present in the bloodstream. It can be due to the side effects of drugs such as chloramphenicol, phenylbutazone and thiouracil. Any patient taking such drugs should tell his doctor as soon as possible if he is feeling unwell or has a sore throat.

Treatment includes the withdrawal of any drug which could be responsible and the administration of antibiotics. Reverse barrier nursing will be needed to protect the patient from further infection and mouth washes given two or three hourly will help to ease discomfort in the mouth and throat. Some patients recover but others will die from overwhelming infections.

The leukaemias

Leukaemia is the malignant overproduction of immature nonfunctioning white cells. The cause is unknown, although it is known that irradiation may result in cell changes which lead to leukaemia. Because leukaemia may affect any type of white blood cell and may also take both acute and chronic forms, there are a number of clinical conditions, hence the collective term 'the leukaemias'.

Whatever the type of leukaemia there are always serious pathological changes in the bone marrow which not only result in the production of a large number of primitive white cells but also in a reduction in the number of red cells and platelets. This means that the patient will develop anaemia and a tendency to bleed in addition to a reduced resistance to infection.

Acute leukaemia

This is usually lymphocytic in type and most commonly affects children.

Clinical features
The onset is generally abrupt. The patient has a raised temperature and looks and feels very unwell. Epistaxis, bleeding gums and purpura (p. 269) soon appear. There is sore throat and ulcers in the mouth because of the lowered resistance to infection. The symptoms and signs of severe anaemia are also present, and muscular and joint pains add to the patient's misery.

Diagnosis is established after examination of the blood which shows anaemia, thrombocytopaenia and usually a vast increase in the number of white cells, all of a primitive type and therefore called 'blast' cells (Fig. 8.5).

Course and complications
Untreated, the patient will develop enlargement of the spleen and liver. Death occurs within a few weeks from anaemia, haemorrhage or severe infection.

Treatment and nursing care
Although no cure has been found for acute leukaemia, modern treatment has induced encouraging remissions of the disease allowing some patients to survive for 5 or more years.

Drug therapy. Cytotoxic agents, such as methotrexate, mercaptopurine and cyclophosphamide, interfere with cell division, but resistance to therapy often develops and side-effects appear. Normal cells in the bone marrow may be suppressed, especially white cells and platelets, increasing the risk of haemorrhage and infection. Damage to the epithelium of the gastrointestinal tract may occur. Mouth ulceration, nausea, vomiting and diarrhoea may be troublesome. Alopecia often follows cyclophosphamide therapy, and although this may be temporary, many patients will be saved anxiety and embarrassment if fitted with a wig before therapy is started.

Singly, drugs are of little use, but the more adventurous use of combinations of drugs has proved effective. These combinations are given in varying cycles to reduce the development of resistance to treatment.

Corticosteroids, in particular prednisolone, reduce the tendency to bleed.

Antibiotics are important to counteract infection.

Blood and platelet transfusions. These are given at intervals as supportive therapy to correct anaemia and restore the blood to as normal a level as possible.

Rest. Rest in bed will be required while the patient is acutely ill. Careful attention should be given to the relief of pressure. Gentle handling and movement of the patient is particularly important to prevent bruising.

Prevention of infection. Because of the possibility of infective complications, isolation nursing is practised for leukaemic patients in some hospitals. To prevent the development of infection while the patient is at a low level of resistance, reversed barrier units have been set up allowing each patient to be nursed in a single room.

Alternatively, if a laminar flow unit is available (Fig. 8.12) the patient can be nursed in a ward beside other patients. This helps to prevent the psychological problems of being nursed in a single room. The patient is now protected by an invisible barrier of positive pressure air which prevents air-borne organisms from coming in to the patient. However, all items which are taken into the unit must be either sterile or scrupulously clean. This method of care is unsuitable if the patient is infected.

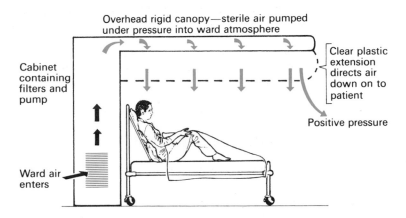

Figure 8.12
Laminar flow isolation unit

Careful attention to personal hygiene on the part of both patient and nurse is important. Any sign of a pyrexia should be reported promptly.

Mouth care. The problems of bleeding gums and mouth ulcers and the risk of superimposed candida infection as a result of antibiotic therapy make regular inspection of the mouth essential. Gentle swabbing may be needed and the patient should be encouraged to rinse his mouth frequently.

Psychological care. The needs and conditions of patients vary and each patient must be considered individually. The decision on whether — and how — to tell an adult patient about his condition requires careful discussion among nursing and medical staff and the patient's relatives. The hospital chaplain or family minister and the family doctor can be of great help in such a situation.

Nursing staff may be faced with difficult questions from the patient, for example on prognosis, and it is important that ways of handling these situations should be discussed. Although junior staff may not feel they have the necessary experience or knowledge to help the patient, they can ensure that questions are not ignored by getting assistance promptly from more senior nursing or medical staff.

The parents of a child suffering from acute leukaemia should be told the prognosis and should be given continued support from the health team at home or in hospital. Every effort is made to enable children to be looked after in their own homes.

Chronic myeloid leukaemia

Chronic myeloid leukaemia affects men and women equally, usually between the ages of 35 and 60.

The onset is gradual and the patient presents with the features of progressive anaemia. Tiredness and weakness may have been present for many months. Abdominal pain may occur and the patient may have noticed swelling in the left flank due to massive enlargement of the spleen.

Haemorrhagic features appear as the disease progresses.

Treatment of chronic leukaemia is often less rigorous than treatment of acute leukaemia. Cytotoxic drugs such as busulphan may induce a remission, allowing a symptom-free period. Blood transfusion is used to correct anaemia, which is assessed by frequent blood examinations. Radiotherapy, by localized irradiation, will reduce the size of the spleen. The combination of radiotherapy and drug therapy allows the blood count to return to normal and may cause a marked increase in well-being for the patient. With treatment the picture of remission and progression of the disease may continue for up to 3 years, although many patients survive even longer.

Chronic lymphatic leukaemia

Chronic lymphatic leukaemia is more common than chronic myeloid leukaemia. It occurs more often in men than women and affects an older age group, usually between 45 and 75 years.

The onset is very gradual, with a very slowly developing anaemia. The disease may go unnoticed until enlarged lymph nodes are found, often in the cervical, axillary or inguinal areas. The liver and spleen enlarge, but the splenic enlargement is not as great as that found in chronic myeloid leukaemia. The combination of mild anaemia, a moderately raised white cell count and enlarged lymph nodes will confirm the diagnosis.

Many patients, especially the more elderly, may be able to lead a normal active life for many years and their life expectancy may not be reduced by the disease. As the disease progresses, treatment becomes necessary. A cytotoxic drug such as chlorambucil is given, and radiotherapy is used to treat enlarged lymph nodes.

Whenever possible, the treatment of patients with chronic forms of leukaemia is supervised by the family doctor. However, as the bone marrow progressively fails, the risks of anaemia, haemorrhage and infection increase, and hospital admission becomes necessary to allow steps to be taken to correct anaemia, control haemorrhage or treat infection.

Disorders involving lymph nodes

Lymph nodes play an important part in the immune mechanism (Ch. 1) and are widely distributed around the body. As a result of this, any disorder present can produce a wide variety of signs and symptoms and the patient's resistance to infection will be much lower than normal.

Although disorders of the nodes such as Hodgkin's disease and lymphosarcoma are not actually disorders of the blood, their management is very similar to that required for the leukaemias.

The glands can also become infected as when a person develops **infectious mononucleosis** (glandular fever, Ch. 1).

Hodgkin's disease

This is a malignant disorder of the lymph nodes which mainly occurs in the 20 to 40 year age range but can occur at any age. The cause is unknown.

Clinical features
In the early stages the disease usually presents with painless enlargement of lymph nodes, especially in the cervical region. On occasion the patient may first present with a pyrexia of unknown origin. As the disease progresses, with other sites being involved, the signs and symptoms may include tiredness, general malaise, anaemia, dyspnoea and weight loss. Resistance to infection is also reduced.

Course and complications
The disease is slowly progressive and eventually fatal but some people survive for many years if treatment is given when signs and symptoms are localized.

Investigations
The diagnosis is made following lymph node biopsy. Lymphangiography will show up the extent of the lymph node involvement.

Treatment and nursing care
Radiotherapy may be used when the disease is localized. Cytotoxic drugs are given, usually in combination to minimize resistance to the drugs, when the disease is

widespread. The nursing problems encountered are similar to those of patients with leukaemia.

Lymphosarcoma

This is another progressive malignant disorder of lymphoid tissue which mainly occurs in the 50 to 60 year age range. Signs and symptoms vary depending upon the sites involved. Treatment is similar to that of Hodgkin's disease.

CARE OF THE PATIENT HAVING A BLOOD TRANSFUSION

Human blood may be transfused in several forms: as whole blood or as a derivative of it, such as plasma, serum, packed cells or platelets.

Plasma and serum can be dried and reconstituted for use by adding specially prepared, sterile, pyrogen-free distilled water. Both are useful substitutes for whole blood when blood volume has to be restored quickly. Packed cells are used when the haemoglobin level is to be raised without greatly increasing blood volume. Before transfusion, compatibility of blood must be established, that is whether the donor blood will mix with the recipient's blood without causing agglutination. The recipient's blood group is determined and, whenever possible, blood of the same group as his own is given (see Table 8.2, p. 262). The donor blood is always cross-matched by mixing it with a little of the recipient's serum to ensure that there is no agglutination. If this is not done and incompatible blood is given, serious transfusion reactions will occur. The early signs and symptoms are fever, rigors, headache, backache, urticarial rashes, vomiting and diarrhoea. Jaundice may follow haemolysis, and in severe reactions oliguria, anuria and uraemia are found.

Blood from volunteer donors is stored in 'blood banks', in special refrigerators maintained at a temperature of 4°C. The domestic ward refrigerator is not suitable for this purpose as its temperature varies. During collection, storage and administration of blood, its sterility must be maintained.

Complications of blood transfusion

Haemolytic reaction
Most of these reactions, in which there is an increased rate of destruction of red cells, are due to blood group incompatibility. This results from either incorrect grouping or cross-matching, or from an error in identification of the blood. Failure to check the labels on the blood or confusion of identity of patients with the same or similar names may result in the wrong blood being given. The following must therefore be checked carefully by two nurses before transfusion is started: the patient's identity, the number of the unit of blood, its group, and whether it has been cross-matched and found to be compatible. If there is any discrepancy the blood must not be given. All clinical features of transfusion reaction may be present.

Allergic reaction
Mild reactions cause slight elevation of temperature and urticarial rashes. Severe reactions may lead to anaphylactic shock.

Febrile reaction
Most reactions are due to pyrogens, but haemolytic and allergic reactions and reactions due to infected blood will also cause pyrexia. The degree of elevation of temperature varies from a slight transient rise to severe rigors with hyperpyrexia or a fever prolonged over several days.

Circulatory overload
Infusion of too much fluid over too short a period may lead to pulmonary oedema and acute heart failure because of the increased work load for the heart brought on by the increase in blood volume. For this reason, packed cells are used in preference to whole blood.

Nurses should be alert to this danger when giving blood to patients with existing heart failure and should ensure that blood is given at the prescribed rate.

Increased pulse rate and sudden dyspnoea are warning features. To compensate for the increased blood volume, the doctor may prescribe a diuretic to be given with each unit of blood.

Specific infections
Blood may be infected due to poor asepsis during collection, storage or transfusion. Septicaemia, profound collapse and shock, or death within hours may follow transfusion of infected blood.

A disease carried by a blood donor may be transmitted by transfusion, for example serum hepatitis, malaria or syphilis. This is prevented by careful screening of blood donors.

Because of the possibility of transfusion complications, the nurse has several responsibilities: ensuring that the correct blood is given to the correct patient at the prescribed rate; careful observation of the patient; hourly recordings of temperature, pulse and respiratory rate; and recording of fluid balance during transfusion. Should reaction be suspected, the transfusion must be slowed or stopped and the doctor informed immediately.

SUGGESTED ASSIGNMENTS
Projects
1. Compare the cost of a 2-month supply of drugs for the following patients:
   a. An elderly man with pernicious anaemia (maintenance dose).
   b. A 5-year-old child with acute leukaemia.
   c. A middle-aged housewife with mild iron deficiency anaemia (note cost of different preparations of the same drug).

2. How is blood for transfusion purposes collected, prepared and stored? If possible find this out from a visit to your nearest centre.

3. Consider what it means in practical terms to be a schoolboy with haemophilia. What facilities are provided by the government to help such a child? What advice and encouragement can be given during the periods that the boy is in hospital?

Discussion topic
To what extent should the formal education of a sick child be pursued if it is known that her prognosis is poor? Consider the implications for the education and health care teams as well as for the child and her family.

FURTHER READING

DHSS Committee of Regional Transfusion Directors 1975 Notes on transfusion, 6th edn. DHSS, London
Hugh-Jones N C 1979 Lecture notes on haematology, 3rd edn. Blackwell Scientific, Oxford

Reference only
Thomson R B 1979 A short textbook of haematology, 5th edn. Pitman, London

9. The Urogenital System

In keeping with tradition, the male genital and urinary tracts will be considered together in this chapter. It should however be noted that, although some structures are common to both, they are two quite separate systems. Female urinary disturbances associated with disorders of the reproductive tract are discussed in Chapter 10; those female urinary disturbances *not* associated with the reproductive tract are included in this chapter.

Because many of the disorders mentioned here are unrelated to each other, a common core of symptoms and signs is not evident; for this reason there is no section dealing with the general features of disease. Some disorders of the urinary tract are found with equal frequency in both sexes and others are not; bladder infection, for example, occurs more often in women than men.

ANATOMY AND PHYSIOLOGY

The kidneys

The two kidneys flank the aorta and the inferior vena cava to which they are joined by stout blood vessels. Figure 9.1 shows the right kidney in section. The most important function of the kidneys is to **maintain constant composition and volume of the body fluids**. This control comprises:

1. Regulation of water content.
2. Regulation of electrolyte content (particularly sodium, chloride and potassium).
3. Maintenance of acid-base balance (pH of the blood).
4. Excretion of waste products of metabolism, drugs and toxic substances.

The kidneys have other functions including the production of the hormone erythropoietin, which stimulates the manufacture of red blood cells, and the hormone renin, which plays a part in vasoconstriction (Ch. 7).

Table 9.1
Normal plasma concentrations of substances referred to in text

Urea	$3.3 - 6.6$ mmol/l
Creatinine	$44 - 150$ mol/l
K^+	$3.5 - 5.0$ mmol/l
Na^+	$135 - 147$ mmol/l
Cl^-	$95 - 105$ mmol/l
Bicarbonate	$21 - 28$ mmol/l
Ca^{++}	$2.1 - 2.5$ mmol/l
PO_4	$0.85 - 1.55$ mmol/l
Protein	$65 - 80$ g/l (6–9 g/dl)

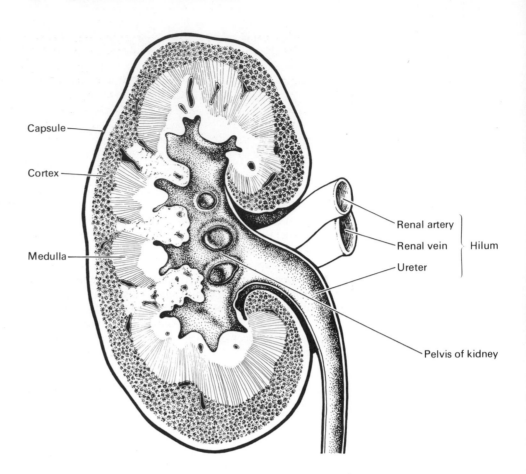

Capsule

Cortex

Medulla

Renal artery
Renal vein   } Hilum
Ureter

Pelvis of kidney

Figure 9.1
Vertical section of kidney
showing normal macroscopic
appearance

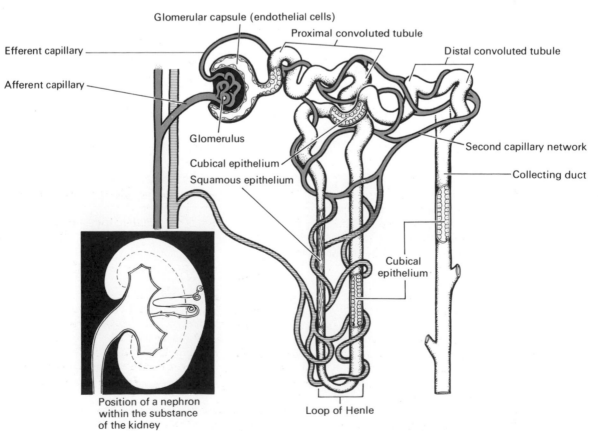

Glomerular capsule (endothelial cells)

Proximal convoluted tubule

Efferent capillary

Distal convoluted tubule

Afferent capillary

Glomerulus

Second capillary network

Cubical epithelium

Collecting duct

Squamous epithelium

Cubical
epithelium

Position of a nephron
within the substance
of the kidney

Loop of Henle

Figure 9.2
A nephron

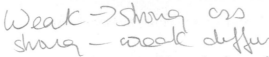

Maintenance of constant composition and volume of body fluids

In health the kidneys carry out this function by the formation of urine, the composition of which can be varied to suit the body's needs. For example, the end-products of protein metabolism are highly acidic, so the urine of a person taking a protein-rich diet would be more acidic than that of a vegetarian; the composition of the blood of the two individuals, on the other hand, would show only very minor differences, if any.

Each kidney is composed of approximately 1 million nephrons (Fig. 9.2), which are the basic functional units responsible for the formation of urine. Urine is derived from the blood by two important processes:

1. **Filtration**, which occurs in the glomerulus of each nephron. Because the diameter of the blood vessel entering the glomerulus is larger than that of the blood vessel leaving it, the blood pressure within the glomerular capillaries is higher than in tissue capillaries elsewhere in the body. For this reason a larger quantity of water and substances dissolved in water pass through into the glomerulus. In a normally functioning kidney substances with large molecules, for instance plasma proteins and the blood cells, are retained within the bloodstream by the capillary basement membrane (Fig. 9.3). In disease, however, protein and red cells may escape into the urine (p. 287). The kidneys have a very rich blood supply and it is estimated that around 170 litres of fluid per day are filtered through the glomeruli.

2. **Selective reabsorption**, which occurs in the renal tubules. Fortunately, under the influence of ADH (Ch. 11), most of the water passed into the glomeruli is reabsorbed leaving only 1·5 litres to be passed out of the body as urine.

Production of ADH is increased during sleep and in consequence the amount of urine produced overnight is reduced. Damage to the distal portion of the tubule on which ADH acts, as in chronic renal failure, leads to a large amount of dilute urine being produced.

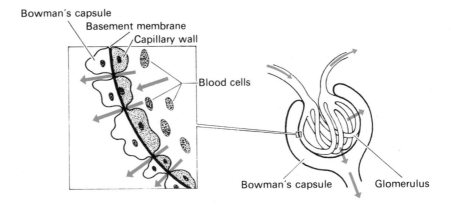

Figure 9.3
Relationship of the glomerulus to Bowman's capsule showing capillary basement membrane

Substances of importance in the nutrition of the body, such as glucose and amino acids, are completely reabsorbed.

Salts, for example sodium, chloride, potassium and calcium, are removed from the filtrate according to the body's needs. Sodium reabsorption is partly controlled by the adrenal cortical hormones (Ch. 11).

Waste substances such as urea and creatinine are not reabsorbed; therefore all appear in the urine.

There is some secretion through the distal parts of the tubule of, for example, drugs and toxic substances. The filtrate continues its passage out of the nephrons and through the collecting tubules where it has the same composition as voided urine.

Healthy kidneys are so efficient that minor variations in the composition of blood plasma are corrected immediately and the proper balance is restored.

From the foregoing it becomes evident that disease of the kidneys may have far-reaching effects and, as the power to eliminate fails, waste substances begin to build up in the blood.

One of the earliest and most important signs of disorder is the inability of the kidneys to concentrate urine, and in the more serious of the chronic disorders the specific

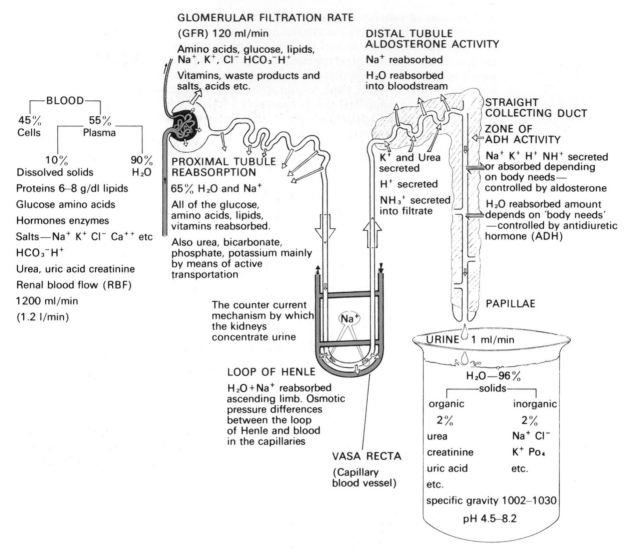

Figure 9.4
Dynamics of kidney function

gravity becomes fixed at 1010. The measurement of specific gravity of urine is sometimes regarded as a chore by busy nurses who may overlook its significance: it is actually very important.

Many of the investigations listed (Table 9.2, p. 284) are concerned with the estimation of renal function.

The ureters

The ureters are two muscular tubes which convey urine from the kidneys to the urinary bladder (Fig. 9.5). Each is continuous with the renal pelvis, which itself is continuous with the hilum of the kidney. The ureters are about 25 cm long and pass down the posterior abdominal wall behind the peritoneum. They pass over the brim of the pelvis and enter the lower posterior surface of the bladder at an oblique angle. The mucous lining of the ureter is of transitional epithelium. Urine is funnelled into the ureter via the renal pelvis and is conveyed to the bladder by peristaltic-like action. The oblique entry of the ureters into the bladder and the arrangement of the bladder muscle normally prevent reflux of urine.

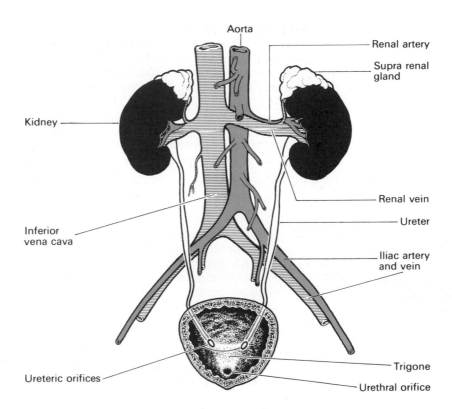

Figure 9.5
Kidneys, ureters and bladder:
relationships

The urinary bladder

The urinary bladder is a hollow, muscular organ which lies in the anterior part of the
pelvic cavity immediately behind the symphysis pubis (Fig. 9.6). The upper surface is
covered by peritoneum in the male. (For details of the pelvic anatomy in the female see
Chapter 10.)

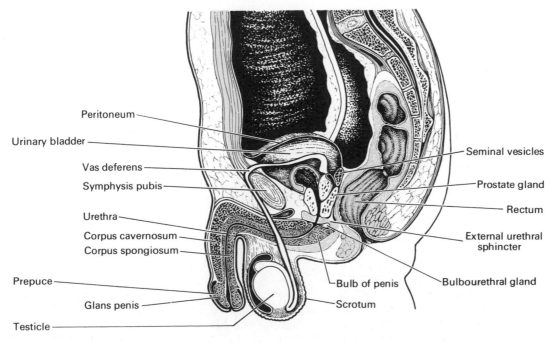

Figure 9.6
Sagittal section of male pelvis
showing bladder only partially
sectioned

The muscle is chiefly made up of interlacing bundles of involuntary muscle tissue. The inner lining consists of several layers of transitional epithelium which allows expansion as the bladder fills with urine. The urethra leaves the bladder at its lowest point. The triangle formed by the openings of the ureters and the urethra is called the trigone. This area does not expand as the bladder fills (see incontinence, p. 308).

The urethra and the penis

The urethra is the passage which conveys urine from the bladder to the outside of the body. In the male it can be divided into three main parts:

1. Prostatic.
2. Membranous.
3. Penile.

The prostatic urethra is about 2·5 cm long and is closely surrounded by the prostate gland. The membranous urethra passes through several layers of membranes and muscles which form the external urethral sphincter. The bulbourethral glands, which secrete a lubricating fluid, lie between these membranes. Their ducts enter the membranous urethra. The penile urethra traverses the length of the corpus spongiosum, which is one of the three cylinders of cavernous erectile tissue comprising the penis (Fig. 9.7). The urethral meatus opens on to the bulbous anterior part of the penis — the glans penis. The glans is covered by a movable cuff of skin called the prepuce or foreskin.

The urethra in the female is very short and for this reason microorganisms gain access to the bladder more readily than in the male (see cystitis, p. 281).

The prostate gland

The prostate gland completely encloses the urethra as it leaves the bladder. It is about the size of a chestnut and produces a watery fluid which is added to the secretions of the testes and seminal vesicles. Also entering the prostate gland are the ejaculatory ducts from the seminal vesicles. The seminal vesicles are, in turn, linked to the testes by the vas deferens, which conveys the spermatozoa from the testes.

The seminal vesicles

These are two small hollow organs; they produce a 'sticky fluid' which is added to that produced by the testes and prostate gland. Spermatozoa are stored in the ampulla of the vas deferens.

The testes

The two testes lie in a small, muscular sac called the scrotum. Each testis is a solid organ and is about 4 cm long. It is surrounded by a serous membrane, the tunica vaginalis, and

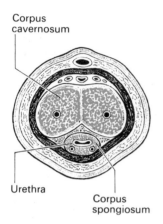

Corpus
cavernosum

Urethra

Corpus
spongiosum

Figure 9.7
Transverse section of penis

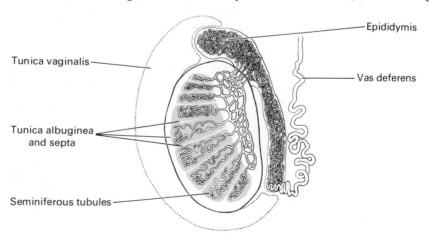

Tunica vaginalis

Tunica albuginea
and septa

Seminiferous tubules

Epididymis

Vas deferens

Figure 9.8
Section of testis

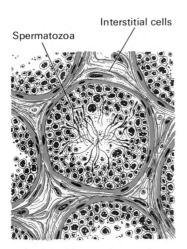

Spermatozoa   Interstitial cells

Figure 9.9
Microscopic appearance of
seminiferous tubule

once this is removed a tough fibrous coat of a whitish appearance, the tunica albuginea, is exposed. The fibrous coat gives rise to septa which divide the testis into about 250 lobules (Fig. 9.8). Each lobule contains from one to four seminiferous tubules. The lining of the seminiferous tubules generates the spermatozoa (Fig. 9.9), which are wafted towards the epididymis and on to the vas deferens. Under the influence of a hormone from the anterior lobe of the pituitary gland the interstitial cells, which lie between the seminiferous tubules, produce testosterone. Testosterone helps maintain the secondary sexual characteristics.

INVESTIGATIONS

An array of tests and examinations may be carried out, particularly in renal disorder, either to pinpoint a diagnosis or to monitor the patient's progress. Table 9.2 shows those most often used.

Minor variations in practice are common so the nurse should be quite certain of local procedure before embarking upon any test. Failure to do so may mean that an entire investigation has to be repeated, which will cause the patient inconvenience and will prolong his stay in hospital.

DISORDERS OF THE URINARY TRACT
Urinary tract infections

Urine provides an excellent medium for the growth of micro-organisms so that infections of the urinary tract are very common, especially in women. The infection may be a complication of some anatomical abnormality but more often than not the urinary tract is quite normal. There is little doubt that most of the urinary tract infections gain access to the urinary bladder by ascending the urethra. In the female the urethra is only about 3 cm long and appears to offer little resistance to invasion by micro-organisms found in and around the entrance to the vagina. Once in the bladder these normally commensal bacteria for example *E. coli* become pathogenic. In males, not only is the urethra longer but the seminal and prostatic secretions are thought to be bactericidal and so create an additional barrier to invading micro-organisms. No similar secretion has been identified as yet in females.

In the past few years doctors have become increasingly aware of the problem of vesico ureteric reflux especially in young girls; in this condition some of the urine passes back into the ureters during micturition. If the urine is already infected the kidney also quickly becomes infected. Often this type of infection is asymptomatic and attempts are now being made to establish screening procedures for girls, when they start school or earlier, so that the problem can be dealt with. It is also becoming increasingly obvious that it is this group of individuals, who have established urinary tract infection by the age of 10 or so, who go on to develop chronic renal disease in adult life. A woman who develops an upper urinary tract infection for the first time in adult life, and whose infection is adequately treated and followed up, rarely develops chronic pyelonephritis. It still however, remains a fact that among women who develop chronic renal failure pyelonephritis is one of the more common causes.

Cystitis and urethritis

Some infections of the urinary tract are confined to the urethra and bladder; in adult women one predisposing factor to recurring bladder infection is sexual intercourse causing mechanical irritation or bruising of the urethra. In this group of patients it is important, when establishing a diagnosis, to enquire about the relationship of symptoms to sexual intercourse.

Clinical features
The features of systemic illness are slight: the patient complains of frequency of micturition which is accompanied by pain in the region of the urethra on voiding urine. In cystitis, although the bladder is empty, there may be an intense desire to pass more urine (strangury) due to spasm of the inflamed wall. In some patients with symptoms suggestive of urethritis and cystitis no organisms can be cultured from the urine.

Treatment

Treatment of urethritis and cystitis is the same as that of infection elsewhere in the urinary tract, namely, the use of antibacterial drugs, for example sulphonamides. The choice of drug should be governed by the sensitivity of the organisms.

Normally a midstream specimen of urine is obtained for culture, and treatment is started immediately with the drug that is most likely to be effective. When the laboratory report is available drug therapy is reconsidered in the light of the organisms found.

Even well-selected drugs, however, cannot be effective if there is an anatomical deformity or obstructive lesion of the urinary tract, so the underlying cause must be sought when infection is persistent or recurrent.

It is common practice to give a 2-week course of drugs followed by a repeat urine culture when treatment is completed. A high urine output is an advantage because frequent emptying of a full bladder voids many organisms and so discourages their multiplication; therefore, the patient should be encouraged to take plenty of fluids.

Doctors exercise care when using some of the antibacterial drugs useful in treating urinary infections because, in patients with impaired renal function, they accumulate in the blood and this may lead to permanent nerve deafness and vestibular damage.

Pyelonephritis

Pyelonephritis is a condition in which there is bacterial infection of the kidney substance and renal pelvis. Of the many predisposing factors obstruction of the urinary tract, diabetes mellitus, pregnancy, ureteric reflux, sexual activity and, in the hospital setting, the introduction of instruments into the renal tract are perhaps the most common. As many as 50 per cent of women will develop a urinary tract infection at some time in their lives. Clinically pyelonephritis may be acute or chronic. The term pyelitis is best avoided as it suggests that the condition is confined to the renal pelvis.

Acute pyelonephritis

This is an acute inflammatory infection of the kidney parenchyma. It nearly always occurs as a result of ascending infection. The most common infecting micro-organism is *E. coli*, 85 per cent of cases, whilst enterobacter, klebsiella, proteus, pseudomonas and enterococci account for the other 15 per cent. The micro-organisms have several major hurdles to overcome before reaching the kidney but once in the kidney the medulla region is very susceptible to infection and the cortex only slightly less so.

Clinical features

All the features of cystitis and urethritis (p. 281) are present. In addition there is pain and tenderness in both loin regions. There will be pyrexia or hyperpyrexia depending on the severity of the infection. Nausea, vomiting, sweating and on occasion rigors are all indicative of considerable systemic involvement. The urine may look cloudy and usually has an unpleasant smell; a 'fishy' odour is associated with infections caused by *E. coli*.

The diagnosis is confirmed by obtaining a midstream specimen (MSU) for culture and sensitivity. A colony count of 10^5 indicates significant bacteruria, counts of 10^4–10^5 are uncertain and counts of 10^4 or below suggest contamination. If the results are in doubt, then the MSU is repeated.

Treatment and nursing care

The medical treatment is to give antibiotics. These are started when a presumptive diagnosis is made and may have to be changed once the results of the culture and sensitivity tests become available. The most common antibiotics used are co-trimoxazole, ampicillin, cephalexin, kanamycin, nalidixic acid, carbenicillin, gentamycin and doxycycline. These patients are often very ill and must be confined to bed during the acute phase until the temperature falls. They will not usually feel like doing much else anyway. The patient will require all the nursing care of a febrile patient. A liberal fluid intake is ensured. A fluid intake and output chart is maintained and the urinary output observed carefully. Any evidence of a decrease in urine output may indicate the beginning of renal failure, as also may a rise in blood pressure.

Four hourly TPR and B/P should be recorded and any changes reported to the medical staff. The midstream specimens of urine are obtained at intervals to find out whether or not the infection has cleared. If the infection is recurrent a full urinary tract investigation is necessary. A micturating cystogram (Table 9.2) may show evidence of vesicoureteric reflux. Sometimes in the case of a child, this may right itself spontaneously as the child grows older, but in other cases the urologist may have to operate on the faulty valve. Failure to treat acute episodes of pyelonephritis adequately may very well lead to the development of chronic pyelonephritis.

Chronic pyelonephritis

As the term implies this is a continuing pyogenic infection of the kidneys. It is usually rather patchy in distribution and ultimately causes distortion of the kidneys due to fibrosis or scarring. (Fig. 9.10B.) The disease may follow an attack of acute pyelonephritis which has been treated inadequately. It may also be caused by infection occurring above an obstruction in the urinary tract, such as stones, urethral stricture or prostatic enlargement.

Clinical features
Often the symptoms are non-specific and the patient may approach the doctor because of lassitude and vague ill health. Symptoms from the urinary tract may, however, be present and include frequency of micturition, dysuria and occasionally loin pain.

The clearest way of demonstrating chronic pyelonephritis is by an intravenous urogram, which may reveal a decrease in thickness of kidney cortex, irregularity of the renal outline and differences in the size of the two kidneys.

Treatment
If treatment is to be really effective it must be started before serious renal damage has occurred. The principles of treatment are the same as for acute pyelonephritis: isolation and efficient eradication of the infecting organism and investigation of the urinary tract for any abnormalities of structure. Where the damage to the kidney tissue is substantial the management is similar to that of chronic renal failure.

Tuberculosis

Tuberculosis of the kidney is always secondary to a primary infection elsewhere in the body and, reflecting the overall pattern of tuberculosis, has diminished in incidence in the United Kingdom over the past few decades.

Clinical features
The patient is often relatively fit, the chief complaint being that of increasing urinary frequency which may become so severe as to be intolerable. Pain in the loin due to obstructive lesions may also be a feature. Diagnosis is confirmed by culturing the tubercle bacilli from specimens of early morning concentrated urine, but as these organisms can take anything up to 12 weeks to culture radiological confirmation of the disease may be sought.

Treatment
Once the diagnosis has been established conservative treatment with the proven antituberculous drugs is commenced. Drugs are used in combination and include the following: sodium aminosalicylate (PAS), isoniazid, ethambutol, rifampicin and streptomycin. Two or three of these drugs are given at any one time, the combinations being changed at intervals to avoid bacterial resistance. The treatment is continued for up to two years. Surgery is only indicated if the disease is very advanced on one side — providing the other kidney is functioning satisfactorily.

Table 9.2
Investigations

Procedure	Purpose and method	Preprocedure, care of patient and notable points	Special postprocedure care	Complications	When used
History and clinical examination	To establish main features of disorder and make provisional diagnosis. To establish base lines.	No special care. Examination performed by doctor.	Nil	Nil	All patients
Urine testing	To detect abnormal constituents, e.g. sugar, albumin, bile, urobilinogen (follow reagent manufacturer's instructions). Observe colour, odour, deposits, specific gravity, osmolality and measure amount	Explain need for specimen of urine. Provide suitable receptacle labelled with patient's name. Specimens should be tested when fresh.	Record results and report to nurse in charge	Nil	All patients as part of routine screening
Midstream specimen of urine (MSU)	To obtain specimens of urine not contaminated with micro-organisms from outside the urinary tract. Specimen is tested in laboratory for presence of micro-organisms and their sensitivity to antimicrobial drugs	Explain procedure to patient. Cleanse genital area around urethra as per hospital policy. Ask patient to start passing urine. Collect specimen in a sterile container before flow ceases. (N.B.: Not the first urine passed.)	Send specimen immediately to laboratory in sterile universal container with relevant forms	Nil	When UTI is suspected or as a screening procedure
Catheter specimen of urine (CSU)	As MSU	See care of self-retaining catheter	As MSU	Nil	As MSU
24-hour urine collection	To measure amount of certain substances excreted in 24-hour period. Results compared with known normal values	Explain procedure to patient. Collect labelled container provided by laboratory (may have preservative depending on test). Start test at 8 a.m. Ask patient to empty bladder and discard specimen. Collect all urine passed during next 24 hours. The last specimen is obtained at 8 a.m.	As in MSU/CSU, above	Nil	In kidney function tests, hormone gland studies, investigation of blood disorders, etc.
Concentration dilution tests	To assess kidney function and posterior pituitary function	For details of these tests consult local procedure manuals, as practices vary considerably	Some patients require close observation to ensure that dehydration does not occur, especially in pituitary studies.	Dehydration	Kidney and pituitary disease
Urea and creatinine clearance tests	Index of kidney damage. Designed to show how much blood is cleared of a substance per min. (Creatinine once filtered into the tubule is not reabsorbed.)	As for 24-hour urine collection. Blood specimens are taken concurrently	Specimens are sent to laboratory in appropriate containers with request forms.	Nil	Kidney disease

Table 9.2
Investigations (Continued)

Procedure	Purpose and method	Preprocedure, care of patient and notable points	Special postprocedure care	Complications	When used
Straight X-ray	To show up tissues of different density	Explanation of procedure	Nil	Nil but caution in pregnancy	Initial screening. Assess kidney size, calculi, suspected chest secondaries
Blood chemistry tests	To measure kidneys' ability to excrete metabolic wastes, e.g. urea, creatinine and electrolytes	No special care	Nil	Rare if properly executed	Routine screening procedure and indicator of direction of disease process
Intravenous pyelogram (IVP) (urogram)	To show an outline of the whole urinary tract on X-ray and indicate kidney function. A radio-opaque compound is introduced intravenously which is then excreted by the kidney	Explain procedure to patient. Consult local instruction manual. Preparation usually includes giving light diet day before and laxative evening before to clear stomach and intestines of gas. Food and fluids are restricted for 6–8 hours before procedure	A cup of tea and toast will be appreciated	May have a reaction to contrast media during the procedure. Patient needs special care if in renal failure.	Any suspected kidney disease. Not normally used during pregnancy
Retrograde pyelography	Used to outline detail of pelvis, calyces, ureter. Contrast media is injected into the kidney via a ureteric catheter inserted through a cystoscope	As for anaesthetic. See cystoscopy below	Observe urinary output and test for blood. Other care as for postanaesthesia.	Haematuria, infection, trauma to the urethra, bladder and ureter	When detail has not been obtained from IVP as in non-functioning kidney. Renal calculi
Voiding cystogram or micturating urethrogram	To show outline of bladder on X-ray, contrast media is introduced into the bladder through a catheter. Patient asked to empty bladder and serial X-ray pictures will show behaviour of lower urinary tract	Explain procedure, patient is catheterized. See catheterization	Observe urinary output. Test for blood. High fluid intake	UT infection, haemorrhage, damage to urethra or bladder	Bladder tumours, bladder diverticul tis, incontinence, vesica ureteric reflux
Isotope renography	To give an indication of renal blood flow. (Hippuric acid labelled with I¹³¹ is injected IV). A Geiger counter placed over the kidneys records the appearance and disappearance of radioactivity	Explain procedure	Nil	Very rarely reaction to the isotope	Suspected obstruction in kidney. Renal transplant
Isotope scanning of kidney	A radioactive isotope of mercury or technetium is given IV. This is taken up by the kidney tubules and a sensor device is passed to and fro over the kidney and a picture of the isotope concentration can be built up	Explain procedure	Nil	None	Renal tumours and cysts

Table 9.2
Investigations

Procedure	Purpose and method	Preprocedure, care of patient and notable points	Special postprocedure care	Complications	When used
Renal biopsy	To remove a small section of the kidney substance for pathological examination. Light, electron and immunofluorescent microscopy techniques are used	Explain procedure. Assess patient and gain co-operation. Obtain written consent. Other care as for any minor operation under local anaesthetic. Kidney is localized by X-ray and surface anatomical landmarks. Blood must be available for transfusion if necessary	Patient must be nursed in bed at complete rest for first 4 hours. Observations of BP and pulse $\frac{1}{4}$ hourly initially. If condition remains satisfactory the frequency of observations can be reduced. All urine is observed for haematuria — bed rest until urine is clear; at least 24 hours of bed rest is advisable	Haemorrhage, shock, infection, pain	Diagnosis of diffuse renal disease, e.g. differentiation of glomerulonephritis. Contraindication perinephric abscess and renal tumours
Cystoscopy and biopsy	To inspect the interior of the bladder, diagnose and treat urethral and bladder disorders by means of an endoscope introduced through the urethra	Explain procedure. As for general anaesthetic (may on occasion be done under local anaesthetic)	As for general anaesthetic depending on whether procedure is for diagnosis or treatment (see postoperative care). Observation of vital signs, and urine for blood	Haemorrhage. Trauma of urethra and bladder. Complications of general anaesthetic. Urinary tract infection.	Diagnosis of bladder and urethral disorders. Treatment of bladder tumours. Transurethral prostatectomy. Taking biopsies for pathology (see retrograde pyelogram)
Renal angiogram	To obtain details of the renal blood supply using X-ray and fluoroscopy techniques. A contrast medium is introduced via a catheter inserted into a major artery, e.g. femoral	As for IVP (see above)	Bed rest 8 hours. Pressure dressing over puncture wound. Observations of vital signs and pulses distal to puncture site.	Haemorrhage from puncture site. Haematuria.	Diagnosis of suspected renal artery stenosis. Renal neoplasms. Abnormal renal vessels
Cystometrogram	To assess the response of the detrusor muscle to filling	As for cystoscopy above	As for cystoscopy above	As for cystoscopy above	Urinary incontinence

DISORDERS OF THE KIDNEYS

A number of pathological disorders may involve the kidneys, among them the group of diseases known to the layman as Bright's disease or nephritis. Nephritis is classified variously by different authorities and the terminology is changed as new discoveries regarding the complex functions of the kidneys and disease processes are made.

The following classification is generally accepted in the Western world:

Acute proliferative glomerulonephritis.
Minimal lesion glomerulonephritis.
Membranous glomerulonephritis.
Chronic glomerulonephritis.

Chronic renal failure may be a sequel to any of these conditions and nephrotic syndrome may follow minimal lesion or membranous glomerulonephritis.

Acute renal failure more commonly arises from some sudden severe disturbance of the circulation than from disease within the kidney itself.

In health the products of metabolism are excreted by the kidneys but in disease of the kidneys their function is impaired allowing urea, creatinine and anions such as phosphate and sulphate to build up in the blood. The concentration of blood urea gives useful indications of the degree of failure; the level only rising when function is reduced by 50 per cent or more. It is for this reason that urea levels are monitored so closely, not because the rise in the amount of urea itself is more harmful than accumulations of other end products of metabolism.

It follows that the clinical features of nephritis and renal failure mostly result from abnormalities in chemical composition of the body or from hypertension and not locally from the site of the diseased kidneys.

The protein in urine when it is present is albumin rather than globulin because albumin is of smaller molecular size and can therefore penetrate the diseased glomerular membrane in larger amounts.

Acute proliferative glomerulonephritis

This is an acute inflammatory disease of the glomeruli. There is often a history of streptococcal infection of the throat or occasionally of the skin some 10 to 14 days before the onset of the renal illness. It can affect any age group but is most likely to happen in childhood.

Clinical features
Because of glomerular damage there is reduced filtration and increased reabsorption of water and salt by the tubules causing the patient to develop generalized oedema. This is most noticeable in the face, which looks pale and puffy. Urinary output is low (oliguria), about 500 ml daily, and small amounts of blood (haematuria) give the urine a smoky appearance. Proteinuria is also present. The patient usually shows features of an acute infection, including malaise, fever and anorexia.

Hypertension, dyspnoea, and pulmonary oedema are often prominent features. Headaches, papilloedema, convulsions and loss of consciousness may follow.

Investigations to confirm the diagnosis include urinalysis, blood chemistry, fluid balance charting and weighing. The antistreptolysin titre may be raised and a throat swab may show the presence of haemolytic streptococci.

Treatment and nursing care
Bed rest and warmth are important during the acute phase and should be continued until haematuria, proteinuria, oedema and hypertension have disappeared. Reduction of protein intake to 20–40 g/day controls the degree of uraemia (that is, when the blood level of urea rises above 6·6 mmol/l). Fluids are restricted to half a litre plus the equivalent of the volume of the previous day's output while the oedema is present and until a diuresis occurs.

A 'no added salt' diet is prescribed in which no salt is used in cooking and no table salt is added to meals; if the oedema is severe a very low salt diet may be given (Ch. 7). The nursing staff should appreciate that this is an extremely unpalatable diet and should do everything possible to tempt the patient to eat. It is important that meals are served attractively.

The original infection, if still present, is treated with an antibiotic. If the hypertension is not controlled by salt and fluid restrictions, drug therapy will be required especially if the dangerous complications of hypertensive encephalopathy (Ch. 7) develops. Pulmonary oedema and acute renal failure (see below) are other complications.

The prognosis for children suffering from this type of glomerulonephritis is good, the majority recovering completely. Recovery is less complete when it occurs in adults, acute renal failure is more common and many progress to chronic glomerulonephritis.

Minimal lesion glomerulonephritis and membranous glomerulonephritis

In minimal lesion glomerulonephritis, as the name suggests, there is very little change in the microscopic appearance of the kidneys but serious functional disorder. In membranous glomerulonephritis histological examination of a biopsy specimen shows thickening of the capillary basement membrane. Some authorities attribute this to an antigen-antibody reaction which results in an allergic response.

The two conditions are described together because they are clinically indistinguishable at the outset. Minimal lesion glomerulonephritis, however, usually occurs in the 5 to 15-year-old age group while membranous glomerulonephritis more commonly occurs in those approaching middle age.

Clinical features

The conditions are associated with an increase in the permeability of the basement membrane leading to proteinuria; it may be only slight and therefore may persist undetected for some time. As the proteinuria increases in severity generalized oedema occurs, which is often the first presenting sign. As much as 30 g of protein per day may be excreted in the urine causing the total plasma content to become greatly depleted.

Diagnosis is established by renal biopsy and histological examination of a specimen of renal tissue.

Treatment

Where minimal lesion glomerulonephritis occurs in children a course of steroid treatment is given.

The prognosis for patients with membranous glomerulonephritis is less favourable and at present there is no form of drug treatment for this condition. One-third of sufferers will recover to complete health but the remainder are liable to develop arterial hypertension (Ch. 7) and progressive renal destruction leading to gradual impairment of renal function and chronic glomerulonephritis.

Chronic glomerulonephritis

This condition may follow either acute proliferative glomerulonephritis or membranous glomerulonephritis. The glomeruli are progressively destroyed and replaced by fibrous tissue. Kidneys so affected are much smaller than normal and have a granular appearance (Fig. 9.10 C).

Often, however, no history of either disease is obtained and the pathological changes in the kidney seem to develop insidiously over many years. The end result is the same, however — chronic failure of renal function.

Nephrotic syndrome

Any patient with heavy proteinuria (more than 5 g/24 h), gross oedema and a low serum albumin is described as having nephrotic syndrome; this is regardless of his age and the cause of his condition.

Causes

The main causes of nephrotic syndrome are glomerulonephritis, renal vein thrombosis, diabetes mellitus, amyloidosis, certain drugs, malaria, connective tissue (collagen) diseases and new growths.

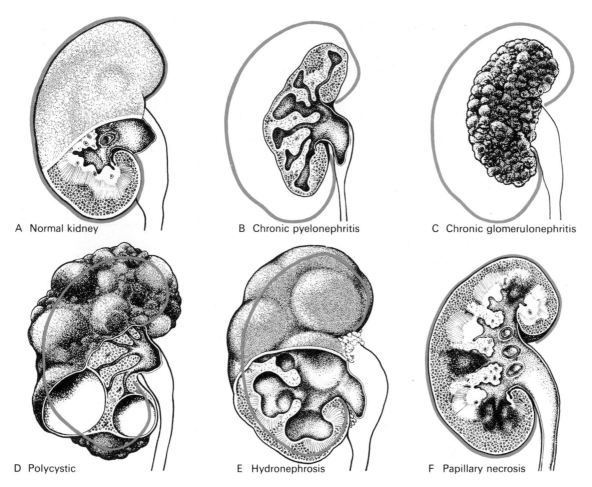

A Normal kidney   B Chronic pyelonephritis   C Chronic glomerulonephritis

D Polycystic   E Hydronephrosis   F Papillary necrosis

Figure 9.10
Kidney diseases

Clinical features

The most striking feature of this syndrome is very heavy proteinuria. Such a loss of protein in the urine is more than can be met by the dietary intake and the result is a low serum albumin (hypoalbuminaemia) which in turn results in a low osmotic pressure and a reduced volume. The low osmotic pressure is responsible for the generalized oedema (anasarca) which is so distressing for the patient. The liver, in an attempt to synthesize enough albumin, manufactures an excess of cholesterol and lipids so that hyperlipidaemia is another characteristic of the syndrome.

Patients with nephrotic syndrome are very prone to infection and premature atheroma.

A variety of other clinical features related to the underlying cause may of course also be present.

Investigations

In addition to investigating the predisposing condition a full urinary tract investigation (Table 9.2) is carried out.

Treatment and nursing care

Treatment is directed towards the relief of oedema and the control of proteinuria. Nursing care of the oedematous patient is described in Chapter 7.

A protein intake of 90–100 g per day is desirable to make good the urinary loss of protein as long as the blood urea is not elevated. Salt intake is restricted by prohibiting salty foods, cooking and table salt. Diuretics may also be used to control oedema.

Corticosteroids such as prednisolone are often effective in young patients whose condition has resulted from glomerulonephritis.

The course of the disease is unpredictable and just occasionally it resolves spontaneously.

Renal failure (uraemia)

Renal failure is a state in which kidney function is no longer able to maintain the body chemistry within normal limits. It can be acute, acute on chronic or chronic.

Acute renal failure (acute uraemia)

A wide range of disorders may cause this condition and it is convenient to classify these as prerenal, renal and postrenal (Table 9.3). The effects produced are similar regardless of cause and even with all the resources currently available there is still a very high mortality

Table 9.3
Causes of acute renal failure

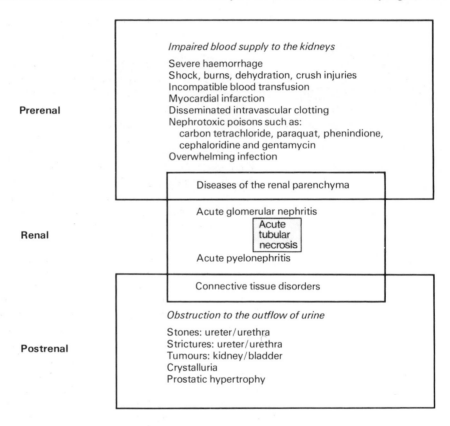

Prerenal

Impaired blood supply to the kidneys

Severe haemorrhage
Shock, burns, dehydration, crush injuries
Incompatible blood transfusion
Myocardial infarction
Disseminated intravascular clotting
Nephrotoxic poisons such as:
    carbon tetrachloride, paraquat, phenindione,
    cephaloridine and gentamycin
Overwhelming infection

Renal

Diseases of the renal parenchyma

Acute glomerular nephritis
Acute tubular necrosis
Acute pyelonephritis

Connective tissue disorders

Postrenal

Obstruction to the outflow of urine

Stones: ureter/urethra
Strictures: ureter/urethra
Tumours: kidney/bladder
Crystalluria
Prostatic hypertrophy

Figure 9.11
Acute renal failure

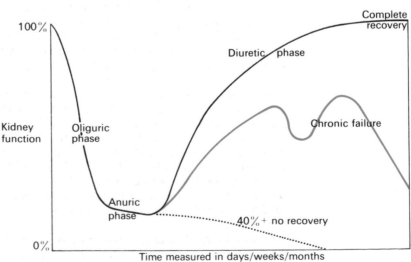

100%

Kidney function

Oliguric phase

Anuric phase

Diuretic phase

Complete recovery

Chronic failure

40% + no recovery

0%

Time measured in days/weeks/months

rate. Acute tubular necrosis (severe damage to the renal tubules due to ischaemia) is a feature of around a third of patients with acute renal failure.

The possible outcomes of acute renal failure are shown in Figure 9.11.

Clinical features

The onset is sudden, the first sign being a marked reduction in urinary output (oliguria) which may progress to complete anuria. The blood urea level rises rapidly especially in patients who are hypercatabolic and using up body proteins for instance following burns. There is also serious disturbance of electrolytes with a dangerous accumulation of potassium (K^+) which in turn produces changes in the electrical conductivity of the heart leading to life threatening arrhythmias. Changes in rhythm may be seen on an ECG.

Investigations

Tests are carried out to establish baselines and to record the response (or lack of response) to treatment. The role of the nurse in monitoring the patient's condition is crucial.

Urinalysis is essential and all urine passed, however small the amount, must be saved and kept in separate containers. Urine volume is often less than 500 ml in 24 hours. In addition to volume, specific gravity (often fixed at 1010) and osmolality measurements are carried out. The urine is tested for blood and other abnormal constituents in the ward whilst specimens are also sent to the laboratory for estimates of myoglobin, sodium and urea. Serial measurements of blood urea, creatinine and electrolytes together with the urine volumes are an essential guide to treatment. The patient should be weighed daily on sensitive bed scales.

Four hourly records of TPR and BP are obligatory.

If a postrenal cause is suspected (Table 9.3) a plain abdominal X-ray may show the presence of calculi (see below) and intravenous urography and/or retrograde pyelography may be necessary to establish the level of obstruction.

Treatment and nursing care

Because these patients are very ill the general nursing care must be of the very highest standard. Treatment is aimed at reducing or minimizing the disturbances due to the renal failure, preventing infection and maintaining nutrition.

Following the initial assessment of fluid and electrolyte balance a planned intake of fluid is given to replace fluids lost as urine and as insensible loss i.e. 400–500 ml plus an amount equivalent to the previous day's urine volume. It is vital therefore that accurate fluid balance charts are maintained. Because of the low urinary output, very little salt is excreted in the urine so that dietary salt must be limited strictly to 1·5 g/day (24 mEq). Dietary potassium must be restricted for the same reason and if plasma potassium levels cannot be controlled in this way, an ion exchange resin such as Calcium Resonium 15 g three times a day may be prescribed. This substance is rather unpalatable so it may be necessary to administer it via a nasogastric tube or per rectum. If the rise is very rapid and the level goes above 6 mmol/1 then other measures such as glucose 25–50 g and soluble insulin 10–20 units via an intravenous infusion may be given. The insulin promotes the transfer of K^+ ions into the cells and so lowers the serum potassium levels. Calcium gluconate 1–2 g i.v. may be given to protect the heart from the toxic effects of hyperkalaemia.

The restrictions in the amount of fluids, salts and proteins which can be given may make it difficult to ensure an adequate Kilojoule intake. However these patients must receive sufficient kilojoules (11·8 MJ–14·7 MJ) with just enough protein (30–40 g) to meet the body's needs and to prevent the breakdown of tissue protein which would cause the serum urea and potassium levels to rise rapidly. Concentrated glucose solutions such as Hycal and Caloreen which are fairly palatable are often used to boost Calorie intake. They are free of electrolytes. If the patient cannot take food orally or if this route is contraindicated for some other reason, then parenteral nutrition may be necessary. Lipids, carbohydrates and amino acid preparations can all be given intravenously.

One of the most serious complications is infection; indeed it is infection that is the cause of the high mortality rate which is still a feature of this disorder.

Nursing measures to prevent the spread of infection (Ch. 1) must be followed carefully. Procedures such as catheterization should be avoided if possible. If nutritional needs are being met parenterally, diligence is required in caring for the infusion site and equipment as infection is often a sequel to this procedure.

Specific nursing measures to prevent pressure sores (Ch. 14), stomatis (Ch. 5), chest infections (Ch. 6) and deep venous thrombosis (Ch. 7) are essential. Antibiotics are not usually prescribed prophylactically but will, of course, be ordered if needed. In general drugs which are excreted by the kidneys are avoided. Nurses need to be watchful for the side effects of drugs and report any such occurrence promptly.

Patients suffering from acute renal failure who are in a hypercatabolic state and those where the measures outlined above have not been successful in keeping the blood urea below 34 mmol/l will require either peritoneal or haemodialysis (see below).

Following the phase of oliguria lasting several weeks the urinary output increases dramatically as the nephrons begin to heal. This second stage is called the diuretic phase but this does not mean that the kidneys have made a complete recovery. It is several weeks or months before the kidneys are able to maintain homeostasis. Therefore during this phase dietary and other measures, even dialysis must continue until there is a definite spontaneous improvement. Some doctors prescribe diuretics such as frusemide during the oliguric phase and it is claimed this shortens this phase.

Chronic renal failure (chronic uraemia)

Chronic failure occurs when the kidneys are progressively and irreversibly destroyed over a period of time.

The renal diseases which most commonly lead to chronic renal failure are glomerulonephritis, pyelonephritis and polycystic disease (see below) of the kidneys. It may also arise as a complication of hypertension, diabetes mellitus and many other diseases. Infections, nephrotoxic drugs and chronic obstruction of the urinary tract are additional causes. In most patients the disorder runs a slow insidious course and is often missed initially.

Clinical features

The clinical picture is seldom clear cut. The early symptoms of lassitude, anaemia, mild depression and so on are all too vague to warrant very active investigations. Other more specific symptoms such as polyuria and nocturia have often become so much a part of the patient's accepted routine that they are not mentioned to the doctor. For these reasons the disease is often well advanced by the time the patient is referred for a full renal investigation.

As the disease progresses to severe renal failure every system and part of the body is affected in some way (Table 9.4). Anaemia caused by lack of erythropoietin, which normally stimulates production of red blood cells by the bone marrow, is responsible

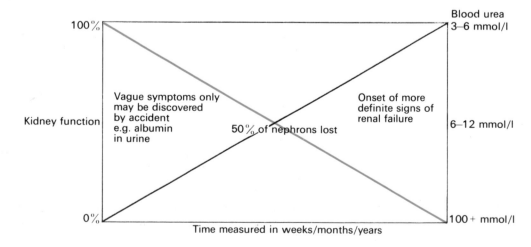

Figure 9.12
Chronic renal failure

Table 9.4
Severe renal failure (After Curtis J R 1978 Chronic renal failure. Practitioner 220:909 June 1978)

	Symptoms		Signs
Neurological	Poor memory		Tremor
	Lack of concentration	uraemic	Twitching
	Drowsiness	encephalopathy	Asterixis
	Fits		Coma
	Paraesthesiae in feet		Hyperreflexia
	Restless legs		Signs of peripheral neuropathy*
Muscular	Cramps		Signs of proximal myopathy*
	Weakness		especially of pelvic girdle
			musculature in renal osteomalacia
Psychiatric	Hallucinations		
	Depression		
	Delusions		
	Mania		
	Anxiety		
Ocular	Sore eyes		Corneal and conjunctival
			calcification*
			'Red eyes'
			Hypertensive retinopathy
			Detached retina
Haematological	Fatigue		Anaemia*
	Dyspnoea		Purpura
	Bruising		Bruises
	Nose-bleeds		
Cutaneous	Itching		Scratch marks
			Pigmentation*
			Purpura
			Dry skin
Skeletal	Bone pains		'Renal rickets' in children*
Joints	'Arthritis'		Gout and pseudogout*
Cardiovascular	Dyspnoea		Hypertension
	Chest pain		Left ventricular failure
	Orthopnoea		Raised jugular venous pressure
	Swelling of the legs		Oedema
			Left ventricular hypertrophy*
			Pericardial effusion
			Pericardial rub*
			Saline depletion and hypotension
Gastrointestinal	Anorexia		Oral ulceration
	Nausea		Foetor (ammoniacal)
	Hiccups		Parotitis
	Metallic taste in mouth		
	Thirst		
	Vomiting		
	Diarrhoea		
Endocrinological	Amenorrhoea		Gynaecomastia*
	Menorrhagia		
	Impotence		

* Suggests chronic rather than acute renal failure

for the lethargy. Polyuria develops because of the impaired concentrating ability of the kidneys and the excess sodium secreted by the diseased tubules. Anorexia, nausea and vomiting are common.

Continuing deterioration in renal function results in an increasing build-up of urea and acid waste products of metabolism. This relative acidity of the blood — in fact the pH indicates that it is still slightly alkaline — is called **acidosis**. Deep, sighing respirations are characteristic of severe renal failure; so too is the almost ammoniacal smell of the patient's breath and sweat. There are other associated features such as hypertension, which may in turn lead to left and then right-sided heart failure.

Distressing hiccups, muscle twitchings and increasing drowsiness precede terminal coma and death.

Figure 9.12 shows the effect of diminishing kidney function over a period of time.

Treatment and nursing care

In most instances the aim is to improve the patient's health and feeling of well-being although the damage sustained by the kidneys cannot be reversed. Just occasionally the underlying condition is amenable to treatment, for example an obstruction of the urinary tract, and this condition will be attended to first. For those patients who sadly do not have a reversible disease process an exacting regime including strict dietary measures will be necessary.

Diet

Protein is usually restricted to 40 or 60 g/day but with no attempt made to exclude second class proteins. The aim is to conserve the patient's own proteins and to keep the production of urea down so that the kidneys can excrete what is produced. If this measure is not successful a much stricter diet of the Giovanetti style may be prescribed. (For details of this diet the student should consult a textbook on dietetics). It is important to provide sufficient kilojoules in the diet to meet the patient's needs because if not the patient will burn up his own proteins and the object of the exercise is defeated. Glucose supplements are useful in chronic failure. Additional iron and vitamin supplements will usually be required to combat anaemia.

Electrolytes. Each patient is an individual and while some who have chronic renal failure retain sodium, most lose it to excess. Salt, then, is restricted or supplemented accordingly. Potassium may be retained so that restriction becomes necessary. The patient must be instructed to avoid foods rich in potassium which would be otherwise permitted in his diet.

Water. Most patients will not need to have their water intake restricted. If, however, the glomerular filtration rate is very low, the kidneys may not be able to excrete extra water. If too much water is taken, this will lead to water intoxication resulting in headaches and possibly fits. It is a fallacy therefore, to instruct the patient to consume large amounts of fluid to 'flush out his kidneys' when he is in renal failure.

Control of acidosis

As the kidney in failure cannot regulate the pH of the blood a metabolic acidosis develops. This is treated by giving sodium bicarbonate or lactate. If the conservative treatment outlined above is not successful haemodialysis and/or kidney transplant is the patient's only hope.

Complications

The complications of chronic renal failure are many. Two of these, anaemia and bone disease are so prevalent as to warrant more detailed consideration:

Anaemia. This is usually a hypochromic normocytic anaemia and is almost invariably a feature of chronic renal failure. The diseased kidneys fail to produce enough of the hormone erythropoietin which stimulates the bone marrow to produce the red blood corpuscles. Also it is thought that the high blood urea levels depress bone marrow function. Patients may have haemoglobin levels as low as 6 to 9 g/dl but have adapted to this and even when requiring dialysis are not invariably given blood transfusions. Blood transfusions in these circumstances reduce the bone marrow's response to the anaemia.

Bone disease. Calcium and phosphorus metabolism are seriously disturbed in renal failure and the development of bone disease is common. The kidney plays an essential role in the metabolism of vitamin D (Ch. 4) converting the biologically inactive 25 — hydroxycholecalciferol — to the active 125 — dihydroxycholecalciferol. This latter substance acts in the gut to promote the absorption of calcium and phosphorus and on bone to increase reabsorption and to mineralize uncalcified osteoid. Children develop rickets whilst adults develop its counterpart osteomalacia (Ch. 4). In renal failure this complication is treated by giving 125—dihydroxycholecalciferol (vitamin D_3)—or a synthetic preparation 1α—hydroxy vitamin D_3.

Plasma phosphate levels increase in renal failure, because the kidney is unable to excrete the absorbed dietary phosphorus. The plasma calcium levels, on the other hand, become low partly because of the vitamin deficiency and partly because of the hyperphosphataemia. The fall in calcium levels causes a secondary hyperparathyroidism which is responsible for the increased reabsorption of calcium from bone resulting in renal osteodystrophy (see also Ch. 11). One way of countering the hyperphosphataemia is to reduce the absorption of phosphorus by giving aluminium hydroxide which binds with the phosphorus in the diet.

Nursing care, like medical treatment, is largely symptomatic. Frequent mouthwashes and mouthcare are essential for the patient with a dry, brown, furred tongue and will help to relieve him of the bitter taste of which he so often complains. A piece of fresh pineapple gently applied to the tongue will usually remove obstinate fur and freshen the mouth. Regular bed-baths help to keep the skin free from sweat, which may cause irritation in chronic renal failure.

Very careful recordings of fluid intake and output must be made and the prescribed diet must be followed unless the patient is unable to tolerate it; this fact must then be reported. Hiccups, restlessness, muscular twitchings and vomiting must also be reported to the doctor since even in the terminal stages it is possible to keep the patient relatively comfortable with correct medication.

Polycystic disease

This is the commonest of the hereditary disorders of the kidney. Most of the patients are well into adult life—40 years or more—before obvious symptoms appear. They may have hypertension, a history of haematuria and renal pain and may already have evidence of renal failure. Both kidneys are enlarged and grossly abnormal with multiple cysts which cause anatomical distortions (Fig. 9.10 D). The onset of renal failure is usually slow so many patients are able to lead useful lives for some years after the diagnosis has been made. Anaemia is often less marked in these patients than in other forms of renal disease. Progression to complete renal failure is however almost inevitable.

Treatment and nursing care are as for patients with chronic renal failure.

Management and nursing care of patients undergoing dialysis

Dialysis is the transfer of solutes across a semipermeable membrane from a solution of high concentration, in this case the blood, to one of low concentration, the dialysate. This process is used to remove waste products, for example urea and creatinine, excess salts and fluid from the blood when the kidneys are failing to do so for some reason. As an 'aide memoire', the principles of diffusion and osmosis are illustrated in Figures 9.13 and 9.14 respectively. There are two types of dialysis namely peritoneal and haemodialysis.

Peritoneal dialysis

Here the patient's peritoneum is used to provide over two square metres of semipermeable membrane. The dialysing fluid is run into the peritoneal cavity (Fig. 9.15) by means of a semirigid plastic catheter such as the McGaw 'Trocath' (Fig. 9.16). The catheter is introduced through the abdominal wall under local anaesthesia and positioned in either the left or right iliac fossa. The catheter is then secured in position by means of a 'purse string' suture. Strict attention to aseptic technique is essential as the patients who require this form of dialysis are very prone to infections. The nurse should ensure that the patient's bladder is empty before this procedure is undertaken to reduce the danger of perforation. Accidental perforation of the bowel is also a potential hazard.

Peritoneal dialysis is very suitable for those patients who require dialysis urgently, for example patients with acute renal failure or those suffering from self poisoning. It

A

Start of experiment   Semipermeable membrane

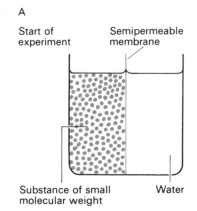

Substance of small molecular weight   Water

B

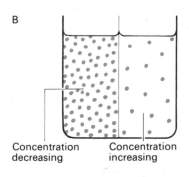

Concentration decreasing   Concentration increasing

C

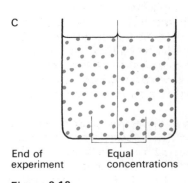

End of experiment   Equal concentrations

Figure 9.13
Diffusion

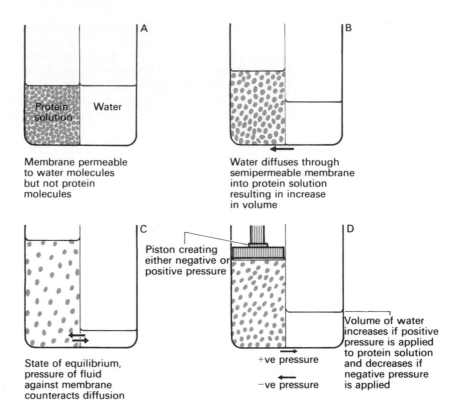

Figure 9.14
Osmosis

A
Membrane permeable
to water molecules
but not protein
molecules

B
Water diffuses through
semipermeable membrane
into protein solution
resulting in increase
in volume

C
State of equilibrium,
pressure of fluid
against membrane
counteracts diffusion

D
Piston creating
either negative or
positive pressure

+ve pressure
−ve pressure

Volume of water
increases if positive
pressure is applied
to protein solution
and decreases if
negative pressure
is applied

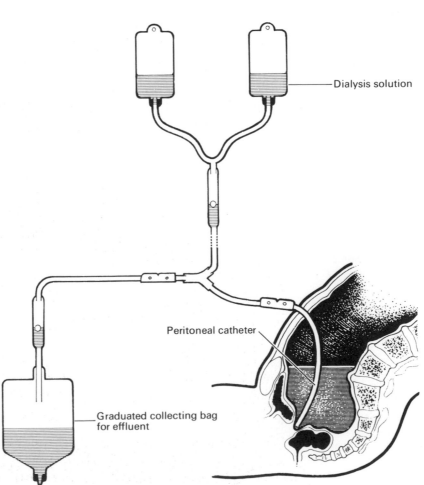

Dialysis solution

Peritoneal catheter

Graduated collecting bag
for effluent

Figure 9.15
Peritoneal dialysis

has a place too in the treatment of patients suffering from chronic renal failure prior to beginning regular dialysis. It is also used on a long-term basis for patients who can no longer be haemodialysed perhaps because they have no accessible veins or are diabetic. Diabetics are very liable to develop retinal bleeding when haemodialysed because of the need to give heparin during the procedure.

After the peritoneal catheter has been secured it is attached to the giving set and two litres of dialysate solution (Table 9.5) are run into the peritoneal cavity. The dialysate must be warmed up to body temperature (38°C) in a hot air oven or lotion cabinet set to that temperature, or passed through a special warming coil. On no account should the dialysate bags be warmed in buckets of hot water because of the risk of introducing infection

The dialysate is left in the peritoneal cavity for $\frac{1}{2}$ to 2 hours to allow the waste products and salts to diffuse into it. It is then drained out into a collecting bag. It may on some occasions prove difficult to get all of the fluid returned but changing the patient's position, for example by sitting him up, will usually be effective. When a

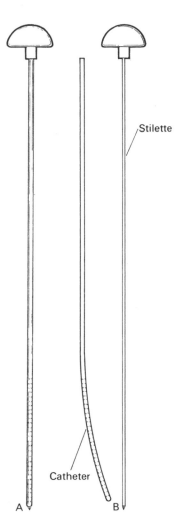

Figure 9.16
Trocath peritoneal dialysis catheter
A. Stilette in catheter
B. Stilette and catheter separated (Note curve of the catheter) (McGaw Laboratories)

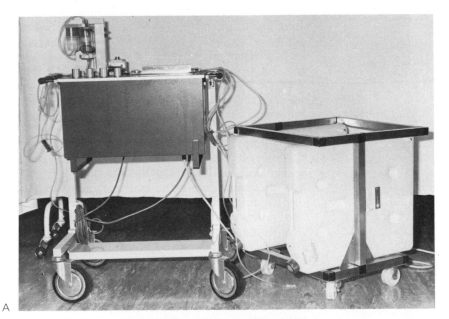

A

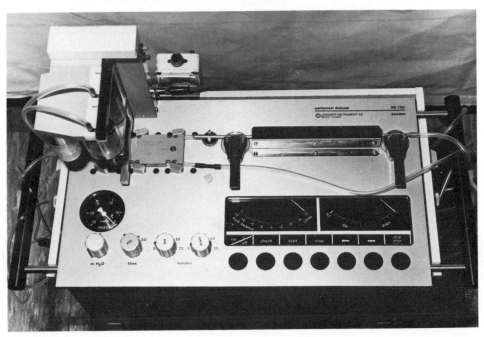

B

Figure 9.17
Automatic peritoneal dialyser
A. Side view
B. Top view

Table 9.5
Typical peritoneal dialysis solutions

Anhydrous dextrose B.P.	1.36 % w/v	6.36 % w/v
Sodium lactate	0.5 % w/v	0.5 % w/v
Sodium Chloride B.P.	0.56 % w/v	0.56 % w/v
Calcium Chloride	0.039 % w/v	0.039 % w/v
Magnesium Chloride	0.015 % w/v	0.015 % w/v
Sodium metabisulphite B.P.	0.005 % w/v	0.012 % w/v
	Water to 100 %	

volume of fluid, equal to that which was run in, is returned the procedure is repeated. It may be necessary to continue this every hour or two hours as prescribed for two or perhaps three days until the patient's condition is stable. Thereafter dialysis for a period daily or on alternate days may be all that is required. If the patient is overhydrated, the stronger dialysate solution will be used. The increased osmotic effect of this solution means fluids will leave the bloodstream and enter the peritoneal cavity so that the amount of fluid returned will be greater than that run in. Regular weighing of the patient will also help keep a check on the effectiveness of dialysis. Most doctors add a small amount of heparin to the dialysate as this prevents fibrin deposition on the catheter tip. During dialysis observations of blood pressure are necessary in case excessive fluids are being lost in which case the patient may become hypotensive. In the longer term specimens of the returned dialysate should be sent regularly for culture and sensitivity. Should infection become evident gentamycin can be added to the dialysate. Systemic antibiotics may also be necessary.

The amount of general nursing care the patient will require during peritoneal dialysis will vary. In acute renal failure very intensive care will be required while long-term patients will be almost self sufficient. Indeed a recent development in this country is the introduction of continuous ambulatory peritoneal dialysis. In this type of programme the patient has a permanent silastic peritoneal dialysis catheter implanted in the abdominal wall and is trained to connect up the dialysate bags himself. Dialysis continues around the clock and is very successful in maintaining a stable body chemistry. Patients have a full check up once a month in the outpatient department. Not everyone is able to carry out the prescribed routines safely and a patient is assessed carefully for his suitability for this form of dialysis.

The introduction of the automatic peritoneal dialysing machines (Fig. 9.17 A & B) in recent years has made the work of the nurse very much easier. The machine, though not yet widely available, will become more so in the next few years. One of its several advantages is that by providing a closed system it reduces the risk of infection very considerably: the machine automatically warms the fluid, controls rate, measures the peritoneal fluid balance and has a built-in alarm should any malfunction arise.

Haemodialysis
Modern management of renal failure would not be possible without the use of the artificial kidney. Artificial kidneys are used in two main ways:

1. For temporary support of patients with acute reversible renal failure whose blood urea cannot be controlled adequately by the use of peritoneal dialysis, or in situations where peritoneal dialysis for such patients would be impracticable, for example the presence of an abdominal wound.

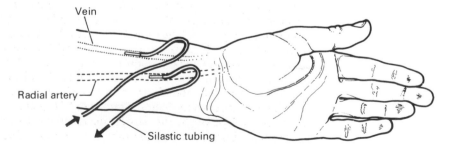

Figure 9.18
External arteriovenous (Scribner) shunt

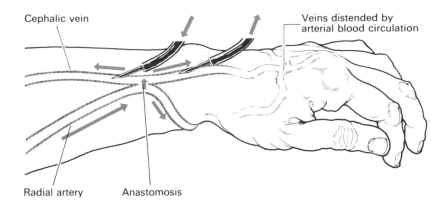

Cephalic vein

Veins distended by
arterial blood circulation

Radial artery   Anastomosis

Figure 9.19
Internal (subcutaneous)
arteriovenous shunt

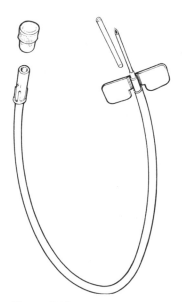

Figure 9.20
Butterfly 14 A.V. fistula set
(Abbot Laboratories)

2. For regular treatment of patients with end-stage renal failure for whom the ultimate goal in most cases is a successful renal transplant.

In order to dialyse a patient repeatedly a method must be available for regular and convenient access to his blood circulation.

One method is a Scribner shunt (Fig. 9.18), which basically consists of a loop of Silastic tubing connecting an artery and a vein. When not in use for dialysis, blood flows continuously through the shunt from artery to vein. To carry out a dialysis the shunt is clamped and taken apart in the middle. The arterial end is connected to the arterial tube of the kidney machine and the venous end is connected to the venous tube of the kidney machine.

Regular care of shunts and connections are nursing responsibilities and it is vitally important that they should be handled skilfully. Shunts should never be tugged, jerked or twisted, and the area of skin around the site of insertion should be kept covered with a sterile dressing. When not being used for dialysis the shunt should be examined at frequent intervals for patency as revealed by a 'thrill' and the temperature of the tubing.

Because of the disadvantages of clotting and infection the Scribner shunt is used mainly in short term dialysis. For long-term dialysis the surgical construction of a subcutaneous arteriovenous fistula, (Fig. 9.19) a technique developed by Cimino of Italy is an alternative. The fistula has to be left for about six weeks before it is ready for use. During this period the veins become distended and thickened and the blood flow is greatly increased. Once established a thin walled silicon coated needle such as in the Abbot Butterfly A.V. Fistula Set (Fig. 9.20) is used. This set allows easy connection to the artificial kidney.

Table 9.6 Typical haemodialysis solution	
Sodium	135–138 mmol/l
Calcium	1·25 mmol/l
Potassium	1·3 mmol/l
Chloride	108·8 mmol/l
Acetate	40 mmol/l
Dextrose	2 g/l

During dialysis blood is taken from the patient's artery (or arterialized vein), passed between layers of cuprophane which are sterile on the blood side and returned to the circulation (Fig. 9.21). The outside of the membrane is bathed by a fast-moving stream of dialysis fluid. The concentration of salts within this fluid is carefully calculated and, since it contains no end-products of metabolism such as urea, uric acid and creatinine, these substances diffuse from the blood into the dialysis fluid. Excess body fluids are removed during haemodialysis by means of ultrafiltration in which a negative pressure is created in the system. Blood is prevented from clotting in the tubes and between the layers of cuprophane by the use of heparin which is given as a continuous infusion or as intermittent injections into the tubing of the machine.

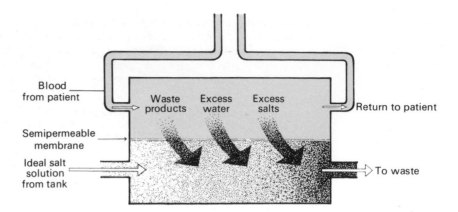

Figure 9.21
The principles of haemodialysis

During dialysis the patient must be carefully observed. Nurses should always be readily available to deal with any emergency or fault which may arise. A patient protection system is incorporated into all dialysis machines which monitors for faults such as leaks or air bubbles. Patients on long-term dialysis who have been trained or are being trained towards independence and who are familiar with the machines will be able to make minor adjustments themselves. In the case of a more serious malfunction the machine must be switched off, the blood lines secured and assistance summoned from staff able to deal with the problem.

The frequency of pulse and blood pressure recordings depends on the circumstances. If the patient is very ill, frequent recordings are necessary. In the case of regular long term dialysis, hourly blood pressure recordings are sufficient. The patient is carefully weighed before starting the dialysis and immediately on finishing.

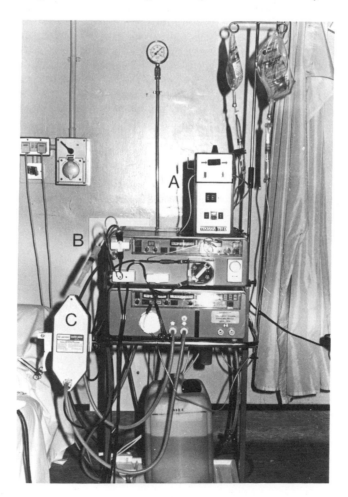

Figure 9.22
Haemodialysis machine. Note small size of exchange unit
A. IV pump
B. Central console
C. Exchange unit.

Ever since haemodialysis became common practice there have been sporadic outbreaks of viral hepatitis among patients and staff. This infection is probably carried and transmitted via the blood and can be a serious and even fatal illness, so care should be taken to reduce the risks by regarding all blood as a potential source of hepatitis. Avoidance of blood spillage and the use of gloves when handling blood are some of the precautions necessary. The incidence of hepatitis in haemodialysis units is now rare because of the very high standard of care in these units and an awareness of the danger. Another important factor has been the reduction in the number of blood transfusions given. Blood transfusions are not given unless absolutely necessary and all blood which is given is of course screened for viral hepatitis antigens. The introduction of small compact disposable dialysis packs has also been a factor in reducing cross infection as well as making the work in these units much easier.

Community care
Because the number of patients requiring dialysis far exceeds the facilities available for them in hospital, it has become necessary for patients to learn to carry out dialysis in their own homes.

Training for home dialysis usually takes 6 to 8 weeks in hospital. If technical problems subsequently prevent the patient carrying out dialysis successfully at home, provision must be made to admit him to hospital whenever the need arises.

Financial outlay for home dialysis is quite considerable, both for the equipment and for alterations to the home. If kidney transplantation is contemplated it is not worth spending a lot of money to establish the patient on dialysis in his own house. Regular haemodialysis in hospital or home has meant that many people continue to lead useful lives who would otherwise be dead, but the degree of rehabilitation achieved is variable and sometimes disappointing.

The nurse must be prepared to give emotional support to the patient and his family, and this she may find psychologically demanding. The dialysis machine, besides being very expensive, imposes restrictions which are often a continuing source of frustration and anxiety; for such a patient a successful kidney tranplant offers a chance to lead an almost normal life: within weeks of operation he will notice a dramatic return of his old strength and vigour.

Unfortunately, enthusiasm for transplantation must be tempered by the realization that mortality is still significantly higher than mortality on regular dialysis; survival rates are between 70 and 80 per cent at 1 year, compared with over 90 per cent at 1 year on dialysis.

Kidney transplant
This consists of removing a kidney from either a living identical twin, sibling or parent or a human cadaver donor and inserting it into a recipient. Usually the patient's kidney which is non-functioning has been removed and he is maintained on a dialysis programme until a kidney from a suitable donor becomes available (see below).

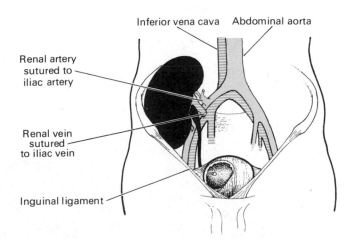

Inferior vena cava   Abdominal aorta

Renal artery sutured to iliac artery

Renal vein sutured to iliac vein

Inguinal ligament

Figure 9.23
Kidney transplant

The donor kidney is transplanted retroperitoneally in either iliac fossa (Fig. 9.23). The ureter of the newly transplanted kidney is transplanted into the bladder or anastomosed to the ureter of the recipient.

The major limiting factor in this procedure is the body's immunological response that leads it to reject the transplanted kidney. The recipient's body recognizes the new kidney as foreign protein and attempts to destroy it. Rejection or threatened rejection of the kidney can occur several hours or several years after the transplant.

Thus the survival of the transplanted kidney depends upon the success of techniques that suppress these immune reactions. In order to minimize or overcome the body's defence mechanism, immunosuppressive drugs such as Imuran and prednisolone are given and continued indefinitely. Because these drugs suppress the immune response of the body's reaction to foreign protein, the patient is more susceptible to infection, making infection a major complication of renal transplant. Therefore, postoperative care should include very strict sterile techniques and aseptic procedures. The nurse must be alert to signs of threatened rejection: fever, swelling and tenderness at the site of transplant, decrease in urinary volume, rise in blood urea and hypertension. Anorexia, malaise and vague feeling of uneasiness may also be experienced by the patient.

Obviously, one of the most important aspects of kidney transplant is the availability of suitable kidneys. In Great Britain, a nationwide scheme has been developed to ensure that each available kidney is matched to the most suitable recipient. The National Organ Matching Service based at Bristol receives and stores data (including tissue type) about all prospective recipients. When a kidney becomes available the donor details are supplied and the matching process is set in action. The most suitable recipient is selected and prepared and arrangements are made to transport the kidney to the recipient hospital.

Calculi

The reason for the formation of calculi or stones in the urinary tract is poorly understood. Several conditions are known to predispose a person to calculi formation, and these are:

1. Excessive loss of water by sweating, for example in hot climates or under certain occupational conditions.
2. Urinary tract infection or stagnation.
3. Hypercalciuria.
4. Prolonged bed rest when calcium is mobilized from the bones.
5. Increased excretion of uric acid as in gout or leukaemia.
6. Dietary factors.
7. Some congenital abnormalities.

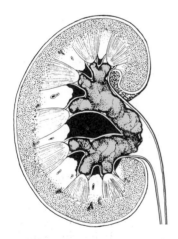

Figure 9.24
Staghorn calculus

Calculi are made up of various combinations of calcium, phosphate, oxalate, ammonia, magnesium and other trace elements and metabolites. The calculi which form vary in size from small particles like sand, to round stones, to staghorn calculi — so named because of their characteristic shape (Fig. 9.24).

Renal calculi are becoming more common in developed countries, while bladder calculi (Fig. 9.25) are becoming less common. This is thought to be due to changes in the standard of living.

Clinical features

The clinical features vary according to the site of the calculi and may be largely asymptomatic in the early years. The patient often complains of a dull pain in the loin area and of being below par. Recurrent kidney infections and haematuria are the main presenting features and always need to be investigated thoroughly.

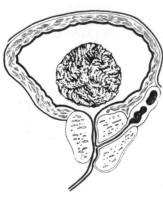

Figure 9.25
Large bladder calculus showing rough spiky surface

Treatment

Surgery is normally indicated in patients who have calculi in the kidney or bladder. Patients who have gout and develop uric acid calculi are given the drug allopurinal to prevent a recurrence following removal. There is no drug which can be given which will dissolve renal calculi. The pre- and postoperative regimes for kidney and bladder operations are described below.

Tumours of the kidney

Some renal tumours are relatively benign, others highly malignant. Two of the latter group are hypernephroma and Wilms' tumour.

Hypernephroma (renal carcinoma)

Hypernephroma is an adenocarcinoma which develops in the kidney tissue.

Clinical features

There may be few signs in the early stages. Later, pain in the loin, a palpable mass in the flank and painless haematuria indicate this serious disorder. A full urinary tract investigation (see Table 9.2) is carried out as painless haematuria is always an ominous sign. Blood-borne metastases occur, giving rise to the so-called 'cannon ball' secondary tumour deposits in the lungs. In some patients the tumour produces an excess of erythropoietin and these patients are found to have polycythaemia. Should this be the case, after removal of the tumour it is likely that there are secondary deposits. Prognosis depends on the degree of malignancy. Not all kidney tumours are equally malignant.

Treatment

After a thorough investigation of the urinary tract the diseased kidney is removed (nephrectomy). A course of X-ray therapy is sometimes given postoperatively depending on the malignancy.

Wilms' tumour (nephroblastoma)

This rare but usually very malignant tumour is one of the few that develops in children. Usually it is discovered in the first 3 years of life. It grows rapidly and gives rise to secondaries, especially in the lungs.

Clinical features

The child is noted to have a large abdomen and to be failing to thrive.

Treatment

In recent years the prognosis for a child with a Wilms' tumour has improved considerably. As with other tumours the earlier it is discovered the better the chances of cure. Treatment consists of surgery and if the tumour is unilateral this usually means removal of the offending kidney. Even if the tumour is bilateral, judicious surgery is assisted by radiotherapy and the use of the cytotoxic drugs—actinomycin D·and vincristine—and the outlook is not as bleak as it used to be.

The parents of these children require considerable emotional support to help them and help the child through the difficult strenuous treatment regimen.

Nursing care of patients undergoing renal surgery

The pre- and postoperative regimen is essentially the same for most kidney and ureter operations with changes in some details only.

Preoperative care

Before any operation on the kidney, and in particular when removal of the kidney is performed, a thorough investigation must be made of both kidneys (Table 9.2). Increasingly the preliminary investigations are being carried out in the out-patient department or in day bed areas, the patient being admitted only a few days before operation for final tests and preparation.

The general care is the same as for any major abdominal surgery including:

1. Skin preparation. The surgeon will indicate whether he intends to use a lumbar or abdominal approach. The appropriate area **and side** will be marked **by the surgeon**, using a skin marker which is not easily rubbed off and does not cause sensitivity reactions.

2. Urine testing.
3. Chest X-ray.
4. Blood transfusion if necessary to correct anaemia.
5. Bowel preparation by evacuant suppositories or enema.
6. Breathing exercises.
7. Consent for operation.

Postoperative Care

The postoperative care of the patient following nephrectomy is similar to that required for other abdominal operations. Particular attention is paid to fluid balance and urinary output.

On return from theatre the patient is usually placed in a lateral position but local practice may vary.

Adynamic ileus occurs in many patients who have had retroperitoneal operations and the surgeon will indicate when oral fluids can be given and the amount. Oral fluids may be withheld for 24 to 48 hours. Adynamic ileus is treated by giving intravenous fluids and by gastric aspiration (p. 168). To prevent chest infections the patient is sat up in bed well supported by pillows and tilted towards the side of the operation to assist in the drainage of the kidney bed. The physiotherapist will continue to assist the patient with breathing exercises and expectoration to keep his lungs clear.

The vacuum drains are maintained for 2 to 3 days, after which time the haemoserous discharge from the kidney bed will become less and the surgeon will indicate when they may be shortened or removed. The dressing should not be changed unless it becomes soaked. In some kidney operations when removal has not taken place a nephrostomy drain may be left in place. This must be managed strictly according to the surgeon's wishes. Great care must be taken to avoid infection gaining entry into the kidney via this form of drain which is asserted into the renal pelvis.

If the patient's condition is satisfactory he is allowed up the day after operation, early ambulation being encouraged as it helps to prevent postoperative complications. All urine should be measured and carefully observed for blood. The kidney is a very vascular organ and following operation haemorrhage is a very likely occurrence. There will always be blood in the urine initially but this should become less over the first 24 to 48 hours. Any obvious continuation of haemorrhage or any reappearance of blood in the urine must be reported immediately. A fall in the urinary output will be evidence that kidney function is becoming impaired. Some simple kidney function tests may be carried out before discharge to ensure that all is well and the patient should be ready for discharge 2 weeks after operation. Some patients may be given a course of radiotherapy.

DISORDERS OF THE URETERS AND BLADDER

Anything which impedes the flow of urine from the kidneys to the outside of the body is likely, sooner or later, to require removal or to be bypassed. Within the genitourinary tract the main causes of obstruction are calculi, tumours, strictures and, in particular, an enlarged prostate gland (p. 319). Outside the urinary tract the most common causes of obstruction are masses within the abdominal and pelvic cavities, for example intestinal tumours, aberrant vessels, ovarian cysts and uterine enlargement. Various disorders of the central nervous system can also cause urinary tract dysfunction. Prolonged back pressure on the kidney eventually leads to impaired kidney function and renal failure. In addition, stagnation of urine almost inevitably leads to infection and to calculi formation.

Ureteric (renal) colic

Sometimes small calculi migrate from the kidney into the ureter and an attack of ureteric colic develops.

Clinical features

In this condition pain is of sudden onset and very severe, reaching a peak 10 to 30 minutes after it begins. The patient is restless and may assume all sorts of positions or may pace up and down the room in agony. Many vomit. Urinary symptoms include frequency and haematuria. The diagnosis is usually made on the basis of the history. If facilities are available an intravenous urogram during an attack will confirm the cause and is useful in the differential diagnosis.

Treatment and nursing care

The patient is confined to bed and an analgesic such as pethidine or morphine is given in addition to an antispasmodic such as atropine. Some surgeons request that all urine passed by the patient be sieved to see if any calculi are passed. This is mainly to confirm the diagnosis. Usually no calculi are observed as they are often very small and difficult to detect. Observations of the patient's temperature, pulse and blood pressure are carried out every half hour. All urine is tested for blood and if this is positive it will tend to confirm the diagnosis.

Bladder calculi

The clinical features are recurrent infections, dysuria, strangury, scalding on micturition and haematuria. The calculi may migrate and block the urethra causing acute retention of urine (p. 306).

Tumours of the bladder

The cause of cancer of the bladder remains elusive but many diverse factors have been implicated, both by observation in animal experiments and by clinical observations of patients. The following are the most common associated factors:

Chemicals used in the manufacture of rubber, plastics, insecticides, cables and dyes.
Cigarette smoking.
Calculi.
Chronic inflammation and diverticulum.
Schistosomiasis.

It is now fairly well established that it is the metabolic products of the various chemicals that cause the cancer, the exact mechanism, as indicated above, being unknown.

The tumours develop in the epithelial lining of the bladder and quite often start as papillary growths. They are relatively benign at this stage and with adequate treatment remain so. Without treatment the tumours become malignant and invade by stages into the superficial muscle layer, the deep muscle, and eventually into the surrounding tissues (Fig. 9.26). Metastasis, especially to bone, is also common. The tumours are often at an advanced stage before discovery.

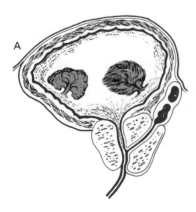

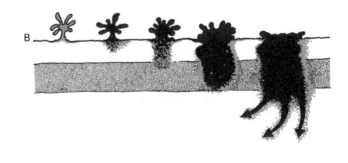

Figure 9.26
Bladder tumours
A. Pedunculated papillomata
B. Stages of bladder tumours showing extension through the bladder wall and invasion of the neighbouring structures

Clinical features

The first evidence of a bladder tumour is often painless haematuria, the blood being bright red. Clot retention may develop. Some patients also have cystitis, frequency of micturition and dysuria. As the tumour spreads it invades the surrounding organs causing relative dysfunction. Involvement of the sacral nerves often results in intractable pain.

Investigations

Diagnosis is usually confirmed by cystoscopy and biopsy. Bimanual examination will give the surgeon some indication of the tumour's stage of development. Other urinary tract investigations include intravenous urogram, micturating cystogram and MSUs (see Table 9.2) Chest X-rays and skeletal surveys along with examination of the blood will also be required.

Treatment

In the early stages when the tumour is seen waving around like a sea anenome when viewed through the cystoscope (Fig. 9.2) the treatment is by diathermy. This procedure has to be repeated at regular intervals as the papillomata have a tendency to recur.

Malignant tumours are treated in various ways depending on the site, degree of malignancy and extent of the tumour.

Tumours which have not invaded deeply into the muscle layer can be treated by radiotherapy. Other more advanced tumours require surgery and several ingenious operations have been devised to cope with this problem. Partial cystectomy is of limited value only, because it reduces bladder capacity and the surgeon cannot be sure he has removed all of the tumour, especially a tumour which has multiple foci.

Usually more radical procedures are called for. One procedure is to remove the bladder and transplant the ureters into the rectum, which then acts as a reservoir for the urine. This operation is only suitable if the anal sphincter is intact. The risks of infection are enormous, as can be imagined. Also, reabsorption of urinary products can give rise to serious electrolyte imbalance.

Another procedure is to isolate a section of ileum and bring it to the surface of the abdomen as a stoma. The ureters are transplanted into the isolated loop of ileum which acts as a conduit (ileal conduit) (Fig. 9.27) for the urine. It is not in any way a storage vessel for urine and a stoma bag has to be worn (see Ch. 5 for care of stoma). The ureters cannot be brought to the surface of the abdomen directly because in this position they become stenosed and within a short while cease to function, hence the need for the ileal loop. Following this operation it is necessary to rest the bowel for a few days until bowel sounds return. In addition to tumours this type of procedure is often carried out where there is lack of bladder function, for example in spina bifida.

Anticancerous Drugs

A number of drugs have been discovered which can be used in the treatment of tumours. They act in various ways but, like radiotherapy, they are all designed to disrupt the metabolism and function of tumour cells to a greater extent than normal cells. With bladder tumours a few of these drugs can be used locally and are introduced via a catheter into the bladder; one such drug is ethoglucid (Epodyl). Others can also be given either orally or by injection. They are now widely used in the treatment of many forms of cancer.

Important features of disordered bladder function

Retention and incontinence of urine are conditions occurring alone or in conjunction with other diseases; for the patient they are distressing and embarrassing.

Acute retention of urine

Acute retention of urine exists when a person is unable to empty his bladder even when it is socially convenient for him to do so.

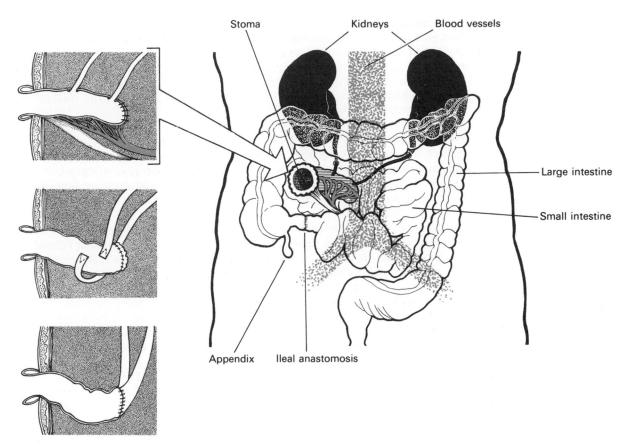

Stoma   Kidneys   Blood vessels

Large intestine

Small intestine

Appendix   Ileal anastomosis

Figure 9.27A
Ileal conduit showing three
different methods of inserting
the ureter into the conduit

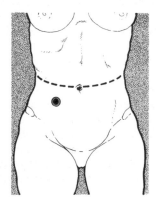

Figure 9.27B
Position of the stoma on the
anterior abdominal wall

Causes

1. Prostatic disease (p. 319).
2. Urethral stricture (p. 316).
3. Bladder tumours (p. 305).
4. Urethral trauma.
5. Stone impacted in urethra.
6. Central nervous system lesion, e.g. paraplegia (p. 117).
7. Postoperative, especially after pelvic operations.

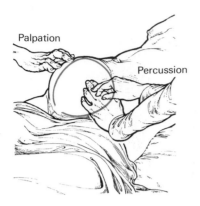

Figure 9.28
Assessing for retention of urine

Clinical features

The onset is sudden, as the name suggests. The patient complains of severe pain in the flank and loin regions. His temperature may be raised and he may be sweating and anxious. If treatment is delayed the patient will become shocked, with a low blood pressure, rapid pulse and a cold, clammy skin. The bladder can usually be palpated and may extend as high as the umbilicus or higher. Figure 9.28 shows the method of palpating and percussing the distended bladder.

Treatment and nursing care

The patient requires catheterization (see below) in most instances except in postoperative retention, which is usually less acute and of psychological origin. Privacy, getting the patient up to the side of the bed, if allowed, running taps in the vicinity and a calm, confident manner in the nurse usually will help the patient to empty his bladder naturally.

If catheterization is required great care must be taken not to precipitate acute renal or cardiac failure by too rapid decompression of the bladder. The sudden release of pressure does produce this effect in some patients. The surgeon will indicate whether he wishes the bladder decompressed over a few hours.

Chronic retention of urine

In this condition the retention is incomplete. The patient may have a distended bladder with overflow incontinence or be unable to empty the bladder completely so that, on voiding, there is a residue of urine left in the bladder.

Causes

1. Prostatic disease.
2. Urethral stricture.
3. Bladder tumours.
4. Bladder calculi.
5. Central nervous system disease.
6. Gynaecological disorder.

Clinical features

The patient feels unwell and is usually aware of having progressive difficulty in passing urine. Urinary stagnation gives rise to infection of the urinary tract. The constant high pressures in the bladder cause changes in the bladder wall in which trabeculae and diverticulae form (Fig. 9.29). In some patients the bladder becomes thin-walled and grossly distended. In addition to increased bladder pressure distortion of the ureters as they enter the bladder causes urine to dam back, resulting in hydroureters and hydronephroses. (Fig. 9.10E). These latter conditions give rise to loin pain and repeated kidney infections. The back pressure on the kidney impairs its function. The blood urea level rises and there is an electrolyte imbalance. It is this and the infection which cause the patient to feel unwell. Many patients, especially the elderly, become confused and disorientated. A full urinary tract investigation is required (Table 9.2).

Treatment and nursing care

Initially catheterization is required and, as in acute retention, if the bladder is grossly distended slow decompression is necessary. It is usually necessary to drain the bladder by catheter for a few days until the blood urea and electrolytes return to normal. This correction of the composition of body fluids often brings about a dramatic improvement in the patient's mental state. (See the section on care of the in-dwelling catheter (p. 314), for management during this period.)

As soon as the patient's condition allows and when the investigations are completed the underlying condition (see below) is treated.

Incontinence of urine

Incontinence of urine is one of the most distressing and troublesome features of a wide variety of disorders. It is a very intricate disorder in which physical, psychological,

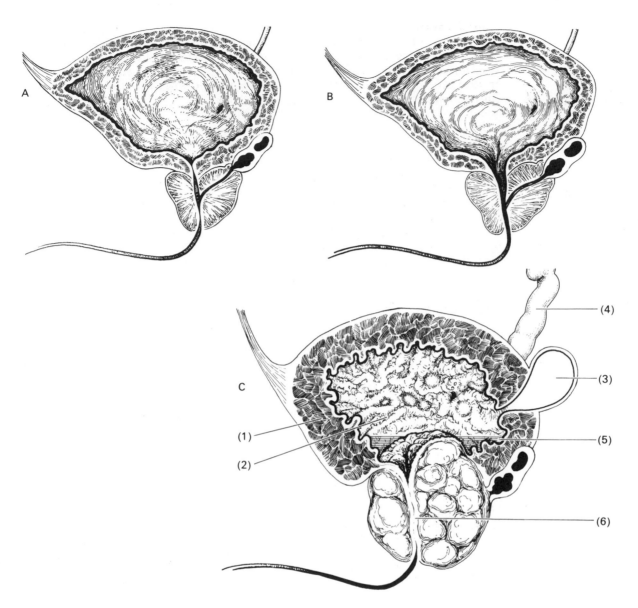

Figure 9.29
Prostate gland
A. Normal structure during
bladder filling
B. Normal bladder emptying
(Note funnelling of bladder neck
into prostatic urethra)
C. Hypertrophy of the prostate
gland showing the changes
resulting from chronic urinary
tract obstruction:
1. hypertrophied bladder wall
2. trabeculae
3. diverticulum
4. hydroureter
5. residual urine
6. urinary tract obstruction

social and economic factors all play a part, either directly or indirectly. One definition
of this complex problem is: any involuntary voiding of urine, per urethra, after the age
at which control of bladder function is usually established.

Applied physiology

The urinary bladder has the function of storing the urine and, by its powerful detrusor muscles, expelling the urine. Urine is retained in the bladder by the sphincter mechanism (Fig. 9.30), which prevents urine from escaping when it should not. This is a passive action most of the time, only becoming active when it is not convenient for micturition to take place.

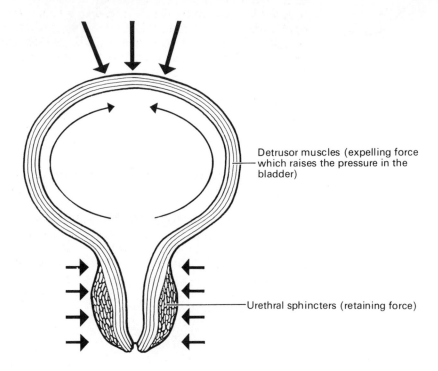

Figure 9.30
Balance of forces between detrusor muscle and urethral sphincters (schematic)

Acquisition of bladder control

Babies and young children up to the age of 18 to 24 months pass urine quite involuntarily, as a purely reflex action. This automatic bladder action is present in every normal child at birth. As the bladder fills up with urine, sensory nerve endings in

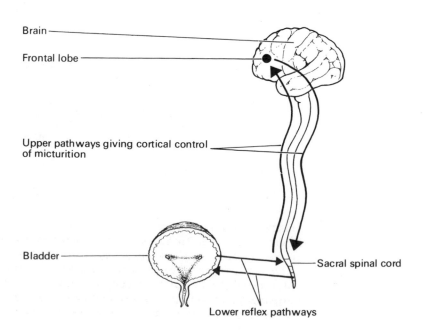

Figure 9.31
Nervous control of bladder (schematic)

the bladder wall respond to stretching and pressure and relay the information to the 2nd, 3rd and 4th sacral segments in the spinal cord (Fig. 9.31). This triggers off a motor stimulus which causes relaxation of the sphincter mechanism and contraction of the bladder muscle, and micturition takes place.

This state of affairs prevails in babies and young children because the central nervous system has not developed to a stage where voluntary inhibition of micturition can be established. Voluntary inhibition is a learned activity in which centres in the frontal lobe, the hypothalamus and the medulla oblongata interact in a complex manner. They enable the external urethral sphincter to be constricted and the reflex response inhibited. Once control is established, the bladder is emptied only when it is socially convenient. For some, however, this 'freedom' is never acquired; for others the system breaks down and control is lost.

Causes

As shown in Table 9.7, a variety of local and generalized conditions may give rise to incontinence of urine.

Investigations

Before any treatment can be started it is important to investigate the problem very thoroughly. Attempts to establish a pattern of voiding are the first steps towards control.

Often the incontinence does not seem to fit readily into any particular category and no one single cause can be isolated. However, unless the disorder is properly investigated and diagnosed, the correct treatment will not be given and the patient may well be labelled 'incontinent' and relegated to a life-style largely determined by his incontinence.

Nurses are often involved in charting patterns of incontinence (Ch. 20) and in observing the patient's behaviour for clues which will help in the diagnosis. Also, various urinary tract investigations may be carried out (see Table 9.2) as suggested by the history and clinical features.

Table 9.7
Causes of incontinence (*After* L E Edwards 1975 Incontinence. The Practitioner 214: 46–55)

Sphincter incompetence	Detrusor abnormalities	Spurious causes
Congenital urethral defects	Neurological lesions of any kind and at any level	Iatrogenic, perhaps following administration of sedatives or diuretics
Urethral trauma, as for instance in fractures of the pelvis	Acute infections	Constipation
Stress incontinence following multiple pregnancy	Chronic infections such as tuberculosis	Locomotor disorder
Bladder neck operations	Postradiation contractures	
Damage at prostatectomy:	Interstitial bladder cystitis	
—damage to sphincter		
—incomplete removal of prostate preventing sphincter closure	Bladder tumours	
—stricture preventing sphincter closure	Psychological enuresis	
Carcinoma of prostate involving sphincter		

Treatment and nursing care

The treatment will depend on the cause of the incontinence. Any underlying conditions are treated, such as urinary tract infections which so commonly afflict elderly women. Obstruction of the urethra is treated, and gynaecological conditions may also be discovered and, if possible, remedied. Various operations have been devised to improve sphincter function when sphincter weakness is the cause of incontinence. One such operation is vesico-urethral suspension in which the bladder and urethra are supported

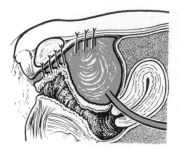

Figure 9.32
Vesico-urethral suspension
('sling' operation)

Figure 9.33
Edwards pubo-vaginal spring
incontinence device
A. About to be inserted
B. In position
(*Illustrated courtesy of Charles
Thackray Ltd., Leeds*)

in a better anatomical position (Fig. 9.32). These and other operations are not always successful but improvements in assessment and new operative techniques are being devised which will benefit those whose lives are made a misery by incontinence. The distressing problem of stress incontinence experienced by so many older women is one such condition for which surgery may bring relief.

External occlusive devices
For women various external occlusive appliances have been invented and are proving successful for some patients (Fig. 9.33). In addition, there are now a number of electronic devices for both internal and external use. These mechanical devices, some of which have to be implanted by surgery, increase the muscle tone of the sphincters. They are still in the early stages of development but will be used increasingly as they become more refined. Figure 9.34 shows two examples of external appliances devised to give indirect stimulation to the pelvic floor. No surgery is required with either device.

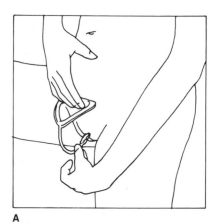
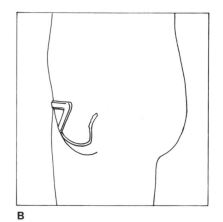

A   B

Treatment of detrusor muscle abnormality
In some patients the cause of the incontinence is a detrusor abnormality (p. 311). If the bladder is atonic some patients will be helped by cholinergic drugs such as carbachol and pyridostigmine bromide. Where bladder function is unstable and uninhibited anticholinergic drugs such as propantheline bromide and emepronium bromide are of benefit. The latter is fairly free of side-effects. Sometimes surgical intervention, in which the bladder above the trigone is denervated, is worthwhile to relieve severe symptoms of urgency, frequency and incontinence. Urinary diversion, where the ureters are transplanted into the sigmoid colon or into an isolated loop of ileum or colon, which is brought to the surface of the abdomen as a urinary stoma, may be the operation of choice (Fig. 9.27, p. 307). These last-mentioned procedures are used where there is a neurological deficit involving sphincter mechanisms of both urinary and faecal outlets.

For many patients, however, the incontinence problem is not readily amenable to any of the treatments described above and other more traditional methods of management have to be used (Ch. 20).

Treatment of non-urethral urinary incontinence
Some patients have non-urethral incontinence via a fistula, for example vesicovaginal or vesicorectal. Very often these patients have urinary tract infections in addition to other pathological conditions. Any such fistula requires surgical repair with treatment of any underlying condition. A full urinary tract investigation will be necessary.

Catheterization
In this procedure a catheter is introduced into the urinary bladder for purposes of:

1. Relieving retention of urine.
2. Emptying the bladder before and after operations on the bladder, prostate or urethra; before some gynaecological operations; and before and after operations on the rectum.

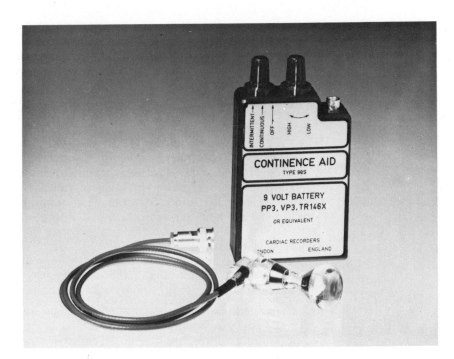

Figure 9.34A
Anal plug stimulator
To give either intermittent or
continuous stimulation

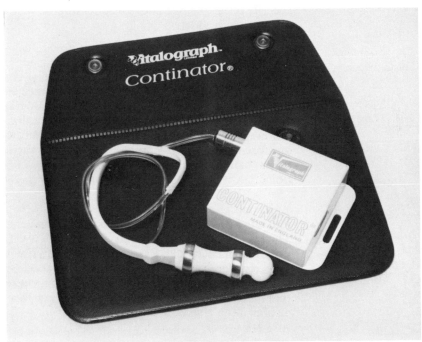

Figure 9.34B
Continator
A stimulator control and
tampon-
shaped vaginal pessary. The
pelvic floor pacing stimulus is
additionally aided by the
mechanical supporting effect of
the vaginal pessary.

3. Facilitating bladder irrigation.
4. Introducing agents which will dissolve calculi (cysteine and uric acid calculi are soluble).
5. Introducing anticancer drugs for bladder carcinoma.
6. Enabling bladder function tests to be done.

It may also be necessary to measure residual urine or urinary output very accurately in some circumstances, for example in patients who have extensive burns. From the above list, which is not exhaustive, it will be appreciated that catheterization is a fairly commonly performed procedure. However, a catheter should not be introduced into a patient's bladder unless a careful consideration of its necessity has been made. The dangers of introducing infection into the urinary tract and of causing injury to the urethra or bladder cannot be stressed too strongly.

A wide variety of catheter types are in use, made from many different materials. The choice of catheter depends on why the patient is being catheterized. Most catheters are packed individually, sterilized and ready for use. Catheters are generally disposable and should be used once only. The best policy is to follow the manufacturer's instructions.

No one should attempt to pass a catheter without having first observed a skilled operator or without having acquired a sound knowledge of the anatomy of the lower urinary tract. The equipment used is usually prepacked and sealed before sterilization in a way which is convenient for use and which lowers the risk of contamination.

If the reason for catheterization does not warrant leaving the catheter *in situ*, the procedure for which it was passed is completed and the catheter is removed. If it is to be retained the appropriate amount of sterile water is injected into the balloon (Fig. 9.37). The catheter is then connected to a sterile, closed drainage system preferably with a non-return valve to help minimize the risk of infection.

Care of in-dwelling catheters
The main problems involved with in-dwelling catheters are the risk of ascending infection and damage to the urethra and bladder.

Infection can get into the urinary tract at various stages in the procedure. These are:

1. By inadequate skin preparation before passing the catheter.
2. By faulty aseptic technique.
3. By injury during passage of the catheter, especially if it is the wrong size.
4. By breaking the closed system of drainage.
5. By lifting the bag above bladder level so that urine flows from the bag or tubing back to the bladder.

The drainage system should be kept closed; the use of spigots, sterile or otherwise, is to be condemned. Bags which can be drained without disconnecting the catheter should be used. Some people advocate putting antiseptic lotion in the drainage bag each time it is drained. The bag must be emptied every 8 hours and strict attention to hand washing is necessary as infection is easily transferred from one bag to the next. The patient must also be warned not to raise the bag above the level of his bladder. The urethral meatal area should be washed twice daily with soap and water. Some surgeons also prescribe the use of an antiseptic cream such as chlorhexidine.

The patient should be provided with plenty of fluids, if there are no contraindications. The aim is to drink at least 1 litre per day—more if possible.

Urine specimens
Patients with in-dwelling catheters all too frequently develop urinary tract infections. The infection often starts off insidiously with few if any clinical features. The patient's urine may have a foul odour or he may have a rise in temperature for a day or two, but little else; hence taking regular catheter specimens of urine (CSU) for culture is advisable. Specimens can be obtained from the catheter using a needle and syringe so that the closed system is not broken. The site on the tubing is cleaned using an isopropyl alcohol swab (Fig. 9.35).

Changing the catheter
If a rubber Foley catheter is used it is recommended that it be changed once a month. However, one of the new silicone, elastomer-type catheters can be left *in situ* for up to 3 months or longer. It should be changed if it becomes encrusted with calcific and other debris or if the urinary tract becomes infected. These complications are much less frequent when a Silastic catheter is used.

Bladder irrigation
There are several ways in which bladder irrigation may be performed.

1. By a **bladder syringe**, which holds 50 ml of fluid. Specially prepared antiseptic lotion is introduced into the bladder via a catheter. There is a very high risk of introducing infection using this method of irrigation. It is useful when local bladder antiseptics such as Noxyflex have been prescribed.

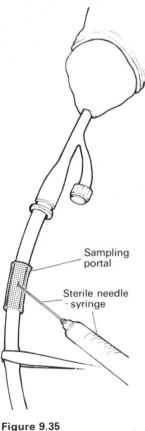

Sampling portal

Sterile needle + syringe

Figure 9.35
Technique of obtaining a urine sample without breaking the closed drainage system

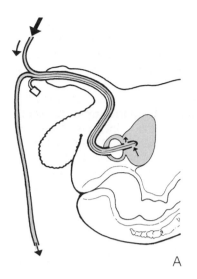
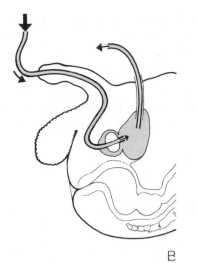
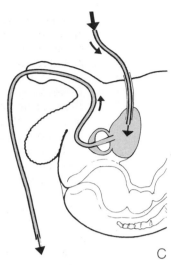

A   B   C

Figure 9.36
Methods of bladder irrigation
A. Three-way Foley catheter
B. Irrigating fluid entering the bladder via a Foley catheter and leaving via a suprapubic catheter to which suction may be applied
C. Irrigation via a suprapubic catheter with drainage via a Foley catheter in the urethra

2. By **continuous closed irrigation**. This entails the use of a three-way Foley self-retaining catheter through which a large amount of sterile water for irrigation is passed into the bladder and, after irrigation of the bladder, is allowed to flow out through the other channel into a closed drainage system (Fig. 9.36A). This form of irrigation is used following prostatectomy and in some bladder operations. The aim is to keep the bladder free of blood clots. The specific regimen and duration will be determined by the surgeon.

3. By **suprapubic cystostomy**. When it is not possible to pass a catheter via the urethra, in order to drain the bladder or for irrigation purposes, the surgeon may have no choice but to perform a suprapubic cystostomy. A catheter is introduced through the stoma (Fig. 9.36B and C). Either a Foley, Malecote or a de Pezzer catheter is used (Fig. 9.36A, B and C). The bladder and abdominal muscles constrict down on to the catheter so that leakage does not occur. The stoma is kept scrupulously clean and dressed as a surgical wound.

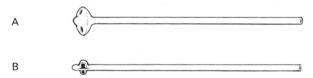

A

B

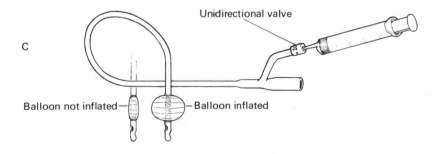

C

Unidirectional valve

Balloon not inflated — — Balloon inflated

Figure 9.37
Three types of self-retaining catheter
A. de Pezzer
B. Malecote
C. Foley

DISORDERS OF THE MALE GENITALIA

Disturbance of structure and function may be congenital in origin or may result from trauma, infection or neoplasm. Only the more common disorders will be described.

Congenital disorders of the urethra and penis

Malformation of the urethra from congenital defects will be seen on neonatal examination (Ch. 17).

Hypospadias

In this condition the urethral meatus does not open on to the anterior tip of the glans but on to the lower surface. Most commonly the abnormal opening is on the undersurface of the glans and is known as glandular hypospadias (Fig. 9.38A). This is fairly easily treated by plastic surgery, as a result of which the urethral meatus is enlarged. Usually the patient experiences no further difficulties either in passing urine or in sexual function (Fig. 9.38B).

Occasionally the openings are further back along the lower surface and, as can be imagined, are much more difficult to treat. Several operations may be required and the urine has often to be bypassed via a temporary perineal urethrostomy. This diversion allows healing to take place following surgery.

Epispadias

In this condition the urethra opens on to the dorsal surface of the penis (Fig. 9.39). As in hypospadias the urethral meatus can be at any point along the penis. It is often associated with another very serious congenital abnormality, namely ectopia vesicae, in which the anterior parts of the bladder and the abdominal wall are imperfectly formed.

These conditions require extensive plastic surgery, quite often with transplantation of the ureters (Fig. 9.27, p. 307). For a discussion of these procedures a more specialized text should be consulted.

Traumatic conditions

Urethral stricture

In modern times urethral stricture is usually a result of trauma, more rarely it is a sequel to gonococcal urethritis. The same sequence of events follows as in obstruction of the urinary flow, but for other reasons. The treatment is dilatation of the urethra using *bougies* and graduated metal sounds. Usually, several treatments are required to dilate the scarred portion of the urethra. An antibiotic drug is often given to prevent infection, which is made likely because of repeated instrumentation and especially if there has been a degree of urinary stasis.

Rupture of the urethra

Occasionally, the urethra is ruptured as a result of trauma, or it may rupture spontaneously because of stricture. This is very troublesome and several operations may be necessary before satisfactory urethral function is established.

Phimosis

The condition of phimosis, which is a narrowing of the foreskin (Fig. 9.40), is usually acquired. It comes about as a result of attempts to retract the foreskin back over the glans before complete separation of the foreskin from the glans has taken place and before the foreskin is big enough to be retracted. The separation is usually complete at about 2 years of age. Retraction before separation is complete splits the adherent areas leaving raw surfaces which cause scar formation and narrowing of the foreskin. This later gives rise to difficulty in retracting the foreskin with consequent problems of hygiene. Infection of the glans (balanitis) is then more common. The operation of circumcision is required. This operation is also done for religious and social reasons.

Phimosis may on occasion be a congenital abnormality.

Paraphimosis

Paraphimosis is a condition where the foreskin has been retracted back over the glans and the patient is unable to replace it. The tight foreskin interrupts the circulation and the glans becomes tense and swollen. (Fig. 9.41).

The condition can usually be treated without anaesthesia by manipulating the glans under the rolled-up foreskin. Cold compresses applied to the penis may help to reduce

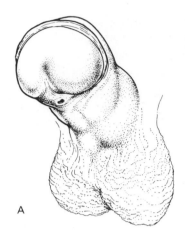

A

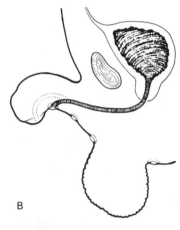

B

Figure 9.38
A. Glandular hypospadias
B. Various sites of urethral opening in hypospadias (schematic)

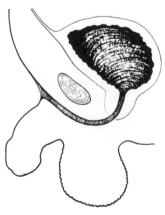

Figure 9.39
Epispadias

the swelling and make manipulation easier. Occasionally, a dorsal slit is made under anaesthesia. A follow-up circumcision may be called for to prevent a recurrence.

Carcinoma of the penis

This is a squamous-celled carcinoma caused by long-standing irritation. It is very rarely, if ever, found in men who have been circumcised before the age of 5 years. It is not a common condition. There is no pain initially and the patient is often late in seeking help. Metastases in the inguinal region are common.

Treatment
The treatment is radiotherapy and/or partial or total amputation of the penis, with block dissection of the inguinal glands. There is no specific preoperative care other than skin preparation. Urine is required for culture and sensitivity. Any urinary tract infection must be treated. The surgeon will give the patient a careful explanation of what is involved and of the need for such radical treatment — if amputation is decided upon.

Postoperatively, attention to hygiene and micturition is important. If surgery is refused one of the cytotoxic drugs such as bleomycin can be used.

Maldescent of the testes

This is a condition in which **one or both** testes fail to pass down the inguinal canal into the scrotum before birth (Fig. 9.42A and B). The embryo testes begin life in the upper coelomic cavity and usually descend around the seventh month of intrauterine life. It is a fairly common disorder, occurring in 30 to 40 per 1000 full-term male births. The reason for the descent of the testes into the scrotum is to keep the testes cooler than would be possible in the abdominal cavity, where the higher temperature would cause germ cell degeneration.

There are three different orders of maldescent:

1. **Retractile testicle**, a normal gonad which has been drawn up into the superficial inguinal pouch.
2. **Ectopic testicle**, where the testicle is prevented from entering the scrotum by a fascial barrier.
3. **Undescended testicle** (also called cryptorchid), where the testicle, which is often abnormal, either partially or completely fails to pass down the inguinal canal to the scrotum.

Treatment
The aim of treatment is to produce a normally functioning testicle. Because the testicle starts to function by the eighth to tenth year of life treatment should be complete by that age at the latest. Two main forms of treatment are used. First, hormones may be given in an attempt to get the testicle to migrate naturally. Some do migrate spontaneously even without treatment, especially in the retractile group. The second form of treatment is surgical. Surgery is always required for an ectopic testicle; an operation called an orchidopexy is performed in which the testicle is brought down and embedded in a pocket of skin in the thigh or anchored by means of a suture to the thigh. In the former operation a second operation is required in 3 months to free the testicle, while in the latter procedure the suture is removed in 7 to 10 days.

In true undescended testes more extensive surgery is often required including removal of the testes and repair of the inguinal hernia which is often present in these patients. There is a high risk of malignancy if the testes are left in the abdominal cavity.

Hydrocele

This is a collection of watery fluid in the tunica vaginalis. There are two types:

1. **Primary hydrocele**, which can occur at any age without obvious cause.
2. **Secondary hydrocele**, which accompanies acute or chronic inflammation of the testes or epididymis, for example gonorrhoea.

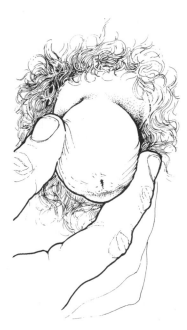

Figure 9.40
Phimosis

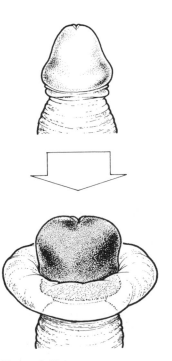

Figure 9.41
Paraphimosis

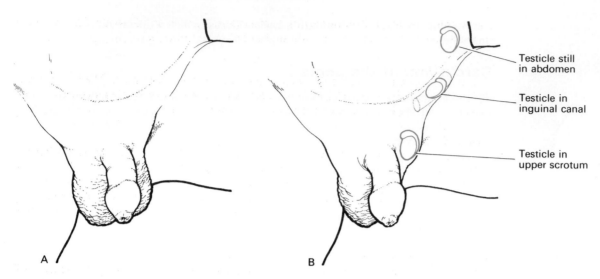

Figure 9.42
Maldescent of testes
A. Normal scrotum
B. Left side of scrotum empty

Testicle still in abdomen

Testicle in inguinal canal

Testicle in upper scrotum

A hydrocele is always translucent unless there has been injury or previous tapping when blood in the vaginal space may render it opaque. They can grow to quite an outrageous size but this is uncommon. Other occasions when scrotal swelling may be extensive include severe oedematous states, for example nephrotic syndrome and congestive heart failure, elephantiasis and inguinal herniation. The latter is the only condition which may be easily reducible though this is not always the case.

Treatment
Most hydroceles, even when quite large, will usually reabsorb. If any persist an operation on the tunica vaginalis is necessary. For elderly patients unable to withstand an operation the hydrocele can be tapped using a fine trocar and cannula introduced into a translucent area. It is not without risk: haemorrhage and infection are common complications.

Varicocele

This is a disorder of the blood vessels draining the testes. The veins from the testes are dilated causing enlargement of the spermatic cord in the upper part of the scrotum and in the groin. It may cause discomfort and an aching pain. In addition, the temperature of the testes is raised which may cause testicular dysfunction in the form of oligospermia. This is a cause of infertility where the wife is normal. Usually no treatment is required; however, in cases of infertility and where discomfort is persistent a small operation to remove a portion of the vein is required. This is not always successful in increasing fertility.

Epididymo-orchitis

Acute epididymo-orchitis is a fairly common cause of acute testicular swelling. It is associated with urinary tract infections so it is necessary to obtain a specimen of urine for microbiological investigation. There is considerable pain and discomfort. The patient will be febrile and should therefore be confined to bed. A scrotal support is necessary. He should have all the care of the febrile patient. A liberal supply of fluids should be provided, and an antibiotic will be prescribed. It is usual, once the acute episode has been treated, to investigate the urinary tract more fully (Table 9.2) so that any underlying disease process can be treated.

New growths of the testes

There are several new growths which arise in the testes; the large majority, however, are either teratomas or seminomas. The former are remarkably complex tumours which arise from embryonic tissues and have areas of tissue of variable origin. The seminomas are more homogeneous tumours and are believed to be derived from spermatocytes. They are less highly malignant than teratomas.

Clinical features
The onset is often gradual, most of the patients being young men. There is a firm, expanding, palpable mass felt in the scrotum. Any young man who presents with a non-translucent mass in the scrotum deserves careful investigation.

Treatment
The scrotum is explored using an inguinal incision and, once the diagnosis is confirmed, the testis, epididymis and cord up to the inguinal ring is removed. A course of radiotherapy is then given as the seminomas are radiosensitive, the teratomas less so. As part of the follow-up review, 24-hour specimens of urine are collected for gonadotrophin estimation: a positive test following removal of the primary is a strong indication that there are metastases.

Nursing care of patients undergoing testicular surgery
The general pre- and postoperative care is the same as for any major surgery. Because of the area's close proximity to the anal region, particular care must be taken with hygiene and skin preparation, as infection is often a troublesome problem. Pain can be quite severe following some operations and analgesics must be given. The area should be closely observed for haemorrhage and swelling. Psychological problems following removal of the testes must be met with understanding and sympathy.

Diseases of the prostate gland

Because the prostate gland closely surrounds the urethra as it leaves the bladder (see Fig. 9.29, p. 309), changes in the size, shape or form of the gland may cause disturbance of bladder and urethral function. Changes in the gland are very common after the age of 50 and surgery on the prostate gland makes up much of the work of most surgical urology units. Because many — indeed most — of the patients are elderly, this condition presents some interesting problems in surgical and nursing management.

Changes in the gland are known collectively as **prostatism**. The changes may be benign or malignant.

Benign growths of the prostate gland

In the benign change a nodular hyperplasia develops. The nodules of glandular and fibrous tissue coalesce to form a large mass which compresses the outer, normal glandular tissue into a false capsule. As the mass grows it compresses and elongates the prostatic urethra making catheterization difficult in some cases. The enlarging gland also pushes up the floor of the bladder causing distortion of the ureters (Fig. 9.29). A complication of the hypertrophy is chronic prostatitis in which the gland substance undergoes inflammatory changes. Acute prostatitis is more usually a complication of gonorrhoea. The malignant changes are described on page 321.

Clinical features
The patient has a history of not feeling well for some time, hesitancy and difficulty in starting to pass urine, a slow stream of urine and dribbling at the end of micturition (see chronic retention, p. 308). Many patients present with acute retention (p. 306).

Investigations
Most of the patients are elderly and a thorough assessment of their physical condition is necessary. A full urinary tract investigation is required (see Table 9.2). A rectal examination is essential in the diagnosis of prostate disease. The urine is tested and a specimen is sent for microbiological investigation.

Surgical treatment and nursing care
The general preoperative care is the same as for any major surgery.

Several routes to the prostate gland are available (Fig. 9.43). The route chosen will depend on the surgeon and on the patient's circumstances. Once the gland is exposed

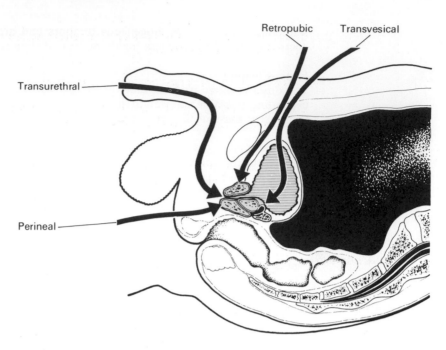

Figure 9.43
Four routes for removal of prostate gland

the nodular hyperplastic area is shelled out, including the prostatic urethra, leaving the false capsule. This leaves a raw area which has a tendency to bleed and which later becomes covered with epithelial tissue.

Postoperative nursing care
The general postoperative care is the same as for any patient undergoing major surgery. The more specific care relating to these patients will depend on the type of operation performed and on the preference of the individual surgeon.

On return from the operating theatre an intravenous infusion will be in progress and, if the patient has lost more than 500 ml of blood, a transfusion may be given. Care must be taken not to overload the circulatory system and so precipitate heart failure.

Provided there are no complications and the patient can take oral fluids in adequate amounts, that is about 3 litres per day, the infusion can be discontinued after 24 hours.

Most patients will have an in-dwelling catheter, which may be a Foley three-way self-retaining type, which facilitates bladder irrigation. Bladder irrigation will reduce the likelihood of clot formation. Even so some patients will develop clots, and this causes severe pain and shock. Clot retention is most likely to occur during the first few hours and most surgeons will prescribe a bladder irrigation regimen.

Clot retention causes severe pain and shock which is not entirely due to blood loss as removal of the clot brings about an immediate improvement in the patient's condition. Sometimes clots form in spite of irrigation.

The catheter can usually be removed after 3 to 5 days or when the urine is clear, except in the case of a transvesical approach when it will be left in position for up to 7 days to enable the bladder wall to heal. On removal of the catheter the patient initially may not have good control of his bladder. He will probably experience frequency of, and considerable discomfort on micturition and will need reassurance that this is only a temporary disturbance. However, if there has been disruption of the external urethral sphincter or other damage at operation, incontinence may be a much greater problem for these unfortunate patients.

If there has been a drain in the retropubic space this is removed after 2 to 3 days. The sutures are removed 8 to 10 days later.

Early ambulation is advisable and, if he is able, the patient will be allowed up the day after operation for a short time. This, along with leg exercises, will help to prevent deep venous thrombosis.

The patient is usually fit for discharge in about 2 weeks. He will frequently admit to feeling better than he has for years. He should, however, be advised to take things easy for a time, gradually increasing his activity back to what for him is normal. Before discharge a specimen of urine is sent for culture and sensitivity tests are made to ensure there is no residual infection.

Carcinoma of the prostate gland

Carcinoma of the prostate is the most common form of neoplasm found in men over 65. The tumour is known to be hormone-dependent.

Clinical features

Like many other cancers found elsewhere in the body it seldom gives rise to symptoms while in a curable stage. Often, the symptoms are indistinguishable from those of prostatic hypertrophy. Dysuria and bed-wetting, flank pain, sciatic pain due to secondaries, anaemia and impotence are the most common presenting features. Many patients present with more wide-ranging symptoms because of secondary deposits.

Investigations

Diagnosis is based on the history, rectal examination, skeletal surveys and blood tests. The latter are not always positive. A biopsy is essential to corroborate the evidence.

Treatment and nursing care

The treatment is removal of the prostate gland and the use of anticancerous drugs and female hormones. Sometimes the prostatic urethra is simply widened a little to allow free passage of urine. The transurethral approach is also used. Some surgeons remove the testes as the tumour is hormone-dependent and this reduces malignant activity. The female hormones used (stilboestrol and its derivatives) also have the effect of damping down malignant activity. They do not bring abour a cure. The pre- and postoperative regimen is the same as that for prostatectomy performed for other reasons.

CONTRACEPTION

Because of the permanency of sterilization as a means of contraception, not all males are willing to undergo such a procedure. There are, however, other methods of contraception, namely coitus interruptus, sheaths and spermicidal agents, although none is as reliable as vasectomy (see below).

Coitus interruptus

This is a widely practised means of trying to prevent conception. In this method the man withdraws his penis from the woman's vagina just before ejaculation in an effort to prevent spermatozoa from entering. The method is not reliable, partly because it requires very careful timing and also because a very large percentage of the spermatozoa are in the first two-thirds of the ejaculation. Because of the uncertainty this is a very unsatisfactory method of contraception. It gives rise to tension between the couple and the fear of unwanted pregnancy is real enough as the failure rate is very high.

Sheaths and spermicidal agents

The use of a sheath (or condom), usually made of rubber, is a commonly used means of contraception. The sheath is placed over the penis and acts as a barrier to the spermatozoa entering the vagina. As a method of contraception it is fairly reliable if used properly. Some agencies recommend the use of spermicidal cream or foam in addition to the sheath as an added protection. The spermicidal agents, which can also be used on their own, are introduced into the vagina directly from their containers via special applicators.

Sheaths and spermicidal agents are available from family planning centres and chemists.

The use of sheaths is thought to help in limiting the spread of sexually transmitted diseases, for example gonorrhoea.

Male sterilization

The most common method of rendering the male sterile at present is by removing a short length of each vas deferens. The procedure is called a vasectomy (Fig. 9.44), and is

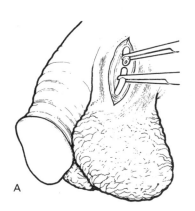

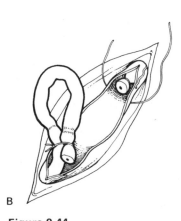

Figure 9.44
Vasectomy
A. Isolation and section of the vas deferens
B. One method ligating the sectioned vas deferens

one of the most effective means of sterilization. It is easier to perform, more free from complications than female sterilization (Ch. 10) and is now becoming an accepted procedure in this country.

Preoperative preparation
A careful explanation of what is involved should be given to both husband and wife, and the wife should also give her consent. The operation is usually performed under a local anaesthetic but a general anaesthetic is given on some occasions. The patient is asked to shave his pubic area and to wash thoroughly.

The operation involves making a small opening into the neck of the scrotum on each side and isolating the vas deferens. A small section is removed and various operations, for example folding ends of the vasa back, have been devised to overcome the problem of recanalization of the vasa. The wound is closed usually with a single silk suture and sprayed with Nobecutane.

Postoperative care and follow-up
The scrotum must be supported and must be observed closely for 15 to 30 minutes in case of haemorrhage. On discharge the patient is advised to seek help if any swelling or haematoma should form. Some pain may be experienced in the testes for a few days. The main complications are haemorrhage, infection and psychological problems.

The man's semen is examined for spermatozoa at regular intervals for 3 months. He must be warned to use some other form of contraception until at least three negative specimens have been obtained. Usually about 3 months has to elapse before the seminal vesicles are completely empty of spermatozoa. The operation does not cause impotence and seems to give rise to very few psychological problems.

SUGGESTED ASSIGNMENTS

1. 'Often the incontinence does not seem to fit readily into any particular category and no one single cause can be isolated.' (p. 311)

Over a specified period of clinical experience in more than one area, do a survey of all the patients whom you nurse who are incontinent and see whether this statement stands up to close examination.

2. Discuss the advantages and disadvantages
    a. to the patient
    b. to the health service

of home dialysis versus hospital-based heamodialysis.

3. Using the nursing process model, devise a home nursing care plan for the parents of a child who is about to be a discharged from hospital having had an ileal conduit constructed. How best may the parents be helped to contribute to such a plan and put it into action? What sort of problems would you anticipate?

Discussion topic
Discuss the merits of different methods of bladder irrigation from the nursing point of view.

FURTHER READING

Anderton J L, Parson F M, Jones D E 1978 Living with renal failure. MTP Press, Lancaster
Blandy John 1979 Lecture notes on urology, 2nd edn. Blackwell Scientific, Oxford
Brundage D J 1975 Nursing management of renal problems. Mosby, St. Louis
Charlton C A C 1973 The urological system. Churchill Livingstone, Edinburgh
Czaczkas J W Karan de Nour A 1978 Continuous haemodialysis as a way of life. Brunel Mazel, New York
Edmondson E 1971 Nursing the incontinent. Butterworth, London
Howells J G 1978 Modern perspectives in the psychiatric aspects of surgery. Macmillan, London

Jameson R M, Burrows K, Large B 1976 Management of the urological patient. Churchill Livingstone, Edinburgh

Newsam J E, Petrie J J B 1975 Urology, 2nd edn. Churchill Livingstone, Edinburgh

O'Hara M 1975 Understanding the causes and treatment of kidney failure. Heinemann, London

Scott R, Deane R F, Callander R 1975 Illustrated urology. Churchill Livingstone, Edinburgh

Uldall R 1977 Renal nursing, 2nd edn. Blackwell Scientific, Oxford

Wing A J, Magowan M 1975 The renal unit. Macmillan, London

10. The Female Reproductive System

THE FEMALE REPRODUCTIVE TRACT

The organs of the reproductive tract are described collectively as the **genitalia** (L. genitalis, to beget). These organs are inactive until the onset of puberty, which usually occurs between the ages of 12 and 17.

The female child is prepared for puberty by the increase in the amount of hormones produced by the pituitary gland, resulting in the secretion of oestrogen from the ovaries and adrenal cortex. At puberty the girl begins to develop the secondary sex characteristics which stamp her as a woman. These are the development of breasts, the enlargement of the genitalia, the growth of pubic and axillary hair and the appearance of deposits of fat on the breasts and hips, resulting in the rounded contours of the body that distinguish the female from the male. This change reaches its climax with the onset of the menarche, the first menstrual period. the girl is now physically able to bear a child.

During the childbearing years most women have a regular menstrual cycle, broken only by pregnancy, until the menopause is reached — between the ages of 45 and 52. At this time menstruation ceases and the woman is no longer able to bear children. Thereafter, because of the decreasing production of the female hormones oestrogen and progesterone, the genitalia and breasts shrink and pubic and axillary hair becomes scanty.

Both puberty and the menopause may be accompanied by psychological changes.

ANATOMY AND PHYSIOLOGY

For purposes of description the genitalia are divided into external and internal organs.

The internal genitalia are housed in the abdominal cavity and are protected by the pelvic girdle, which forms a basin-shaped structure with an outlet in its base. This is known as the **true pelvis** and is important in obstetrics.

The outlet of the pelvis is spanned by muscles and ligaments which form a sling to support the pelvic organs. There are three perforations or openings, permitting the passage of the urethra in front, the vagina in the middle, and the rectum at the back. They are all sites of potential weakness in the pelvic floor.

A wedge of muscle between the vagina and rectum is known as the **perineal body**. It has attachments to eight muscles and is the corner-stone of the pelvic floor. If it is damaged in childbirth or weakened by slackening of the muscles in old age, the whole pelvic floor ceases to function adequately. The skin covering this area is known as the perineum.

External genitalia

The external genitalia are shown in Figure 10.1.

Internal genitalia

These organs are illustrated in Figure 10.2.

The vagina

The vagina is the link between the internal and external organs. It is a muscular canal which begins at the introitus, passes upwards and backwards and ends at the uterus. Its

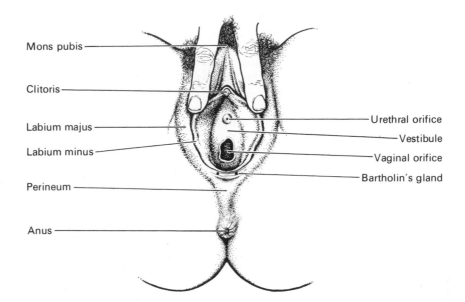

Figure 10.1
The external genitalia

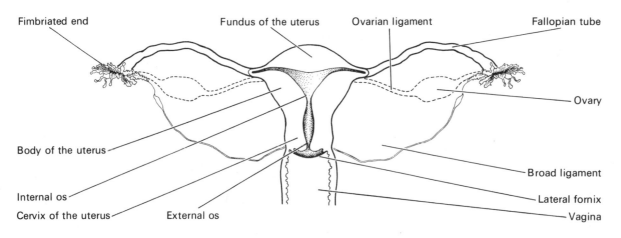

Figure 10.2
The internal genitalia

lining is in folds allowing it to expand easily. The vaginal walls secrete a cleansing and lubricating fluid which is acidic during the childbearing years and alkaline before puberty and usually after the menopause.

The uterus
The uterus is a hollow, muscular, pear-shaped organ lying almost at right angles to the vagina and bent over the urinary bladder. Its lower end, the cervix, projects into the vagina for about half of its length. The opening of this part into the vagina is called the **external os**. The upper end of the cervix opens into the body of the uterus at the **internal os**. The area between the points of entrance of the uterine (Fallopian) tubes is domed and called the **fundus**.

The uterus has an outer covering of peritoneum, a middle muscular layer (myometrium), and an inner lining of epithelium (endometrium), which alters in thickness during each menstrual cycle. It has the ability to expand to accommodate a 40-week fetus and to contract again after childbirth to its normal length of approximately 7·5 cm.

The uterine tubes

These are two thin muscular tubes which provide a passageway directly from the uterus into the peritoneal cavity. At the distal end of each tube are finger-like processes called **fimbriae**, one of which is a little longer than the others and is attached to the ovary. The uterine tubes are like long arms flopping at the sides of the uterus.

The uterine supports

The uterus is supported in the pelvic cavity by the surrounding organs, the muscles of the pelvic floor — particularly the levator ani muscles — and ligaments, which are derived from folds of peritoneum and connective tissue.

The **broad ligaments** are formed by double folds of peritoneum on either side of the uterus. They hang down over the uterine tubes and are attached to the sides of the pelvis. They contain the round and ovarian ligaments.

The two cardinal ligaments are attached to the sides of the cervix and extend laterally to the walls of the pelvis.

The two uterosacral ligaments are attached to the posterior wall of the cervix and extend backwards, on either side of the rectum, to the sacrum.

A deep depression between the vagina and rectum formed by peritoneum is known as the **pouch of Douglas**.

The ovaries

The ovaries are the female gonads (sex glands) which secrete the hormones oestrogen and progesterone.

They are approximately 3 cm long and 1·5 cm wide and lie in the peritoneal cavity on the back of the broad ligament near the fimbriated ends of the uterine tubes.

The medulla or central part of the ovary is composed of fibrous tissue and contains blood vessels, lymphatic vessels and nerves.

The cortex or outer layer is composed of connective tissue called stroma which contains follicles in various stages of development. The appearance of the cortex depends on the age of the individual and the stage of the menstrual cycle.

Before puberty the surface of the ovary is smooth. The follicles in the stroma, called primordial follicles, are small and immature. During the childbearing years at each menstrual cycle, one or more follicles are stimulated to grow. Each follicle contains a maturing ovum and, during each cycle, one of these follicles matures, rises to the surface of the ovary, ruptures and releases the ovum into the uterine tube. This process is known as ovulation. The remainder of the follicle develops as the corpus luteum.

If the ovum is not fertilized, towards the end of the cycle the corpus luteum degenerates into a scar-like white body called the corpus albicans.

After the menopause there is a gradual disappearance of the follicles but there are numerous white bodies throughout the stroma.

The menstrual cycle

Menstruation and the events leading up to it are termed the menstrual cycle (Fig. 10.3) and are under the control of hormones.

The anterior pituitary gland secretes the follicle stimulating hormone (FSH) which stimulates a primordial follicle to grow and mature.

As the follicle develops it secretes oestrogen which eventually inhibits the secretion of FSH and stimulates the release of the luteinising hormone (LH), also from the anterior pituitary. Oestrogen causes the endometrium to begin to thicken.

When it is sufficiently mature the follicle ruptures and releases an ovum which is then carried slowly along the uterine tube towards the cavity of the uterus. Ovulation has now taken place.

The remainder of the ruptured follicle develops into the corpus luteum which secretes progesterone. Progesterone prepares the breast and uterus for *gestation* and is only present in the circulation after ovulation, unlike oestrogen which is secreted throughout the cycle.

If the ovum is not fertilized, about 12 days after ovulation the corpus luteum degenerates and the secretion of progesterone and oestrogen ceases. Lack of

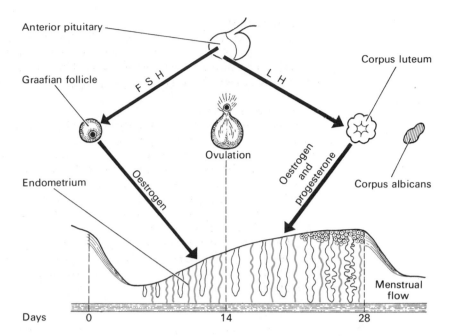

Figure 10.3
The menstrual cycle

progesterone causes the endometrium to break down giving rise to the menstrual flow which normally lasts from 3 to 5 days.

This entire process is under the control of the hypothalamus.

Related structures lying in close proximity to the reproductive organs are shown in Figure 10.4.

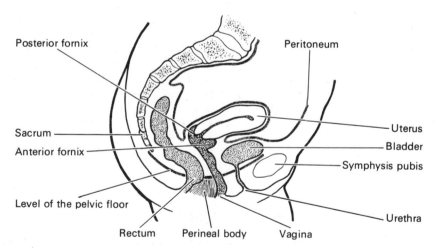

Figure 10.4
Sagittal section of pelvis

Fertilization of the ovum (Fig. 10.5A-D)

Spermatozoa are formed in the testes (Ch. 9) and are contained in a fluid known as semen, which is deposited in the posterior fornix of the vagina during sexual intercourse or coitus.

The number of spermatozoa deposited in one act of intercourse is about 300 000 000, although only one spermatozoon is needed to fertilize the ovum.

Each spermatozoon has a head, which carries genetic material, and a long tail, which enables it to move in a fluid medium. Many spermatozoa perish during their passage through the cervical mucus into the body of the uterus; those that reach the outer third of the uterine tubes are able to survive there for approximately 36 hours.

Fertilization occurs when the head of a spermatozoon penetrates an ovum and the genetic material of both mix. The fertilized ovum is propelled along the uterine tube by

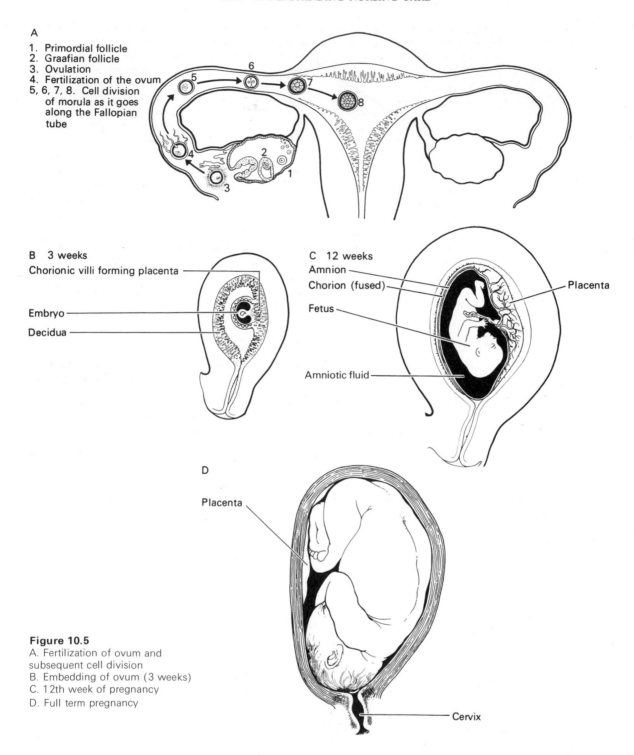

A
1. Primordial follicle
2. Graafian follicle
3. Ovulation
4. Fertilization of the ovum
5, 6, 7, 8. Cell division of morula as it goes along the Fallopian tube

B   3 weeks
Chorionic villi forming placenta
Embryo
Decidua

C   12 weeks
Amnion
Chorion (fused)
Fetus
Amniotic fluid
Placenta

D
Placenta
Cervix

Figure 10.5
A. Fertilization of ovum and subsequent cell division
B. Embedding of ovum (3 weeks)
C. 12th week of pregnancy
D. Full term pregnancy

gentle peristaltic movements; during this time it begins to divide; it finally reaches the uterine cavity as a small mass of cells. About 6 to 8 days after fertilization this mass becomes embedded in the endometrium, which has been specially prepared to receive the fertilized ovum. The endometrium is now known as the decidua.

Chromosomes
Each cell in the body contains 46 chromosomes **arranged in pairs**. Two of these are the sex chromosomes; the remaining 44 are called autosomes. At fertilization the

reproductive cells — the ovum and the spermatozoon — each contain 23 chromosomes, so that when they unite the resulting embryo has 46 chromosomes. The new individual is different from both parents but has some characteristics of both.

Genetic abnormalities
Some abnormalities seen in babies at birth or in later life are caused by chromosomal abnormalities. The diagnosis is made by examining cells from the body under a microscope. An example of such a disorder is Down's syndrome (Ch. 15).

Genetic counselling
Couples can now have genetic counselling when there is a history of hereditary disease in the family. They will be told the chances of recurrence of the abnormality before embarking on a pregnancy. Alternatively, a pregnant woman can be investigated and counselled at an early stage in gestation.

It must be remembered, however, that many congenital abnormalities in the newborn are caused by viral infection and by the effects of drugs taken by the mother before the 12th week of pregnancy. At this time the placental barrier, which protects the growing embryo, is not fully developed. The rubella virus is particularly dangerous. Care must be taken to ensure that the mother avoids all drugs except those prescribed by her doctor.

Signs and symptoms of pregnancy

1. Amenorrhoea occurring when hitherto the cycle has been regular. The expected date of delivery (EDD) should always be estimated from the first day of the last normal period, to which 9 months and 7 days are added. For instance:

Last menstrual period (LMP)	– 1st March
Expected date of delivery (EDD)	– 8th December

The immunological pregnancy diagnosis test will be positive about 2 weeks following the LMP — that is at the 6th week of pregnancy.

2. Breast changes. The breasts become enlarged, tense and tender. The veins around the areolar area of the breast become prominent and pigmentation of this area occurs. The Montgomery follicles enlarge (Fig. 10.6).

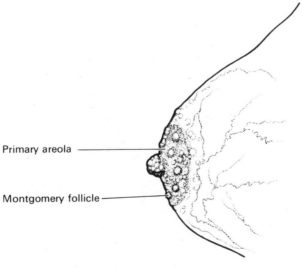

Primary areola

Montgomery follicle

Figure 10.6
Enlargement of the breast in pregnancy

3. There may be nausea and occasionally vomiting, which can be troublesome during the early months.
4. Frequency of micturition may also occur. This is principally due to displacement of the bladder and subsequent reduction of the bladder capacity by the growing uterus.
5. The uterus is palpable per abdomen by the 12th week of pregnancy (Fig. 10.7). *Quickening* or 'feeling life' is experienced about the 18th week of pregnancy — earlier in *multipara*.

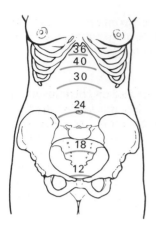

Figure 10.7
Growth of uterus showing the
fundal heights at the 12th, 18th,
24th, 30th, 36th and 40th week

The fetal heart may be heard by using an *ultrasonic* device called the *Doptone* after 12 to 14 weeks of pregnancy and by using an ordinary fetal heart stethoscope from the 20th week. Fetal parts can be palpated at 26 to 28 weeks.

Antenatal care

As antenatal care has improved throughout the years so have the chances of survival for the mother and the baby.

Antenatal care from the beginning of pregnancy is essential and all babies should be born in hospital where expert care can be given by obstetricians, paediatricians and midwives, who have available all the sophisticated equipment and facilities of a modern

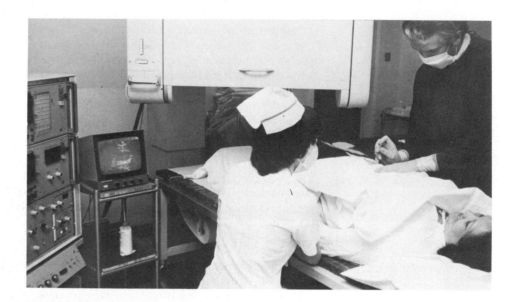

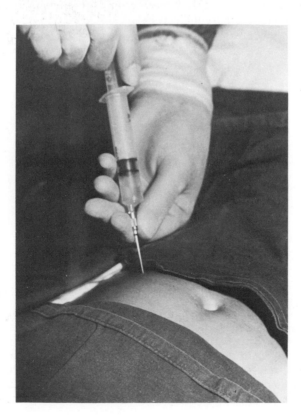

Figure 10.8

Amniocentesis being carried out in the scan room. Scan result is shown on the screen (left) to locate placental site. Amniocentesis detail. (By courtesy of Dr J. B. Scrimgeour, Consultant Obstetrician and Gynaecologist, Western General Hospital, Edinburgh)

obstetric hospital. It is essential to include instruction on parentcraft during the antenatal period and to prepare both parents for labour and the subsequent care of the baby.

Antenatal screening for congenital abnormalities

Recent research has evolved a method of detecting neural tube defects, such as major degrees of spina bifida, by estimating the *alpha-feto* protein level in the blood at the 16th week of pregnancy. If the level is raised above normal limits the test is repeated and, if still raised, a specimen of amniotic fluid is withdrawn (amniocentesis) (Fig. 10.8). From this specimen the diagnosis is made and termination of pregnancy is offered to the patient and her husband. Amniocentesis may also be offered, in an increasing number of centres, to patients who are over 35 years of age to exclude Down's Syndrome (Ch. 15). This is carried out at the 16th week of pregnancy. Other genetic abnormalities may be diagnosed in this way (see p. 329).

Ultrasonography

Ultrasonography is used in all fields of medicine as a diagnostic aid. In obstetrics the ultrasonic scan, (Fig. 10.9) which has no radiation hazards, has almost totally replaced the X-ray examination (Fig. 10.10).

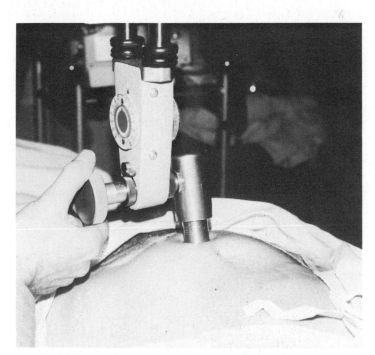

Figure 10.9

Ultrasonic scan in process showing probe passing over abdominal wall (By courtesy of Dr J. B. Scrimgeour, Consultant Obstetrician and Gynaecologist, Western General Hospital, Edinburgh)

Scans are particularly useful for:

1. Diagnosis of pregnancy as early as 6 weeks.
2. Estimating fetal growth and maturity by measuring the fetal biparietal diameters.
3. Locating the placental site prior to amniocentesis and in antepartum haemorrhage.
4. Diagnosis of multiple pregnancy in the early weeks of pregnancy.
5. Diagnosis of breech presentation.

To carry out this procedure olive oil is applied to the abdomen and the probe which is connected to the ultrasonic machine is 'run over' the abdomen (Fig. 10.9). The uterine contents show up on the screen (Fig. 10.8). This result is photographed by a polaroid camera and the photograph is placed in the patient's records.

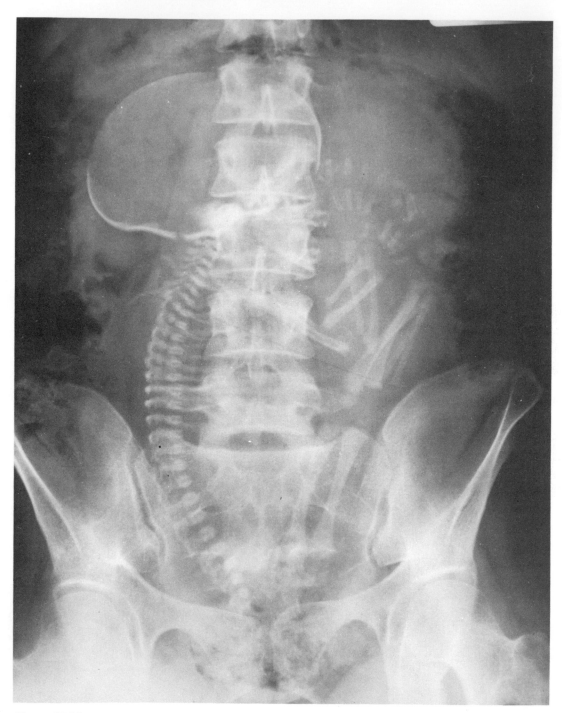

Figure 10.10

X-ray of unusual breech presentation

Labour

This is the process by which the baby is born.

Signs of onset of labour
1. Rupture of the membranes (Fig. 10.11).
2. Appearance of a blood-stained mucus discharge. During pregnancy the cervical canal contains a plug of mucus which is discharged at the onset of labour and is known as *show*.

3. Onset of painful uterine contractions which may begin with general abdominal discomfort and backache. The contractions of true labour can be timed by the clock and occur at 15–20 minute intervals, gradually becoming more frequent and of longer duration.

Labour may begin with any of the above signs in any order or all signs may be present.

Labour may be induced (*induction of labour*) or spontaneous in onset. The mother-to-be requires sympathetic encouragement and support especially from the midwives in attendance. Labour is divided into three stages.

The **first stage** (Fig. 10.11) is from the beginning of dilatation of the external cervical os until its full dilatation. The membranes or bag of *forewaters* may rupture at any time before the onset of labour, during the first stage or at the beginning of the second stage of labour. This is the longest stage of labour but its duration has been reduced by modern obstetric practice, such as using intravenous syntocinon. Drugs such as pethidine and diamorphine may be prescribed by the doctor for the relief of pain.

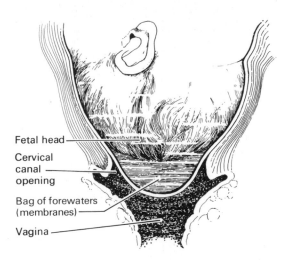

Fetal head

Cervical canal opening

Bag of forewaters (membranes)

Vagina

Figure 10.11
First stage of labour

In the **second stage** (Fig. 10.12), during which the baby is born, the mother 'bears down', assisting the action of the uterus in expediting the birth of the baby. (The care of the baby is described in Ch. 17.)

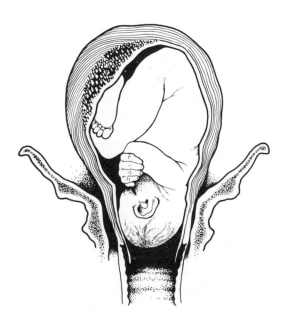

Figure 10.12
Second stage of labour

The **third stage** (Fig. 10.13) is concerned with the expulsion of the placenta and membranes. The contraction during which the shoulders and body of the baby are born detaches the placenta from the wall of the uterus and the uterus contracts and retracts, causing a reduction in its size. The placenta is pushed into the lower part of the uterus and during the next contraction it appears at the vulva and is expelled.

Haemorrhage is a grave risk at this stage and *ergometrine* or *syntometrine* is used to prevent and control haemorrhage if it occurs.

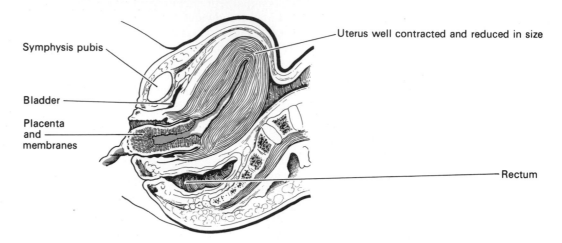

Figure 10.13
Third stage of labour

Symphysis pubis

Bladder

Placenta and membranes

Uterus well contracted and reduced in size

Rectum

False labour

False labour may occur towards the end of pregnancy. The uterine contractions, though painful, are irregular and there are no other signs of labour present. The doctor or midwife may carry out an examination per vaginam to differentiate. If the patient is in true labour the cervix will be dilated and in false labour no dilation will have occurred.

Puerperium

The puerperium begins when the placenta is expelled and ends 6 weeks later. During this time the uterus, ligaments, pelvic floor and vagina return to their pregravid state. Lactation is initiated (p. 359) and the mother recovers from the physical and emotional stress of childbirth.

Great patience and tact are required at this time in handling the new mother and her baby. The mother may have frequent spells of weeping over apparently trivial incidents, particularly in association with her baby. This emotional instability is part of the normal pattern of the puerperium and an experienced midwife and health visitor can give invaluable support.

Planned early discharge

This may be requested by the patient who would have preferred a home confinement but is willing to come into hospital for delivery and return home as soon as possible, usually within 2 or 3 days. Agreement to this request must be reached between the consultant obstetrician and general practitioner and the domiciliary midwife who will make an assessment of the home conditions.

Domiciliary midwifery

Although Scotland has a 99·38 per cent hospital delivery rate (1977 figure) the option still remains open for a home confinement.

There are women who prefer to remain at home but maternal and perinatal statistics have indicated that hospital provides the maximum safety for the mother and baby. Serious complications may arise in labour which cannot be forecast such as post-partum haemorrhage endangering the mother's life or an asphyxiated baby who may not survive or survive with a risk of brain damage.

Emergency flying squad (emergency obstetric service)

This service is based at a hospital providing cover for the surrounding area and is available to the medical practitioner and midwife to deal with obstetric emergencies at home. The service provides resuscitation for the mother and baby if necessary and may transport them to hospital for further treatment. It is equipped however to carry out forcep deliveries in the home. Although the Emergency Flying Squad service is very effective, there could be considerable delay in reaching the patient and this might prove fatal; because such a service is necessary it lays emphasis on the dangers of confinement in the home.

Emergency delivery

Delivery of a baby in the street or in an ambulance, private car or aircraft, perhaps en route to the hospital usually hits the newspaper headlines. Although this does not occur frequently, the nurse may be faced with this emergency. Occasionally the expectant mother experiences no discomfort or pain and reaches the 2nd stage of labour without being aware of what is happening. The 2nd stage can progress to delivery of the baby very rapidly, especially in a multiparous patient.

Dealing with emergency delivery

1. The nurse should ask a responsible person to dial 999 explain that an ambulance is required urgently and what it is required for.

2. As the mother-to-be will be very upset and afraid, the nurse must comfort her and endeavour to promote confidence and keep calm.

3. It is essential to ensure as much privacy as possible and all onlookers must be sent away firmly.

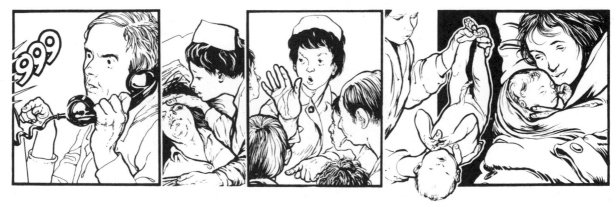

Figure 10.14

Emergency delivery

4. The mother should be placed flat on her back lying on newspaper, a coat or anything clean to protect her from cold and contamination from the ground or floor. Clothing from the lower part of her body should be removed and she must be encouraged to keep her legs widely open. The baby will be expelled and the nurse should gently hold him head down by supporting the head and shoulders with one hand and with the other grasping the ankles to allow mucus to drain away from the naso pharynx so that he can breathe. A clean tissue or handkerchief, if available, could be used to wipe the eyes, nose and mouth. The baby's colour is blue at birth but when respiration is established it becomes pink. If the baby fails to breathe, gentle skin stimulus by flicking the soles of the feet may initiate respiration. A newborn baby loses heat very quickly and should be placed against the mother's body so that heat will be transmitted, lying on its side to promote drainage of mucus. Clothing can be tucked around mother and baby. If the cord is long enough the mother may hold the baby in her arms. It is much safer to leave the baby attached to the placenta as sterile materials will not be available to cut the umbilical cord. If the placenta appears at the vulva it should be gently lifted out and placed in close proximity to the baby. It is essential that no traction is put on the cord or any effort made to hasten the delivery of the placenta as severe haemorrhage could occur. If however there is excessive bleeding from the vagina

the fundus of the uterus should be palpated and gently massaged with a circular movement of the hand which will stimulate uterine contractions and thus control bleeding.

The mother and baby should be transported to hospital accompanied by the nurse as soon as possible.

CONTRACEPTION

The best method of preventing unwanted births is to prevent pregnancy from occurring by the judicious use of contraception. Advice and literature on this subject are readily available from family planning services.

Methods

Various methods are available:

1. Mechanical methods, the vaginal diaphragm (Fig. 10.15) and the condom (see Ch. 9) are commonly used. Neither is completely effective.

The vaginal diaphragm is a dome made of fine latex or plastic and attached to a circular wire spring giving the appearance of a cap hence its other name, cervical cap. It fits across the upper vagina to provide a barrier preventing the ejaculated spermatozoa

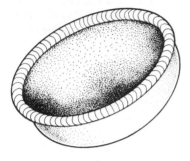

Fig 10.15

Vaginal diaphragm

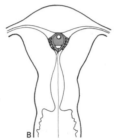
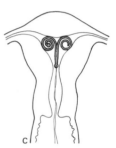

Figure 10.16
Intrauterine devices A. Lippes loop
B. Dalkon shield C. Saf-t-coil
D. Copper 7

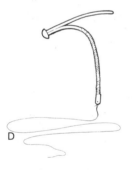

from reaching the cervix. It is made in various sizes and every woman using it is individually fitted.

Women using this method of contraception are advised to insert the diaphragm routinely every night after cleaning it and smearing the rim and the dome with a spermicidal cream.

It should be left in position for at least 6 hours after coitus.

2. Intrauterine Devices (IUDs, Fig. 10.16) in a variety of shapes are also widely used. They are made of inert radio-opaque plastic and must be fitted into the uterus by a skilled practitioner. Threads are attached to them so that the woman can check regularly that her IUD is in place.

IUDs are simply foreign bodies in the uterus. They have a contraceptive effect but are not completely reliable. They have recently been modified to include copper or zinc which allows smaller devices to be used without loss of effectiveness.

Another device, the Progesterat (Fig. 10.17) is T shaped and releases a small amount of progesterone daily which increases the efficiency of the method. This particular device must be replaced once a year.

3. The most effective method, if used correctly, is oral contraception. The contraceptive pill usually contains some form of oestrogen and progestogen. It works mainly by inhibiting ovulation but also has an effect on the endometrium and the cervical mucosa which can prevent implantation occurring. Clear instructions for use are given with each packet.

Oral contraceptives regulate the menstrual cycle and shorten the length of flow of each menstrual period. Initial side effects sometimes experienced by women are:

Nausea.
Sore and swollen breasts.
Slight weight gain.

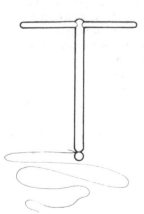

Figure 10.17
Progesterat

These are of short duration. More serious complications, such as deep venous thrombosis, are comparatively rare, but all women who take the pill should have regular medical examinations every 3 to 6 months.

4. Natural forms of contraception such as coitus interruptus (see Ch. 9) and those which make use of the 'safe period' are the forms recommended to people who are opposed to artificial means of contraception. The life spans of spermatozoa and ova are short and fertilization occurs near the time that the ovum is released. Both these methods are based on calculating the time of ovulation and avoiding intercourse during the fertile period, that is for approximately 10 days. The remaining days of the cycle are termed the 'safe period'. Special calendars and the calculation of body temperature are used to determine the time of ovulation.

This method known also as the 'Rhythm Method' has obvious disadvantages and is not recommended to women with irregular cycles, but it can be used effectively by those determined to do so.

The Billings method is also based on the calculation of the time of ovulation. According to Billings every woman has a mucus loss from the cervix and vagina whenever she ovulates. Billings maintains that by teaching a woman to recognise her own cervical mucus pattern she can then calculate her infertile and possibly fertile days by daily charting of her cervical mucus loss. To be safe coitus should not take place for three 'dry' days following mucus loss.

Sterilization
The ultimate resort in contraception is sterilization. Both male and female sterilization should be regarded as irreversible.

Male sterilization
The operation of vasectomy is not effective immediately. Only after 3 months can the couple dispense with alternative forms of contraception (see Ch. 9).

Female sterilization
Female sterilization is effective immediately but involves an operation under general anaesthesia and normally a short stay in hospital. Usually the uterine tubes can be cauterized through the laparoscope. Failing this, laparotomy, involving an 8 to 10 day stay in hospital, is performed to cut and tie the uterine tubes.

Following sterilization intercourse can be enjoyed normally by both sexes.

INFERTILITY

The term 'infertility' is preferred to 'sterility'. Infertility is the state in which a couple who desire conception are unable to achieve it. During the early years of marriage many couples practice contraception; therefore a marriage cannot be considered infertile until the couple have performed regular coitus without the use of contraceptives for a period of 2 years.

Infertility may be either primary, when the wife has never conceived, or secondary, when there has been either one child or an aborted conception of the marriage.

Initially, when a couple decide to have their infertile marriage investigated, they should be seen as a unit by one person such as the family doctor. Often during these preliminary discussions erroneous ideas are corrected and the couple can be instructed in techniques of sexual intercourse and in the most suitable time for coitus in relation to conception. In many cases this 'treatment' is sufficient and pregnancy soon follows. If it does not then ideally the couple should be investigated at the same time, the husband by a urologist and the wife by a gynaecologist.

Infertility in the female is commonly caused either by some factor preventing the spermatozoa from having free passage to the uterine tubes where the ovum is fertilized, or by the woman failing to ovulate so there is no ovum to be fertilized.

Investigations

Vaginal examination.
Laparoscopy with insufflation of the uterine tubes.
Hysterosalpingogram.

These investigations should confirm or eliminate anatomical deformities of the tract and patency of the tubes.

If one or both uterine tubes are found to be obstructed, further tests may be performed to exclude tuberculosis.

Ovulation is confirmed by:

Charting daily basal body temperature.
Vaginal cytology.
Ferning of cervical mucus.
Endocrine assays for progesterone.
Endometrial biopsy performed during the second half of the menstrual cycle.

In some couples it may be possible to perform a postcoital test. An hour or two following coitus a specimen of mucus from the cervical canal is examined under a microscope for the presence of motile spermatozoa. If large numbers of live and active sperms are present the husband is considered normal and intercourse satisfactory. It may be that some secretion in the vagina is killing the sperm.

Most of these investigations involve only a short stay in hospital or may be performed on an out-patient basis. The nurse has a valuable role to play. She can offer reassurance and guidance to the patient and should have sufficient knowledge of the subject to be able to answer questions intelligently.

Investigations of husband and wife may be ineffective and no cause may be found for the couple's infertility. Psychiatric assessment may then be necessary. This may, for example, disclose that the wife has an abnormal fear of pregnancy itself or of the responsibilities of motherhood.

New hope has been given to many childless couples by the recent successes of Artificial Insemination of the Husband's semen (AIH), Artificial Insemination of an unknown donor's semen (AID), fertility drugs, and the 'test tube babies'.

AETIOLOGY OF DISORDERS

There are four main groups of causes of disease of the female reproductive tract:

1. Anatomical deformity.
2. New growths.
3. Hormone imbalance.
4. Infection.

Anatomical deformity may be congenital, for example malformation or absence of one or more organs, or it may be acquired by trauma to organs, muscles, ligaments or other structures. This trauma may be associated with childbirth, surgery, obesity, old age or disordered bladder and bowel functions.

New growths may be either benign or malignant and may involve the reproductive organs or the pituitary gland.

Hormone imbalance may be due to disordered function of the ovary or the pituitary, or disturbance of the hypothalamus, which is the nerve centre controlling the pituitary gland. Hormone imbalance is common at the onset of puberty and at the menopause.

Infection in the pelvic area may follow childbirth or abortion. It is usually associated with ignorance regarding personal hygiene or it may be transmitted from the sexual partner. During the childbearing years when the woman is more exposed to infection she is afforded some protection by the acidic vaginal secretion. After the menopause this safeguard no longer exists because the vaginal secretions become considerably less acidic.

GENERAL FEATURES OF DISORDER

Vaginal discharge

In health there is a white mucoid discharge from the vagina which increases in amount and thickens in consistency immediately before and after a menstrual period, at ovulation and during sexual excitement.

Abnormal or excessive vaginal discharge takes various forms. It may be merely an excess of the normal secretion or it may contain micro-organisms that cause it to become mucopurulent or purulent. Discharge containing pus is greenish-yellow in colour, offensive and accompanied by itching.

Other causes of vaginal discharge are the presence of foreign bodies in the vagina, such as radium implants and occasionally tampons which have been left in place more than 48 hours. These produce a foul-smelling discharge and vaginal toilet is essential following their removal.

Carcinoma of the cervix in its later stages causes a bloodstained, fetid discharge. Frequent baths and the use of bidets should be encouraged. The patient will need sensitive management because she may feel extremely embarrassed by the constant foul smell which surrounds her.

Advice on the use and disposal of sanitary napkins is also essential, especially in the prevention of spread of infection.

Pruritus vulvae

Itchiness of the vulva is commonly associated with vaginal discharges, particularly those produced by the organisms *Candida albicans* and *Trichomonas vaginalis*. It may also be a feature of skin diseases, allergies, diabetes and psychosomatic disorders. It disturbs sleep and is both a distressing and socially embarrassing condition.

Menstrual disturbances

Menorrhagia
This term is used to describe a menstrual period occurring at the normal cyclical time but accompanied by heavy and prolonged bleeding.

Metrorrhagia
This is intermenstrual bleeding — that is bleeding which occurs between the normal menstrual periods and in addition to them.

Polymenorrhoea
This term refers to unusually frequent menstruation.

Oligomenorrhoea
This defines infrequent menstruation.

Amenorrhoea
The absence of menstruation is known as amenorrhoea. It may be either primary or secondary.

Primary amenorrhoea is the term used when menstruation has never occurred. It may be described as 'real amenorrhoea', in which case there is usually some endocrine abnormality, or 'apparent amenorrhoea' because, although the girl has developed all the secondary sex characteristics and experienced the symptoms of menstruation, she has never had a menstrual flow. This is because the membrane occluding the vaginal opening has no perforation and therefore the flow cannot escape. It is simply treated by making a hole in the hymen with the patient under general anaesthesia.

Secondary amenorrhoea may be defined as the absence of menstruation for a period which is twice that of the normal menstrual cycle of a woman who has menstruated previously. This state is normal during pregnancy.

Dysmenorrhoea
This is the word used to describe pain associated with menstruation. There are two recognized types of dysmenorrhoea.

Primary or spasmodic dysmenorrhoea is colicky pain experienced on the first day of menstruation. There is usually no organic cause and it is common in young girls.

Secondary dysmenorrhoea occurs in older women and is secondary to pelvic abnormality such as pelvic congestion, uterine colic or endometriosis.

Premenstrual tension
Irritation and lability of emotions are experienced to a lesser or greater extent by most women in the days prior to menstruation.

Bleeding per vaginum

Dysfunctional uterine bleeding
This is the term used to describe abnormal bleeding following any of the above patterns for which no organic cause can be found.

Postmenopausal bleeding (PMB)
This is vaginal bleeding which occurs in women who have stopped menstruating. Such bleeding is only called PMB when it has been established that the woman has not had a menstrual period for approximately 1 year.

Postcoital bleeding
This is bleeding after sexual intercourse.

Pain

Low back pain and low abdominal pain are common features of disorder in the pelvic area. Referred pain is a feature when nerve pathways are disturbed.

Dyspareunia
This is pain during or after sexual intercourse.

Urinary symptoms

These are commonly associated with gynaecological disease because of the close proximity of the bladder and urethra to the uterus and vagina.

Urinary incontinence is very distressing. A particular symptom of gynaecological disease is stress incontinence. Increased abdominal pressure such as coughing, laughing and sneezing causes a small amount of urine to escape involuntarily from the bladder. It is common in pregnancy and uterovaginal prolapse and is associated with a congenital weakness of the internal sphincter of the bladder.

Large bowel symptoms

These include, for example, constipation, which may occur as a result of pressure on the bowel due to a retroverted or prolapsed uterus or the presence of a fistula.

Abdominal swelling

The presence of tumours or ascites in the abdominal cavity may give rise to an increase in the size of the abdomen.

Anaemia

Iron deficiency anaemia is a common accompanying feature of disorders of the female reproductive tract.

INVESTIGATIONS
History

History taking is an important preliminary to diagnosis of gynaecological diseases, particularly in relation to menstrual bleeding, vaginal discharge and urinary symptoms.

General physical examination

General physical examination is essential prior to surgery, particular attention being paid to the patient's blood picture.

Pelvic examination

Examination of the pelvic organs via the vagina enables the gynaecologist to detect any obvious disorder, such as the presence of polyps, tumours or uterine displacements, and to estimate the gestation of a pregnancy.

Figure 10.18A, B and C show the positions which are commonly used and referred to in gynaecology.

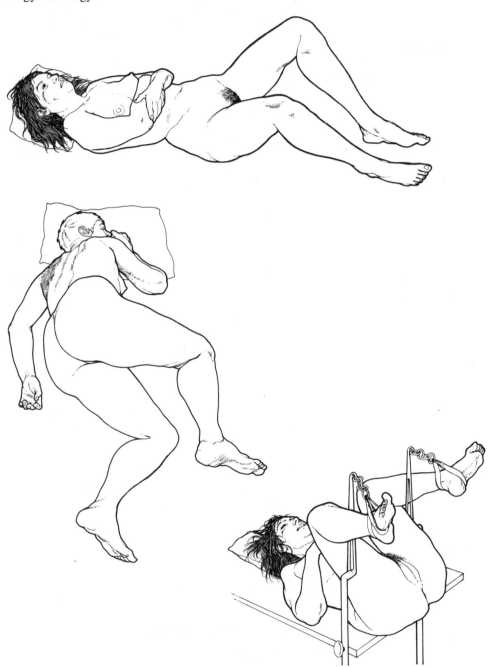

Figure 10.18A
Dorsal position

Figure 10.18B
Sims' position

Figure 10.18C
Lithotomy position

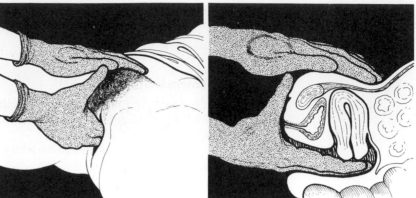

Figure 10.19
Bimanual examination

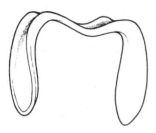

Figure 10.20
Sims' speculum

Vaginal examination

Vaginal examination may be performed in a variety of ways:

1. **Bimanual examination.** Two fingers of one hand are inserted into the vagina while the other hand is used to palpate the abdomen (Fig. 10.19).
2. **Speculum examination.** Insertion of a vaginal speculum such as a Sims' speculum (Fig. 10.20) or more commonly Cusco's speculum (Fig. 10.21), allows the cervix to be inspected visually.

Rectal examination

It is possible but more difficult to palpate the cervix, uterus and appendages via the rectum. Rectal examination may be used in conjunction with vaginal examination to determine the presence or to assess the extent of a lesion.

During vaginal and rectal examination the nurse plays a vital role. She preserves the patient's modesty by ensuring that she is correctly positioned and adequately draped. She reassures the patient by her presence, by guiding her into the positions required by the doctor and by her repeated exhortations to relax. The muscles of the abdomen and pelvic floor must be relaxed if the doctor is to gain any information from the examination.

Examination under anaesthesia

A diagnosis can sometimes be confirmed by vaginal examination under anaesthesia and by dilatation and currettage whereby scrapings are obtained from the cervix and lining of the uterus. Biopsy may also be performed by this route.

Laparoscopy

Laparoscopy is performed under general anaesthesia. Approximately 4 litres of gas (carbon dioxide or nitrous oxide and air are used) are injected either through the abdomen or via the cervix to inflate the peritoneal cavity, giving the surgeon a wider area in which to work. A large trocar and cannula are inserted into the abdominal cavity through a small incision made just below the umbilicus. A special endoscope, called a laparoscope, which has a fibreoptic lighting system is passed through this cannula allowing the pelvic organs to be examined visually. Using forceps attached to the cervix the uterus can be manipulated during the procedure.

There are a variety of attachments available which allow biopsies to be taken from the ovaries, dye to be inserted to test the patency of the uterine tubes, and diathermy to cauterize the tubes.

This procedure has largely superseded laparotomy as a means of investigation and tubal ligation as a means of sterilization.

Nursing care

Preparation of a patient for this procedure may include abdominal and pubic shave, administration of suppositories or disposable enema and the usual preparation prior to general anaesthesia.

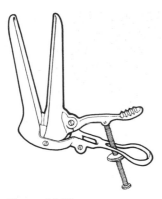

Figure 10.21
Cusco's bivalve speculum

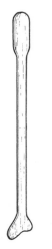

Figure 10.22
Ayre's spatula

One or two clips are used to close the abdominal incision; they are usually removed within 48 hours. Following this procedure many patients experience shoulder tip pain which is pain referred from the diaphragm due to the distension of the abdomen by CO_2. Oral analgesics and reassurance are normally all that is required.

Hysterosalpingogram
A hysterosalpingogram is an X-ray of the genital tract following the injection, through the cervix, of a radio-opaque fluid to demonstrate intrauterine abnormalities and to test the patency of the uterine tubes.

Cervical smear
A cervical smear is an aid to the diagnosis of cancer. To take a cervical smear a Cusco's bivalve speculum (Fig. 10.21) is inserted into the vagina. An Ayre's spatula (Fig. 10.22) is passed through the speculum to take scrapings from the neck of the cervix. The scrapings are deposited on a glass slide, fixed with pure alcohol and sent for cytological examination.

Clinics offering this service to women are available in most cities in the Western hemisphere. All patients attending gynaecology or antenatal clinics have a cervical smear taken routinely.

High vaginal swab
A swab may be taken from the vagina to test for the presence of micro-organisms so that the correct treatment may be administered.

Immunological pregnancy test

This test requires the collection of an early morning specimen of urine. It is used to confirm a diagnosis of suspected pregnancy 2 weeks after a missed period. It may also be used to indicate the level of human chorionic gonadotrophin (HCG) in the urine of a woman who has recently aborted a hydatidiform mole.

Other tests

Blood tests, radiography and skin tests are used to confirm that the patient is not suffering from tuberculosis and are also used in conjunction with 24-hour collections of urine to investigate endocrine abnormalities. The haemoglobin estimation is also very important.

DISORDERS OF THE FEMALE REPRODUCTIVE TRACT

Cervical erosion (ectropion or eversion)

The vaginal portion of the cervix is normally covered with squamous epithelium similar to that lining the vagina. Oestrogen stimulation may cause this lining to be replaced by columnar epithelium similar to that lining the cervical canal, giving rise to the appearance typical of cervical erosion. This condition is more properly named cervical ectropion or eversion.

The erosion appears as a red, circular area covered with mucus surrounding the external os. It is common in women taking the contraceptive pill and during and after pregnancy.

Clinical features
Mucopurulent discharge.
Intermenstrual bleeding.
Postcoital bleeding.
Irritation and discomfort.

Treatment
Cautery of the cervix using diathermy is performed under general anaesthesia. This may be carried out in a day bed area. The patient should be warned that the healing process

takes about three weeks and that during this time she will have an increased amount of vaginal discharge which may be bloodstained.

Cryosurgery (application of extreme cold) is becoming increasingly popular in the treatment of this condition. It can be performed in an out-patient department since it does not require general anaesthesia.

Pain, similar to that experienced in dysmenorrhoea, may occur during the freezing process. The treatment is usually followed by a vaginal discharge, severe enough to require the wearing of sanipads, for 2 to 3 weeks. Postcoital bleeding may occur in a few cases therefore patients are usually advised to avoid intercourse for two weeks.

Infections

Infections within the female reproductive tract are very common.

Vulvitis

Lower genital tract infections are usually first seen and treated by the patient's general practitioner. Alternatively, the patient may be referred to an out-patient clinic. Admission to hospital may be required for treatment of a more serious condition to which the infection is secondary.

The vulva is covered with skin and is subject to any skin disorder. It is also the primary site of some sexually transmitted diseases. Discharges from the bladder, vagina and rectum make the vulval area moist and lack of hygiene may allow the vulva to become infected by a variety of organisms. A chronic condition may develop with constant irritation, tenderness and ulceration. This condition may be self-inflicted by the indiscriminate use of deodorants, talcum powders and soaps to which a woman may develop an allergy. The wearing of tights and pantee girdles, particularly if not changed frequently, capture heat and moisture causing sufficient irritation for the skin to break down. These are very difficult conditions to treat and, although not serious, cause considerable discomfort.

Clinical features
In the acute stages of infection the vulva becomes very moist from discharge, inflamed, swollen and tender. The inguinal glands may also become swollen and tender.

Treatment
The aim of treatment is to keep the area clean and dry. Warm baths and vulval toilet and mild, non-irritating antiseptic lotions are useful as well as applications of powders that do not contain deodorants or perfumes. Ointments should never be applied as they make the area more moist and therefore more susceptible to infection.

In some instances vulvitis may be secondary to another condition, such as thrush or diabetes mellitus, and the vulval irritation should improve when the primary condition is treated. If necessary the irritation can be controlled by the administration of mild sedatives.

Bartholinitis

Infection of Bartholin's gland and duct is usually due either to *E. coli*, staphylococcal infection or gonorrhoea. It may however be caused by any pathogen.

Clinical features
A reddened swelling appears on the vulva in the vicinity of Bartholin's gland and the patient complains of acute discomfort.

During the acute stage an abscess may form and once the infection subsides a cyst may develop.

Treatment
In the acute stage treatment is bed rest, analgesia, and a broad spectrum antibiotic.

If an abscess forms, then surgery is necessary to drain the pus. Blockage of Bartholin's duct or gland by an abscess or cyst is an extremely painful condition often requiring emergency admission to hospital. Often the condition is too painful to allow shaving of the area prior to a general anaesthetic being administered for surgery.

Surgery involves suturing the wall of the abscess or cyst to the vaginal wall following incision to drain the pus or fluid. This procedure is called marsupialization and is preferable to incision of the abscess or excision of the cyst.

Postoperatively, vulval toilet is performed every 4 hours during the day. On discharge home the patient is advised to continue regular bathing of the vulva either by use of bidets or baths, and to complete her antibiotic therapy. She may also be advised to avoid any factor which might have contributed to the cause of the condition such as wearing tight trousers or cycling.

Vaginitis

Most female genital tract infections affect the vagina, causing it to become inflamed. The descriptive term used is vaginitis.

These conditions are characterized by pruritus and by the presence of a vaginal discharge possibly causing skin excoriation (Table 10.1).

Table 10.1
Vaginitis

Type	Organism	Discharge	Special points	Treatment
Monilial vaginitis	*Candida albicans*	White and creamy	Associated with diabetes mellitus, oral contraceptives, pregnancy.	Nystatin vaginal cream or Nystatin pessaries, one into vagina each night for 14 nights.
Trichomonas vaginitis	*Trichomonas vaginalis*	Greenish-yellow, frothy; offensive	Transmitted during coitus	1. Of patient: Metronidazole (Flagyl) 200 mg orally t.i.d. for 1 week. Vaginal pessaries such as Locan and Penotrane, one nightly for 2 to 3 weeks. 2. Of sexual partner: Metronidazole 200 mg orally t.i.d. for 1 week. Abstinence from coitus.
Senile vaginitis	Coliform bacilli streptococcus	Brown	Minute ulcers on vaginal walls	Oestrogen Lactic acid: 1. Orally, usually stilboestrol 2. Locally—creams, pessaries such as Dienoestrol cream, Tampovagen pessaries.

A low grade non-specific vaginitis will result if the normal bacteria found in the vagina become pathogenic.

Cervicitis

It is difficult to differentiate cervicitis from other lower genital tract infections. However if the cervix is chronically infected then the affected area should be removed by cautery or cryosurgery. The latter would seem to be the more successful method.

Salpingitis

Infection ascends in the genital tract and ultimately organisms may reach the uterine tubes causing salpingitis. Infection may also reach the tubes directly from:

1. The uterus after childbirth or abortion.
2. The bowel.
3. The peritoneal cavity.

Causative organisms
Staphylococcus
Streptococcus
Gonococcus
E. coli
Tubercle bacillus

The resulting infection is usually bilateral and may be either acute or chronic.

Acute salpingitis

The patient suffering from acute salpingitis may be very seriously ill.

Clinical features
Sudden onset.
Pyrexia.
Tachycardia.
Purulent vaginal discharge.
Tenderness and intense pain felt in one or both sides of the lower abdomen.
A mass felt in the same area.
Associated urinary tract infection.

Treatment
A cervical smear may be taken to find the causative organism and appropriate chemotherapy commenced. Complete bed rest is essential to allow the inflammation in the uterine tubes to resolve, if possible, without thickening the walls of these very narrow tubes. Thickening is accompanied by a narrowing or complete blockage of the lumen, a cause of sterility.

Peritonitis may develop, therefore the nurse should observe and report any changes in temperature, pulse and respiration (TPR) or in the site and character of the pain. Surgery is usually contraindicated, because of the risk of infection.

After treatment of a mild infection the inflammatory process affecting the tubes should resolve and the vital structures should revert to normal. In some cases the tubes become blocked. If this occurs at the fimbriated end of the tube the ovary may also become involved.

Chronic salpingitis

Chronic salpingitis may develop after repeated mild infections which have never been completely irradicated.

Clinical features
Pallor due to latent sepsis.
General malaise.
Lower abdominal pain which worsens premenstrually and after exercise.
Backache.
Increased vaginal discharge.
Menstrual irregularities.
Dyspareunia.

The patient is often in and out of hospital having her symptoms investigated.

Treatment
For the young woman rest and chemotherapy are the basis of treatment. Hysterectomy and bilateral salpingo-oöphorectomy may be performed on an older woman once the infection has been controlled by antibiotics and provided she wants no more children.

Abortion

Abortion is the word used to describe termination of pregnancy. It may occur spontaneously or be induced artificially.

Spontaneous abortion

It is estimated that one in four pregnancies abort spontaneously. This commonly occurs about the 12th week of gestation but may occur anytime during pregnancy.

It is thought that more than half the abortions occurring spontaneously are caused by fetal malformation and the remainder are due to some abnormality in the mother, such as progesterone deficiency, uterine fibroids or an incompetent cervix.

It is also possible that a defect in the chromosomes from the spermatozoa may also give rise to defects which may result in abortion.

Threatened abortion

When a woman with a confirmed (or suspected) pregnancy presents with slight vaginal bleeding and, on examination, the cervix is found to be closed she is diagnosed as 'threatening to abort'. If cared for the pregnancy may be able to continue normally.

Treatment

Complete bed rest in hospital is the only form of treatment. The patient is reassured and given sedation orally or intramuscularly as required. Constipation is avoided by ensuring that the patient takes roughage in her diet and, if necessary, by the regular use of mild aperients or suppositories.

She is discouraged from stretching, bending, vigorous movement and smoking. Visitors are asked not to excite her.

Vaginal examination is not performed for 48 hours, to allow the pregnancy to settle. during this time all sanitary towels and bedpans are saved for inspection in case some placental tissue has been passed. If, on examination, the external os is found to be closed, the patient can be allowed up once the bleeding has stopped.

A positive immunological pregnancy test reassures that all is well and the woman is discharged home. Many authorities advocate rest and all recommend that coitus should be avoided because of the risk of introducing infection.

Inevitable abortion

If the patient presents with lower abdominal pain and vaginal bleeding which is red and contains clots, abortion is usually inevitable.

On examination the external os is usually dilated, which means that the pregnancy cannot continue. If diagnosis needs to be confirmed the Doptone (p. 330) may be used to prove that the fetus is dead, although an immunological pregnancy test should already have produced a negative result.

Complete abortion

In some cases the fetus and placenta are passed complete in the amniotic sac, hence the term 'complete abortion'.

Following a complete abortion rest at home for 1 week is necessary during which time the vaginal discharge is observed. It should be a normal *lochia* lasting from 7 to 10 days.

Complete abortion usually occurs about the 6th or 8th week of gestation.

Incomplete abortion

If the fetus and placenta are not delivered in their entirety the abortion is said to be incomplete.

The vaginal loss may be quite heavy causing the patient to become shocked. The vagina must be evacuated of clots as quickly as possible. The os is inspected using a Cusco's speculum and the products of conception are removed from the cervix and vagina. At this stage ergometrine (0·5 mg i.m.) is given if bleeding is heavy. The patient's haemoglobin should be estimated and blood should be cross-matched in case transfusion is required.

The uterus is evacuated under general anaesthesia as soon as possible and the patient should be able to be discharged home within 2 days.

At the time of the abortion the patient may be considerably upset emotionally and may require sedation as well as reassurance. Both she and her husband should be informed of the facts as they occur and advised to attempt another pregnancy as soon as they wish.

Habitual abortion

The term habitual abortion is used when a woman aborts three or more consecutive conceptions.

Causes
Incompetent cervix.
Uterine abnormalities.
Abnormality in the chromosomes of one or other parent.

For many patients no cause can be found.

Treatment
Correct the cause when possible, for instance an incompetent cervix; it can be treated simply with Shirodkar's suture.

Under general anaesthesia and using the vaginal route, an unabsorbable suture is placed and tied round the cervix at the level of the internal os (Fig. 10.23).

The patient is nursed in bed for 3 to 5 days before being discharged home. She is encouraged to rest as much as possible during the remainder of her pregnancy. The suture is removed 7 to 14 days prior to term and she is permitted to deliver normally.

If abortion becomes inevitable the stitch must be removed.

If the cause is unknown the patient once pregnant should be advised to avoid travel, exertion and coitus, to take a nutritious diet and rest in bed for 2 hours each afteroon.

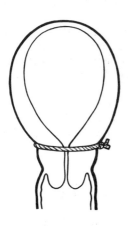

Figure 10.23
Shirodkar's suture

Ectopic pregnancy

In this condition the fertilized ovum becomes implanted outside (ectopic) the uterine cavity. The commonest site is the uterine tube where it is impossible for a pregnancy to continue much beyond the 10th week of gestation.

Tubal abortion

The fertilized ovum dies. It may be absorbed completely or aborted completely into the peritoneal cavity. It may be absorbed incompletely or it may become surrounded by blood clot thus forming a tubal mole.

Clinical features

The main features of tubal abortion are colicky pain in the lower abdomen followed by a small amount of dark coloured vaginal bleeding. On vaginal examination a small tender lump may be felt to one side of the uterus. Referred pain to the shoulder may be another feature. The patient may be severely shocked. Diagnosis, which may be difficult, can be aided by the patient's history but can only be confirmed by surgery.

Tubal rupture

Ruptured ectopic pregnancy is fortunately rarer than tubal abortion but is easier to diagnose.

Clinical features

The woman experiences sudden severe lower abdominal pain following which she quickly becomes shocked due to haemorrhage into the peritoneal cavity.

Treatment

Sedation and analgesia are required immediately and on admission to hospital blood transfusion is usually necessary prior to surgery.

Both tubal abortion and ruptured ectopic pregnancy are treated with immediate surgery. Either partial or total salpingectomy is performed. The tube is conserved if at all possible, especially if the woman wishes to conceive again.

The postoperative care is that given routinely to a patient following laparotomy. The patient is usually discharged home within 8 to 10 days.

The nurse's most important duty is accurate observation of the patient to assist in diagnosis of this potentially dangerous condition.

Induced abortion

Abortion may be induced criminally by the backstreet abortionist. Most of these abortions are infected and the unfortunate woman is usually eventually admitted to hospital, or at least treated by a doctor, for pelvic inflammation.

Legally in the U.K., the fetus is said to have become viable at the 28th week of gestation. The 1967 Abortion Act allows termination of pregnancy to be performed up to this period of gestation in hospital or licensed nursing homes for therapeutic reasons. It is also required that all terminations of pregnancy are notified on a prescribed form to the Health Department.

In hospital it is preferred that termination of pregnancy be performed before the 12th week of gestation. After this time the placenta is fully developed and the fundus too high in the abdomen to allow the gynaecologist to be certain that he has removed all the products of conception.

Termination techniques: 0 to 14 weeks

The commonest technique used to terminate pregnancies at this period of gestation is **vacuum aspiration** using a special suction machine (Fig. 10.24).

This is a short procedure performed in theatre under general anaesthesia; it is accompanied by minimal blood loss. The patient may be discharged home the day following operation. This technique may be used to treat patients on an outpatient

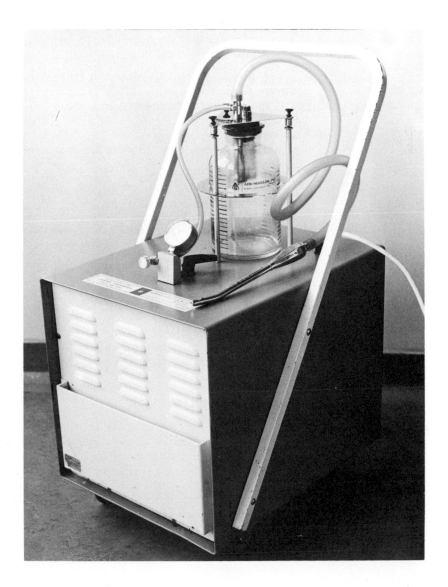

Figure 10.24
Vacuum suction apparatus

basis during the early weeks of pregnancy. A small amount of bright red blood loss from the vagina for a few days is normal.

If vacuum suction apparatus is not available **dilatation and curettage** (D & C) may be performed.

Menstrual regulation which can effectively terminate pregnancy up to the seventh week of gestation is becoming increasingly popular. Three to ten days following an overdue period a woman who has been at risk of becoming pregnant can have her uterus emptied of endometrium. Thus her menstruation is regulated whether or not she was pregnant.

The uterus is emptied either by aspiration using a 50 ml syringe attached to a narrow catheter, or, by inserting high into the vagina pessaries containing prostaglandins.

Termination techniques: after 14 weeks
Intra-amniotic administration of prostaglandins. This method involves a miniature labour which can be distressing not only to the individual patient but to others in the ward.

Hysterotomy carries a high mortality and is seldom advocated.

Nursing care and observations
Nursing duties include reassurance to all patients distressed by the condition. Observations to be made of the patient undergoing termination are:

Type and site of pain; normally it is in the lower abdominal region and is intermittent.

Type and quantity of vaginal discharge, including inspection of used sanitary towels and bedpans.

When the uterine contents are expelled they should be examined to see if abortion is complete. If incomplete, evacuation of the uterus under general anaesthesia is necessary before the patient can be discharged home.

Complications
Complications which may follow termination of pregnancy are:

Pelvic inflammation.
Salpingitis.
Ruptured uterus.
Secondary infertility.
Psychological disturbance which often manifests itself as a phantom pregnancy.
Death.

The earlier during pregnancy that termination can be carried out the less likelihood there is of any of these complications occurring.

Tumours

New growths other than those originating from endometriosis are commonly found in the female reproductive tract.

Ovarian tumours

A variety of cysts may form on the ovary. Some are small benign cysts which are symptomless. Others may grow very large and disturb ovarian function. The commonest is the pseudomucinous multilocular cyst which has numerous compartments containing a sticky substance. These cysts have a tendency to become malignant.

A bizarre type of tumour is the dermoid cyst which is usually benign. It may contain a variety of structures such as hair, teeth, cartilage, sebaceous glands, brain, bowel or thyroid tissue.

Small benign cysts in young women usually disappear in time without treatment. All other cysts should be excised since, if left, malignant changes may occur.

The operations performed are:

Ovarian cystectomy	Cyst removed and ovary reconstituted
Oöphorectomy	Ovary and tumour removed when it is impossible to save the ovary
Total hysterectomy and bilateral salpingo-oöpherectomy	Removal of uterus, both tubes, vault of vagina, both ovaries and tumour

The last operation is performed in women who have completed their families and who are near the menopause. This extensive operation is undertaken to safeguard against carcinoma of the ovary, which may remain undetected until the late stages of the disease when the signs and symptoms of pelvic cancer appear.

Malignant changes

Ascites is a prominent feature in the later stages and is accompanied by loss of weight and abdominal distension. Severe pain may be experienced when the growth spreads into the peritoneal cavity.

Postoperatively either radiotherapy or cytotoxic drugs may be administered to reduce the rate of growth of the residual tumour. Neither of these methods may be successful and with either the patient is subjected to a number of unpleasant side-effects to add to her discomfort.

Prognosis is poor. The patient may linger for a comparatively long time. Frequent abdominal paracentesis with consequent loss of protein may be necessary to relieve the ascites. The patient is terminally ill and should be allowed as much activity as she feels capable of and must never be expected to follow a strict timetable. A high protein diet should be encouraged and use made of proprietary foods to tempt the patient. Skin care is essential. The patient becomes emaciated and lethargic and will spend a great deal to time in bed. The abdomen will frequently be distended with ascites, therefore the skin will alternate between being taut and lax. She can be advised to wear maternity clothing which will adapt to her frequent changes in girth.

Patient comfort is essential. All questions asked by the patient and her relatives should be answered as honestly as possible to form a basis for psychological support.

Benign uterine tumours

Polypi are small benign tumours which grow on the wall of the uterus and are attached to it by a stem or peduncle. They cause vaginal discharge and menorrhagia and are treated by cautery.

Fibroids

Fibroids are benign new growths of the uterus common in women who have no children; symptoms are commonly produced in the 35 to 45 age group.

They originate within the myometrium as small, encapsulated structures composed of fibrous and muscle tissue. They are classified according to site (Fig. 10.25):

Intramural (interstitial): within the muscle wall.
Submucous (extramural): projecting into the uterine cavity.
Subserous (subperitoneal): growing outwards into the peritoneum, sometimes becoming pedunculated.
Cervical (within the cervix): a rare fibroid which ultimately may occlude the cervical canal.

Clinical features

Fibroids may be symptomless for many years. They grow slowly but eventually tend to grow large, causing increased girth and pressure symptoms such as frequency of micturition, stress incontinence, retention of urine, constipation, haemorrhoids and varicose veins. Menorrhagia is common with consequent iron deficiency anaemia, and sometimes the patient complains of metrorrhagia. A submucous fibroid will cause a foul-smelling vaginal discharge. Many women with fibroids are infertile and often their presence is discovered during investigations of infertility.

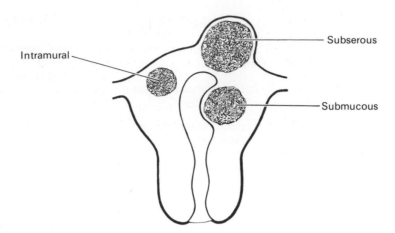

Figure 10.25
Sites of fibroids

If symptomless, fibroids should be left alone; otherwise treatment depends on the age of the patient. If she is near the menopause hysterectomy is performed. Myomectomy, cutting the capsule and shelling out the tumour is performed if possible on women who still desire conception.

Carcinoma of the uterus
Body and fundus

Malignant tumours in this area are slow growing and occur most commonly in nulliparous women after the menopause.

They are characterized by postmenopausal bleeding which is always investigated by dilatation and curettage. If the curettings show signs of malignancy, hysterectomy and bilateral salpingo-oöphorectomy are performed. Younger women may present with metrorrhagia. In this instance dilatation and curettage is performed and scrapings are always sent for cytological examination. If malignant cells are present similar radical surgery is performed on the younger woman.

Cervix

Carcinoma of the cervix is the second commonest form of cancer found in women. It can occur at any age but is most commonly found in the 40 to 50 age group and in women who have had a large family early in their lives.

Malignant changes in the cells of the cervix spread locally very quickly. The bladder and rectum are soon involved and metastases to bone and lungs follow rapidly.

Classification
Carcinoma of the cervix is classified as follows:

Stage 0   Nothing abnormal on visual examination of the cervix, but cytological examination shows presence of some malignant cells.

Stage I   Tumour is localized to the cervix. Erosion apparent on naked eye inspection of the cervix.

Stage II   Local spread of the tumour.

Stage III   Invasive cancer involving vagina and pelvic wall.

Stage IV   Bladder and rectum involved. Possibly liver metastases.

Clinical features and diagnosis
In stage 0 there are no symptoms. Routine cytological examination has been of great value in detecting this state described as 'carcinoma *in situ*' or the 'preclinical state'. A positive cervical smear is further investigated by the removal of a cone biopsy from the cervix. In some younger women this often removes the whole area of malignant cells and

no further surgery may be necessary. Close follow-up is maintained, cervical smears being taken at frequent intervals.

The most important symptom of invasive carcinoma is vaginal bleeding, which is due to ulceration of the lesion. The examining finger of the gynaecologist may be sufficient to cause bright red bleeding. The bleeding may manifest itself as a brown offensive discharge, as postcoital bleeding, as intermenstrual bleeding or, in the case of the older woman, as postmenopausal bleeding. Diagnosis is confirmed by biopsy. This disease must be diagnosed early to be treated satisfactorily.

Treatment
If the tumour is localized, surgery followed by radiotherapy to destroy residual tumour is the treatment of choice. The extent of the surgery depends on how far the tumour has invaded the tissues. For many patients total hysterectomy and bilateral salpingo-oöphorectomy would be sufficient. In some cases more radical surgery involving removal of the fatty tissue in the pelvis, including the lymph glands, may be necessary. This operation is known as Wertheim's hysterectomy.

Pain is experienced when the nearby organs become involved and may become excruciating when bone metastases develop. Anaemia, loss of weight and emaciation are present as in all carcinomata. Bladder involvement may give rise to symptoms which range from dysuria to leakage of urine from a fistula. Similarly rectal involvement may cause alteration in bowel habit and ultimately may lead to a rectovaginal fistula. In these later stages radiotherapy alone is the treatment of choice.

Prognosis in stages III and IV is poor. In the early stages when it is possible to remove all of the tumour and surrounding tissues prognosis is good.

Carcinoma of the vagina

Carcinoma of the vagina is very rare. It is characterized by post-menopausal bleeding and on examination a firm, hard, ulcerated area is felt in the vagina. It is treated with radiotherapy.

Benign tumours of the vulva

The commonest area of the vulva on which a benign tumour grows is the urethral meatus. It is thought to result from chronic or recurrent infection and is commoner in parous postmenopausal women.

It is very painful, causing dysuria and possibly bleeding. It is treated surgically by excision of the tumour and cauterization of the area from which it grew. Some dysuria must be expected for a few days following this procedure.

Malignant tumours of the vulva

These are relatively uncommon tumours which are usually seen in women over 60 years of age.

Clinical features
The tumour appears as a small, hard, painless ulcer on the labia which, if untreated, will eventually spread to involve the whole of the vulva and will travel, via the lymphatics, to the inguinal and femoral glands.

Such a tumour is preceded by leukoplakia, which is considered to be a premalignant condition. The skin of the vulva becomes white in patches and very itchy, causing the patient to scratch the area. Eventually the skin cracks and malignant change in the cells may follow.

Surgical treatment
Treatment is to excise the diseased area. The operations performed are simple vulvectomy or, more often, radical vulvectomy, which is a very mutilating operation involving removal of the vulva and the inguinal nodes on both sides.

Nursing care

The patient must be prepared for a long stay in hospital and complete bed rest following surgery. She should be encouraged to bring into hospital with her some work or hobby to occupy her during this time.

Routine preparation for major surgery is followed, particular attention being paid to shaving and cleansing the skin of the abdomen, perineum, buttocks and thighs.

Routine postoperative care is required immediately after return to the ward. After 24 hours she is nursed first in the semirecumbent and then in the upright positions. A urinary catheter drains the bladder until the surrounding tissue heals. Bowel movements are controlled by the use of suppositories.

This is not a painful operation but it is a distressing one, particularly as the wound is in an area which can be easily seen by the patient when it is exposed for dressings.

Sterile petroleum jelly impregnated gauze covered by large sterile pads is used to dress the wound. Initially there may be a considerable amount of soakage from the wound necessitating frequent changes of dressing.

As the wound begins to heal the patient is encouraged to move the area to avoid developing skin contractures. In approximately 6 weeks she will be mobile again.

Physiotherapy and general nursing care are vital during the prolonged period of bed rest. Probably most important is the psychological support which can be given by all staff in an effort to make the patient's stay in hospital as pleasant as possible.

Endometriosis

Endometriosis has been mentioned already as a possible cause of infertility. It is described as functioning endometrium outwith the lining of the uterus and has been found in a variety of sites, the commonest of which are the ovary, the myometrium and the pouch of Douglas.

It is subject to the same changes during the menstrual cycle as the endometrium lining the uterus, but the blood flow from this endometrium cannot escape via the vagina. As a result cysts and adhesions form, such as the chocolate cyst on the ovary and the adenomyoma in the muscle layer of the uterus, giving rise to a variety of gynaecological complaints, notably dysmenorrhoea.

The aberrant endometrium ceases to function during pregnancy and the menopause. Endometriosis may therefore be treated by suppressing oestrogen function, so inducing an artificial menopause. In young women it may be possible to remove the areas of endometriosis surgically without damaging healthy tissue. Total hysterectomy and bilateral salpingo-oöphorectomy are performed as the alternative and more radical treatment.

Uterine displacements

The accepted normal anatomical position of the uterus is that it should lie at right angles to the vagina and curve forward over the bladder in a position of anteversion. It is, however, a mobile organ and may adopt a variety of positions within the pelvis.

The commonest abnormal positions in which the uterus may be found are **retroversion**, which is backward displacement, and some degree of **uterovaginal** prolapse, which is downward displacement.

Retroversion (Fig. 10.26)

There are two types of retroversion: mobile and fixed. The former is an uncomplicated condition in which the uterus can be manipulated easily into the position of anteversion; it is usually symptomless.

A fixed retroverted uterus is often complicated by the presence of chronic pelvic inflammation or endometriosis, which causes the uterus to adhere to the pouch of Douglas.

Clinical features

The patient may complain of dyspareunia, backache, dysmenorrhoea and menorrhagia.

To assess whether or not the symptoms are due to retroversion, a pessary test is performed. The uterus is manipulated into the anteverted position, if necessary under

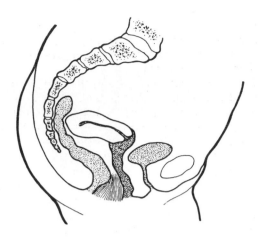

Figure 10.26
Retroversion

general anaesthesia, and a Hodge pessary (Fig. 10.27) is inserted to hold it in this position. The pessary is left in position for 4 to 6 weeks.

If the symptoms are relieved by this measure but recur when the pessary is removed, the uterus falling back into the retroverted position, it can be assumed that the symptoms are caused by retroversion.

Treatment

A ventrosuspension operation is usually performed. This consists of shortening the round ligaments and pulling the uterus forward into the anteverted position.

This operation is performed via the abdominal route and pre- and postoperative care is similar to that required by the patient undergoing abdominal hysterectomy.

Some women with retroverted uteri are infertile and following correction of the retroversion conception may result.

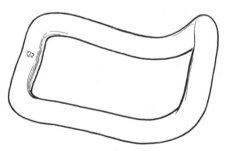

Figure 10.27
Hodge pessary

Uterovaginal prolapse

Many older women experience some degree of descent (prolapse) of the uterus through the vagina because of laxity of the vaginal walls and weakening of the muscles and ligaments which support the uterus.

Commonly affected are postmenopausal parous women whose muscles have been stretched during childbirth and in whom lack of oestrogen following the menopause has caused the pelvic organs to shrink and the muscles to lose tone. Prolapse sometimes results when there is a condition present which raises intra-abdominal pressure such as tumours, ascites or obesity.

This condition may present simply as herniation of the walls of the vagina causing swellings in the urethra (urethrocele), bladder (cystocele), rectum (rectocele) and pouch of Douglas (enterocele) (Fig. 10.28).

The cervix may descend through the vagina until the uterus lies completely outside the vulva. This type of prolapse is called procidentia (Fig. 10.29).

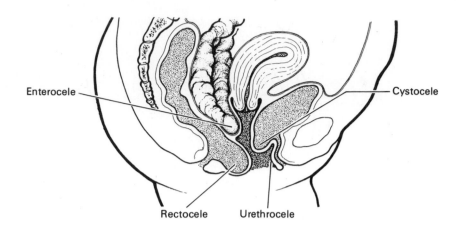

Figure 10.28
Prolapse of the uterus

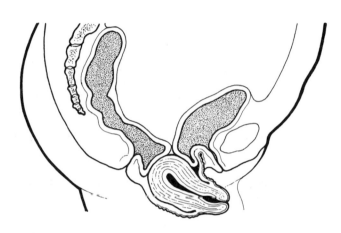

Figure 10.29
Uterovaginal prolapse
(procidentia)

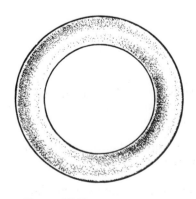

Figure 10.30

Ring pessary

Classification
Three degrees of prolapse are recognized:

1. First degree: cervix still inside the vagina.
2. Second degree: cervix appears outside the vagina.
3. Third degree: uterus lies completely outside the vulva — complete procidentia.

Clinical features
These features may appear in a variety of combinations and are dependent on the site of the prolapse (Table 10.2). Common to all is the sensation of 'something coming down'. In third degree prolapse the displaced uterus can be seen. Other possible features are:

Stress incontinence.
Frequency of micturition.
Retention of urine.
Difficulty in micturition or defaecation.
Vaginal discharge or bleeding due to ulceration of the prolapse.

Treatment
The aim of treatment is to replace the prolapse and keep it in position. Physiotherapy to tighten the muscles of the pelvic floor is sufficient in a few early cases. As a temporary measure, for instance until after a pregnancy or until a patient is fit for surgery, a ring pessary (Fig. 10.30) may be inserted to distend the vaginal walls. The pessary is usually made of polythene and is available in a variety of sizes. The size is chosen according to the length of the vagina, and if it is fitted properly the woman should experience no discomfort and it should not interfere with coitus. Every 4 to 6 months the pessary is removed and the vaginal wall inspected. Any signs of ulceration are treated before the pessary is reinserted.

Table 10.2
Types of prolapse

Name	Area involved	Main symptom	Operation
Urethrocele	Lower anterior vagina	Stress incontinence	Anterior colporrhaphy
Cystocele	Upper anterior vagina	Dysuria Frequency of micturition	Anterior colporrhaphy
Rectocele	Posterior vagina Perineum	Difficulty in defaecation	Colpoperineorrhaphy
Enterocele	Posterior vagina Small intestine	Pelvic discomfort	Colpoperineorrhaphy and removal of the peritoneal sac
Procidentia	Vagina, uterus, pelvic muscles and ligaments	Protrusion of cervix at vulva	Manchester repair and amputation of cervix *or* vaginal hysterectomy

The most usual form of treatment is surgery to restore the organs to their correct anatomical positions by removing the excess tissue which forms the herniae and repairing the stretched muscles and ligaments. Surgical treatment of procidentia requires shortening of the cardinal and uterosacral ligaments and possibly amputation of the elongated cervix. In some areas vaginal hysterectomy is performed routinely but in others only if there is some other indication, such as fibroids or postmenopausal bleeding.

NURSING CARE OF PATIENTS UNDERGOING MAJOR PELVIC SURGERY
Via the abdominal route

Female patients undergoing pelvic surgery through the abdominal route require similar nursing care regardless of the precise nature of the operation.

These patients are admitted routinely 2 days prior to surgery. This allows the usual preoperative investigations to be carried out and also gives the patient an opportunity to familiarize herself with her new environment and to see other patients in the different stages through which she will progress. Routine admission procedure is followed during which it is important that the doctor explains the nature of the operation to the patient and, if at all possible, to her husband. This is partly so that the consent form may be signed but primarily to reassure the couple and correct any erroneous ideas about the effects the operation may have on the patient and on their marital relationship.

Preoperative nursing measures
  Midstream specimen of urine.
  Pubic and perineal shave.
  Evacuant enema.
  Light diet.
  Night sedative.

A major complication of pelvic surgery is deep venous thrombosis. To counteract this is an intravenous infusion of *dextran 70* injection (Macrodex) is often administered during and after the operation. Blood transfusion may also be necessary.

Postoperative care
Routine postoperative care is required. The patient may have an intravenous infusion, a urinary catheter, and, in the case of a Wertheim hysterectomy, vacuum (Redivac) drainage.

Once the patient has settled in bed, her face, hands and perineum are sponged; then she is helped into her nightdress and her hair is combed. This procedure helps to make her feel more comfortable and boosts her morale considerably.

Pulse and blood pressure are charted every half hour initially. If the pulse rises and the blood pressure falls, the foot of the bed should be elevated immediately and the change in the patient's condition reported. The wound site and the perineum are both inspected in case haemorrhage is responsible for the fall in blood pressure. If there is external haemorrhage, pressure in the form of sterile pads is applied to the area. These measures are usually sufficient; rarely is a patient required to return to theatre.

The morning after the operation the patient is usually able to tolerate fluids and a light diet, so the intravenous infusion is discontinued.

If an in-dwelling urinary catheter has been inserted, it is allowed to drain freely for 48 hours; after this time the patient usually has no difficulty in passing urine normally. If a catheter is not in position the patient should be helped up to the commode from the first morning after the operation. Usually little difficulty is experienced in passing urine.

Strong analgesics are required regularly for the first 48 hours. The administration of these drugs should be timed so that the patient is comfortable but not sleepy at meal times; she will be able to eat, get up to the commode and take a short walk round her bed after eating. To prevent the development of deep venous thrombosis the patient is encouraged to exercise her calf muscles while in bed and to get up for short frequent walks.

By the third or fourth day after the operation, the patient should be allowed up for a bath and a walk round the ward. Deep venous thrombosis is still a danger so she must be discouraged from sitting with her legs dependent for any length of time. A dry dressing on the wound prevents the material of the nightdress from catching on clips and stitches. Clips are usually removed on the fifth day following operation and stitches on the seventh day.

On the second postoperative day the administration of two suppositories helps to disperse the flatus which causes many patients considerable discomfort.

If all goes well the patient should be discharged home 11 or 12 days after operation. She is given an out-patient appointment for 6 to 8 weeks after the operation and she is advised not to do any lifting for at least 3 months, to take plenty of exercise and to resume marital relations as soon as she wishes.

Complications
    Chest infection.
    Urinary tract infection.
    Wound infection.
    Wound dehiscence (burst abdomen).
    Deep venous thrombosis.
    Pulmonary embolism.
    Death.

Via the vaginal route

Preoperative measures
The usual preoperative measures are required but particular attention must be paid to shaving the vulval and perineal areas.

An ulcerated prolapsed uterus must be treated prior to surgery. In order to do this the patient must be admitted to hospital 1 or 2 weeks prior to the operation. Each day the patient has an immersion bath following which her procidentia is replaced manually. A vaginal pack soaked in magnesium sulphate and glycerine is inserted.

The patient remains in bed with the foot of the bed elevated to allow gravity to aid the process. The following morning the procedure is repeated. Physiotherapy and general nursing care are important since the patient is confined to bed.

Postoperative care
Postoperative care is similar to that required by those undergoing abdominal hysterectomy.

A urinary catheter draining freely will be in position for 48 hours. The patient is encouraged to drink plenty of fluids and her urinary output is carefully measured and recorded. It may be necessary to recatheterize for a further 48 hours if urinary retention develops. Bladder control is usually regained quite quickly.

A vaginal pack may be inserted in the operating theatre to control bleeding. A written order is normally given by the surgeon to remove the pack, usually between 8 and 24 hours after insertion. If left in longer, there is danger of infection developing and the pack will become hard and stick to the vaginal walls, causing trauma when it is eventually removed.

It is essential that vulval toilet be performed 4 hourly for the first 2 days. A soon as her condition permits, the use of bidets, if available, is encouraged. By the third or fourth day the patient should take baths twice daily with salt in the water to promote healing. She should be encouraged to move around as freely as possible and to adopt a normal posture. A cushion or an air ring to sit on greatly aids her comfort.

Stitches inserted in this area are usually of the absorbable type. If not they are removed within 5 days.

Ten to 14 days after the operation vaginal examination is performed to break down adhesions. If satisfactory the patient can be discharged home with an out-patient appointment in 6 to 8 weeks and advice to avoid constipation, heavy lifting and coitus for 3 months.

THE BREAST

The breasts play an important part in a woman's body image. Some women pay large sums of money for surgical operations that either enlarge their breasts, make them smaller or improve their shape. It follows that removal of a diseased breast will have a profound psychological effect upon a woman.

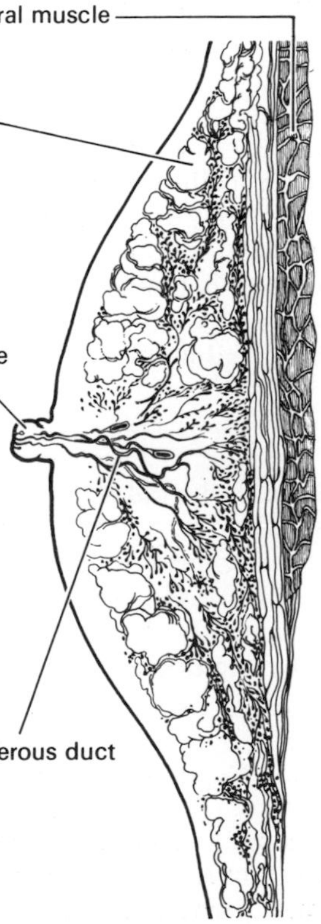

ANATOMY AND PHYSIOLOGY

The anatomy of the breast is illustrated in Figure 10.31. It is important to note that blood and lymphatic supplies to the breast are liberal; this is of particular significance in relation to some disorders and their treatment.

Blood supply is via the mammary branches of the axillary, internal thoracic and intercostal arteries.

Venous drainage takes place through veins following similar routes to those of the arteries.

Lymphatic drainage is through vessels distributed all over the breast which drain mainly into the axillary lymph nodes.

The breasts develop at puberty under the influence of the ovarian hormones to which they continue to respond throughout reproductive life. Each menstrual cycle therefore brings changes within the breasts. Premenstrually there is an increase in blood supply and in growth of glandular tissue, which gives rise to the discomfort experienced by many women. The slightly nodular feel of the breasts at this time is also regarded as physiologically normal. The breasts resume a resting phase after menstruation (Fig. 10.31). The cyclic changes continue throughout reproductive life unless pregnancy intervenes, but cease at the menopause with the decline in the production of the ovarian hormones.

Pectoral muscle

Fat

Nipple

Lactiferous duct

Figure 10.31
Section showing breast in resting phase

Lactation

During pregnancy the secretory cells and duct system develop under the influence of oestrogen and progesterone (Fig. 10.32). About 2 to 3 days after delivery of the baby the blood levels of oestrogen fall. When a certain level is reached the anterior pituitary gland releases prolactin, which is the lactogenic hormone, and the alveoli produce milk.

The milk is propelled along the lactiferous ducts and is stored in the ampullae. When the baby sucks he draws the nipple and areola into his mouth. The action of his jaws empties the ampullae and lower ducts. The sucking stimulus initiates a neurohormonal reflex and the postpituitary gland releases oxytocin, causing the myoepithelial cells in the alveoli to contract, and the milk is propelled along the ducts. This process is called the draught reflex and the mother is often aware of the flow of milk towards the nipple.

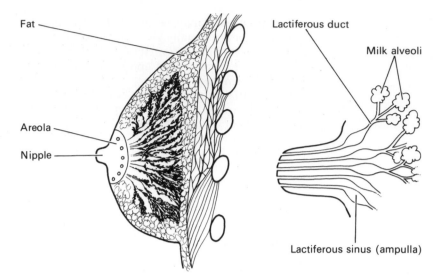

Figure 10.32
Section showing lactating breast

Suppression of lactation

There are many indications for suppressing lactation, some of which are beyond the scope of this chapter. the commonest reasons are:

1. Medical conditions of the mother, for example diabetes mellitus, tuberculosis or cardiac disease, in which the extra demands made by lactation may adversely affect her health.
2. Malformation of the mother's nipple such that the baby is unable to grasp it.
3. Abnormalities of the baby, for example a preterm baby or a baby with a congenital abnormality that affects sucking and swallowing: cleft lip or palate or poor development of the lower jaw.

Method
Oestrogen was widely used to inhibit lactation until quite recently, but because of the risk of thromboembolism it is now prescribed only in selected cases. A firm supporting binder is applied to the breasts; no attempt should be made to express milk even if the breasts become hard and uncomfortable, as more milk will be produced. The patient needs reassurance, and a fresh binder should be reapplied frequently. An analgesic such an Panadol or pentazocine (Fortral) may be prescribed by the doctor.

DISORDERS OF THE BREAST

The breasts may be affected by a variety of pathological conditions including congenital abnormalities, infections, tumours and diseases that affect the skin. By far the most common and important disorder is cancer, which is, therefore, considered in more detail.

Chronic mastitis

This is a condition in which there is dysfunction of the breast; it is **not** an inflammatory state. The normal cyclic changes that occur during menstruation become out of phase. As a result part or all of the breast becomes fibrous or cystic and the patient experiences pain and discomfort.

Of the various treatments which may be prescribed, reassurance and a well-supporting brassiere are probably the most useful. Should a large cyst form it may require surgical removal. The condition regresses at the menopause.

Acute mastitis

This is an inflammatory condition generally associated with childbirth but rarely occurring before the first 7 to 10 days following delivery. The patient complains of pain and tenderness in the affected breast and on examination there is a clearly defined flushed area. The patient's temperature may be elevated and she feels generally unwell. The infection may be blood-borne or introduced through a fissured nipple.

Early diagnosis and antibiotic therapy have greatly reduced the possibility of abscess formation and in most cases breast feeding may be continued once the local symptoms have cleared up.

Tumours of the breast

These may be either benign or malignant.

Benign tumours

The tumour is most commonly a fibroadenoma, the result of an overgrowth of fibrous and glandular tissue from the linings of the ducts. As the tumour grows it presses on the healthy tissue around it, which becomes flattened to form an envelope or capsule. The tumour is round or oval, smooth and mobile and easily removed. (Fig. 10.33).

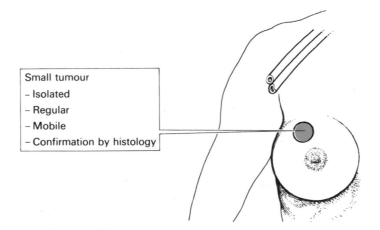

Small tumour
- Isolated
- Regular
- Mobile
- Confirmation by histology

Figure 10.33

Benign tumour of the breast

Malignant tumours

Breast cancer is the most common cause of death in middle-aged women in the Western world. The patient is generally around 50 years of age and often has a family history of the disease, for example a mother or a sister who has had cancer of the breast. It has been found that most breast cancers occur following the menopause and charts show a peak in the 85-year-old age group.

Clinical features

1. The earliest symptom is a painless lump (Fig. 10.34) or thickening in the breast. Usually this is noticed by the patient herself, but with improved facilities for diagnosis it is becoming more common for tumours to be recognized first by a doctor.

2. Alteration in the shape of the breast or retraction of the nipple suggest that the tumour has begun to infiltrate locally.

3. Dimpling of the skin, which is said to look like the peel of an orange (*peau d'orange*), indicates that the small lymphatics beneath the dermis have become blocked.

4. Ulceration through the skin is a late feature. If left untreated the tumour will become a fungating mass.

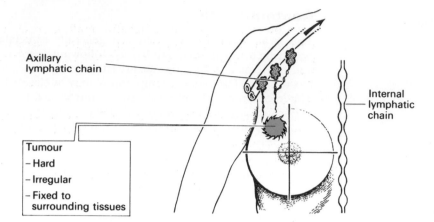

Figure 10.34

Malignant tumour of breast

Malignant tumours spread by the lymphatics and the bloodstream. Metastases will be found in the lymph nodes of the axilla on the affected side initially and later elsewhere. Metastases spread via the blood and invade bones, lungs, liver and other organs. A comparison of the features of benign and malignant tumours is given in Table 10.3.

Table 10.3
Features of benign and malignant tumours

Benign tumour	Malignant tumour
Well-defined lump	Usually a lump or thickening
Smooth and either firm, cystic or soft	Irregular and hard in consistency
Round or oval	Irregular in shape
Often tender	Painless in early stages
Slow-growing	Rate of growth variable, often rapid
Mobile when examined	Fixed to surrounding tissues; tentacles of tumour grow out in all directions
No spread within body	Metastases spread to various other organs

Investigations

Clinical examination
In addition to a full physical examination the doctor will take a history of the patient's past and present symptoms. In particular he will note the date of the last menstrual period (in order to assess the patient's present state in the cycle) and will perform a detailed examination of both breasts.

Thermography
This is a means of recording the infra-red radiation from the body by the use of special cameras.

The patient sits for 10 minutes in a room with air temperature of 19°C, with the upper part of her body unclothed in order to lower her skin temperature. Films are then taken.

A black area of the film indicates a higher than normal temperature (a 'hot spot') and suggests a malignant tumour.

Xerography
Images of breast tissues can be obtained on selenium-coated metal plates. This investigation requires a reduced dose of radiation and enables identification of small tumours 0·5 cm in size which may not be detectable by self-examination or palpation.

Ultrasound

Cosgrove (1979) suggests a hopeful application of localisation of breast tumour through the use of ultrasound. Early reports indicate a good success rate in the early detection of breast tumours. This technique may prove of value for mass screening because of its lack of toxic effects.

Radiology

X -ray mammography. A special technique for soft tissues is necessary to X-ray the breast and this is expensive. A mammogram is therefore taken only on patients considered to be at special risk or not pronounced clear on thermography. A malignant tumour shows up as an irregular mass.

Chest and axial skeleton. Ordinary X-rays of various parts of the body will show metastases of malignant tumours if present.

Treatment of early disease

If there is no evidence of metastases the surgeon will perform either of the following:

1. Simple mastectomy: excision of the breast. This is often followed by a course of radiotherapy.
2. Radical mastectomy: removal of the breast together with the underlying pectoral muscles and the axillary lymph nodes.

Where there is doubt as to the diagnosis the surgeon usually removes the lump only and asks the pathologist for an immediate frozen section examination. This is carried out while the patient is under the anaesthetic; once the surgeon knows the result he will either suture the wound or carry out mastectomy.

Nursing care

On admission to hospital the patient will be frightened regardless of whether or not the diagnosis has been established. Fear of death and its consequences to her family may be uppermost in her mind. Preoperatively she may become aggressive or depressed and tearful. Whatever the manifestations of her anxiety, the thoughtful nurse will afford opportunities for the patient to talk about her fears in privacy and will explain the preoperative routine in simple terms. She is most likely to give way to her emotions when consent for the operation is obtained, when the skin is being prepared or during the night if sedation has not been effective. The nurse should be alert to these possibilities and ready to deal with such a situation sympathetically and with sensitivity. The hearty 'jollying along' approach is wholly inappropriate. It may help to comfort the preoperative patient if the nurse cites examples of women well known in public life who have had a breast removed and yet continue to look attractive and keep active. During the preoperative period the patient may also be upset by what she hears from other patients in the ward, and, therefore, it is essential that the nursing staff give correct and reassuring information. Each patient should be treated as an individual, and emotional support given relevant to her specific needs at that time.

Two days are generally sufficient to enable the investigations and routine procedures prior to major surgery to be carried out. Unless visiting is encouraged or the nursing staff make a particular effort to get to know the patient, it can be a time of great loneliness for her.

Steps should also be taken to keep the husband informed and prepared for the change he will find in his wife.

At operation the surgeon will have taken great care to seal the severed blood vessels, but because the breast is so vascular some postoperative bleeding is inevitable. Drainage tubes will have been placed in separate stab wounds to prevent blood and serum from collecting under the skin flaps as this would delay healing. It is usual to apply suction to the drains by means of Redivacs (Fig. 10.35) which should be changed at least daily. The drainage must be measured and recorded and the bottles checked at regular intervals in case excessive loss should occur.

On regaining consciousness the patient will immediately feel to see if her breast has been removed, and if the diagnosis was in doubt she will ask what was found. The patient's anxiety will be heightened if no explanation is forthcoming and the nurse should be prepared to give an explanation, which she has ascertained from the surgeon.

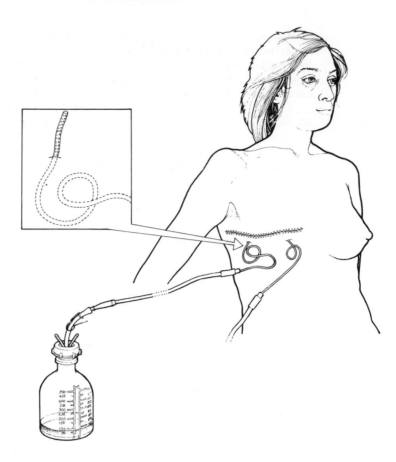

Figure 10.35
Mastectomy showing position
of vacuum (Redivac)
drains

The usual postoperative regime for major surgery will be followed. The patient is allowed to sit up gradually and to drink and eat within the limits of nausea.

The dressing should be inspected regularly and is normally left undisturbed for three days unless there is evidence of abnormal bleeding or soakage. If the dressing is wet it should be replaced using a strict aseptic dressing technique. Vacuum (Redivac) drains are inspected for patency and the amounts of fluid in the Redivacs measured accurately and recorded on the patient's fluid balance chart.

Care of the arm on the affected side
As soon as the patient has recovered from the effects of the anaesthetic, she should be placed comfortably with sufficient pillows in a semirecumbent position. The arm on the side of the mastectomy incision must be slightly abducted and the forearm supported by a pillow. If the patient is not correctly advised she will tend to hold the affected arm in a rigid position and this may lead to muscle contracture and consequent restriction of arm movement.

Observation of the arm should be made at regular intervals in order that the presence of lymphoedema may be detected. A woman who has had a radical mastectomy will be more likely to develop this distressing complication, but it may also occur following simple mastectomy or in women who have had radiotherapy. If lymphoedema should occur, the use of the Flowtron machine (an inflatable sleeve which utilises intermittent compression) may give some subjective relief initially, although very seldom is there a marked improvement in arm volume for a significant period. Elevation of the swollen arm as often as possible will also provide relief.

Precautions should be taken by the nursing staff not to apply a blood pressure cuff to the affected arm, and no subcutaneous or intramuscular injections should be administered in this arm. Doctors will not use this arm for routine venepuncture or the administration of intravenous drugs or fluids.

When the patient is being lifted in bed or getting out of bed, the nurse should be particularly careful not to compress or grip the axilla especially where there has been lymph node removal during surgery. This will be painful for the patient and may cause dehiscence of part of the incision.

The nursing staff must encourage the patient to maintain good posture once the patient is mobile. She may develop a tendency to hunch her shoulders, or to hold one shoulder higher than the other. Adequate support in a suitable chair and correct support with pillows when the patient is sitting up, and tactful verbal reminders when the patient is walking will help to eliminate bad posture.

It is advisable for the patient not to wear rings or other jewellery on the affected arm in case lymphoedema develops, and care should be taken when cutting or manicuring fingernails to prevent infection developing in the arm.

Exercises

Providing there are no contraindications to exercise of the affected arm, the surgeon will permit the physiotherapist to commence a regime of gentle exercises on the first postoperative day if the patient is maintaining normal progress. It is beneficial if a nurse is present while the physiotherapist is instructing the patient in her initial exercises so that the nurse may encourage the patient to persevere with the exercises when the physiotherapist is not present.

On the first postoperative day, the physiotherapist will attempt to achieve increasing abduction of the affected arm, gradually obtaining abduction of 90°. The patient is encouraged to use her 'good' arm to help to support the affected arm during these exercises. The physiotherapist and the nurse may also perform the exercises with the patient and, therefore, help the patient to feel that she is not doing all the work, but that a team effort is being made to help her.

When the patient is able to attain abduction of the affected arm, encouragement should be given to move the forearm backwards, and this exercise should be performed bilaterally. This is particularly important if the patient is to receive subsequent radiotherapy as this position has to be maintained during treatment (Fig. 10.36).

Grasping both hands together in front of the abdomen and gently raising both arms upwards as far as the patient is able is another helpful exercise. These exercises should be encouraged every hour while the patient is awake and supervised by the physiotherapist or nurse. Privacy should be maintained at all times so that the patient does not feel embarrassed or self-conscious.

Once the Redivac drains have been removed, the patient should hold on to the back of a chair with her good arm and practise swinging the affected arm in a pendulum movement. Brushing and combing her hair with the affected arm also assists mobilisation of the affected arm. The provision of a full length mirror in the bathroom will assist the patient to correct any defects in her posture with the help of the physiotherapist. The nurse may help the physiotherapist by unobtrusively watching the patient's posture as she moves about the ward, and report her observations to the physiotherapist.

If the patient is very apprehensive about performing these exercises, other aids may be used. Pulley attachments are available which may be attached to the head of the bed, and the patient instructed to use the pulley in a 'see-saw' motion using the good arm and the affected arm alternately. Education and support of the patient are of paramount importance if good movement is to be obtained following mastectomy.

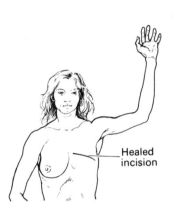

Figure 10.36

Position of arm during radiotherapy treatment following mastectomy

Radiotherapy

Patients who have carcinoma of the breast with the involvement of lymph nodes will probably be given a course of 20 treatments by irradiation in the course of one month. Treatment is usually begun once the mastectomy incision has completely healed. Consultation between the patient, the surgeon and the radiotherapist is essential during this period. The treatment is usually now carried out on an out-patient basis, the patient being given radiotherapy for five days in the week with a period of rest at weekends. Side effects are few with modern treatment, but occasionally the patient may complain of tiredness and slight blistering of the skin in the irradiated area.

It is important for nurses working in the radiotherapy wards or treatment areas to be aware of aspects of skin care appropriate to patients having treatment to the breast area, and to be able to explain the care necessary both verbally and with the use of appropriate leaflets.

During treatment and for some weeks after treatment, the skin of the area being treated may require special care. Some reaction in the skin as a result of treatment is to be expected in all patients and this will be discussed as treatment progresses. During treatment it is desirable to keep the skin as dry and cool as possible. Sensible light, loose-fitting clothing and the use of a mild starch dusting powder, combined with the avoidance of wetting during washing and bathing are all that are required. Heavily perfumed talcum powder, deodorants, scents or creams are to be avoided.

Any reaction to treatment by the skin is likely to begin towards the end of the course and to continue to develop for some days after treatment stops. It will then begin to regress and should be almost completely settled by the time of the patient's first return appointment.

It is important to instruct the patient that once the skin has apparently returned to normal, it remains more sensitive than normal skin to ultra-violet light. Sunbathing to a degree liable to cause sunburn must, therefore, be avoided. The use of medical lamps, such as ultra-violet or infra-red lamps, is not advised.

Hair washing or hair dressing is permitted providing adequate precautions are taken to avoid wetting the area being treated, for example backwards washing is preferable.

There is no contraindication to vaccination or innoculation in the future but the injections should never be given into the arm on the treated side.

Physiotherapy should be continued throughout the period of radiotherapy treatment and classes are held in many departments of physiotherapy once a week to demonstrate suitable exercises.

Prosthesis

Initially a light weight prosthesis will help to improve the patients appearance if it is worn with a well-fitting brassiere and will help her to become less self-conscious about her body image. It will exert no pressure on the area of excision until wound healing is complete. Expert advice may be sought from the appliance specialist in the hospital.

Once healing of the mastectomy site is complete, there is a tendency for the shape of the remaining breast to change and there may be slight contracture of the operated site. It is often wise to delay the fitting of a permanent prosthesis until the size of breast has been established. Many types of permanent prostheses are now available and may be demonstrated by the surgical appliance specialist. An artificial breast made of silicone gel has been found to be most satisfactory by the majority of the patients.

Rehabilitation

It is essential to ensure that once the patient returns home she is encouraged to begin to lead as normal a life as possible. Support should be given by family, relatives and friends when necessary. The Mastectomy Association can also help with many problems or queries.

A woman who has had a mastectomy may experience periods of depression and apprehension after she has returned home, and may become acutely aware of feelings of loss and disfigurement. It is important to encourage her to perform light household tasks initially such as dusting using a circular motion with her affected arm. She should be encouraged to take pride in her personal appearance and grooming, and develop a positive approach to life so that her initial depression will rapidly disappear and she will feel she has a meaningful contribution to make to her own life and that of her family.

Gradually she will be able to resume driving, sewing and most domestic tasks. It is of great encouragement if each achievement is praised without overemphasis. Activities such as tennis and swimming will soon be resumed and the latter is particularly beneficial both physically and psychologically.

The patient must be reassured that she will be able to resume a normal sex life with no loss of libido on her part as a result of her mastectomy. Good communication between partners is essential, and if the husband is not able to accept what he considers his wife's disfigurement, help may be obtained from the general practitioner or the Marriage Guidance Council.

Where lymphoedema persists in the arm, the woman must be particularly careful to avoid burns to that arm for instance long oven gloves should be worn and care taken to avoid burns from cigarettes or matches. She should take care not to prick her fingers while sewing or when manicuring her nails and cuticles.

Treatment and care of the patient with advanced disease

Breast cancer is considered advanced if a large local tumour cannot be removed or if metastases are found in other organs. Cure by this time is impossible and treatment is aimed at either containing the rate of growth of the tumour or relieving distressing symptoms.

Sometimes treatment will also cause a temporary remission of the disease. Various treatments may be used.

Alteration of the hormone environment
Oöphorectomy. In the premenopausal woman this will create an artificial menopause and a big decrease in the production of oestrogen.

Administration of oestrogen, on the other hand, will be suitable for the postmenopausal patient, whose own production of oestrogen will be minimal.

Major endocrine surgery
Hypophysectomy. Removal of the pituitary gland or alternatively its destruction by radiotherapy (Ch. 11).

Adrenalectomy. Removal of the adrenal glands. Reference is made to the effects of endocrine surgery in Chapter 11.

Prevention

Health education is vitally important. There are still many misconceptions about breast cancer and fear prevents some women from consulting a doctor when they have reason to be suspicious of a lump. Breast cancer kills and unless it is treated early there is little hope of cure. Early detection may be achieved in the following ways.

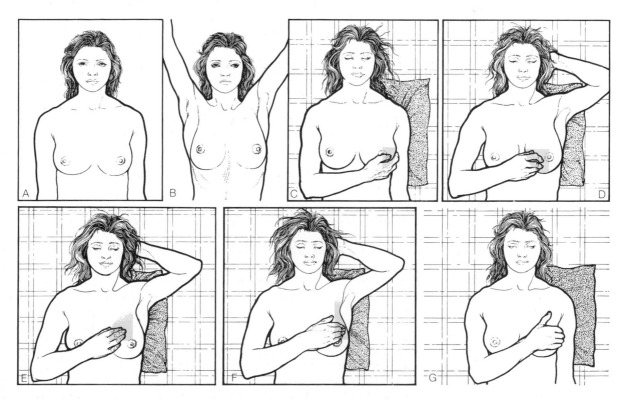

Figure 10.37
A and B Inspection by looking into a mirror C.–G. Systematic self-examination by palpation

Self-examination
Ideally every woman should be taught how to examine her own breasts and be encouraged to do this regularly every month of her reproductive life, and in particular when she is at a vulnerable age. Any change in shape or any puckering of the skin in the

breast is noted preferably by performing the examination while standing in front of a mirror (Fig. 10.37A and B).

The routine for self-examination by palpation is to lie on a flat surface with a folded towel under the left shoulder. Using the fingertips of the right hand the left breast should be examined systematically (Fig. 10.37C–G). The right breast should be palpated in the same way using the left hand.

Examination is best carried out immediately after menstruation when the breast is resting and easiest to palpate.

Screening

In many countries there are clinics which aim to detect cancer at a very early stage in women who are symptomless. The service provided in these clinics or diagnostic centres is usually free and is becoming more widely available.

Facilities include those for:

Clinical examination.
Thermography.
X-ray mammography.

For those at special risk screening should be carried out annually. Patients and members of the public often seek advice from nurses. The nurse must therefore be familiar with the technique of self-examination and with screening facilities available within her area. Any woman who confides that she has an abnormality of her breast must be urged to go to her own doctor or to the appropriate clinic immediately.

SUGGESTED ASSIGNMENTS

1. What cancer screening facilities are available for women of child-bearing years in your vicinity? Are they adequate? How can women of varying social backgrounds be educated to use such services?

2. Infertility is a grave social and psychological problem of many marriages. How can the infertile couple be helped to cope with their difficulties?

3. Isotopes in implants used for treating carcinoma of the cervix have a very long half-life.

    a. Discover what provisions are made in your hospital to prevent such materials being lost.

    b. What routine steps would be necessary if a radio-active isotope is spilt or lost?

4. The protection of people in radiotherapy units is based on three well-known principles. These are that the dosage of radiation absorbed is dependent on:

1. The duration of exposure.
2. The distance from the source.
3. The use of shielding.

Make a list of those people whom you consider would require protection and ascertain how in your hospital these principles are employed to provide this.

5. Find out how antenatal care is organized in your area. What provisions are made to encourage attendance and what scheme is in use for follow-up of 'defaulters'?

FURTHER READING

Garland G W, Quixley J M E, Cameron M D 1971 Obstetrics and gynaecology for nurses, 3rd edn. English Universities Press, London

Garrey M M, Govan A D T, Hodge C H, Callander R 1978 Gynaecology illustrated, 2nd edn. Churchill Livingstone, Edinburgh

Hector W, Bourne G 1979 Modern gynaecology with obstetrics for nurses, 6th edn. Heinemann, London

Jeffcoate Sir Norman 1975 Principles of gynaecology, 4th edn. Butterworth, London

Kleinman R L 1971 Family planning handbook for midwives and nurses. International Planned Parenthood Federation, London

Kleinman R L 1974 Family planning handbook for doctors. International Planned Parenthood Federation, London

Law B 1973 Family planning in nursing. Crosby Lockwood Staples, London

Llewellyn-Jones D 1978 Fundamentals of obstetrics and gynaecology. Gynaecology Volume 2, 2nd edn. Faber, London

Marchant J 1978 Rehabilitation of mastectomy patients. Heinemann, London

Robinson N, Swash I 1977 Mastectomy. A patient's guide to coping with breast surgery. Thorsons Wellingborough, Northants
Scottish Health Education Unit 1979 The book of the child. SHEU, 21 Lansdowne Crescent, Edinburgh

For Reference
Cosgrove D 1979 Radiotherapy ultrasound in tumour localisation. Nursing Times (24th May): 13–14
Myles M F 1981 Textbook for midwives, 9th edn. Churchill Livingstone, Edinburgh
Scottish Health Education Group 1980 The book of the child. SHEG, Edinburgh
Walker J, MacGillivray I, Macnaughton M C (eds) 1976 Combined textbook of obstetrics and gynaecology, 9th edn. Churchill Livingstone, Edinburgh

11. The Endocrine System

The glands comprising this system have in common the fact that they all secrete chemical substances called hormones which are discharged directly into the blood or lymph. The hormones are carried in the circulatory system to a target organ or tissue which responds to the hormonal stimulus. The word hormone means 'to arouse' or 'wake up to' activity.

The endocrine glands which will be considered in this chapter are:
The pituitary.
The thyroid.
The parathyroids.
The pancreas.
The adrenals.

Other glands and tissues produce hormones too, for instance the skin and the kidneys; and one of the glands listed above, the pancreas, secretes pancreatic juice as well as the hormone insulin. Pancreatic juice, however, is discharged via the pancreatic duct into the duodenum (Ch. 5). Insulin is secreted directly into the blood.

Endocrine hormones are synthesized in the endocrine glands, metabolized in the liver and excreted.

There are three main types of hormone:

1. Small proteins composed of amino acids.
2. Amines.
3. Steroids.

Control of endocrine function. The hypothalamus and pituitary together control most of the functions of other endocrine glands, exceptions being parathormone and aldosterone secretion. The pituitary is stimulated by the hypothalamus of the brain, which passes releasing factors and nervous stimuli to the pituitary whose hormones then act on target glands and tissues. The hypothalamus, in turn, is influenced by higher centres of the brain.

Maintenance of normal hormone levels in the body is achieved through negative feedback mechanisms. A good example of such a mechanism in everyday life is a thermostat which controls a central heating system. This device ensures that when the room temperature drops below a predetermined level, the source of heat is switched on, and when the temperature rises above the desired level, the source is switched of.

In the endocrine system, when the level of a hormone rises above or falls below the normal level, the pituitary gland responds by releasing less or more of the appropriate stimulating hormone.

THE PITUITARY GLAND

This small but vitally important structure is sometimes called the master gland because of its influence on other endocrine glands.

STRUCTURE AND FUNCTION

The pituitary gland (Fig. 11.1) lies in the sella turcica of the sphenoid bone. A stalk connects it to the hypothalamus just behind the optic chiasma, and pituitary enlargement can, therefore, damage vision (Ch. 12). Below are the sphenoidal air sinuses (Fig. 13.1, p. 422). The gland has three lobes, anterior, intermediate and posterior; the intermediate lobe is rudimentary in man.

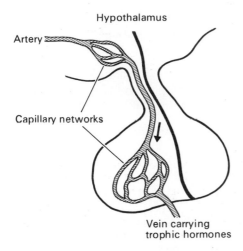

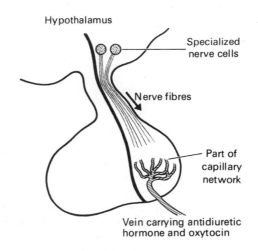

A. Relationship of anterior pituitary to hypothalamus. A portal venous system carries releasing and inhibiting factors from the hypothalamus to the anterior pituitary, stimulating or inhibiting its release of trophic hormones into the bloodstream.

B. Relationship of posterior pituitary to hypothalamus. Oxytocin and antidiuretic hormone are produced by special cells in the hypothalamus, travel along nerve fibres, are stored and released by the posterior pituitary into the bloodstream.

Figure 11.1
The pituitary gland

The anterior lobe

This part of the gland consists of two cell types:

1. Chromophobes — precursors of secretory cells.
2. Secretory cells — either eosinophil or basophil.

Anterior pituitary hormones (Table 11.1)

These secretions (Fig. 11.2) regulate:

1. Growth and activity of the whole body.
2. Other endocrine secretions.

Hypothalmic releasing and inhibiting hormones, which enter the anterior lobe via blood vessels in the pituitary stalk, control the synthesis and secretion of anterior pituitary hormones.

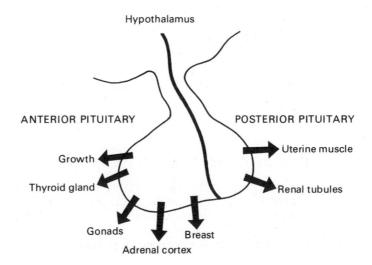

Figure 11.2
Targets of principal groups of pituitary hormones

Table 11.1
Anterior pituitary hormones

Hormone	Regulation of hormone	Action of hormone

1. Growth hormone (GH)
   a. Somatogenic
 	
   b. Diabetogenic
		Mainly development of skeletal and connective tissue;
		
		Opposes the action of insulin

2. Thyroid stimulating hormone (TSH)	Regulated by levels of circulating thyroxine	Controls thyroid activity
3. Adrenocorticotrophic hormone (ACTH)	Regulated by corticosteroid concentrations in blood	Regulates adrenal cortical activity and release of corticosteroids
4. Prolactin	During pregnancy, ovarian hormones inhibit secretion of prolactin	Stimulates milk production post-partum; prolactin released during suckling stimulates milk production for the next feed; the baby 'orders' his next meal
5. Gonadotrophic hormones a. Follicle stimulating hormone (FSH)	FSH stimulates the ovarian follicle to produce oestrogen; as oestrogen levels rise, FSH is suppressed	Necessary for normal development of male and female reproductive organs; FSH stimulates ripening of the ovarian follicle in the female and spermatogenesis in the male
b. Luteinizing hormone (LH)	The corpus luteum secretes progesterone; as progesterone levels in the circulation rise, LH production is reduced	LH stimulates the development of the corpus luteum in the female and testosterone secretion in the male

Table 11.2
Posterior pituitary hormones

Hormone	Regulation of hormone	Action of hormone
Oxytocin (Greek for sharp birth)		Contracts the uterus at term, inducing labour. It is used in obstetrics to stimulate uterine contractions. During lactation oxytocin facilitates milk ejection from breast ducts.
Pitressin (vasopressin) (antidiuretic hormone—ADH)	Plasma volume receptors in the great veins of the thorax send impulses to the hypothalamus which responds to (1) increased plasma volume by reducing ADH secretion thus increasing urinary output; (2) dehydration by increasing ADH causing greater reabsorption of water in the kidney. Water balance is maintained, 14 to 18 litres daily being reabsorbed from the kidney, under the influence of ADH.	1. Antidiuretic effect 2. Contracts smooth muscle of intestine, urinary bladder and blood vessels. Effect on blood pressure is negligible.

The posterior lobe

In this lobe hormones which have been synthesized in the hypothalamus are stored.

Posterior pituitary hormones (Table 11.2)
These secretions (Fig. 11.2) stimulate:

1. The renal tubules, causing reabsorption of water (Fig. 11.3).
2. The uterine muscle at the end of pregnancy, causing contraction.

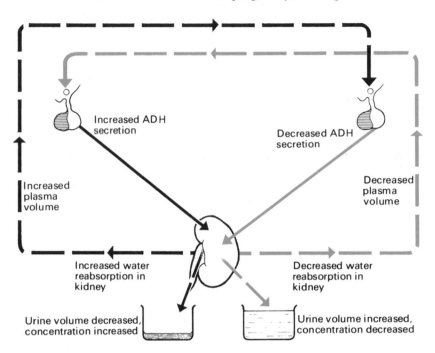

Figure 11.3
Role of ADH in maintaining water balance

PITUITARY DISORDERS

Disordered function may result in undersecretion (hyposecretion) or oversecretion (hypersecretion) of one or several groups of hormones. If there is undersecretion of all of the anterior pituitary hormones the condition is called hypopituitarism.

There are three main groups of causes of pituitary disorder.

Tumours. If the new growth is of secretory tissue hypersecretion occurs. A craniopharyngioma, on the other hand, is of non-secretory tissue and its presence may limit normal function and cause hyposecretion.

Pituitary destruction. This may be the result of a catastrophe, such as a fractured base of skull, or it may follow an infection such as encephalitis. Destruction of the pituitary gland or its removal (hypophysectomy) may be undertaken for therapeutic reasons (p. 375).

Disordered function. This may occur with no demonstrable organic cause.

Signs and symptoms vary according to the nature and extent of the endocrine dysfunction and the age of the patient. If the cause of the disorder is a tumour there may also be pressure symptoms, for instance headache and vomiting, and visual disturbance if the optic chiasma is involved (Fig. 12.5, p. 402).

ANTERIOR PITUITARY DISORDERS

These may be summarized as follows:

Hypofunction	Hyperfunction
Bodily growth and activity understimulated	Bodily growth and activity overstimulated
Target glands understimulated	Target glands overstimulated

Hypofunction

Growth hormone (GH)

Insufficient growth hormone during childhood results in failure to grow to normal height. The condition is called dwarfism and the person is normal in all respects except that of stature.

Adrenocorticotrophic hormone (ACTH)

Hyposecretion of this hormone causes ill effects resulting from lack of stimulation of the adrenal cortex and the thyroid. The result is either sexual immaturity if this deficiency occurs in childhood or regression of sexual activity in an adult.

Total deficiency

All anterior lobe hormones may be deficient and the effects vary. The principal conditions are:

Fröhlich's syndrome

The cause is usually progressive destruction either of the anterior pituitary or more often of the hypothalamus caused by an expanding tumour such as a craniopharyngioma. The condition is characterized by obesity, diabetes insipidus (p. 376), sexual immaturity and drowsiness. Typically it develops at puberty. Depressed sexual function, for instance absence of menstruation in girls, is one of the earliest symptoms. Mental dullness is common. The syndrome is comically illustrated by the fat boy in Dickens' *Pickwick Papers* who was always falling asleep and had an enormous appetite and a sluggish mentality.

Simmonds' syndrome

Atrophy or destruction of the anterior lobes of the pituitary may result from:

1. Trauma, associated with a fractured base of skull.
2. Tumour, such as a chromophobe adenoma.
3. Infection, including tuberculosis.
4. Postpartum haemorrhage and, in consequence, impaired blood supply to the pituitary gland. If the syndrome results from this mishap it is called **Sheenhan's syndrome**.
5. Surgery, as in treatment of hormone-dependent breast cancer.

If the condition develops in childhood, growth ceases and the child looks older than her years (women are more likely to be affected than men). When this deficiency occurs in an adult, there is loss of sexual function, amenorrhoea, atrophy of the genital organs and loss of axillary and pubic hair. Blood pressure is low, energy diminished and thought processes slow. A young woman may, within 5 years, show all the features associated with old age. Since the normal endocrine response to environmental changes is absent in hypopituitarism coma may follow infection, stress or injury (Table 11.2).

Hyperfunction

Growth hormone

Hypersecretion is usually due to an adenoma. If it occurs in childhood, that is before the bony epiphyses have fused, gigantism results. Untreated individuals may reach 2 to $2\frac{1}{2}$ m (7 to 8 feet) in height with proportionately large muscles and organs. At maturity, however, giants become prone to infection. Pressure from the adenoma may cause headaches, vomiting and blindness. If hypersecretion starts after the epiphyses have fused growth in length cannot take place; instead bone thickening occurs. This is especially noticeable in the jaws, hands and feet, hence the name given to the condition, **acromegaly** (Fig. 11.4).

Adrenocorticotrophic hormone

Hypersecretion is the cause of Cushing's syndrome (p. 396).

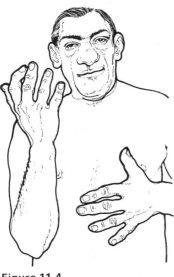

Figure 11.4
Acromegaly

Investigations

1. Radioimmunological assay of pituitary hormones such as ACTH and TSH.

2. Measurement of target organ response to pituitary hormones. No response indicates disease of the target organ, not of the pituitary.

3. Insulin tolerance test. GH, ACTH and prolactin are secreted in response to hypoglycaemia. The test can be dangerous when metabolic responses are below normal because of hypopituitarism. Careful supervision is necessary and injectable glucose should be available at the bedside to correct severe hypoglycaemia, should it occur.

4. Growth hormone investigation. Levels rise after strenuous exercise and during the early period of slow wave sleep.

5. X-rays. These may show enlargement of the sella turcica due to an expanding tumour and the bony abnormalities characteristic of acromegaly.

Methods of treatment

Radiotherapy
A tumour may be destroyed or removed by radiotherapy emanating either from: *yttrium 90 implants* inserted via the nose and sphenoidal sinus, or *conventional radiotherapy*, usually after surgery.

Hypophysectomy
This method of treatment may be chosen, and is usually preferred if the tumour is pressing on the optic chiasma. It is performed through a frontal craniotomy or through the sphenoidal sinuses (Fig. 11.5).

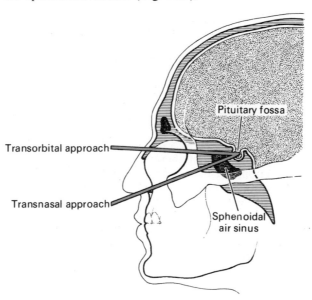

Figure 11.5
Hypophysectomy

Liquid nitrogen freezing
The pituitary is approached through the nose and a cryoprobe is used to apply liquid nitrogen, so damaging the gland.

Drugs
Bromocryptin has been found to reduce levels of growth hormone and may have a place in the treatment of acromegaly in the future.

Replacement therapy
The replacement may be of one hormone only or of several. When hyposecretion of TSH or ACTH is affecting thyroid and adrenalcortical function, the secondary hormones — thyroxine, cortisone and oestrogen or testosterone — are usually administered instead of giving pituitary trophic hormones.

POSTERIOR PITUITARY DISORDERS

The only condition which is likely to be encountered is diabetes insipidus. It may occur alone or in combination with other pituitary deficiencies.

Diabetes insipidus

The cause is usually hyposecretion of vasopressin (or, rarely, failure of renal tubules to respond to the stimulus of the hormone).

Causes of hyposecretion
1. Pituitary tumour.
2. Infection such as meningitis.
3. Fractured base of skull.
4. Surgery.
5. Idiopathic malfunction.

Either sex and any age may be affected.

Clinical features
These stem from the fact that water is not reabsorbed by the distal renal tubules (Fig. 11.3). In consequence abnormally large quantities of filtrate enter the urinary bladder and the patient may void 5–20 + litres of urine daily. The continuing loss of fluid results in frequent drinking (polydipsia) to assuage thirst. The unconcentrated urine has a specific gravity of 1000–1004; serum electrolyte levels may vary, and hydronephrosis (p. 289) may result from polyuria.

Investigations
1. Records of fluid intake and output.
2. Water deprivation test. The patient does not drink for a specified period such as 8 to 12 hours and must be supervised during this time. In diabetes insipidus, polyuria continues, and dehydration, weight loss and rising serum electrolyte levels ensue.
3. Pitressin tannate injection. This results in decreased urinary output with a higher specific gravity in most instances. There is, however, no response if the disease is nephrogenic.

Treatment
1. Replacement therapy, either by: (a) pitressin tannate in oil by intramuscular injection, the suspension being shaken and warmed first, or by (b) lypressin (synthetic pitressin derivative) in a nasal spray. The spray is absorbed from the mucous membrane of the nose and the effect lasts about 3 hours. It may be preferred for children and may also be used, between injections, by others.
2. Chlorpropamide. This substance enhances the action of any endogenous antidiuretic hormone.
3. Chlorothiazide. This reduces polyuria, but the mechanism by which it is achieved is not understood.

NURSING CARE IN PITUITARY DISORDERS

Disturbances in function are shown in many ways and prolonged or continuing treatment may be needed. Abnormalities of stature and appearance may result in much distress. In dwarfism, for instance, the small person may be handicapped socially, psychologically and physically. The developing mind is imprisoned in a child's body. Anxiety about slow growth is often greatest in boys: a youthful appearance with delayed pubertal development may add to embarrassment and lead to much unhappiness. It is important to accord the small person the same respect one gives other individuals.

In dwarfism, the child and his parents should be told about the expected pattern of growth and advised that adult stature may be greater than expected. Learning and social and athletic activities at which they may excel should be suggested. The person should be encouraged to dress and behave in accordance with his age.

Sensitivity, too, should be displayed to the patient with acromegaly who has become unhappily aware of his altered appearance and speech.

Special aspects of preoperative management

The gland is often approached via the nose, and nasal swabs are taken to ascertain if antibiotic therapy should be started. Antiseptic nasal creams may also be prescribed to control organisms, and the nose may be packed with cocaine and adrenaline 1:1000 to prevent bleeding.

Special aspects of postoperative management

Any activity leading to an increase in intracranial pressure should be avoided. The patient is nursed lying flat and measures are taken to prevent vomiting or sneezing: he should be warned not to blow his nose.

In all procedures for pituitary destruction cortisone is prescribed to prevent symptoms of adrenal cortical deficiency from developing.

Nursing observations and records

Complications which are of particular importance after this type of operation are intracerebral compression and bleeding, leakage of cerebrospinal fluid and infection.

Particular attention is paid to observations relating to:

1. Intracranial pressure.
2. The nose, for CSF leakage.
3. Temperature, pulse and respiration, for signs of infection.

Continuing supervision

Following an operation for pituitary destruction the patient is readmitted, after an interval of 3 months, and cortisone therapy is stopped to see whether it is necessary to continue the drug. Pituitary destruction or hypofunction, from any cause, may demand the replacement of one or several hormones.

Cortisone may have to be taken for life. The patient will be advised to increase the dose in times of infection or stress and always to carry a card bearing the diagnosis and details of current drug therapy in the event of an emergency.

Thyroxine is given if hypothyroidism is detected.

Sex hormones. Oestrogens for women, testosterone — by implants in the abdominal wall — for men, and gonadotrophins to restore fertility, may be needed.

Pitressin is prescribed to treat diabetes insipidus. Should the patient be a diabetic his insulin requirements will probably become less.

THE THYROID GLAND
STRUCTURE AND FUNCTION

This gland lies in the neck, in front of the trachea (Fig. 11.6). It has a very rich blood supply. Embedded in its **posterior surface** are four parathyroid glands. Passing very close to the thyroid is the recurrent laryngeal nerve, supplying the muscles of the larynx. These anatomical relationships are important in surgery of the gland, because of the danger of accidental damage.

Microscopically the gland is composed of spherical vesicles made up of thyroid cells. Thyroid hormone secreted by these cells is stored in the form of colloid in the vesicles and is released into the bloodstream when required. Iodine is necessary for the formation of the hormone and must be supplied in the diet. Production of the hormone is controlled by the hypothalamus operating through the anterior pituitary. Regulation of production is by means of a feed-back system described on page 370.

The main functions of thyroid hormone are summarized below:

1. It controls the basal metabolic rate.
2. It is essential for normal mental and physical development of children.
3. It influences the functioning of the nervous system, deficiency of the hormone causing slowing down and sluggishness, excess causing overactivity and excitability.
4. It potentiates the effects of adrenaline and sympathetic nervous activity. An excess is seen as features of overactivity

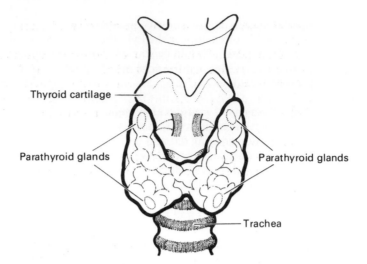

Figure 11.6
Thyroid gland showing position of parathyroids

5. It is necessary for the formation of vitamin A from carotene.
6. It lowers levels of blood cholesterol.
7. It increases the absorption of glucose from the intestines.

Tests of thyroid function

These are carried out to determine whether the gland is over- or underactive. Since most of the tests presently in use are of a sophisticated biochemical type and do not involve the nurse to any great extent, only a brief description is provided.

1. ^{131}Iodine (I) uptake test. A measured dose of ^{131}I is given, and the proportion taken up by the thyroid gland is measured by a counter. Provided patients are not suffering from iodine lack, an increased uptake indicates hyperthyroidism, a decreased uptake, hypothyroidism. In the latter a greater than normal amount of ^{131}I is found in the urine, which must be collected for specified periods after the initial dose.

2.   Direct measurement of circulating thyroid hormone can be carried out. This test has largely replaced the protein-bound iodine (PBI) test, which was easily disturbed by a number of factors.

3. Tests of the function of hypothalamus-pituitary-thyroid interrelationship. Normally the administration of thyroid releasing hormone (TRH) stimulates the pituitary to produce thyroid stimulating hormone (TSH). If hyperthyroidism is present the feed-back mechanism activated by high levels of thyroid hormone prevents this response. The test involves measuring blood levels of TSH after administration of TRH.

4. Basal metabolic rate. This test is not often used, as it is an inexact indicator of thyroid function. It is based on the patient's utilization of oxygen under controlled circumstances, from which his energy consumption can be calculated. The result is compared with normal people of the same age, size and sex.

DISORDERS OF THE THYROID GLAND

Goitre

The term goitre refers to enlargement of the thyroid gland. A simple goitre is not associated with excess secretion of thyroid hormone. Normally these patients are euthyroid or have degrees of hypothyroidism.

Aetiology

1. Iodine deficiency. This limits the amount of thyroid hormone made. As a result, enlargement. Endemic goitre is found in areas remote from the sea, where diet is deficient in iodine. Some 'fad' diets also lack iodine, while in pregnancy there can be a

relative iodine deficiency because of increased urinary excretion and the demands of the fetus.

2. Goitrogens. Certain substances inhibit the uptake of iodine by the gland, bringing into play the mechanism described above and leading to goitre. Among these substances are the thiouracils, carbimazole, potassium perchlorate (all used in the treatment of hyperthyroidism), sodium aminosalicylate (para-aminosalicylate — PAS), lithium compounds and phenylbutazone.

Clinical features

As a rule, there is only a painless swelling in the neck. Gross enlargement may press on the trachea causing cough and dyspnoea, and on the oesophagus leading to dysphagia.

Treatment

The administration of iodine in the form of potassium iodide to children suffering from deficiency prevents further enlargement. It does not reduce the size of the gland. Adults are given thyroxine 0·1 to 0·25 mg daily, which has a similar effect and may reduce the size of the thyroid. Goitrogens are, of course, avoided. Surgery (subtotal thyroidectomy) is carried out when the gland becomes unsightly or causes difficulty in breathing or swallowing (see below for further details). Following surgery, thyroxine may be given to prevent symptoms of hypothyroidism.

Hyperthyroidism

Sometimes referred to as thyrotoxicosis, or exophthalmic goitre, the main features of this condition (except exophthalmos, see below) are caused by increased secretion of thyroid hormone. Although the cause is uncertain, it is thought that a form of antibody, a long-acting thyroid stimulating substance (LATS) found in the blood, may be responsible.

Clinical features

Increased heat production, sweating and excitability are typical. Patients suffer weight loss, although they usually have a good appetite. Heart rate is increased even while sleeping. In a long-standing condition, disturbance of heart rhythm and heart enlargement may result. Exophthalmos (protrusion of the eyeballs) is often the most obvious sign. The cause of this is still uncertain. Mood disturbance can resemble acute anxiety states, with restlessness, agitation and tremor. Varying degrees of elation may also be seen.

Treatment

The results of treatment are extremely satisfactory though the distressing exophthalmos is not usually eliminated. Three well-established methods are used. Each is more suitable than the others in certain circumstances.

Antithyroid drugs. These interfere with the production of thyroid hormone in various ways. One of the most widely used drugs is carbimazole. Its side-effects are not common but, if they occur, propylthiouracil can be used instead. Higher doses are given for up to 4 months to reduce hormone production to normal, then lower maintenance doses are given. After a year or two it is possible to see if remission has occurred by gradually withdrawing the drug. Another drug which may be used is potassium perchlorate. In severe hyperthyroidism, disturbances of cardiac rhythm may be controlled by propranolol. Drug therapy is most suitable for young children, for adults with smaller goitres and for pregnant women.

Radioactive iodine therapy. This method is most suitable for people of older age groups on recurrence of symptoms after partial thyroidectomy, or in cases of pre-existing debilitating disease such as rheumatic heart disease. It is never used in pregnancy and is undesirable for persons of reproductive age. The treatment consists of administering, orally a radioactive isotope of iodine (^{131}I). This is taken up by the thyroid gland, where the emitted radiation is concentrated on thyroid cells, destroying some of them. The risk of producing hypothyroidism is a significant complication. The use of such radioactive materials requires special handling facilities and staff trained in the necessary precautions.

Surgery. Partial thyroidectomy is used mainly in adults and particularly where drug therapy has not controlled the condition. About seven-eighths of the gland is removed. Prior to operation, drugs are used to reduce thyroid function to normal. Potassium iodide is given for 14 days to reduce the vascularity of the gland. This makes operation easier and safer.

Nursing care

One of the principles which must be uppermost in the nurse's mind is that her attitude towards her patient must not be coloured by those features of the disease, such as mood elevation, anxiety and restlessness, which can be demanding and difficult to deal with.

Rest. The maximum provision for rest is essential. This includes a quiet, non-stimulating environment and a quiet, calm approach by staff. A limited amount of activity is useful to minimize boredom and frustration. Restriction on the number of visitors may also help by reducing stimulation. Extreme restlessness may require the use of sedatives. Other patients in the ward, who may be disturbed by a restless, overactive patient, must not be forgotten.

Diet. There are a number of reasons why diet is important. The overactive patient with increased metabolic rate requires increased amounts of carbohydrate to meet his energy requirements. Weight loss may indicate a need for increased protein. Sweating results in greater than normal fluid loss, which must be replaced by increased intake. A few patients will not have good appetites and will require special consideration. Stimulating drinks such as coffee and even tea may need to be avoided.

Observation. This should include:

1. Pulse rate (radial and apex) including rate when asleep.
2. Temperature and respiratory rate. An increased temperature may indicate infection, particularly if drug therapy has caused leucopenia.
3. Weighing, which should be carried out at least weekly.
4. Rashes due to drugs, which should be noted and reported at once.
5. Mood and behaviour.

Comfort. To a great extent, the patient's comfort depends on allowing for his extra sensitivity to heat. Adequate ventilation is helpful, and very light bedclothes should be used. Frequent changes of clothing and linen and frequent baths help to cope with excess sweating.

Nursing in surgery of the thyroid

A period of medical treatment is always given to ensure that no signs of hyperthyroidism are present when the operation is carried out. Electrocardiography is also carried out to detect any cardiac abnormality. Preparation for surgery is essential, as for other forms of operation. It must be remembered that reassurance about the cosmetic result is of importance, especially to younger women. A full explanation of what patients may expect postoperatively is necessary. Preoperative administration of potassium iodide or Lugol's iodine for 2 weeks prior to operation renders the gland firmer and less vascular, thus minimizing the risk of postoperative complications.

Except in cases of malignancy, about five-sixths of the gland is removed. Sufficient gland tissue is thus left to provide an adequate supply of hormone. The incision is made along a natural skin fold in the neck and is closed with stainless steel clips. There are often small wound drains — these are usually removed after 24 hours, and all the clips in about 3 days.

There is a normal tendency for patients to be frightened to move their heads after this operation. They should be reassured by careful support of the head, protecting the wound from strain, whenever position is changed. During the first day, patients will not feel like eating, but frequent small drinks should be encouraged. These will help the sore throat, which is a normal feature. From the second day on, increasing mobility is allowed and the diet progresses from soft to normal.

Postoperative observations

Observation after operation is for the purpose of detecting complications: these are, fortunately, uncommon.

1. *Haemorrhage.* In the early postoperative period pulse and blood pressure readings should be taken every 15 minutes. Dressings should be examined for signs of bleeding and, since blood may run round behind the neck and shoulders, these areas should also be examined. Blood may not escape from the wound but may collect in the tissues. Nurses should therefore be alert to breathing or swallowing difficulties caused by pressure of blood on the trachea and oesophagus. In cases of serious respiratory difficulty, the wound should be reopened with clip removers, which should be kept at the bedside. Blood vessels will have to be religatured in theatre, and if the degree of respiratory difficulty warrants it, a tracheostomy may be performed.

2. *Damage to nerves.* Because of the proximity of the recurrent laryngeal nerve, temporary signs of interference may appear. Permanent damage is rare. Hoarseness and sore throat are to be expected after operation, but if they increase in severity or if respiratory difficulty occurs, nerve injury may be indicated. *Dysphonia* (difficulty in speaking) can also occur, as a result of vocal cord paralysis. If both cords are paralysed, breathing difficulties may require tracheostomy.

3. *Tetany.* Accidental removal of parathyroid glands leads to depression of blood calcium levels. The features of this rare but serious complication may take up to a week to appear. Severe cases are manifest within 24 hours. Paraesthesia of extremities develops, with painful muscle contractions. Painful flexion of wrists and ankles also occurs (p. 384). The condition is quickly relieved by intravenous calcium gluconate.

4. *Thyroid crisis.* This is now extremely rare because of improved preoperative preparation. It is heralded by a rapid increase of pulse and temperature occurring within 24 hours of operation accompanied by restlessness and delirium.

5. *Hypothyroidism.* This long-term complication occurs in a few cases. Treatment is by administration of thyroxine.

Hypothyroidism

This term implies underactivity of the thyroid gland. Causes include ^{131}I therapy and surgery. Primary hypothyroidism associated with a goitre (Hashimoto's thyroiditis) is of autoimmune origin.

Cretinism

Hypothyroidism in children is known as cretinism. Maternal hormones supply a baby's needs for up to 3 months after birth. Then, if the baby is hypothyroid, features due to deficiency begin to appear. These are a general stunting of mental and physical growth. If left untreated the child becomes a mentally retarded dwarf with coarse facial features. Early detection and administration of the deficient hormone leads to great improvement in physical growth and, in some cases, mental development. In others, mental retardation persists.

Myxoedema

This term refers to the clinical state resulting from prolonged severe hypothyroidism. As would be expected, many of the features are the converse of those of hyperthyroidism. These include lack of energy, apathy, sensitivity to cold, reduced sweating and a slowed pulse rate. Accumulation of mucin in tissues gives the appearance of oedema, especially around the eyes. Mental slowness is obvious. Hair becomes dry and brittle and may be thin. Amenorrhoea may develop and anaemia may also be present. Treatment by the administration of thyroxine must be given for life. Careful adjustment of dosage is necessary to avoid symptoms of hyperthyroidism.

Nursing care

To a large extent this depends on the symptoms. The patient's slowness of thought and action requires much patience and understanding. Sensitivity to cold indicates the need for a warm environment and adequate clothing and blankets. Dry skin is helped by using bath oil and suitable lotions. Constipation, which is common, suggests the need for more roughage in the diet and, if necessary, suitable aperients. In general, what makes the patient comfortable is a good guide. If thyroxine is being administered, watch should be kept for signs of hyperthyroidism. Diet should have adequate protein and iron content, but excessive carbohydrate should be avoided.

THE PARATHYROID GLANDS
STRUCTURE AND FUNCTION

The four parathyroids lie behind the thyroid gland (Fig. 11.6); branches of the thyroid arteries provide their blood supply. In the embryo, the parathyroids occasionally migrate elsewhere, for example to the mediastinum. Their number can also vary. They secrete **parathormone**, which maintains plasma calcium levels within a narrow range despite the large daily exchanges of calcium between intestines, bloodstream, kidneys and bones.

Parathormone secretion is not regulated by the anterior pituitary but varies inversely with plasma concentration. Plasma phosphate concentration is inversely related to that of calcium.

The main functions of parathormone are:
1. To mobilize calcium and phosphate from bones into blood (Ch. 4).
2. To reduce renal excretion of calcium.
3. To promote intestinal absorption of calcium aided by vitamin D. (These actions raise the plasma calcium.)
4. To reduce phosphorus reabsorption by the kidneys, thus promoting its excretion and lowering plasma phosphate. This is necessary, since calcium and phosphate together tend to precipitate out of solution and could thus damage tissues and especially arterial walls.

PARATHYROID DISORDERS

Hyperparathyroidism

This term denotes excessive parathyroid activity; the condition is uncommon, the highest incidence being among females and between the ages of 30 and 50. The disease may be familial.

Primary hyperparathyroidism. The cause is usually a benign adenoma or adenomas (90 per cent of cases), occasionally hyperplasia and more rarely cancer. There is oversecretion of parathormone, regardless of plasma calcium concentration. Calcium and phosphorus are mobilized from bone, renal absorption of calcium is increased, plasma calcium levels rise and urinary phosphate excretion is increased.

Secondary hyperparathyroidism. In some diseases where there is depression of the plasma calcium, there is compensatory enlargement of the parathyroids. The underlying disease may be intestinal, causing malabsorption of vitamin D and calcium, or renal, where there is excess calcium excretion.

Clinical features of primary hyperparathyroidism
Raised plasma calcium causes lethargy and anorexia. It weakens and eventually paralyses muscles. The paralysing effects of excess calcium on the gut wall may cause abdominal pain and constipation. Polyuria occurs, since the kidneys are filtering and excreting excess mineral salts. The nauseated patient may be reluctant to drink, but he should be encouraged to do so to prevent dehydration and formation of renal stones. Renal disorders are common, with formation of calcium-containing kidney stones due to high urinary calcium. Calcium-depleted bones become brittle. Osteitis fibrosa (replacement of bone by fibrous tissue) causes vague pains, which may be mistaken for rheumatism and can lead to bone deformities. Cyst formation in bones adds swelling to deformity. Calcium 'ring' deposits can occur in the cornea, and effects on nervous tissue may cause agitation, confusion or depression.

Nurses should ensure that patients whose bones are so fragile are protected from accidents.

Investigations

1. Measurement of plasma calcium with the patient at rest and fasting. (Calcium absorption following meals would affect the readings.) Plasma calcium is raised and plasma phosphorus reduced in primary hyperparathyroidism.

2. Measurement of parathormone levels by radioimmunoassay when possible.

3. Bone X-rays. These may reveal cysts and low bone density.

4. Bone biopsy. This may show reabsorption of trabeculae by osteoclasts and replacement by fibrous tissue (oesteitis fibrosa).

5. Intravenous urogram. This may demonstrate calcium deposits in the renal tract.

6. Urinary calcium, measured on a normal diet, is increased because the increase in the amount filtered overwhelms the effect of renal reabsorption under the influence of parathormone.

Treatment

Secondary hyperparathyroidism. Oral vitamin D will raise plasma calcium levels by enhancing absorption and so remove the stimulus to parathyroid hyperplasia. Operative treatment is seldom indicated.

Primary hyperparathyroidism is treated by surgical removal of abnormal parathyroid tissue. If hyperplasia of all four glands exists, three and a half are removed.

Preparation for operation
Preoperatively, the patient may be infused with methylene blue to facilitate recognition of parathyroid tissue. This procedure causes skin and mucous membrane to develop a greenish tinge. The patient should be warned about this beforehand and assured that the colour will disappear quickly. Ward staff without experience of this operation should also be prepared for this change in appearance.

Postoperative observations
Hypoparathyroidism occurs if much parathyroid tissue is removed and because calcium-depleted bones take up free calcium. Plasma calcium levels are monitored by:

1. Taking blood samples.
2. Frequent observation of the patient for signs of latent tetany, using Chvostek's and Trousseau's signs (p. 384) and noting any tingling sensations in the limbs.

Should signs of hypocalcaemia develop, an intravenous injection of 10 per cent calcium gluconate is given. Dihydrotachysterol (DHT), an analogue of vitamin D, is sometimes given in large doses postoperatively (8 mg daily for 2 days). Because they act more slowly than DHT, vitamin D preparations are less satisfactory for immediate postoperative management. Aluminium hydroxide may be given orally with meals to reduce phosphorus absorption. (Since blood calcium levels are now reduced phosphorus levels rise.) Later, a high calcium diet is given, the calcium usually consisting of calcium salts, because these patients often have renal disorders and milk is inadvisable because of its high protein and phosphorus content.

Postoperative complications
These are similar to those which may follow thyroidectomy (p. 381), for example a slipped blood vessel ligature resulting in a haematoma which compresses the trachea. Clip removers should be available for such an eventuality, so that pressure on the trachea may be relieved. If the surgeon has explored the mediastinum chest complications may arise.

Rehabilitation
Maintenance therapy with DHT is continued, with out-patient supervision of dosage, until bone healing occurs. If hypocalcaemia persists, the patient may require life-long calcium supplements and vitamin D_2. Existing stones do not dissolve so renal function may be impaired permanently.

Hypoparathyroidism

Hypoparathyroidism may either arise spontaneously or follow disease or injury, but more often it results from accidental removal of the parathyroids during thyroidectomy.

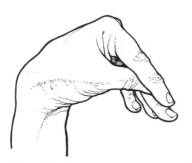

Figure 11.7
Carpal spasm

Clinical features

1. **Tetany** develops when plasma calcium falls below 7–8 mg/100 ml. There is increased excitability of nerves and muscles. Motor and sensory nerve impulses fire off spontaneously. Abnormal sensory impulses cause tingling sensations (paraesthesiae), while the motor impulses cause involuntary muscle twitches. These twitches are most obvious in the muscles of the inner forearm and hand supplied by the ulnar nerve. There is flexion of wrist and knuckles with extension of the fingers (carpal spasm, Fig. 11.7). Because of defective muscular control, the patient is more liable to fall and requires careful observation. Two signs of latent tetany are:

Chvostek's sign. Tapping the facial nerve at the jaw angle produces twitching of facial muscles.

Trosseau's sign. Applying a blood pressure cuff to the arm causes muscular spasm of forearm and hand.

2. **Laryngospasm** may be severe enough to obstruct the airway.
3. **Epileptic convulsions**, due to increased excitability of nerve cells in the brain, may be the first symptom.
4. **Psychological disturbances** may range from minor disorders to major psychoses.

Investigations

These are carried out when the patient's condition permits.
1. Fasting plasma calcium (normally 9–11 mg/100 ml).
2. Serum inorganic phosphate (normally 4–6 mg/100 ml).
3. Renal phosphate clearance (normally 6–15 ml/minute).
4. Twenty-four-hour urine collection to measure urinary calcium excretion. Nurses must explain to the patient the importance of an accurate 24-hour urine collection and of fasting before certain blood specimens are taken. It may also be necessary to collect faeces. Some investigations may make it imperative that the calcium intake is known and, if this is so, a special diet will be supplied.
5. Electrocardiograph may demonstrate variations in cardiac muscle function.

Treatment

Emergency treatment
Calcium salts such as 10 ml of 10 per cent calcium gluconate are given intravenously to raise the plasma calcium level when symptoms are severe and require urgent relief. If epileptic convulsions occur, the patient must be protected from injury.

Replacement therapy
Parathormone injections are ineffective since the patient soon produces antibodies neutralizing their action. Vitamin D_2 (calciferol) can be given daily to increase calcium absorption or, alternatively, DHT 0·5 mg–1 mg daily.

The inverse relationship between calcium and phosphorus means that phosphorus levels fall as calcium levels rise. A low phosphorus diet may be given initially, to reduce the work of the kidneys in excreting excess phosphorus. As these two minerals are found in the same foods, calcium-rich foods are restricted at first.

Aftercare

Out-patient supervision will be needed to carry out the following:
1. Periodic serum calcium estimations to monitor drug dosage.
2. Periodic observation of renal function. Overdosage of vitamin D can cause hypercalcaemia with consequent risk of renal calculi.

Serious intellectual impairment cannot be restored by treatment, hence the need for early diagnosis to prevent such complications.

THE PANCREAS
STRUCTURE AND FUNCTION

The endocrine secretions of the pancreas are produced by groups of cells called the islets of Langerhans. They contain two cell types:

1. Alpha (α) cells secreting **glucagon**. This promotes glycogen breakdown, thereby raising the blood glucose.
2. Beta (β) cells (75 per cent of the islets) secreting **insulin**. This lowers the blood glucose by:

   a. Promoting glycogen synthesis particularly in liver and muscles.
   b. Increasing cellular utilization of glucose in many tissues.
   c. Inhibiting gluconeogenesis from protein.

Both hormones are secreted in response to changes in blood glucose levels. Insulin is produced when levels are rising and glucagon when levels are falling.

PANCREATIC DISORDERS

The only condition which will be discussed results from the failure of the pancreas to secrete sufficient insulin to meet the body's requirements. This failure may be either partial or total. The disorder is called diabetes mellitus.

Diabetes mellitus

Diabetes mellitus is the commonest endocrine disorder. Prevalence in urban societies is 2 to 6 per cent, many people being unaware of their condition. The disease is commoner in prosperous societies and among certain races.

Aetiology
1. Genetic endowment is important in those contracting diabetes. In all age groups environmental factors may determine which of the genetically predisposed develop clinical diabetes.
2. Age: 80 per cent of cases occur in those over 50 years.
3. Obesity and diabetes are associated but uncertainty exists as to whether obesity causes or results from diabetes.
4. Physical stress may induce diabetes in susceptible people, mainly by increasing corticosteroid production. Corticosteroids are antagonistic to insulin.
   A few cases result from:

1. Pathological processes such as carcinoma of pancreas.
2. Certain treatments, for example with corticosteroids.
3. Increase of hormonal insulin antagonists. This may occur during pregnancy or because of overproduction of pituitary growth hormone (an insulin antagonist).

Clinical features
Diabetes affects the metabolism of proteins, fats, carbohydrates, water and electrolytes. Without the secretion of a sufficient amount of insulin, glucose cannot pass into tissue cells and instead accumulates in the circulation, with the following results:

1. The blood glucose level rises (**hyperglycaemia**).
2. The kidneys are unable to reabsorb all the glucose passing through them and glucose appears in the urine (**glycosuria**).
3. The high concentration of glucose in the filtrate exerts an increased osmotic pressure which hampers the reabsorption of water by the renal tubules, so that a much larger volume of urine than normal is formed (**polyuria**).
4. Polyuria leads to dehydration and thirst. The patient drinks large quantities (**polydipsia**).
5. Fat is utilized for energy production instead of carbohydrate, but is incompletely metabolized since for its total combustion, carbohydrate must be metabolized simultaneously. Toxic acid products of incomplete fat metabolism (**ketones**)

accumulate in blood and urine and are also excreted in breath, giving it a characteristic smell.

6. Ketoacidosis causes vomiting and drowsiness and may lead to coma and death.
7. Increased gluconeogenesis occurs, causing weakness and wasting of muscles.

Investigations

Urine tests. Glycosuria suggests diabetes.

Blood glucose tests. High blood glucose levels (over 150 mg/100 ml) indicate diabetes in anyone displaying other symptoms of the disease.

Glucose tolerance tests (GTT). Glucose 50 g is given orally to the fasting patient and blood samples are taken half hourly. Venous blood glucose levels of 130 mg/100 ml or more with failure to return to fasting levels in 2 hours are diagnostic of diabetes mellitus. Nurses must ensure that the glucose is properly dissolved and diluted to the same strength since the concentration affects absorption rate. The patient must drink all of the mixture and he should not reduce his carbohydrate intake in the days prior to GTT since the test should reflect insulin response under normal dietary conditions. Urine may be tested hourly during GTT but little extra information is gained.

In Figure 11.8, the GTT shows a comparison of blood glucose and insulin levels in normal people, mild diabetics needing only diet therapy, moderately severe diabetics needing diet and oral hypoglycaemic drugs (OHD) and severe diabetics needing diet and insulin therapy.

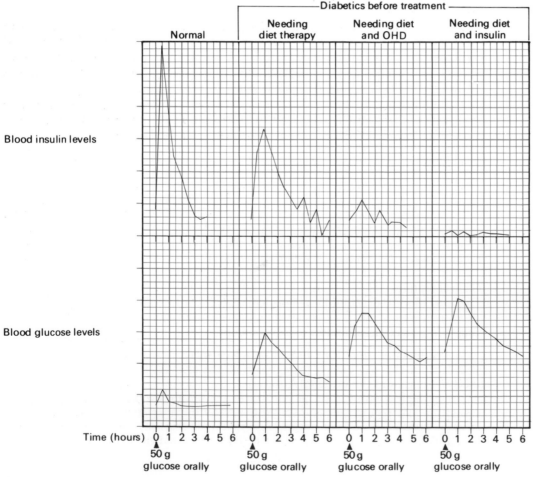

Figure 11.8
GTT showing comparison of blood glucose and blood insulin levels

Methods of treatment

For treatment purposes, diabetics form two groups:

1. Juvenile onset diabetics.
2. Mature onset diabetics.

Juvenile onset diabetes usually develops within the first 40 years. These are insulin-dependent diabetics. If insulin therapy is withheld they rapidly develop fatal ketoacidosis.

Mature onset diabetes usually appears in the middle-aged or elderly who are often obese. Most of these patients produce some insulin and are less prone to developing ketosis. However, complications associated with long-standing diabetes can occur in both types: many mature onset diabetics have histories of mild symptoms which have been overlooked, thus delaying treatment. The aim of treatment is to re-establish normal metabolism. There are three methods:

1. Diet alone.
2. Diet and an oral hypoglycaemic drug.
3. Diet and insulin.

Diet alone

Dietary control alone is suitable for most mature onset diabetics. Weight reduction is important and a diet ranging from 3400 kJ to 5000 kJ daily is prescribed according to individual needs. The carbohydrate allowance is about 40 per cent of the total. Research shows that small snacks spread over the day are more effective for weight reduction than three large meals, since there is adequate insulin response to smaller meals. Often the patient must learn new eating habits, especially if he has a 'sweet tooth'. The diet is reviewed regularly.

Oral drugs and diet.

Oral hypoglycaemic drugs are prescribed for the few mature onset diabetics who cannot be controlled by diet alone. Hypoglycaemic attacks are less likely on oral therapy than on insulin therapy, but are still possible. In times of illness, these drugs may be inadequate to control diabetes, insulin being required until diabetes is stabilized. The principal groups of drugs are:

The sulphonylureas (Table 11.3) (sulphonamide derivatives) reduce the release of glucose from the liver: the duration of action varies. Serious side-effects are rare. Chlorpropamide can cause jaundice. All can cause hypoglycaemia.

Table 11.3
The sulphonylureas

Action	Pharmaceutical name	Proprietary name	Daily dose
Short	tolbutamide	Artosin	0.5–3 g
		Rastinon	0.5–3 g
Intermediate	acetohexamide	Dimelor	500–1500 mg
	glibenclamide	Daonil	
	glymidine	Gondafon	
	tolazamide	Tolanase	100–500 mg
Long	chlorpropamide	Diabinese	100–500 mg

The biguanides (Table 11.4) lower the blood glucose level possibly by increasing glucose uptake in the tissues. Side effects are nausea, vomiting and diarrhoea.

Table 11.4
The biguanides

Pharmaceutical name	Proprietary name	Daily dose
metformin	Glucophage	0.5–3 g
	Obin	0.5–3 g
	Diguanil	0.5–3 g
phenformin	Dibotin	50–250 mg

If a patient becomes resistant to sulphonylureas alone, a biguanide may be added. Diabetics on sulphonylureas tend to gain weight, although their diabetes is well controlled. Obesity is a health risk. Another danger is that individuals may come to depend on drugs rather than diet to control diabetes.

Insulin and diet
Juvenile onset diabetics require insulin injections and diet prescribed to match their physical activities and to maintain their weight. Blood glucose and urine tests indicate whether a balance between carbohydrate intake and insulin dosage is being achieved. Weight loss, hyperglycaemia and high glycosuria indicate the need for more insulin, while hypoglycaemia demonstrates that too much insulin is being injected for the carbohydrate ingested. (A scale balance is the symbol of the British Diabetic Association; their motto is 'Balance is life'.)

Stabilizing diabetes
Injected insulin cannot eliminate the glycosuria which occurs after meals in severe diabetes. Insulin dosage is adjusted to keep blood glucose levels as near normal as possible between meals.

1. Urine testing for glycosuria in insulin dependent diabetics is performed immediately before meals since glucose levels should then be nearly normal if insulin therapy is adequate.

2. In the case of patients on oral therapy or diet, blood glucose is lowest after overnight fasting and rises during the day, peaking after meals. A urine test performed 2 hours after the largest meal reflects the highest blood glucose level of the day. Satisfactory control exists when tests are persistently negative or show only occasional glycosuria. When the patient is receiving low doses of tablets or none at all, testing urine thrice weekly suffices, provided that the diabetes remains stable.

3. Testing for ketones is important during illnesses and when over 2 per cent glycosuria exists.

Urine testing: the nurse's role
The test specimen must be urine which has been recently formed. The patient should empty his bladder, and half an hour later the test specimen should be obtained. If this is not done test results will relate to urine that has been in the bladder for some time.

Coping at home
Stabilization of diabetes is best achieved on an out-patient basis; otherwise, when the patient returns to a more energetic routine than in hospital, increased energy output will cause insulin requirements to fall. The patient may learn to adjust his insulin dosage when necessary (Fig. 11.9). Generally, he should reduce his insulin when

Figure 11.9
The need to adjust insulin dosage

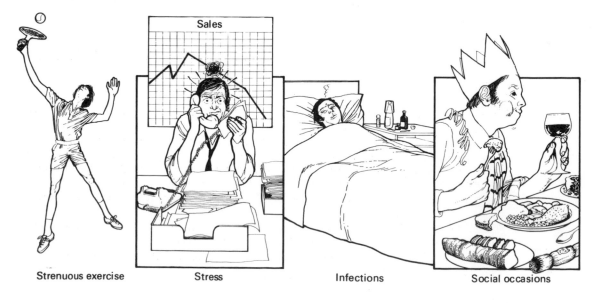

Strenuous exercise   Stress   Infections   Social occasions

hypoglycaemia occurs and increase his insulin when glycosuria occurs over a similar period, but if in doubt medical advice should be sought.

The daily dose of insulin must **never** be missed even if food intake is reduced.

Types of insulin

Insulin is prepared from cattle or pig pancreas. The various types differ in speed and duration of action.

Soluble insulin is quick-acting but short-lasting. At least two injections daily are needed when used alone. Soluble insulin alone is often prescribed until acute illness has subsided and diabetes has been stabilized. Some people remain healthier using soluble insulin, particularly if they have suffered any complications of diabetes.

Modified insulins (Table 11.5) are combined with other substances to prolong their action.

Mixing insulins

1. Incompatible insulins:

a. Soluble and lente insulins should not be mixed. The more acidic soluble insulin alters the reaction of lente, disturbing its timing.

b. Protamine zinc and soluble insulins should not be mixed in a syringe as the excess protamine combines with the soluble insulin and increases the amount of protamine zinc insulin with risk of night-time hypoglycaemia.

2. Insulins which can be mixed are:

a. Isophane and soluble insulins, Isophane, which contains just sufficient protamine to bind insulin in preparation, can be mixed with soluble insulin.

b. Lente insulins can be mixed together.

Table 11.5
Modified insulins

Action	Type	Onset time (hours)	Duration (hours)
Long	rapitard (biphasic) protamine zinc	3–6	24–36
	insulin zinc suspension (ultra lente)	6–8	30–36
Intermediate	globin zinc insulin	2–4	18–24
	insulin zinc suspension (amorphous semilente)	less than 1	12–16
	insulin zinc suspension (lente)	less than 1	24
	isophane	2–4	24–30

Injections

As insulin is a polypeptide hormone, and would be inactivated if taken orally, it must always be given by injection.

The patient learns to inject himself on the outer parts of the thighs, the upper arms and the lower abdomen (Fig. 11.10). Automatic injectors (Fig. 11.11) can be used with one hand, thereby increasing the number of potential injection sites. Repeated use of the same site may lead to fat atrophy and interfere with insulin absorption.

Antibodies are produced after prolonged injection with insulin, and in time larger doses may be required.

Highly purified or 'monocomponent' insulins such as Actrapid, Semitard and Monotard should overcome problems of insulin resistance and skin allergies. The patient should in any case know the animal source of his insulin, since hypoglycaemia may occur if this is changed.

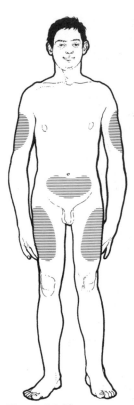

Figure 11.10
Injection sites for
insulin

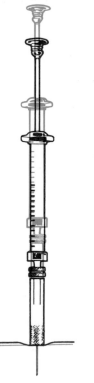

Figure 11.11
Automatic injector

Glass syringes, non-disposable needles and urine testing kits are available on prescription. Syringes, preset to inject a certain insulin dose, are available for blind diabetics. The setting should be checked frequently by a sighted person. Equipment, especially syringes and needles, should be kept out of reach of children to avoid accidents.

Cleanliness of equipment is essential to avoid infection.

Insulin concentrations

Insulin is measured in units, and strengths of insulin preparations are expressed as units per millilitre. Soluble insulin is available in the basic strength of 20 units (u)/ml, so insulin syringes are marked in units of 20 per ml (Fig. 11.12).

20 u/ml strength. If this insulin is ordered, 1 mark is equal to 1 unit. If 10 units are ordered, 10 marks or 0·5 ml are drawn in the syringe.

40 u/ml strength. Every mark denotes 2 units of insulin. If 10 units are required, 5 marks or 0·25 ml are drawn in the syringe.

80 u/ml strength. Every mark denotes 4 units of insulin. The more concentrated insulins are preferable for large doses since the latter can be injected in a smaller volume.

(In the United States and Canada, an insulin concentration of 100 units/ml is available.)

Two sizes of syringe are available on prescription in Great Britain: the 1 ml model has 20 marks, the 2 ml model has 40 marks. The syringes are made to BS1619.

Diets and nutrition

Foods labelled 'diabetic' cannot be taken freely. Their kilojoule value and carbohydrate content must be considered.

Diets should meet bodily needs for energy, repair and growth. A manual worker will require a larger diet and more insulin than a sedentary worker. For insulin-dependent diabetics, dietary fat and protein may be unrestricted but are sometimes specified to ensure adequate intake; also glucose taken alone raises blood glucose to higher levels than when taken with protein and fat.

Dietary carbohydrate must be measured accurately to balance the dose of insulin taken.

Nurses, and diabetic patients, should be able to adjust diets to avoid monotony and provide maximum freedom; this adjustment requires a knowledge of carbohydrate exchanges.

Foods with a carbohydrate content which cannot be estimated should be avoided, for instance thickened soups and sauces. Where no choice of menu is likely to be available, say, in a friend's home, prior consultation is advisable.

Energy sources not derived from protein, fat or carbohydrate are:

1. **Alcohol.** Dry wines and spirits have a high kilojoule count because of their alcohol content and are restricted for those on reducing diets.

2. **Sorbitol** contains no carbohydrate but has a high kilojoule content.

Diabetes and pregnancy

There is no reason why a diabetic should avoid pregnancy if she receives adequate medical care. Genetic counselling is advisable. Pregnancy carries certain risks — in particular there is a greater risk of stillbirth or neonatal death. Induction of labour or Caesarian section is usually necessary. The chances that a diabetic mother will have a diabetic child are increased.

Elective surgery

The patient is admitted about 3 days preoperatively to assess his diabetes. Intravenous glucose may be given if fasting blood glucose levels indicate it is needed. Postoperatively, insulin is given according to the degree of glycosuria and blood glucose concentration.

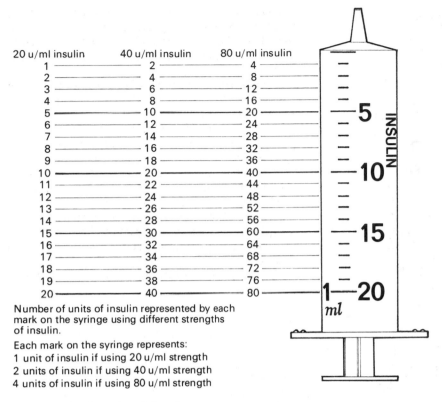

20 u/ml insulin	40 u/ml insulin	80 u/ml insulin
1	2	4
2	4	8
3	6	12
4	8	16
5	10	20
6	12	24
7	14	28
8	16	32
9	18	36
10	20	40
11	22	44
12	24	48
13	26	52
14	28	56
15	30	60
16	32	64
17	34	68
18	36	72
19	38	76
20	40	80

Number of units of insulin represented by each
mark on the syringe using different strengths
of insulin.

Each mark on the syringe represents:
1 unit of insulin if using 20 u/ml strength
2 units of insulin if using 40 u/ml strength
4 units of insulin if using 80 u/ml strength

Figure 11.12
Calculation of insulin dosage

Diabetic ketoacidosis

Other terms used include diabetic coma and severe hyperglycaemia.

When there is insufficient insulin for glucose metabolism, the sequence of events shown in Table 11.6 occurs.

The severity of the crisis is proportional to the acidosis, not to the blood glucose level.

Possible causes
1. Neglect of treatment through ignorance or carelessness.
2. Illness or stress which increases insulin requirements.

Table 11.6
Ketoacidosis

Biochemical changes	Symptoms and signs
1. Glucose accumulates in the blood in large quantities (hyperglycaemia)	Thirst
2. Hyperglycaemia causes osmotic diuresis with excess loss of water and electrolytes in urine	Polyuria Low BP Raised pulse Dehydration Dry tongue Inelastic skin
3. Body cells use fat as an alternative fuel. Fat is incompletely metabolized and ketones appear in blood and urine (ketosis). Ketones affect the brain—causing drowsiness and eventual coma—and the respiratory centre—stimulating rapid, deep breathing	Anorexia Vomiting Drowsiness Loss of consciousness Deep respirations Acetone smell on breath

Treatment

Analysis of blood samples enables blood glucose, electrolytes and carbon dioxide combining power (an indication of the degree of metabolic acidosis) to be measured.

1. Precipitating causes are treated when known (for example antibiotics are given for infections).

2. Dehydration is corrected by intravenous infusion (for example, normal saline followed by 5 per cent dextrose to prevent further breakdown of fat and protein).

3. Carbohydrate metabolism is re-established by giving soluble insulin intravenously or intramuscularly. The subcutaneous route is ineffective due to circulatory collapse. Insulin doses are calculated 3 to 4 hourly according to blood glucose level. Insulin can also be given by continuous intravenous infusion when much smaller doses are required, for example, six units per hour.

4. Intravenous sodium bicarbonate or lactate is occasionally given to correct acidosis.

5. After insulin therapy and correction of acidosis, potassium begins to enter the cells, depleting blood potassium levels. This may cause cardiac arrhythmias, therefore potassium is given intravenously.

Nursing care involves all the techniques employed in care of the unconscious patient (Ch.3). A nasogastric tube may be inserted to minimize risk of inhaling vomitus. When conscious, the patient is allowed oral fluids containing carbohydrate. Later, he progresses to a solid diet.

Aids to nursing observations

1. An oscilloscope to detect cardiac arrhythmias.
2. A self-retaining catheter to facilitate urinalysis.

Records

It is an important nursing responsibility to maintain accurate records. Special charts (Fig. 11.13) on which all information is correlated should be provided; entries should always be made promptly and clearly.

Hypoglycaemia

A diabetic learns to recognize symptoms of hypoglycaemia. Onset is rapid when the blood glucose level falls below about 50 mg/100 ml.

Clinical features

Clinical features result from abnormal brain function due to shortage of its vital 'fuel' — glucose. Unlike other body tissues, the brain can use only glucose as its energy source. Symptoms vary and include rapid heart rate, sweating, hunger, unsteadiness of gait, truculent behaviour and alterations in consciousness. If hypoglycaemia develops more slowly there is usually lethargy, reduction of spontaneous activity, conversation and movement, and behaviour similar to that produced by alcohol intoxication. This type of hypoglycaemia occurs more commonly in patients treated with 'long-acting' insulins or oral hypoglycaemic agents.

Treatment

Treatment must be prompt. Blood glucose levels fall below those necessary to maintain metabolism of brain cells and prolonged attacks may produce irreversible cerebral changes. The underlying cause of hypoglycaemia can be determined later. The hypoglycaemic diabetic should have carbohydrate, such as glucose sweets or a glass of milk. If he loses consciousness, intravenous glucose or intramuscular glucagon is injected. (Glucagon raises the blood glucose level by increasing glucose release from the liver. By giving a child glucagon, parents are often able to restore consciousness sufficiently to give glucose orally.)

The diabetic should always carry a card (Fig 11.14) indicating his condition and insulin regime to anyone who may find him in a distressed condition. An unconscious diabetic should be treated as if he were hypoglycaemic unless proved otherwise. Incorrect treatment of hypoglycaemia with insulin can be fatal, whereas permanent damage is unlikely to result from giving glucose to a patient in a hyperglycaemic coma.

DIABETES MELLITUS

UNIT No.
NAME

Diabetic Ketosis Chart

TIME	INTAKE				OUTPUT		P.	R.	B.P.	URINE		Blood Sugar mg%	Sol. Insulin Units	BLOOD CHEMISTRY				COMMENTS
	ORAL		INTRAVENOUS		Urine ml.	Stomach ml.				S.	A.			Na	K	Cl	HCO₃	
	Nature	Volume ml.	Nature	Volume ml.														

Figure 11.13
Diabetic ketosis chart

When a diabetic is about to undertake unusually strenuous exercise, he should reduce his insulin dose or take an extra 10 g carbohydrate to prevent hypoglycaemia.

Continuing care

Diabetes mellitus may be controlled, but not cured. People living with this disorder may be confronted with difficulties and complications.

Emotional problems
It is difficult to accept cheerfully the need for daily insulin injections and to struggle with a rigid diet. Knowledge will help the diabetic achieve greater flexibility and confidence in his diet and other features of his life-style, hence the importance of education about all aspects of his condition. This means team work, involving doctors, nurses, dieticians, the patient and his family. The British Diabetic Association (BDA) provides information on self-help and includes advice about diets, the life of a diabetic, holidays and car insurance. The organization finances research into diabetes and helps to dispel prejudice against diabetics, for instance among employers.

Most occupations are open to diabetics. Those where there may be injury to themselves or others if hypoglycaemia occurs, such as driving public vehicles or working on scaffolding, are unsuitable.

Adolescents may resent the 'discipline' of diabetes and fluctuating control may result. The adolescent may not always be at fault since nervousness, fear and infection can cause hyperglycaemia.

A child's emotions and activities fluctuate more than an adult's. This may cause instability. Children should not constantly be made to feel different from their peers. Provided they are taught the necessity of dietary control, they should be allowed to choose from the full range of foods for which a reliable carbohydrate value is available.

I am a diabetic

If I am found ill or fainting please

read the instructions overleaf . . . .

I am a diabetic

If I am found ill or fainting please give me two tablespoonfuls of sugar in water. If this does not revive me please call a doctor or an ambulance immediately.

Name _____

Address _____

_____ Telephone No. _____

Name of Doctor or Hospital _____

Address _____

_____ Telephone No. _____

My usual dose of insulin is _____ units of _____

brand _____ *(type of insulin)* _____

given at _____
          (time(s) of day)

Figure 11.14
Diabetic card

Early complications
Blurred vision may result from instability of blood glucose levels. This condition is transient.

Tingling of feet due to **neuropathy** (nerve damage) also resolves once diabetes is stabilized.

Infections may occur since hyperglycaemia and glycosuria provide an ideal growth medium for bacteria. Common infections are vulvovaginitis, urinary infections, pyelonephritis, infections in skin creases of the obese person and conjunctivitis.

Long-term complications
These occur more often but not exclusively in poorly controlled diabetics.

Visual defects
Three visual defects resulting from diabetes are cataract, retinal disease and vitreous haemorrhage (Ch. 12).

Neuritis
This usually causes paraesthesia (pins and needles) of extremities and pain. Ankle and knee reflexes may disappear. Diarrhoea, postural hypotension and impotence may occur due to autonomic neuropathy.

Cardiovascular disorders
Poor circulation, especially in the elderly, means that injury or infection to blood-starved limbs can quickly lead to gangrene. Diabetics should take special care of their feet, which need to be washed, dried, and inspected daily for any sign of damage. Those with poor circulation should not cut their toe-nails themselves but should attend a chiropodist. Shoes and stockings should allow toe movement. New shoes need to be broken in gradually. The diabetic should be discouraged from walking barefoot, especially on wooden floors or other potentially rough surfaces.

The risk of coronary artery and cerebral vascular disease is increased in diabetics.

Renal changes
Nephrosis (p. 288) may occur in diabetics of long standing and result in death from renal failure.

THE ADRENAL GLANDS

These two glands are located on top of the kidneys.

STRUCTURE AND FUNCTION

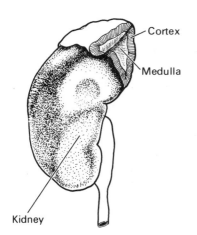

Figure 11.15
Section of adrenal gland

Each consists of two separate functional parts, the cortex and the medulla (Fig. 11.15).
The adrenal cortex. Three groups of hormones are secreted:

1. Glucocorticoids. Of these, the most important is cortisol (hydro-cortisone). This is secreted in response to the adrenocorticotrophic hormone (ACTH) from the anterior pituitary. In turn, ACTH secretion is brought about by a releasing factor secreted by the hypothalamus and controlled by a feed-back mechanism based on blood levels of cortisol. Cortisol stimulates gluconeogenesis (the formation of glucose) from protein. It antagonizes the action of insulin. It is important for the excretion of water by the kidneys, for the manufacture of red blood cells, to help maintain blood pressure and for the body's ability to respond to stress. Excess cortisol inhibits the inflammatory reaction, interferes with protein synthesis causing muscle and bone weakness and leads to hyperglycaemia.

2. Mineralocorticoids. Aldosterone, the most important of these, is concerned with maintaining normal levels of sodium in the body. A fall in body sodium leads to increased secretion of aldosterone. The effect of this is to increase the kidney's reabsorption of sodium from the urine, thus conserving it.

3. Androgens. These are sex hormones produced in both sexes which are concerned with muscular development and the growth of pubic and axillary hair.

The adrenal medulla. Functionally separate from the cortex, medullary activity has much in common with sympathetic nervous activity. The hormones secreted are noradrenaline and adrenaline which have the effect of preparing the body for physical exertion. Thus, when the need arises, heart rate increases, blood pressure rises, blood is diverted to essential organs (heart and muscle), energy is made available by converting liver and muscle glycogen to glucose, the bronchial smooth muscle is relaxed to allow greater air entry and the metabolic rate is increased.

DISORDERS OF THE ADRENAL GLANDS

These may result from abnormalities of either the cortex or the medulla.

Underactivity of the adrenal cortex

Addison's disease is a chronic condition of underactivity. It may be the result of tuberculous destruction of the gland or of atrophy.

Clinical features
These derive from the failure to secrete the necessary hormones. Serious loss of sodium occurs in the urine. Low blood pressure is characteristic, and patients may faint on

standing up. There is also a tendency to develop hypoglycaemia and a raised blood urea. Skin pigmentation will develop. Tiredness, anorexia and nausea are common. Weight loss and menstrual disturbances may occur. Response to stress is impaired and patients may succumb to infections, injury or exposure to cold.

Treatment and nursing care

Management of Addison's disease is mainly the replacement of the missing hormone. Initially cortisol 20 mg is given twice daily. It may also be necessary to give fludrocortisone to maintain fluid and electrolyte balance. Monthly follow-up sessions are necessary to monitor and adjust the dosage if necessary. Patients must be instructed on what to do if a minor illness occurs, for example a heavy cold or influenza. In such circumstances, the daily dose of cortisol should be doubled by the patient. Each patient should have a supply of intramuscular hydrocortisone to be given by his doctor in an emergency. A card should be carried at all times, indicating that the bearer is taking corticosteroid therapy.

Acute adrenal failure

This crisis calls for urgent and intensive treatment. A severe degree of shock develops with a dramatic fall in blood pressure. Oliguria or anuria may result. Vomiting may occur with weakness, apathy and confusion. Unless treated quickly and adequately, coma and death will follow. Measures to combat the fall in blood pressure should be taken. The patient is nursed flat, with the foot of the bed elevated. Intravenous fluids are given to maintain water and sodium balance; up to a litre of normal saline may be given quickly. It may also be necessary to give intravenous glucose. Cortisol is administered intravenously for up to 48 hours. In most cases remarkable improvement will occur within 24 hours, and once the patient's progress is certain and gastrointestinal disturbance has settled, cortisol may be given orally.

During the initial period the patient remains very ill and much depends on the accurate observation and recording of vital signs. Particularly important are blood pressure readings, observations of level of consciousness and measurement of fluid intake, urinary output and amount of vomitus. In addition, the patient's comfort depends on thoughtful nursing care. Such episodes are very frightening for patients, so a quiet, reassuring and confident approach by the nurse is essential. Nursing should be carried out in a quiet atmosphere with the minimum of stimulation. Patients will benefit from the reduction of emotional and physical disturbance. Once the crisis is over, management continues as described for Addison's disease.

Overactivity of the adrenal cortex

A variety of syndromes may result from overproduction of the various hormones of the cortex. Among these is Cushing's syndrome, the result of excess quantities of circulating cortisol.

Cushing's syndrome

This complex disorder is usually the result of bilateral adrenal hyperplasia, which may be caused by a tumour of the adrenals or by a tumour of the pituitary secreting excess ACTH (p. 374). The syndrome is uncommon but merits some discussion because its symptoms may easily be produced by the therapeutic use of corticosteroids, a not uncommon means of treating a variety of disorders.

Clinical features

Clinical features of Cushing's syndrome include muscle wasting and symptoms of diabetes mellitus (glycosuria, polyuria and thirst). Obesity of the trunk is marked, the contrast with the thin legs and arms giving a characteristic appearance (Fig. 11.16). Obesity is contributed to by sodium and water retention, which also leads to hypertension. Patients develop a moon-shaped face, women grow facial hair and may cease menstruating. In men, impotence may develop. The skin bruises easily and shows striae (purple markings). Osteoporosis leads to fractures and the collapse of vertebrae.

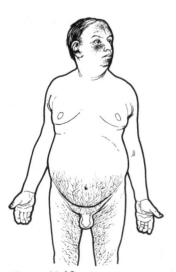

Figure 11.16
Cushing's syndrome

Methods of treatment

The approach clearly depends on the cause. If the syndrome was induced by corticosteroid therapy, the dosage is adjusted. Pituitary tumours may be removed or irradiated (p. 375). Adrenal hyperplasia may be treated by total adrenalectomy (rendering life-long replacement therapy a necessity). Total adrenalectomy can be a serious operation, since it removes the patient's ability to respond to stress. This effect is minimized by administering cortisol intramuscularly for a day or two before operation, and continuing for a period after surgery.

Preparation for surgery

As in any form of surgery, it is necessary to explain to the patients the full details of his treatment before operation, the aim being to allay high levels of anxiety.

Postoperative therapy

Following operation, an intravenous infusion is necessary to prevent electrolyte imbalance. Sodium and potassium levels in the plasma will be monitored in order to decide on the appropriate intravenous regime. Once the condition has stabilized, cortisol may be administered orally, together with fludrocortisone to regulate sodium and water balance.

Postoperative nursing care

The patient is nursed lying flat for a period to prevent hypotension and circulatory failure. Blood pressure recordings are necessary at least every 15 minutes, until it is certain that his condition is stable. Observation of other vital signs, skin colour and urinary output are essential, as well as of the wound and any drainage. Coughing and deep breathing are painful because of the wound, so a great deal of encouragement, together with chest physiotherapy, is necessary. Note should be taken of any chest pain or dyspnoea. When the patient is ready for mobilization, a frequent check of his blood pressure must be made once he gets up. If hypotension occurs he should be returned to bed and the doctor notified. The nurse must also note any signs of hypoglycaemia (p. 392), which may necessitate intravenous glucose. **Adrenal crisis**, the most serious complication of this form of surgery, is most likely to occur between 9 and 12 hours after operation. Symptoms of this complication are nausea, weakness, abdominal pains and signs of shock. The administration of a vasoconstrictor drug such as metaraminol will be necessary, and patients should be managed as described for acute adrenal failure (p. 396).

Overactivity of the adrenal medulla

This is usually caused by the presence of phaeochromocytoma, a rare tumour of the medulla which secretes large quantities of the medullary hormones.

Clinical features

Effects are hypertension, which may be sustained or intermittent, features of increased metabolism or hyperglycaemia and glycosuria. Serious consequences such as heart failure and cerebrovascular accident may result from the hypertension.

Treatment

As most tumours are benign, removal usually results in cure. Surgery carries with it a serious risk of severe hypotension once the tumour has been removed.

Surgical management

Before surgery, drugs which counteract the effect of adrenaline are given. Included in these is propanolol which blocks the effect of adrenaline on the heart. During surgery, bouts of hypertension are controlled by intravenous phentolamine, while after removal of the tumour, hypotension is controlled by metaraminol. This is continued into the postoperative period. Careful observation of blood pressure is crucial after surgery.

SUMMARY AND IMPORTANT NURSING CONSIDERATIONS IN ENDOCRINOLOGY

Treatment of any endocrine disorder consists of the following:

1. Decreasing hormonal output of hyperactive glands by, for example, surgery or radiotherapy. If the pituitary is stimulating the secretions of an overactive gland it may be destroyed surgically or by other means.

2. Supplementing hormones of underactive glands or stimulating the gland to produce the hormone by, for example, giving pituitary trophic hormones.

If any endocrine glands are completely removed or destroyed, essential hormones must be supplied for life.

It must be remembered that all patients are different, and contributing to these differences are the endocrine glands. Malfunction of these glands produces changes in behaviour or appearance, the basis of which the nurse should understand. Features of the disease are often very obvious and may be a source of embarrassment to the individual, one example being exophthalmos in thyrotoxicosis. Endocrine disorders can profoundly affect a person's life and the lives of those around him, as in the early senescence induced by hypopituitarism.

Education of the patient and of others involved is a vital part of treatment of endocrine disorders. The greater the understanding of the situation by all concerned, the more assured the patient will be of his ability to cope with his disorder and the more flexible can be his way of life. The patient must know that his treatment does not usually provide for excessive hormonal demands resulting from physical and emotional stress. He should try to avoid such situations and should know how to cope of they arise inadvertently.

Probably the most significant part of the nurse's role is her observation of the patient for complications resulting from his disease, his surgery or hormone replacement therapy. Of special importance are appearance, sweating, pulse rate, blood pressure, respirations, urinary output and symptoms such as headache, vomiting and pain. Prompt recognition of any abnormality can be life-saving. It should be remembered that not only are individual readings of pulse rate and blood pressure important, but also the upward or downward trend observed over a period.

The continuing scientific advances in endocrinology and the plethora of tests and equipment that results should never be allowed to lessen the nurse's sensitivity to her patient. Through all the drama of caring for such seriously ill patients, it must never be forgotten that the patient's basic needs must be attended to — his skin, diet and comfort. He needs reassurance and information about his condition, as do his relatives.

SUGGESTED ASSIGNMENTS

1. Patients having long-term hormonal replacement therapy may, from time to time, experience problems. Explain how in the case of (a) thyroid hormone replacement and (b) cortisone replacement these problems can be detected early.

How should patients be helped to recognize the early symptoms?

2. A diabetic must be knowledgeable about his condition if he is to lead a normal and active life. Investigate the education of diabetics in your hospital, in particular:

a. Which personnel are involved?

b. What is taught to diabetics?

c. How are allowances made for patients of differing abilities to understand what is being taught?

3. What associations for diabetics are there in your locality? As an exercise, find out how such an organization endeavours to meet the special needs of diabetics.

4. Explain how thyrotoxicosis might come to be confused with a particular psychiatric illness.

When a patient is being treated for thyrotoxicosis in a medical ward, some of the clinical features of the illness are liable to affect fellow patients and staff. What do you think the effects might be, and how as a nurse can you seek to minimise them?

FURTHER READING

Borthwick L. J. Stowers J. M. 1979 Oral hypoglycaemic agents. The Practitioner (March): 358–366

British Diabetic Association 1972 The diabetics handbook. The British Diabetic Association, London

Edmondson E 1972 Nursing the diabetic patient. Butterworth, London

Lewis J G 1973 The endocrine system. Penguin Library of Nursing Series. Churchill Livingstone, Edinburgh

Montgomery D A D 1979 The insulins. The Practitioner (March): 349–356.

Oakley W G, Pyke D A, Taylor K W 1978 Diabetes and its management, 3rd edn. Blackwell Scientific, Oxford

Sheldon J. 1979 Diabetic coma. The Practitioner (March): 333–340

Small J C, Clarke-Williams M 1972 Endocrinology. Heinemann, London

Ventura E 1978 Footcare for diabetics. American Journal of Nursing (May): 884–888

Wellcome Foundation 1972 Living with diabetes. Wellcome Foundation, London

12.   *The Eye*

The study of the eye and its disorders is called ophthalmology, a fascinating and intricate specialty. This chapter is not, however, written for those intending to specialize in ophthalmic nursing but for students who, as part of their basic training, may spend a month or two working in an eye hospital or ophthalmic clinic of an out-patient department. It may help the student with a patient admitted to a general or mental hospital who, by chance, happens also to have an eye condition.

The aim is, therefore, to provide an introduction to some common eye disorders and to the principles which underlie their treatment and nursing care.

ANATOMY AND PHYSIOLOGY

Figures 12.1 to 12.3 show the structure of the eyeball and the associated parts of the eye.

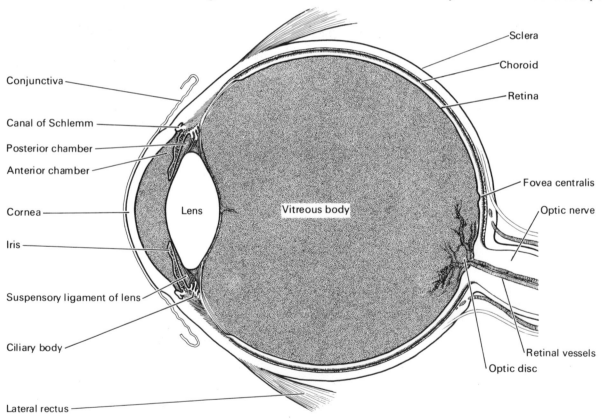

Figure 12.1
Section through eyeball

The eyeball

The eyeball is an almost spherical structure which has three layers:

1. The outermost coat consisting of the transparent **cornea** and the tough, strong, opaque **sclera**. It protects the delicate structures within the eye.

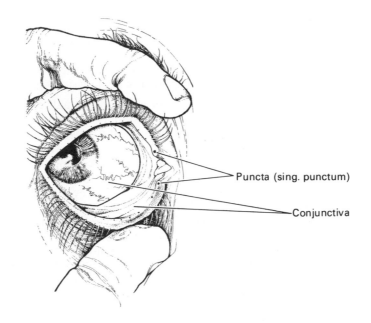

Figure 12.2
Eyelids and conjunctiva

Puncta (sing. punctum)

Conjunctiva

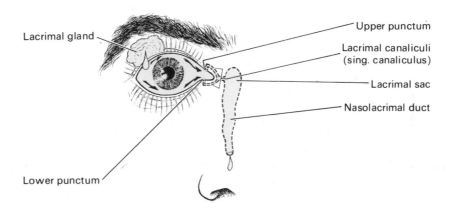

Lacrimal gland

Upper punctum

Lacrimal canaliculi
(sing. canaliculus)

Lacrimal sac

Nasolacrimal duct

Lower punctum

Figure 12.3
Lacrimal apparatus

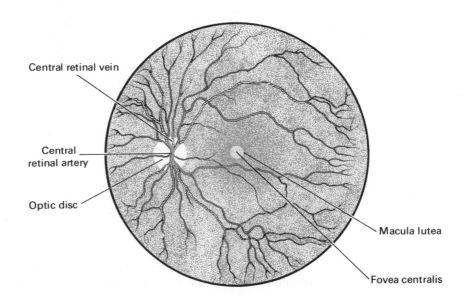

Central retinal vein

Central
retinal artery

Optic disc

Macula lutea

Fovea centralis

Figure 12.4
Optic disc, macula and retinal
vessels (ophthalmoscope view)

2. The middle layer consisting of the vascular, pigmented **choroid** which is continued forwards as the **ciliary body** and the **iris**. Together these structures form the uveal tract.

3. The innermost, nervous layer, the **retina**, containing the light-sensitive cells, the rods and cones. In the centre of the retina is the **macula lutea** (yellow spot), within which lies the **fovea centralis**, an area of acute vision where cones are very numerous.

The entry point of the optic nerve and retinal vessels, the **optic disc** (Fig. 12.4), lies to the side of the macula lutea. The retina is the only place in the body where blood vessels can readily be seen and can show abnormal changes in generalized diseases such as hypertension, some disorders of the nervous system and, of course, in diseases of the eye itself. In each **optic nerve** two sets of fibres supply the visual fields on opposite sides of the body; for example, the left temporal and right nasal fibres combine to form the right half of the right visual field (Fig. 12.5). The diagram also shows how pressure on the **chiasma**, for example from a tumour of the pituitary gland, can cause loss of half the field of vision from each eye (bitemporal hemianopia).

Within the eyeball the lens divides the **anterior chamber** containing aqueous fluid from the **vitreous body** which lies behind.

Aqueous humour is secreted by the ciliary body; it circulates around the anterior chamber and is drained away via the **Canal of Schlemm**.

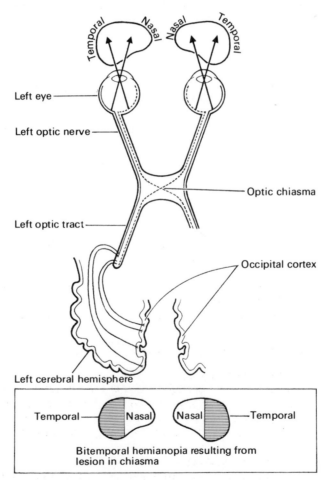

Figure 12.5
Visual pathways and visual fields

Associated structures

The accessory parts of the eye are the **eyelids, lacrimal apparatus** for production and drainage of tears and the **conjunctiva**, a fine mucous membrane which lines the lids and continues over the eye as the corneal epithelium. All of these structures function to protect the eye and to facilitate vision.

Each eye is rotated within the orbit by means of the six extrinsic muscles which are inserted into the sclera.

Normal vision

The design of the eyeball allows light reflected from objects within the range of vision to fall on to the retina. Light from distant objects travels in straight lines so that, in order to fall exactly on to the retina, these rays of light must be refracted (bent). Refraction occurs as light rays pass from one medium to another, for example from air to water or vice versa. Light entering the eye is refracted in the same way, starting with the anterior surface of the cornea.

The parts of the eye through which light must pass before reaching the retina are called the **refractive media**. They are: the cornea, the aqueous, the lens and the vitreous body.

The cornea plays the greatest part in refraction; the lens, however, has an important role because by accommodation, that is, alteration in its shape, the degree of the refraction can be varied.

In a normal eye both near and distant objects can be focused (Fig. 12.6A and B). This normal refractive power is termed **emmetropia**. To be able to see detail of an object clearly, an inverted image must be brought into exact focus on to the macula lutea. The cones in and around this area are sensitive to daylight and enable us to see colour and detail of objects (central vision). The rods situated nearer the periphery of the retina enable us to be aware of our surroundings (peripheral vision) in the daytime and to permit some night time vision.

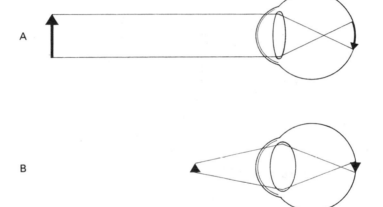

Figure 12.6
A. Normal eye focusing a distant object (over 20 feet away)
B. Normal eye focusing a near object (note alteration in shape of lens)

The formation of a nerve impulse for transmission to the brain is the result of a biochemical process in the retina. Once formed the impulse is conveyed via the optic pathways (Fig. 12.5) to the visual area of the occipital cortex for interpretation as sight.

Vision with errors of refraction

Myopia (short sight)
The length of the eyeball is greater than normal, therefore light rays are brought to a focus at a point which falls short of the retina. The person can see by holding objects close to the eyes, but objects at a distance appear blurred. Correction is achieved with a concave lens which focuses the image on to the retina (Fig. 12.7).

Hypermetropia (long sight)
The length of the eyeball is shorter than normal, therefore light rays are brought to a focus at a point behind the retina. Objects are seen clearly at a distance but appear

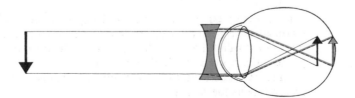

Figure 12.7
Myopia

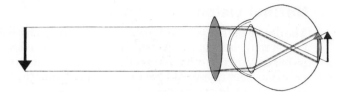

Figure 12.8
Hypermetropia

blurred close to the eye. Correction is by a convex lens which brings the image forward on to the retina (Fig. 12.8).

Astigmatism
In this condition the eye is optically oval, so that horizontal and vertical planes of light are brought to a focus at different points. Correction is with a cylindrical lens.

Presbyopia (old sight)
This occurs in normal aging and should not be confused with failing vision. From approximately 45 years of age onwards the lens gradually loses its elasticity so that its ability to alter its shape to accommodate for near and distant objects gradually diminishes. The person sees more clearly at a distance where only passive accommodation is required; so objects are held further away from the eye in order to see detail. A common example is an older person who needs to have a newspaper at arm's length in order to be able to read the small print (Fig. 12.9). Correction is achieved by means of a convex lens.

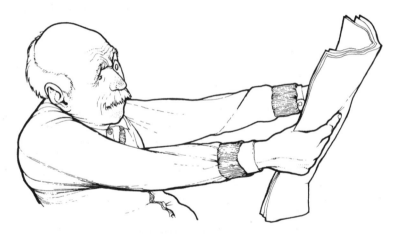

Figure 12.9
Presbyopia

Effect of drugs on the eye

There are a number of drugs which, apart from their general effects, also cause changes in the eye, notably those which stimulate the parasympathetic nervous system. Patients heavily sedated with opiates have constricted pupils; conversely, persons intoxicated with alcohol will have pupils which are widely dilated. Some antidepressants and powerful analgesics such as pethidine produce unwanted side-effects on the eye which can be a nuisance to the patient.

There are two very important groups of drugs used in the treatment of eye conditions:

Mydriatics
These drugs dilate the pupil (Fig. 12.10A). They work by paralysing the muscle which constricts the pupil thus leaving the dilator muscle unopposed. Some mydriatics also paralyse the ciliary muscle which controls the shape of the lens so that the individual cannot focus for near vision.

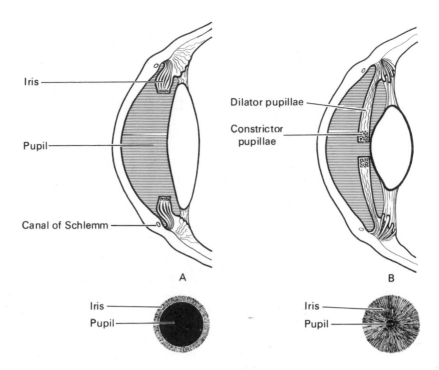

Figure 12.10
A. Effect of mydriatics B. Effect of miotics

Examples of mydriatics are:

1. **Atropine sulphate** $\frac{1}{2}$–2 per cent. It takes about 30 minutes to dilate the pupil fully and its effects, which cannot be counteracted, last for 10 days. It is used to limit the formation of adhesions between the iris and the structures which lie behind in, for example, inflammatory conditions involving the iris or following intraocular operations such as cataract extraction. Occasionally people are hypersensitive to atropine. The eye becomes red and irritable and an allergic-type rash develops on the lids and conjunctiva.

2. **Mydrilate** (cyclopentolate hydrochloride) 1 per cent is a recent preparation and is used in many departments for examination purposes. This drug has maximum effect in 30–60 minutes, and recovery occurs in 24 hours.

3. **Phenylephrine hydrochloride** 10 per cent. This drug takes about 20 minutes to dilate the pupil and lasts for several hours. Mydrilate and Phenylephrine may be used in combination to dilate the pupils for examination purposes. Their action can be counteracted by Pilocarpine 1 or 2 per cent.

Miotics

These constrict the pupil. They have a stimulating effect on the constrictor and ciliary muscles so that in addition to constriction of the pupil the lens accommodates for near vision (Fig. 12.10B). Miotics increase the drainage of aqueous humour by some unknown mechanism and because of this they are of particular use in the treatment of glaucoma (p. 411). Examples of miotic drugs are eserine $\frac{1}{4}$–$\frac{1}{2}$ per cent and pilocarpine 1–4 per cent.

AETIOLOGY OF DISORDER

As most of the tissues within the orbit are similar to those found elsewhere in the body — skin, hair, vessels, nerves, muscles and mucous membrane — it follows that the eye and its associated structures can be affected by many of the same disorders that affect other organs.

The highly specialized tissues of the eye, the cornea, the lens and the complex that makes up the iris, the ciliary body and the choroid are unique in their structure and behaviour. The cornea contains no blood vessels and is dependent upon tears and aqueous to keep it healthy, while the lens depends solely on aqueous for its nourishment. The presence of toxins in aqueous can give rise to haziness of the cornea or opacities in the lens, which will in turn affect vision. Trauma will also cause opacities. The iris, ciliary body and choroid are contiguous vascular structures, the former having no power of regeneration if partially removed, as in iridectomy. The ciliary body is involved in the phenomenon of *sympathetic ophthalmitis*.

FEATURES OF DISORDER

1. **Diminution of visual acuity.** Loss of sight can be so gradual that the patient does not notice it until the disease is well advanced; this is typical of chronic glaucoma. There can, of course, be sudden and complete loss of vision.

2. **Pain** may arise within the eye or be associated with pain of the face as in disease of the trigeminal nerve.

3. **Lacrimation** (formation of tears) may be excessive and cause watering of the eye. If the tear duct is blocked and lacrimal secretion is unable to pass down and into the nose in the usual way, it will overflow down the cheek. Alternatively if there are too few tears the eye becomes dry and the cornea is endangered.

4. **Double vision**, in which the patient does literally see 'two of everything'.

5. **Cosmetic defects**, for example ptosis (drooping) of the lid.

EXAMINATION AND INVESTIGATIONS

Enquiry is made into the patient's general health and detailed examination of other parts of the body is carried out as required. The ophthalmologist will make a systematic examination of the eye from the eyelashes to the optic disc. Investigations may include the following:

Tests of visual acuity

The ability of the eye to perceive the shape of objects is assessed for both near and distance vision.

Near vision
Ordinary printer's types are used in testing near vision.

Distance vision
Special test-types are used, with the patient placed at a standard distance for testing distance vision.

In the Snellen test-type letters are arranged in rows of diminishing size (Fig. 12.11A). The normal eye would see the top letter at 60 metres and subsequent lines at decreasing distance. For convenience the patient stands 6 metres away from the vision board and his visual acuity is measured according to the number of lines of letters he can read accurately. This is then expressed as a fraction, the upper 6 being the test distance in metres. Thus $\frac{6}{6}$ is normal vision, but if it is $\frac{6}{36}$ then he can only see at 6 metres what he should be able to see at 36 metres. Ability to see to top letters only is $\frac{6}{60}$. If the patient is unable to see the top letters even when moved closer to the board, his ability to count the examiner's fingers or see hand movements is tested and, failing this, his perception of light. The person is regarded as totally blind if he is unable to perceive light.

The vision of each eye is tested separately with and without glasses, if worn. The eye which is not being tested is occluded.

For children or non-English speaking adults the 'E' Test (Fig. 12.11B) can be used. The person is given a wooden E which he moves to correspond with the position of the E on the test-type. For the very young child a test involving recognition of simple objects on the test-type (Fig. 12.11C) is more suitable.

Ophthalmoscopy

An ophthalmoscope (Fig. 12.12) is an instrument which permits a view of the fundus of the eye. The examination can be carried out on any patient without prior preparation, but it is preferable for the pupils to be dilated and a darkened room is ideal. The nurse should always screen the patient from direct sunlight which makes examination impossible.

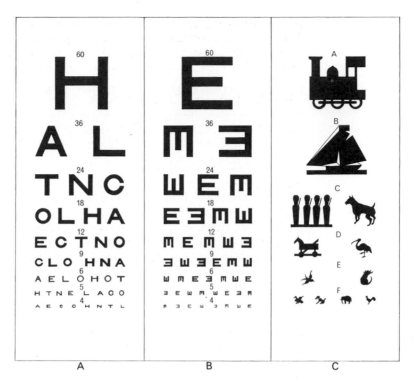

Figure 12.11
A. Test type—Snellen B. Test type—'E' test C. Test type—recognition of objects

The very specialized technique of indirect ophthalmoscopy is particularly useful in retinal detachment surgery.

Slit lamp examination

The aim is to allow examination of the structure of the eye magnified by means of a narrow beam of light. The patient is seated with the head fixed in a suitable rest with a forehead bar and adjustable chin rest (Fig. 12.13). The examiner is seated opposite the

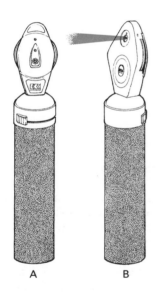

Figure 12.12
A direct ophthalmoscope
A. Back view (held to examiner's eye) B. Side view

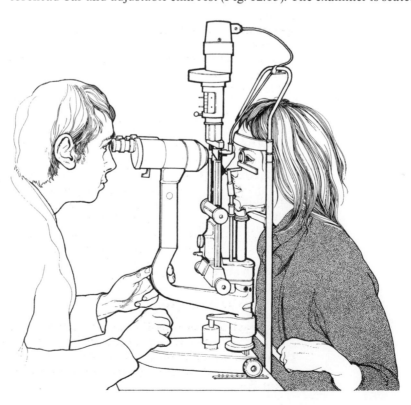

Figure 12.13
A slit lamp

patient, looking through a binocular microscope. Light from the slit lamp is condensed into a narrow sharp band which will show up the parts of the eye to be examined, for example the cornea, anterior chamber, lens, iris detail and anterior vitreous.

Measurement of intraocular pressure

In health the pressure within the eye is maintained by the flow of aqueous into and out of the anterior chamber at approximately 15 to 20 millimetres of mercury. A rough estimation can be made by palpation. Accurate measurement is achieved by a tonometer attached to the slit lamp and is important in the diagnosis of glaucoma.

Estimation of the visual fields

This is done either by using a special apparatus called a perimeter or more simply by comparing the patient's fields with that of the examiner, one eye at a time. With the open eye fixing on the examiner's eye the patient's ability to see hand movements is compared with that of the examiner.

Perimetry is essential for determining the loss of vision in certain eye conditions, notably chronic glaucoma, and also for localizing an intracranial lesion which involves the visual pathway.

Staining the eye

A dye such as fluorescein sodium dispensed in liquid or strip form (Fig. 12.27, p. 417) will stain the cornea a bright, luminous green where there is loss of corneal epithelium as in corneal abrasion from an ulcer or foreign body. If a Fluoret strip is used it should first be moistened with sterile normal saline and then applied to the inside of the lower lid. Fluorescein drops are instilled in the usual way but should be followed by one or two drops of normal saline. Multidose bottles of fluorescein are highly dangerous because the dye harbours and promotes the growth of pyocyanaeus.

Bacteriological investigation of lacrimal secretion

A sample is taken from the lower conjunctival sac and sent to the laboratory for culture. This is carried out routinely before many operations and is used to find the causative micro-organisms and their sensitivity where there is infection of the eye, for example in conjunctivitis. The lower lid should be well everted so that the specimen is taken only from the conjunctival sac. Care must be taken to label the specimen indicating right or left eye.

COMMON DISORDERS OF THE EYE

Conjunctivitis

Inflammation of the conjunctiva has many causes including bacterial infection by the *Staphylococcus aureus*, the pneumococcus and occasionally the gonococcus and allergic reactions to eye make-up, drugs, dyes, and so on. It may also occur in association with general illness such as measles, asthma and some skin conditions.

Clinical features
The patient will complain of gritty pain but usually **no visual loss**. The whole of the conjunctiva is red and sore and possibly oedematous. In severe cases there is a purulent discharge which causes the lids to stick together especially after sleep. The cornea is always clear and the pupil normal.

Treatment
The cause is removed where possible. Local antibiotics are prescribed in cases of infection and a culture may be taken of the discharge. The eye is left uncovered.

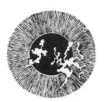

Figure 12.14
Dendritic ulcer

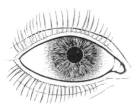

Figure 12.15
Circumcorneal injection

Keratitis

Inflammation of the cornea is fairly common at all ages and can be serious. It can be a recurring condition thus causing the patient a good deal of misery as well as visual loss. There are many causes of keratitis including infection, response to allergy and injury.

The most usual sequence of events leading to keratitis in one eye is an abrasion caused by a foreign body or superficial injury which has become infected causing corneal ulceration. A virus infection due to the Herpes Simplex ('cold sore') virus characteristically gives rise to a dendritic ulcer (Fig. 12.14) which is not easily seen unless stained with fluorescein. Occasionally keratitis is due to some endogenous illness such as syphilis in which case the condition is non-ulcerative and both eyes are affected.

Clinical features
There is pain in the eye, excessive watering, loss of vision and spasm of the lids. The redness is classically circumcorneal (ciliary injection) due to engorgement of the deep blood vessels (Fig. 12.15). An accompanying iritis is common and the patient may have general malaise. Severe keratitis of any type can cause extensive destruction of the cornea; if perforation follows then aqueous humour will leak out and the infection spreading inwards will cause further damage to internal ocular structures.

Treatment
This depends on the cause and on the severity of the condition. The patient may require hospital admission.

The sensitivity of any organism present should be determined by culture. The doctor may prescribe antibiotics to be given locally either by drops or, if there is severe infection, by subconjunctival injection and systemically. A mydriatic such as atropine 1 per cent will be ordered (see iritis below).

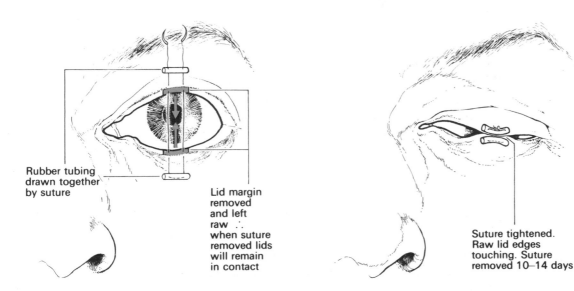

Rubber tubing drawn together by suture

Lid margin removed and left raw ∴ when suture removed lids will remain in contact

Suture tightened. Raw lid edges touching. Suture removed 10–14 days

Figure 12.16
Tarsorrhaphy

Local heat usually by hot spoon bathing or by electric eye pad affords some relief of pain. Between treatments, the eye is kept closed and covered with a pad for the patient's comfort and to protect the vulnerable cornea. If the infecting agent is the herpes virus, then IDU (5-iodo-2-deoxyuridine) drops or ointment is used intensively. Sometimes cauterization is indicated. This may be done by a qualified ophthalmic nurse on medical instruction, by application of pure carbolic on the tip of a sharpened orange stick. If the cornea has lost its sensation a tarsorrhaphy may be carried out. In this operation the lids are joined together centrally over the cornea to give it protection. (Fig. 12.16). Extensive corneal damage may require corneal grafting (keratoplasty), the donor material having been taken from a cadaver eye. Exposure keratitis (Ch. 3) is preventable and, if it occurs in hospital, it should be regarded as a lapse in nursing care.

Iritis

Iritis, inflammation of the iris, is usually associated with inflammation of the ciliary body (**cyclitis**) and therefore often referred to as **iridocyclytis**.

As the layer of the eye involved in this process is called the uveal tract the inflammation may also be called **uveitis**.

Anterior uveitis is inflammation of the iris and ciliary body.

Posterior uveitis or choroiditis is inflammation of the choroid.

A combination of anterior and posterior uveitis is known as **pan-uveitis**.

The causes include trauma, local infection and systemic conditions like rheumatoid arthritis, gonorrhoea, ankylosing spondylitis or sarcoidosis, but in most cases no underlying cause is found. The course of the inflammation parallels the behaviour of inflammation elsewhere; it may be acute, clearing away as quickly as it came, or it can wear on with fibrotic replacement of specialized tissues and adhesions between the iris and the lens (posterior synechiae). This latter course can obviously disturb vision and, less obviously, block the flow of aqueous causing a secondary glaucoma.

Clinical features

The redness resembles that of keratitis and indeed iritis can well be secondary to keratitis. The cornea is clear and the pupil may be small (due to inflammatory spasm or distortion by inflammatory adhesions). There is blurring of vision, pain and photophobia.

In severe iritis the exudate from the inflamed iris, consisting of cells and protein, any sink to the bottom of the anterior chamber to form a layer of pus, known as **hypopyon**. Secondary glaucoma may arise due to interference with the aqueous flow.

Treatment

Guttae (G) atropine 1 per cent is prescribed twice daily because the pupil must be dilated to lessen the risk of anterior synechiae (adhesions between the iris and cornea). Dilating the pupil also lessens the pain by preventing sphincter spasm.

Provided the cornea has no abrasion and infection does not contraindicate their use, steroids such as G. betnesol 0.5 per cent are given locally to suppress inflammation. The appropriate antibiotics are given for any obvious infection.

Secondary glaucoma is treated with systemic Acetazolamide 250 mg: this reduces the flow of aqueous.

If the condition persists or does not respond to treatment subconjunctival injection of steroids and mydricaine may be necessary. Oral steroid therapy is indicated in choroiditis and the usual precautions with these drugs must be adhered to.

Sympathetic ophthalmitis

This is inflammation of the uveal tract of one eye following a perforating injury involving the uveal tract of the other eye causing similar inflammation. The injured eye is called the 'exciting eye' and the subsequently affected eye is called the 'sympathizing eye'.

This condition does not usually arise until 10–14 days after the injury has occurred but it can occur after several years have elapsed. In some circumstances the removal of the exciting eye may be necessary especially if the eye is not likely to regain useful vision. Local and systemic steroids are used in treating the sympathizing eye and prognosis has been improved by the use of these drugs.

Panophthalmitis

This is an intense, purulent inflammation of the uveal tract usually following a penetrating injury. Pus accumulates within the eyeball with eventual destruction. The only treatment is early and adequate systemic antibiotics, but once vision is lost evisceration is indicated.

Glaucoma

This term means a raised intraocular pressure causing hardness of the eye. Untreated it will reduce the blood supply to the optic nerve with resulting progressive loss of visual field. Any circumstance which blocks the flow of aqueous through the pupil or out of the eye will cause glaucoma. All types of glaucoma have serious consequences for the patient.

Acute glaucoma (closed angle or congestive glaucoma)

Characteristically acute glaucoma affects middle-aged, edgy women with long sight. Because long-sighted eyes are small the anterior chamber is shallower than usual and the filtration angle consequently narrower. With increasing age the lens increases in size thus giving less room for the filtration of aqueous into the canal of Schlemm.

Some precipitating factor, either local or general, which causes the pupil to dilate is all that is required for such persons to develop acute glaucoma. Since the pupil normally dilates in the dark or in response to stimulation of the sympathetic nervous system, watching a horror film could provoke an attack in susceptible individuals.

As shown in Figure 12.17 contact between the iris and cornea results in complete blockage of the filtration angle.

Clinical features
There is a sudden onset of severe pain which radiates out from the eye. The patient becomes generally ill with nausea and vomiting, the latter feature very occasionally being responsible for misdiagnosis. The eye is deeply engorged. Vision is markedly decreased. **The cornea is steamy and the pupil fixed and dilated.** A considerable increase in intraocular pressure will be found on examination.

Treatment
The tension is reduced as a matter of urgency; if it is left for as long as 4 hours the patient may well become blind.

Medical
Conservative treatment is started on admission using:

1. Acetazolamide (Diamox) 500 mg intramuscularly or intravenously. Apart from its diuretic properties (Ch. 7), Diamox decreases the production of aqueous by the ciliary process.

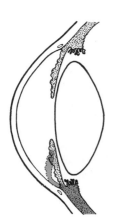

Figure 12.17
Blockage of filtration angle in acute glaucoma

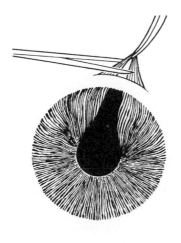

A

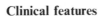

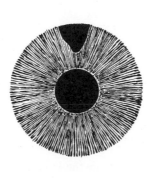

B

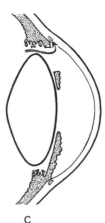

C

Figure 12.18
A. Broad iridectomy
B. and C. Peripheral iridectomy

2. Miotic drugs such as G. eserine ¼ – ½ per cent and G. pilocarpine 1–2 per cent are instilled intensively until the pupil is a pinpoint. As a result the iris is drawn away from the cornea and the angle which was closed is opened, allowing some drainage of the aqueous. G. pilocarpine is usually prescribed 6 hourly for the unaffected eye as a

prophylactic measure. Systemic administration of drugs which alter the osmotic balance between the plasma and the aqueous, for example intravenous infusion of mannitol, may be used.

Surgical
Afterwards surgery is carried out on both eyes. First a drainage operation (Fig. 12.8A) is performed on the affected eye to allow aqueous to flow through a permanent fistula to the subconjunctival space.

Later a peripheral iridectomy (Fig. 12.18B and C) is performed on the second eye to allow aqueous to reach the drainage angle despite a dilated pupil.

Chronic glaucoma (simple or open angle glaucoma)

A gradual rise in pressure in the eye causes symptomless but progressive loss of visual fields. This is one of the most common blinding diseases in the Western world.

Clinical features
The patient is usually over 50 years. As the retina is destroyed slowly and progressively from the periphery the patient can still read until the condition is well advanced. For this reason the disease tends not to be noticed in the early stages. It is usually picked up on casual examination.

Treatment
The patient is usually treated as an out-patient, miotic drugs being instilled into the eyes.

The response to miotics is noted by checking the intraocular tension, the visual fields and the optic disc. Failure to respond to medical treatment is an indication for a surgical drainage operation similar to that performed for acute glaucoma.

Secondary glaucoma

This is a rise in pressure due to disease or injury to the eye, for example in iritis where cells and exudates are thrown off into the aqueous, slowing or stopping drainage at the angle of the eye. Treatment is to deal with the cause.

Congenital glaucoma (buphthalmos or 'ox eye')

This is glaucoma occurring in a baby due to a developmental defect of the aqueous drainage system. The tissues in a young child are so elastic that the whole eye enlarges as the result of pressure within the eye.

There is a risk of reduced vision if the condition is neglected and in some eyes it is part of a malformation for which no satisfactory treatment may be possible.

Cataract

A cataract is any opacity of the lens; some types may give rise to gradual loss of vision.

Types of cataract
Cataracts are classified according to their various causes.

Senile cataract
Degenerative changes occur in the lens with advancing age, starting from about 55 years. It may take several years for the lens to become completely opaque.

Diabetic cataract
Patients with diabetes mellitus have an increased tendency to cataract. The changes are similar to those of senile cataract but tend to start earlier (45 to 50 years).

Young diabetics are prone to develop cataracts, particularly if their diabetes is not well controlled.

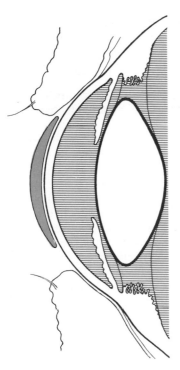

Figure 12.19
Corneal contact lens

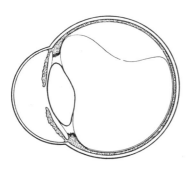

Figure 12.20
Detached retina

Figure 12.21
Example of operation for retinal
detachment

Congenital cataract
If a mother contracts rubella during the 9th to 12th week of pregnancy the baby may be born with congenital cataracts. Rubella vaccine (Ch. 1) has reduced the incidence.

Traumatic cataract
A penetrating injury or blunt injury which causes rupture of the lens capsule will allow aqueous to seep in, thus causing opacity of the lens.

Treatment
Treatment is surgical extraction of the lens and replacement of the lost focusing power by a suitable spectacle or contact lens (Fig. 12.19). In an adult the lens is generally removed in its capsule using forceps or a cryotherapy probe. (Details of care before and after the operation are given on p. 417).
In younger patients (under 35) the lens and its capsule are broken up and aspirated piecemeal.

Detachment of the retina

Detachment occurs when the innermost layer of the retina containing the rods and cones becomes separated from the pigment epithelium layer below (Fig. 12.20). A breach in the retina allows fluid to accumulate beneath it so causing further separation. The hole or tear usually occurs at the periphery then extends backwards.
Detachment occurs most commonly in myopic eyes because the myopic retina becomes especially thin and is liable to develop breaks; it is also common after cataract extraction. It may be secondary to some other condition such as inflammation or, less commonly, presence of a malignant growth in the choroid. Retinal detachment may occur at any age.

Clinical features
The patient complains of seeing flashing lights as the retina tears, and then a feeling of a curtain across the vision. There is no pain but serious loss of vision if the retina is not returned to and secured in its normal position.

Treatment
Some kind of surgery is usually indicated because the hole needs to be sealed off and the sub-retinal fluid removed. The patient may be admitted for a period of complete bed rest, with the head positioned to allow the retina to fall back into place and the subretinal fluid to be absorbed. Once the retina is as flat as possible, surgery is undertaken to secure it. Various methods may be employed, depending on the surgeon and on the type of detachment for example if there is just a hole or a tear with no sub-

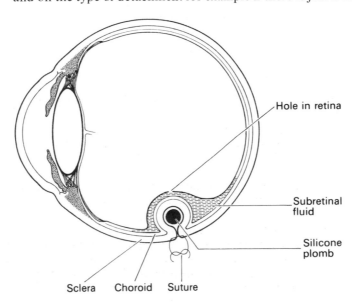

Hole in retina

Subretinal fluid

Silicone plomb

Sclera   Choroid   Suture

retinal fluid present then light coagulation or cryotherapy may be used to seal the edges of the hole. If, however, the detachment is more extensive, a ridge is formed opposite the hole by a band of silicone sewn over the sclera altering the shape of the eye and bringing the sclera and choroid into contact with the hole (Fig. 12.21). The edges of the hole may be sealed and the sub-retinal fluid can be drained or left to absorb.

In photocoagulation of the retina a powerful beam of light is focused through the pupil on to the retinal pigment epithelium, which turns the light into coagulating heat. It may be used in flat retinal tears.

Trauma

Foreign bodies

Particles may enter the conjunctival sac and give rise to irritation. Usually they are easily removed but occasionally one may become impacted in the conjunctiva of the upper lid. If so, eversion of the upper lid is necessary in order to remove it. The competent first aider can generally dislodge the particle using a corner of the patient's handkerchief. Irrigation using a household eye bath is usually effective if the foreign body is loose.

Foreign bodies which embed in the cornea are much more serious and require prompt specialist attention. After removal of the particle, the eye must be stained to ascertain the extent of corneal abrasion. Atropine is then instilled and if necessary an antibiotic. The eye is covered with an eye pad and the patient is asked to return for a check-up, usually the following day. Should a particle of metal be left in the cornea for more than 4 hours, rust will appear which is difficult to remove.

Perforating injuries

Any sharp instrument may perforate the cornea or sclera and damage the structures within the eye. Young children may stick knives, darts or arrows into the eye. Fireworks are a hazard and road traffic accidents where there is shattering of the windscreen may cause a perforating injury.

The first aid treatment is to put a sterile dressing over the injured eye and transport the patient to hospital as quickly as possible, keeping him flat and his head still.

A history is taken in the accident and emergency department, and the patient is admitted and sent to the operating theatre for examination under general anaesthetic as soon as is practicable. Consent for an anaesthetic and also consent for removal of the eye, if necessary, is required.

In theatre the eye is carefully examined and assessed, then cleaned and sutured.

If the eye is too badly injured to have any useful vision and if it is likely to act as a source of inflammation to the other eye (sympathetic ophthalmitis) then the eye is enucleated (removed).

Non-perforating injuries

Direct violence

A severe blow from a fist or a kick from a booted foot close to the eye or to the eye itself may not perforate the eyeball but will probably cause damage to the delicate structures within. If the small blood vessels of the iris are torn, blood will collect in the anterior chamber giving rise to the condition of hyphaema (Fig. 12.22). Treatment is to admit the patient to hospital for a period of complete bed rest to allow the blood to be absorbed. If the blood is not absorbed it may interfere with the drainage of the aqueous, thus causing pain in the eye and a rise in intraocular pressure (secondary glaucoma). A cataract can also result from this type of injury.

Burns

Burns may be thermal or chemical (Ch. 14).

Thermal burns often involve other parts of the patient's body, but a firework may cause damage mainly to the eye and lids.

Chemical burns are more common and arise because an acid or alkali has entered the eye. Of these lime burns, occurring frequently at building sites, are among the most serious. The pain is so severe that the patient is often quite unable to co-operate with any first aid measures designed to remove the lime.

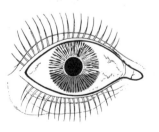

Figure 12.22
Hyphaema

The most important duty of the first aider is to get the patient to hospital with the minimum delay. Copious lavage using water or normal saline from whatever utensil is at hand, for example, a jug or teapot, will help if this treatment is possible. In the accident and emergency department the eye will be irrigated immediately with disodium versenate 1 per cent (anaesthetic drops having first been instilled to relieve pain and reduce spasm of the lids). Particular care is taken to see that no particle is retained within the upper or lower conjunctival sac where it would continue to cause tissue necrosis.

Following medical treatment the patient is likely to require surgery to deal with the scarring which results.

Burns caused by caustic soda should be irrigated with normal saline.

Strabismus (squint)

In normal vision the two eyes are used together; two images are formed, one on each retina, and they are fused by the brain so that one image is seen in three dimensions. This is called binocular vision.

If during development of vision in the young child there is failure to fuse the two images because of weakness of one of the eye muscles, then one eye deviates or squints. To prevent double vision the brain suppresses the image formed by the wandering eye, which begins to lose its acuity. Eventually the squinting eye will lose its central vision altogether, and for this reason it is important that treatment is carried out before the child is 5 years of age.

Treatment
A combination of both medical and surgical treatment may be necessary.

Medical
Conservative treatment involves correction of refractive errors, occlusion of the 'good eye' to make the 'lazy eye' work and exercises supervised by the orthoptist. If the child's eye is covered, co-operation of the mother is essential as the child will need almost constant supervision in order to prevent him from removing the patch.

Surgical
This involves either weakening or strengthening one or more of the eye muscles, for example a muscle may be severed and reinserted into the sclera behind its original point of attachment, thus in effect lengthening the muscle.

Because the operation is extraocular, little preparation is necessary. Since it is not always carried out on the squinting eye and several operations may be necessary, the parents should be forewarned and reassured.

Recovery is usually speedy and uneventful. A baby or very small child may rub his eye but this does not usually cause any damage. In older patients with long-standing squints the operation is carried out mostly for cosmetic reasons.

CARING FOR OPHTHALMIC PATIENTS

It is not within the scope of this book to describe nursing procedures which, in any case, require to be demonstrated and practised in the clinical situation. There are, however, some principles of care which will be considered.

General care

Ophthalmic nursing is in many ways very different from general nursing. Eye patients often do not feel ill but nevertheless may be required to lie still for some time. For example, a patient with a retinal detachment may have to be nursed postoperatively in a particular position where he is unable to amuse himself or watch television. The hours will pass very slowly. Since some patients have well-founded fears of loss of sight the period spent in hospital is likely to seem long, tedious and anxious. The nurse can help such patients by talking to them, keeping them informed of what is going on in the ward and in the world outside and encouraging them to talk about their worries. The ward should be kept quiet and patients should be protected from sudden noises, but the atmosphere should be cheerful and optimistic. Newly admitted patients are likely to be nervous, as are many of those the nurse meets in out-patient or accident and emergency departments. A quiet, calm, confident nurse will help them to feel more at ease and to co-operate.

Before local procedures are carried out the patient must have his head well supported. If the patient is not in bed then he is best placed on a couch with his head slightly raised for any but the most minor undertakings. The nurse can then work from behind with the aid of a good light (Fig. 12.23). Since the patient should be discouraged from contracting his facial muscles, flinching or making unexpected movements while care is being given, it is sensible to start with him in as comfortable a position as possible and to spend a little time in helping him relax.

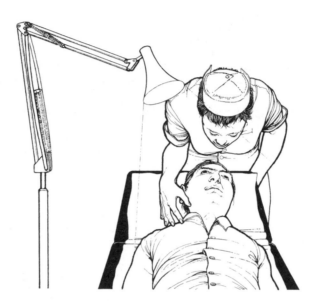

Figure 12.23
Positioning patient and light prior to giving eye care

Local care

When carrying out treatment to the eye the nurse must:

1. Use flawless, aseptic techniques at all times.
2. Be gentle and precise in her movements.
3. In all cases of infection or inflammation, care for the unaffected eye first. In this way she will avoid contamination from the infected eye and the patient will know what to expect before his painful eye is touched.
4. Remember that the cornea is the most sensitive part of the eye. She will therefore avoid touching it in any way. If, for example, drops are to be instilled she will ask the patient to look up and allow the drops to fall gently into the lower conjunctival sac (Fig. 12.24). If she is going to remove a foreign body from under the upper lid she will ask the patient to look down to his toes before attempting to evert the lid and so avoid pressure on the cornea.
5. Check carefully any preparation to be instilled in or applied to the eye (correct patient, correct drug, **correct eye**, correct time).
6. Ascertain whether ointment is to be placed in the conjunctival sac or applied to the lid margins.
7. Ask the patient to close his eye before placing an eye pad in position. This is particularly important if the eye has been anaesthetized as the pad could rub the cornea without the patient's knowledge.

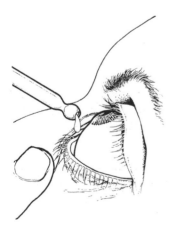

Figure 12.24
Instillation of drops into lower fornix

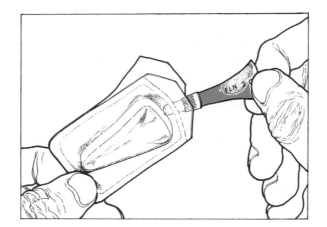

Figure 12.25
Individual preparations—minim drops

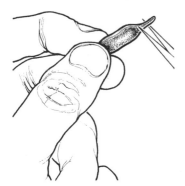

Figure 12.26
Individual preparations—Aplicaps

Figure 12.27
Individual preparations—Fluoret strip

Local preparations
These include:

1. **Drops** (guttae) which may be dispensed in either aqueous or oily solutions. The patient should have his individual bottle if individual doses (Fig. 12.25) are not dispensed.

2. **Ointments** (occulenta). These are usually dispensed in single dose containers (Aplicaps) (Fig. 12.26). If the ointment is contained in a multidose tube the risk of contamination is considerably increased.

3. **Fluoret strips** (Fig. 12.27). See the section on staining the eye, page 408.

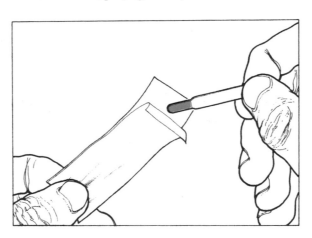

Care of the surgical patient

Until recent years most intraocular operations were performed using a local anaesthetic. This was because a general anaesthetic carried the risk of postoperative vomiting and the subsequent danger of hyphaema (p. 414) and iris prolapse.

Preoperative care of a patient having an intraocular operation
For the elective operation requiring an incision into the eyeball, such as cataract extraction, a patient is admitted 2 nights before the operation. This allows time for orientation, examination and investigations.

Orientation
This includes measures taken for any surgical patient, but an elderly patient, especially if in hospital for the first time, needs extra care and fuller explanation. If he is not familiar with the use of a bedpan, urinal or feeding cup before the operation, then he is likely to become agitated and confused when confronted with such things for the first time immediately after it and his recuperating eye will be endangered. Time should

be taken to show him how to lift himself up the bed gently and also how the nursing staff will lift him.

Explanations of the postoperative programme and its restrictions may need to be repeated several times.

Examination and investigations

A general physical examination is carried out by the doctor. Should the patient have a cough the operation may have to be postponed not only because of possible respiratory complications but because of the risk to the eye wound. Haemorrhage within the eye is more likely if the patient's blood pressure is high, so measures may have to be taken to reduce it. As part of the campaign to prevent infection the patient must be generally clean. If the hair has been neglected it should be washed during this period. The nurse can explain that it would be inadvisable for the hair to be washed for a week after the operation. Urine will be tested as a matter of routine; the presence of sugar or albumin is of particular significance and should be reported without delay.

At the time of obtaining consent for the operation, reassurance can be given that it will be the operated eye only which will be covered after the operation. The relatives should be seen and their co-operation sought in such matters as approaching the patient very quietly on their first postoperative visit and bringing in soft, in preference to hard, sweets or biscuits.

Smears are taken from the conjunctival sacs for culture. Afterwards antibiotic drops are usually prescribed for instillation as a prophylactic measure. The lashes of the eye for operation are trimmed short using sharp-bladed but blunt ended scissors. A calm, relaxed manner, a steady hand and some petroleum jelly on the blades of the scissors (so that the lashes adhere to them) are prerequisites for success. Some surgeons like the lacrimal sacs to be syringed preoperatively to ensure patency.

On the morning of the operation the routine is similar to that for any patient about to have a general anaesthetic.

Postoperative care

While the patient is in theatre, the bed area is cleared, the oxygen and suction points are checked and the bedside locker is placed on the side of the unoperated eye. Once he comes round from the anaesthetic, the patient is nursed in the dorsal position with one pillow for approximately 6 hours. At the end of this time, provided the patient's condition is satisfactory, he will be sat up gradually with more pillows and supported with a back-rest.

It is necessary to make sure the patient has a bell to call a nurse for anything which is needed as it is important that the head is kept fairly still following an intraocular operation. Hands and face will be washed gently postoperatively, but he will be left in his operation gown until the following morning to avoid unnecessary movement.

The patient will need reassurance that the operation went according to plan and that, provided he keeps reasonably still and avoids touching his eye, there is every chance it will be successful. He may need to be reminded that he should not try to reach anything from his locker. Careful observation is needed during the night because he is more likely to become confused if he wakes.

On the first postoperative morning the first dressing is carried out usually with the surgeon present. Stitch cutters may be required to remove the lid suture so that the eye can be examined. The eye is gently swabbed with sterile normal saline solution and compared with the unoperated eye. The lids, wound, conjunctiva and the anterior parts of the eye are all inspected and any abnormalities are noted in the nursing records. The doctor will usually prescribe a local antibiotic and a steroid to counter postoperative inflammation and mydriatic drops to prevent this inflammation from causing adhesions with a constricted pupil.

If the first dressing is satisfactory, the patient is given a bed-bath and allowed to sit out of bed. He may be helped to the toilet if he is sufficiently recovered from the anaesthetic. Provided the meal is cut up and placed well within reach so that he has no need to bend his head down, he is usually allowed to feed himself.

Dressings are carried out daily and treatment is given as prescribed. On the second postoperative day the patient can be given a general bath with help and he can walk to the toilet unaided. A male patient may shave from the second day taking a little extra

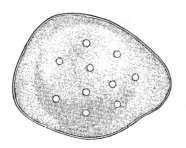

Figure 12.28
Cartella shield

care around the operated eye. He needs to be warned not to bend down to pick things up, such as slippers out of his locker, not to rub his eye or make sudden jerky movements of his head. From the second or third postoperative day, dark glasses are worn by day. A pad or Cartella shield (Fig. 12.28) is applied over the eye at night to avoid damaging it while asleep. Providing there are no complications he is ready for discharge on the fifth to seventh postoperative day.

On discharge, drops are still generally required and it is important that the person who will instill the drops at home is instructed as necessary. If he is worried about rubbing his eye the patient can be given a supply of eye pads to wear at night only. If the patient already has his own glasses the lens for the operated eye is occluded so that he can use his spectacles to see with his non-operated eye.

An out-patient appointment is made for some 2 weeks after discharge. If he is discharged to his own home arrangements may have to be made to provide a home help, 'meals on wheels' and possibly visits from a district nurse. If it is impossible to provide such help and if there is no one with whom the patient can stay, a period of convalescence may be required. Advice includes reminders not to bend, stoop or lift heavy weights. Normally about 2 months following lens extraction the eye will be sufficiently quiet to permit refraction for the necessary spectacles. The patient's name will be placed on the waiting list so that extraction of the lens from the other eye may be carried out when required.

CARING FOR THE VISUALLY HANDICAPPED

A patient may be completely blind, that is to say he cannot distinguish light from dark, or he may be partially sighted but have such limited vision that it is of little use to him. Whether or not he qualifies for registration as a blind person is a decision for an ophthalmic specialist to make.

Blindness may arise in a variety of ways from either injury or disease. In old age it is most often due to disease of the blood vessels within the eye or to disease of the retina. Initially loss of sight causes the patient to become profoundly depressed and in some instances he may develop suicidal tendencies.

If blindness develops quickly and unexpectedly in an elderly person he may become literally too terrified to move and be found wretched and immobile in a chair. Young people, given time, skilled supervision and encouragement, usually come to terms with their blindness and it is well known that some develop increased acuity of their other senses such as hearing and touch. While some remain bitter and resentful there are many more who acquire such serenity and optimism that they are sources of inspiration to their sighted friends and relatives.

Blind persons often manage to move around unaided in their own homes or in familiar surroundings, but when admitted to hospital they become upset and afraid to venture about the ward. The nurse must therefore take time to explain the geographical layout and the location of the things the patient needs to use. He must be warned of any hazards, for example equipment in the ward over which he could trip or hurt himself. This is of particular importance if blindness is incidental to some other condition for which the patient has been admitted and he is therefore being nursed in a general ward not specially geared to his needs. Doors which are left half open, and this includes locker doors, are dangers to the blind; so too is anything left out of its accustomed place. Orderliness is important.

Provided that he is well enough and safety precautions have been taken, the blind patient should be encouraged to walk about. When guiding him it is best if, having first offered him a bent arm to hold, the nurse then walks slightly ahead.

At meal times he should first be told what is in the meal; then the clock face can be used to describe the whereabouts of the various portions of food — for example potatoes at 12 o'clock, peas at 8 and meat at 5 o'clock.

A sighted person who is dozing should be approached by quietly saying his name and then by a gentle touch on his head or arm; it is the same with a blind person. Failure to give adequate warning may startle the patient who may 'jump'. The imaginative nurse will realize that unless she uses the patient's name and speaks to him directly when in the company of others he is unlikely to realize that it is he who is being addressed.

Similarly, when about to leave the room, she should say that she is going and thus avoid the embarrassment of leaving the patient talking to himself. Unless the patient is known to be deaf it is not only unneccessary but shows a lack of sensitivity to shout. She must always remember to tell him first what she is about to do. Sympathy and understanding are essential when caring for the blind but to offer pity is unkind. The nurse will do the patient the greatest service by encouraging him to be independent.

Services for the visually handicapped

The services available to blind and partially sighted persons vary from country to country. In Great Britain some are provided by welfare services and others through a number of voluntary organizations. It is only upon registration that the full range of facilities become available in Britain so that, although it is not obligatory for the visually handicapped to register, it is to their advantage to do so.

The register for blind and partially sighted persons is maintained in Britain by the local authorities. If a person wishes to become registered he must first obtain a certificate from an ophthalmic specialist, who will examine him free of charge. Responsibility for the visually handicapped is shared between the health, education and social work departments. The services provided by them and the voluntary organizations collectively include:

Special primary and secondary education in either day or residential schools.
Various training facilities, for example in Braille, typewriting or handcrafts.
Industrial rehabilitation and sheltered workshops.
Personal services such as home visits and individual advice.
Financial benefits and special concessions, for example reduced rates on public transport, income tax and radio licence relief.
Free loan tape recorders, radios and books in Braille and Moon type.
Social clubs.
Holiday homes.
Guide dogs and training facilities.
Special equipment including white walking sticks, Braille clocks, watches and controls for stoves.

SUGGESTED ASSIGNMENTS

1. Ask a friend to cooperate in the following exercise.
Blindfold yourself (no cheating!) for a whole evening and carry out as many of your normal activities as you can without help (ask your friend to intervene only if you are in real danger of harming yourself). Try to imagine that your inability to see is permanent and then consider how this would affect your life.
If possible visit a special school for the blind to find out how they teach people recently blinded to live with their handicap.

2. What are the commonest causes of accidental injury to the eye in your area? Are there any industries or sports played which put the eyes at special risk? Without being too restrictive, suggest practical safety measures to reduce the incidence of injury in either of the above.
Make a simple list of precautions suitable for young boys using an adventure playground.

3. Plan a programme for a week to help to relieve the monotony and boredom for partially sighted elderly patients in a hospital ward.

4. How would you advise someone who wishes to donate his eyes for medical use after death? For what purposes can cadaver eyes be used?

FURTHER READING

Bedford M A 1971 A colour atlas of ophthalmological diagnosis. Wolfe Medical Books, London
Chawla H B 1975 Simple eye diagnosis, 2nd edn. Churchill Livingstone, Edinburgh

Duguid I M, Berry A 1971 Ophthalmology. Oxford University Press, London
Percy E, Smith W A M 1973 Modern Practical Nursing, Series 14 Part 1. Heinemann, London
Rooke F C E, Rothwell P J, Woodhouse D F 1980 Ophthalmic Nursing. Churchill Livingstone, Edinburgh
Trevor-Roper P D 1974 The eye and its disorders. Blackwell, London
Wilson P 1976 Modern ophthalmic nursing. Arnold, London

13. The Ear, Nose and Throat

Ear, nose and throat (ENT) surgery and nursing, in common with other fields, have benefited from advances in science and technology.

The introduction of antibiotics and other chemotherapeutic agents has revolutionized the treatment of many formerly troublesome ENT affections, with a subsequent reduction in morbidity. Also, radiotherapy and cytotoxic drugs are being used increasingly in the treatment of malignant conditions as an adjunct to surgery. The use of the operating microscope has opened up new frontiers for ear, nose and throat surgeons and, of course, for their patients. To improve or re-establish a person's hearing is indeed a rewarding exercise. The scope of ENT surgery is very wide, ranging from microscopic reconstruction of the middle ear, to emergency life-saving tracheostomy. These two procedures have implications for nurses in terms of both basic nursing care and more technical nursing skills, as do most other procedures undertaken by the ear, nose and throat surgeon.

Some of you may still be puzzled as to why ear, nose and throat surgery should be a comprehensive speciality; a discussion of the anatomical relationships between these three areas will perhaps convince you of the rationality of the specialism.

The ear, nose and throat make up a large, irregular cavity in the skull (Fig. 13.1) which has openings into the middle ear via the auditory tube, into the larynx and hence into

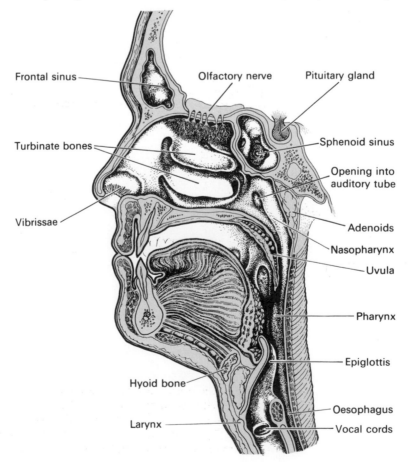

Figure 13.1
Saggital section through nose, nasopharynx and larynx

the lungs. The pharynx is continuous with the oesophagus and so there is an opening into the stomach. Openings are also found leading from the sinuses, to allow drainage of mucus, and from the orbits, so that tears can drain into the nose.

This complicated cavity (or cavities) is lined with epithelial tissue. Most of the epithelial lining is of ciliated columnar epithelium, while in the pharynx and leading into the oesophagus it is of the stratified variety.

THE NOSE AND PHARYNX

The nose and the upper part of the pharynx form the upper section of the respiratory tract; the lower part of the pharynx is common to both the respiratory and alimentary tracts.

Anatomy and physiology

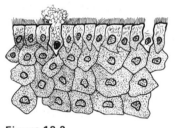

Figure 13.2
Ciliated epithelium showing goblet cells which produce mucus

The ciliated columnar epithelium lining the nose (Fig. 13.2) is interspersed with 'goblet' cells which secrete mucus. The mucus traps bacteria and other foreign particles that impinge on the mucous membrane; the actions of the cilia are to sweep this unwanted material to the natural orifices. The mucous membrane has another role besides preventing the entry of foreign bodies into the respiratory system: to warm and moisten the incoming air. The structure of the nose, with its various bones projecting into it, presents a large surface area with a rich blood supply, enabling this function to be performed adequately. The sensory nerve endings of smell (olfactory nerves) protrude into the attic of the nose (Fig. 13.1).

The sinuses, which are lined with ciliated epithelium, are normally filled with air. They give resonance to the voice and lighten the weight of the skull. Because of the very small and sometimes awkwardly placed openings from them (Fig. 13.3) and because the mucous membrane can easily become swollen and congested, acute and chronic sinusitis are fairly common disorders.

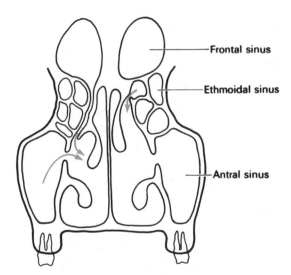

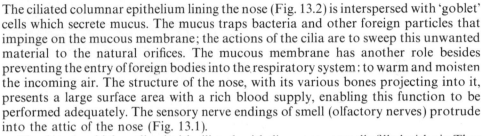
Frontal sinus

Ethmoidal sinus

Antral sinus

Figure 13.3
Ostia draining paranasal sinuses

DISEASES

Epistaxis

Bleeding from the nose is a very common form of haemorrhage, especially in children and the elderly. It is not a disease in itself but may be a sign of disease. The bleeding may be spontaneous from any area but especially from Little's area. The nose has a very rich, blood supply (Fig. 13.4). Any blow on the nose may obviously result in bleeding as may fractures of the nasal bones, facial bones or base of skull. Also new growths in the nasal cavity such as polyps, benign haemangiomata and carcinomata may bleed. Various inflammatory disorders, for example, acute and chronic rhinitis and sinusitis and perhaps more rarely syphilis and tuberculosis, may be responsible for the bleeding. Of the more general disorders cardiovascular diseases, such as hypertension and telangiectasis, are likely causes the former being a common reason in the more elderly person. Blood diseases such as leukaemia, thrombocytopenia and agranulocytosis should also be excluded if the epistaxis is recurrent.

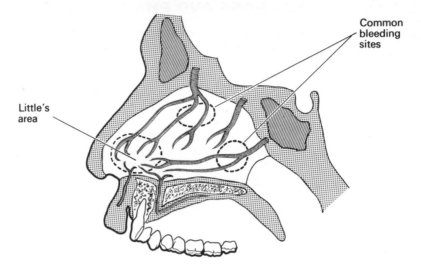

Figure 13.4
Blood supply to the nose showing common bleeding sites

Clinical features
The onset of bleeding is sudden in most cases and may be from one small area or from several. As was mentioned, Little's area is very often the bleeding site. If bleeding is profuse and prolonged the patient will exhibit signs of shock. The patient may also vomit quite large quantities of blood if the bleeding point is at the back of the nose and the blood is swallowed

Treatment and nursing care
The patient should sit down with the head slightly forward over a basin and the clothing well protected. The nostrils should be cleared by blowing one at a time; using a good light the nasal passages should be inspected. If the bleeding area is at the front the nostrils should be pinched for 10 minutes exactly. A pledget of cotton wool may be placed in the nostril before applying the pressure. It may be necessary to pack the nose if pressure does not stop the bleeding or if the bleeding is far back in the nose. The arrangement of the packing is shown in Figure 13.5. Before packing, the nasal passages

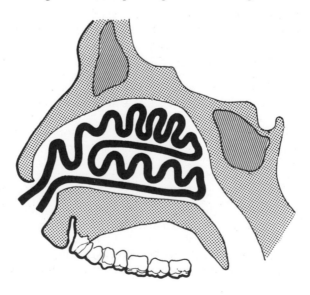

Figure 13.5
Nasal pack in position

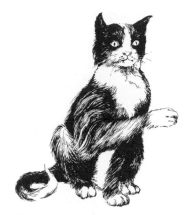

A Domestic cat

B House dust mite

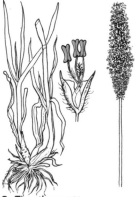

C Timothy grass

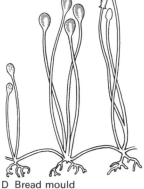

D Bread mould

Figure 13.6
Some common allergen sources

are first sprayed with a local anaesthetic such as 5 or 10 per cent cocaine or, more often, 4 per cent lignocaine in an equal amount of 1:1000 adrenaline. The success of packing depends to a large extent upon adequate anaesthesia of the nasal mucosa. Twenty-five mm ribbon gauze which has been soaked in BIPP (bismuth iodoform paraffin paste) or Calgitex is inserted under direct vision.

Various forms of packs and epistaxis balloons such as Simpson's and Brighton's are available, although some ENT surgeons favour the use of Foley catheters to stop an epistaxis. Systemic antibiotics must be given if packs are to remain in for 24 hours or more because of the danger of infection. The surgeon may also use chemical cautery agents, for instance silver nitrate stick or trichloroacetic acid, administered under a local anaesthetic; for more persistent and recurrent bleeding, electrocautery may be needed. Following cautery there may be a degree of local infection and crusting and some surgeons therefore prescribe Neomycin cream to be applied to the area.

If no local cause for the bleeding is found the patient will usually be referred to a physician for further investigation.

Hay fever—allergic rhinitis

This is a very common condition: an estimated 3 million people in Britain are afflicted to a greater or lesser extent. Each year around half a million patients require medical attention. Many also suffer from some degree of asthma. The condition is often due to an allergic response to a foreign protein in pollen (Fig. 13.6). In this case it will be seasonal being worst in spring and especially during the summer. It may also be a reaction to various animal proteins when it is usually more dramatic in its course.

Clinical features
There are bouts of sneezing, eyes water and are itchy and nasal linings are red and swollen causing blockage of the nose.

The condition is a fairly typical antigen-antibody reaction. The pollen acts as a an allergen stimulating the susceptible individual to produce specific antibodies. These antibodies become fixed on to the tissues of the eyes, nose and lower respiratory tract. When this happens the patient is said to be sensitized; when he is next exposed to pollen he develops the signs and symptoms described above.

Prevention and treatment
Various centres perform pollen counts to give potential sufferers an early warning of when they will be most at risk. Individuals who are known to be allergic should take precautions to prevent overexposure to the pollens. Wearing spectacles or sunglasses keeps pollen out of the eyes and reduces the discomfort of photophobia. Doors and windows should be kept shut. The doctor may prescribe a simple antihistamine, which may be effective in relieving the symptoms. Patients should be discouraged from using decongestants continuously and should use them only in urgent situations to relieve severe congestion. Once the nasal passages are clear they can be kept dry using a powder called sodium cromoglycate. This substance is thought to stabilize the 'mast' cells preventing their degranulation and hence the liberation of spasmogens which cause the mucosa to become oedematous and to produce large amounts of serous and/or mucoid secretions in the nasal cavity, a prominent feature of allergic rhinitis. Sodium cromoglycate used topically has a mainly preventative effect.

Nurses are often involved in investigating the cause of the hay fever and other causes of chronic rhinitis, of which there are many. Investigations include skin tests to find possible allergens. If the causative allergen is isolated a course of desensitizing injections is given over a period of several weeks. In the case of pollen sensitivity the course is best given in the weeks before the pollen season begins.

The outlook for patients whose lives are made miserable by allergic rhinitis has improved considerably over the last few years and is likely to improve even more.

Sinusitis

This is an inflammation of the mucosal lining of one or more of the sinuses. In children the sinus most commonly involved is the ethmoid whilst in adults it is the maxillary sinuses. Like inflammation elsewhere it can be acute or chronic. Repeated attacks of acute sinusitis will eventually lead to the chronic condition. (Fig. 13.7).

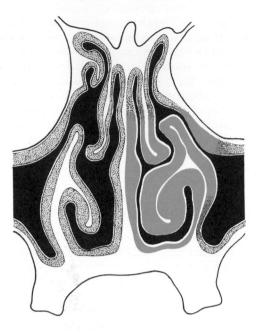

Figure 13.7
Normal and congested mucous membrane in nasal cavity

Clinical features

The majority of cases are secondary to acute rhinitis or the common cold or, more rarely, to measles and influenza. A child will often get an attack of acute sinusitis following swimming if he has been jumping into the water without holding his nose, this is especially so if the child has an infection. Infection may also spread from an infected tooth socket or be a sequel to fractures of the facial bones. The signs and symptoms, dependent to some extent on the sinuses involved and usually appearing a few days after the primary infection has apparently cleared, are:

Increasing nasal obstruction.

Purulent nasal discharge if the sinuses are draining, which causes irritation in the throat and halitosis.

A sense of fullness in the cheek if a maxillary sinus is infected.

The patient feels toxic and has a headache, especially in the morning, which may clear as the day goes on.

The temperature may be raised.

The nasal mucosa is congested and the anterior nostrils are excoriated. In children with ethmoidal involvement a degree of orbital cellulitis may be present.

The diagnosis can be confirmed by *transillumination of the sinuses* in a darkened room; by X-ray pictures or proof puncture (see below).

Treatment and nursing care

During the toxic and febrile stage the patient should have all the nursing care of the febrile patient (Ch. 1). If possible, nasal swabs should be obtained for culture and sensitivity tests. Strict attention should be paid to nose blowing and, if necessary, instructing the patient on the proper method, which is to blow one nostril at a time. Paper handkerchiefs should be provided and a disposal bag conveniently placed for collecting them. The room temperature and humidity should be kept fairly constant as changes in either affect nasal mucosa. Moist inhalations are helpful for adult patients but should not be given to children because of the danger of scalding. Specific medical treatment includes the administration of nasal decongestants. Antibiotics will also be prescribed according to the results of bacteriological investigations. Analgesics such as soluble aspirin and paracetamol will give symptomatic relief. Some patients may require antral puncture and lavage. This procedure is described below.

In the majority of cases the inflammatory changes clear up completely with adequate treatment and the ciliated columnar epithelium recovers its functions. Sometimes the condition becomes more chronic, especially when the maxillary (antral) sinuses are infected, because of their poor drainage (Fig. 13.3).

Antral puncture and lavage

This is the introduction of a special trocar and cannula (Lichtwitz) into the antral sinus (Figs. 13.8 and 13.9). It is a common procedure in ENT departments and is used in both diagnosis (proof puncture) and the treatment of sinusitis. The procedure, which is carried out by the doctor, is usually done under local analgesia, the anaesthetics of choice being either lignocaine 4 per cent with adrenaline 1 in 1000 (coloured pink) or cocaine 5 to 10 per cent with adrenaline. Cotton-tipped probes are soaked in the anaesthetic and inserted under the inferior turbinate bone for 10 to 15 minutes. Some doctors prefer 2 per cent lignocaine by injection because it gives a more profound anaesthesia. In children a general anaesthetic may be required. Specimens of the sinus contents are usually sent for bacteriological examination or, if cancer is suspected, for cytological studies.

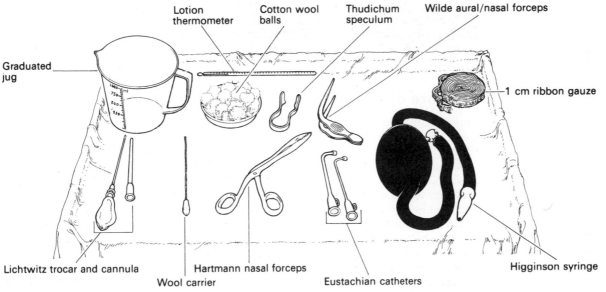

Figure 13.8
Instruments for use in antral puncture and lavage

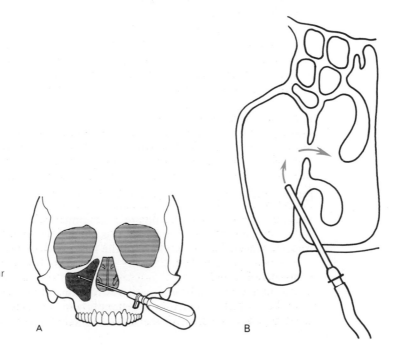

Figure 13.9
Antral puncture A. Lichtwitz trocar inserted into antral sinus below inferior turbinate bone B. Antral lavage

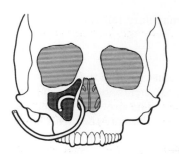

Figure 13.10
Polythene tube in antral sinus

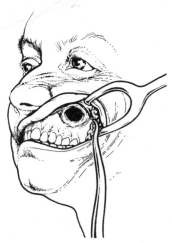

Figure 13.11
Caldwell-Luc intranasal antrostomy

For some patients the doctor may leave a fine polythene tube in position in the antral sinus (Fig. 13.10), which greatly facilitates repeated lavage. Repeated lavage may be necessary in chronic sinusitis to clear sinuses of debris, giving the mucosa a chance to recover. This procedure is often carried out by an experienced ENT nurse. The complications of antrum puncture are fainting — it is not a pleasant experience — other more rare complications include perforation of the orbit, cellulitis, surgical emphysema and osteomyelitis.

In some unfortunate patients the condition does not respond to repeated lavage and chemotherapy. These patients require more radical surgery in the form of an intranasal antrostomy or Caldwell-Luc operation (Fig. 13.11). In this procedure the antral lining is removed. For more details of this procedure a more specialized text should be consulted.

Complications of sinusitis

Various complications can arise from acute and chronic sinusitis. These include spread of infection to the orbits and osteomyelitis of the frontal and maxillary bones. Infection can also spread by various routes to the cranium, causing a variety of intracranial complications. For a discussion of these complications a more specialized text should be consulted.

Fracture of the nose

This usually follows a blow on the nose. The nasal bones, which are not very robust, break easily. Depending on the force of the blow the sinuses and facial bones may also be involved.

Bruising and swelling are seen on examination, and bleeding from the nose may be profuse.

No active first aid treatment should be given other than cold compresses to relieve pain and swelling and to stop bleeding.

The extent of bony injury is confirmed by X-ray. If the bones are out of alignment the fractures are reduced by manipulation. This is best done as soon as possible. The nasal area, being vascular, is prone to haematoma formation, which separates the fragments of broken bone. If this is allowed to develop fully it is more difficult to stabilize fragments in position after manipulation. Fractures of nasal bones heal fairly quickly, which is an important consideration for the surgeon in deciding when to reduce the fracture. If bone and cartilages heal in an abnormal position, the free flow of air may be obstructed and this may give rise to difficulties.

Most patients will be admitted to hospital if reduction is necessary. The patient is nursed in the upright position supported by pillows. If there is a history of loss of consciousness the patient should be observed for changes in conscious level (Ch. 3). The nurses should also observe for cerebrospinal fluid rhinorrhoea.

Analgesics will be required for relief of pain. Antitetanus prophylaxis and antibiotics are also prescribed.

If there are no complications only a short stay in hospital is necessary. In the case of more extensive damage to the facial bones referral to a plastic surgeon may be necessary. The patient may also require correction of any deformity at a later date, for example, to relieve nasal obstruction or for cosmetic reasons.

Deviations of the nasal septum

Deviations of the nasal septum are quite common. The fault may lie in the cartilaginous septum, turbinate or palate bones. It is often congenital; there is unequal growth of the bones giving rise to asymmetry of the nasal cavities or it may be a sequal to trauma.

Clinical features

These include complaints of nasal obstruction, frontal headaches and recurrent attacks of sinusitis. The obstruction is generally worse in one side than the other but is not usually so bad as to affect the sense of smell.

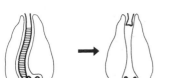

A Submucous resection

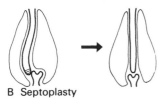

B Septoplasty

Figure 13.12

Treatment and nursing care
The treatment is surgical and the two operations most commonly performed are:

1. submucous resection (Fig. 13.12A)
2. septoplasty (Fig. 13.12B).

Preoperative care
The general care is the same as for any operation. X-rays are taken of facial bones. Any active infection is treated before operation. In the period immediately before the operation the surgeon may wish the nasal cavities to be anaesthetized. One method of achieving this is by Moffat's procedure. This consists of instilling 5 ml equal parts of adrenaline 1:1000 and lignocaine 4 per cent in each nostril. The patient has to hold this solution in the nasal cavity for 20 minutes. Alternatively if the patient is not able to cooperate the nasal cavities can be packed with 25 mm ribbon gauze (Fig. 13.5) which has been soaked in equal parts of adrenaline 1:1000 and lignocaine 4 per cent. The aim of these procedures is to reduce the amount of bleeding at the operation.
The patient is warned that there will be packs in the nose after the operation.

Postoperative care
Special attention is paid to the airway as packs will be *in situ*, these are left in for two days and then removed. Packs are of two types either, 'finger cot' packs with a 'bullring' nose pack or nose pad. Alternatively 25 mm ribbon gauze which may be impregnated with petroleum jelly. Observation for bleeding either post nasally or anteriorly is essential. The patient is discharged following removal of the packs and instructed to return if there is any bleeding and not to pick or blow his nose.

Acute tonsillitis

Acute inflammation of the tonsils and adenoids is a common disease. The condition is seen more often in children than adults, as the tonsils atrophy with age. Chronic tonsillitis and infectious diseases such as measles and scarlet fever predispose to acute tonsillitis. The causative organisms vary, but the haemolytic streptococcus is the most common.

Clinical features
The severity of the condition may range from a mild catarrhal inflammation to a severe septic infection. A feeling of fullness in the throat, leading to soreness and pain on swallowing, is the usual sequence. Earache, with enlargement and tenderness of the lymph nodes, is also common. The patient has all the signs of a febrile illness, and in severe cases he feels very ill.

Treatment and nursing care
The patient is usually under the care of a physician rather than an ENT surgeon. Because the condition is infectious he should be isolated. He will require all the nursing care of the febrile patient (Ch. 1). Gargles are given to keep the mouth and throat clean. Analgesics provide symptomatic relief. In severe cases an antibiotic is prescribed after ascertaining sensitivity of the causative organism. The condition usually clears away completely, but in some cases a peritonsillar abscess (quinsy) develops and more active antibiotic treatment is required after incision of the abscess to allow drainage of the pus. This relieves the pain almost immediately and recovery is speeded up. Strict attention to oral hygiene is necessary.

Chronic tonsillitis

This condition may follow acute tonsillitis and can cause considerable general ill-health due to the absorption of toxic substances from the tonsils. The tonsils are persistently reddened as are the pillars of the fauces. A caseous substance accumulates in the crypts, which are ulcerated, and liquid pus can be expressed from them with a spatula. There is often a bad taste in the mouth and the patient has foul breath. Some patients experience persistent soreness of the throat with acute exacerbations. There is swelling of the lymph nodes and the patient feels vaguely unwell. The toxic substances absorbed from the infected tonsils are thought to be a factor in causing many diseases such as rheumatic diseases, nephritis, chest infections, fibrositis, neuritis and iritis.

There is much controversy as to whether tonsillectomy is always necessary. The appearance of the tonsils themselves is not a reliable criterion. Nevertheless, it is a very commonly performed procedure, the details of which are given below.

Hypertrophied nasopharyngeal tonsils or adenoids

The adenoids, which, like the tonsils, are composed of lymphoid tissue, lie on the posterior wall of the nasopharynx. They atrophy as immunity develops. The adenoids often become inflamed, resulting in hypertrophy of the glands, and because of their position various signs and symptoms arise. These include mouth breathing and snoring and frequent prolonged head colds. Complications can and do frequently follow, the most serious being sinusitis and blockage of the auditory tubes leading to secretory otitis media (glue ear). The same general ill-health found in chronic tonsillitis occurs. Depending on the frequency and severity of the attacks conservative treatment is tried first. If the child develops complications and fails to thrive, removal of the adenoids is indicated.

Treatment and nursing care

In children both tonsils and adenoids are usually removed at the same time (adenotonsillectomy). In adults, only the tonsils are removed, the adenoids having atrophied.

The general preoperative care is the same as for any other operation under a general anaesthetic. Should there be evidence of upper respiratory tract infection or should the tonsils be acutely inflamed, the operation may be postponed as infection increases the risk of postoperative bleeding. For details of the operations performed — dissection and, now much more rarely, guillotine — a textbook on ear, nose and throat surgery should be consulted.

Postoperative care
Patients are nursed in the post-tonsillectomy (semi-prone) position (Fig. 13.13) so that any blood from the tonsil bed can drain freely from the mouth. If bleeding is suspected, evidence being swallowing and an increase in pulse rate, a careful inspection of the tonsil area is made using a good light, unless bleeding is profuse, cold compresses are applied to the cheek in the hope that the clot will stabilize. If the bleeding is profuse the nurse must maintain a clear airway, clear blood by gentle suction and inform the surgeon. Maintenance of a clear airway is vital and it is important to pull the tongue forward if this falls back. There is no use in giving oxygen if the airway is obstructed. The patient's colour will show signs of improvement as soon as the airway is properly cleared. Half hourly pulse and blood pressure readings are recorded. The normal postoperative care and attention are given. Some surgeons prescribe soluble aspirin or paracetamol to relieve pain. The latter drug does not interfere with the blood clotting system and is preferred by some surgeons, to relieve pain. The routine of different units varies considerably, but most units encourage patients to take a normal diet as soon as possible following operation. Gentle but firm insistence is often required. The length of stay in hospital also varies. As most tonsillectomy patients are children, extended visiting periods are allowed to enable parents to be with their child as much as possible. A very small number of patients do have a bleeding episode so that nurses must be alert at all times for this possibility.

Before discharge the child's parents should be given instructions regarding diet, schooling and what to do in the event of bleeding from the tonsil bed.

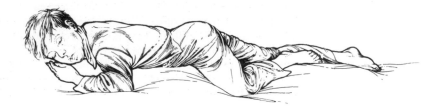

Figure 13.13
Post-tonsillectomy position

THE EAR

The ear is concerned with hearing and balance.

Anatomy and physiology

As can be seen from Figure 13.14, the ear can be conveniently divided for descriptive purposes into three areas, the external, middle and internal ear. The **auricle** of the ear directs sound waves along the **external auditory canal**, where the waves cause the **tympanic membrane** to vibrate. This vibrating membrane in turn causes the three auditory **ossicles** to oscillate. The footplate of the **stapes** is fitted into the **oval window** of the vestibule (Fig. 13.15) and the vibrations transmitted by the ossicles pass into the fluid in the **cochlea**.

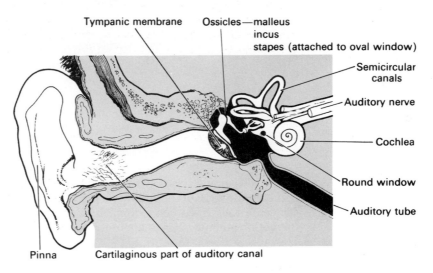

Figure 13.14
External, middle and internal ear

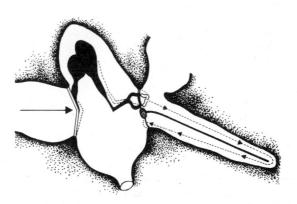

Figure 13.15
Transmission of sound. Sound waves cause the tympanic membrane and ossicles to vibrate enabling the sound to pass into the endolymph of the cochlea. The sound waves are magnified about 20 fold by this mechanism

The effect of conducting sound waves through this elaborate structure of canals, membranes and ossicles is to amplify the sound waves bombarding the pinna. This is necessary in order to stimulate the sensory nerves. Any congenital or acquired disruption of these structures causes conductive deafness (Table 13.1).

Sensory nerves arising from a structure within the cochlea — the **organ of Corti** — are thus stimulated and sensations of sound are transmitted along the cochlear division of the auditory nerve to the temporal lobe in the brain, where sounds are interpreted.

Congenital and acquired abnormalities of the auditory nerves give rise to a type of deafness known as sensorineural or perceptive deafness (Table 13.1).

Closely approximate to the cochlea is another very complex arrangement of canals and caverns, the **utricle, saccule** and **semicircular canals**, which make up the **labyrinth**. The semicircular canals are arranged in three planes. The whole complex arrangement is filled with fluid, and specialized nerve endings project into this fluid. Some of the nerve endings have **otoliths** attached to them which move with any currents set up in the fluid.

Table 13.1
Main causes of deafness

Conductive deafness		Perceptive deafness	
External ear	Middle ear	Inner ear	Intracranial
Congenital atresia	Congenital deformities	Hereditary cochlear defects	Tumours in cerebellopontine angle
Acquired atresia	Otosclerosis	Presbycusis	Multiple sclerosis
Accumulation of cerumen	Perforated eardrum	Intrauterine causes	Encephalitis
Foreign bodies	Dislocation of ossicular chain	Labyrinthitis	Meningitis
Inflammation—otitis externa	Acute otitis media	Ménière's disease	Cerebral tumours
Furuncle	Chronic suppurative otitis media	Meningitis	Psychogenic
New growths	Secretory otitis media	Viral infections	
	Cholesteatoma	Trauma	
	New growths	Noise-induced	
		Allergy	

The sensations caused by stimulating these nerve endings are conveyed along the vestibular division of the auditory nerve to the cerebellum and other parts of the brain. The sensations arise when movements of the head cause the fluid to flow and so provide the brain with information about the position and movements of the head and body.

DISEASES

Foreign bodies in the ear

All general practitioners and casualty departments are accustomed to dealing with foreign bodies in the external canal of the ear. Often there are few symptoms except perhaps slight deafness.

Treatment
The canal is inspected using an auriscope (Fig. 13.16). Provided the foreign body is not impacted and is not organic in nature, syringing will usually remove it.

Wax

Wax or cerumen is a normal secretion from wax glands in the cartilaginous part of the meatus (see Fig. 13.14). In some patients wax accumulates and causes such symptoms as deafness, earache, discharge, tinnitus and vertigo. If the wax is soft it is easily removed using a Jobson Horne probe tipped with cotton wool. Hard wax must first be softened, for which various preparations are used. They are usually in the form of drops and include 10 per cent soap solution, sodium bicarbonate solution and various proprietary cerumenolytic agents. These agents are used prior to syringing the ear. In some patients where the wax has become very hard and covered by a layer of keratin it may be necessary to give a general anaesthetic in order to remove it.

Syringing the ear
This is generally a safe and simple method of removing wax and other foreign bodies from the external auditory canal (Fig. 13.17). It is well within the competence of the nurse but should not be done without prior instructions from the doctor. The procedure should not be carried out if the patient is known to have a dry perforation of the tympanic membrane or where there is an acute inflammation of the external or

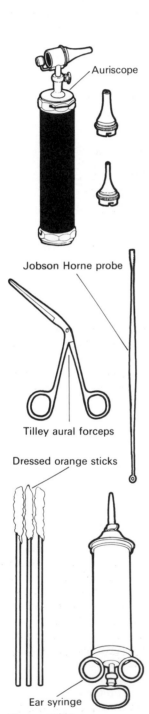

Auriscope

Jobson Horne probe

Tilley aural forceps

Dressed orange sticks

Ear syringe

Figure 13.16
Instruments for removing wax

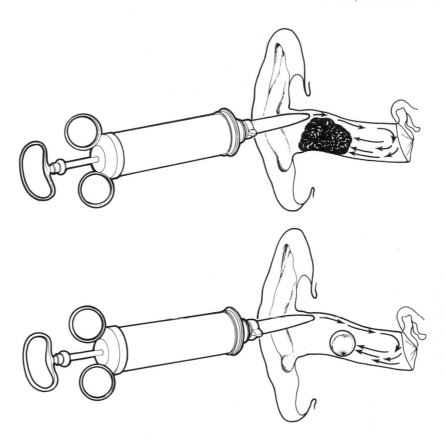

Figure 13.17
Ear syringing

middle ear. The main solutions used are normal saline for irrigation, 1 per cent sodium bicarbonate solution or, most frequently, plain tap water. The doctor will advise on the lotion to be used.

The lotion should be at 37°C when it is in the external canal; otherwise convection currents will be set up in the labyrinth and the patient will become dizzy. The nurse should not undertake this procedure before:

1. Having observed an experienced person perform it.
2. Having performed it herself under supervision.

Complications are giddiness, perforations of the tympanic membrane, trauma from the syringe nozzle and otitis externa.

Otitis externa

This may be either localized or diffuse.

Localized external otitis

This is usually due to infection of a hair follicle (furunculosis) in the cartilaginous part of the external canal (see Fig. 13.14).

Clinical features
There is severe earache, a red and swollen orifice and an increase in pain especially over the tragus when the ear is touched.

Treatment
Various forms of packing are used, such as wicks of glycerin and magnesium sulphate BP paste. Symptomatic relief is obtained from analgesics. An antibiotic may be prescribed for some patients.

Diffuse external otitis

This condition can occur in one or both ears. It is often associated with the scalp condition seborrhoeic dermatitis or dandruff. The inflammation results in intense irritation; the patient tries to relieve the irritation by poking in his ears, which only exacerbates the condition.

Treatment

If dandruff is thought to be a predisposing factor, the patient should use a medicated shampoo. Various drugs are used locally, including antibiotics and steroid preparations. The condition is very difficult to cure and the patient should be discouraged from poking in his ears. (Similarly, mothers should be warned of the risks of unnecessary use of cotton wool buds when caring for their infants.)

Acute otitis media

Acute inflammation of the middle ear is a very common complaint; to avoid serious sequelae it must be promptly and adequately treated.

Predisposing factors

These include blocked auditory tubes, enlarged adenoids, stomatitis, rhinitis of any origin, sinusitis, faulty nose blowing, tumours of the nasopharynx, diving into infected water and perforations of the tympanic membrane.

Clinical features

It follows from what has just been said that infection of the middle ear is nearly always via the auditory tube. The auditory tube becomes blocked and the air normally in the middle ear and mastoid cells is absorbed; mucus collects which later becomes purulent. On examination of the ear the tympanic membrane is seen to be inflamed and bulging. The patient has earache, is deaf and, if a child, becomes febrile. There may be a discharge of blood and pus from the ear with immediate relief of pain if the tympanic membrane ruptures.

Treatment

If the inflammation does not respond to antibiotics or if perforation of the membrane seems likely, the surgeon may perform a myringotomy (an incision of the tympanic membrane) to allow drainage of pus. This avoids the laceration of the membrane which occurs should it rupture spontaneously. This procedure, which necessitates a general anaesthetic, is not often required because of the effectiveness of antibiotics in resolving the infection. Nasal decongestants are prescribed to relieve congestion and to allow drainage via the auditory tube. This also allows air to pass up the tube and so equalizes the pressure on either side of the tympanic membrane.

Complications of acute otitis media

These are always serious, the most dangerous being chronic suppurative otitis media with mastoiditis, destruction of the ossicles and perforation of the tympanic membrane.

Secretory otitis media

This condition arises because of blockage of the Eustachian tubes, often by enlarged adenoids. It is mainly a disease of childhood. The middle ear cavity becomes filled with a thick mucinous material hence the alternative name of 'glue ear'. The child becomes deaf, a fact which may not always be readily appreciated by parents and teachers.

Treatment and nursing care

The surgeon makes a small incision in the tympanic membrane (myringotomy) and sucks out the mucinous material using a **Zollner** sucker. This is often quite difficult to accomplish as the material is very tenacious. Once cleared a grommet (Fig. 13.19) is fitted into the incision and this ensures adequate ventilation of the middle ear cavity.

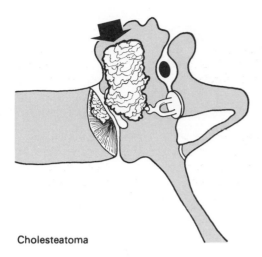

Cholesteatoma

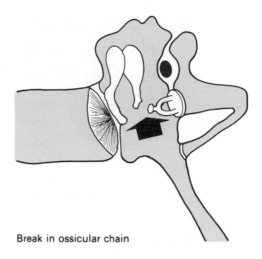

Break in ossicular chain

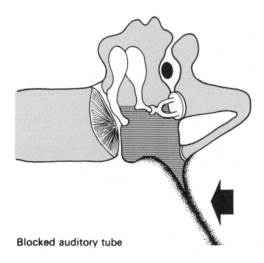

Blocked auditory tube

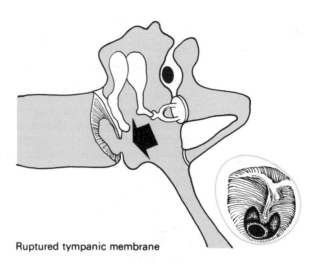

Ruptured tympanic membrane

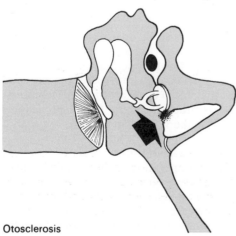
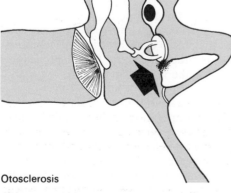

Otosclerosis

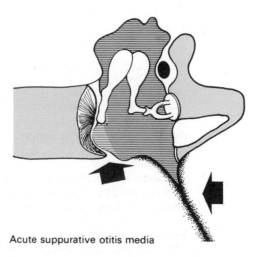

Acute suppurative otitis media

Figure 13.18
Common causes of middle ear
deafness

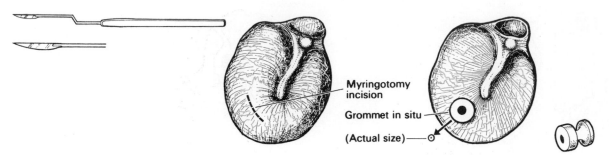

Myringotomy
incision

Grommet in situ

(Actual size)

Figure 13.19
Grommet inserted into typanic
membrane following myringotomy
and clearance of secretions

The pre- and postoperative care is essentially the same as for other ear operations (see below) only in this instance there are usually no packs or external dressings. Only a short stay in hospital is needed. On discharge the child's parents are advised to avoid getting the external auditory canal wet, hence no swimming until it is healed. Flying is also prohibited. The grommet gets pushed out by the healing tympanic membrane, by which time normal ventilation and drainage via the Eustachian tube should be re-established. Regular follow-up is arranged as the disorder may recur.

Chronic suppurative otitis media

This is a chronic inflammatory disorder in which pus is produced. There are two types, namely simple and dangerous chronic suppurative otitis media (CSOM).

Most patients come to surgery with a long history of chronic middle ear disease relating a sad story of progressive deafness and a foul smelling aural discharge. The discharge is often intermittent and the patient will report periods when the ear has been dry especially following treatment.

In the more dangerous form there is cholesteatoma formation (Fig. 13.18) with destruction of the ossicular chain. As with any chronic inflammatory process there is always the danger of extension to neighbouring tissues and structures. Chronic mastoiditis, lateral sinus thrombosis, cerebral abscess, meningitis and facial paralysis are all possible serious complications of this disorder.

Treatment and nursing care

Better primary health care and the advent of antibiotics have reduced the incidence of chronic ear disease. Nevertheless the busy otorhinolaryngology department still sees many patients with chronic ear disease. The introduction of the binocular operating microscope has enabled the ENT surgeon to perform more reconstructive surgery instead of the radical surgery of the past.

The main operations performed are cortical mastoidectomy, modified radical mastoidectomy and radical mastoidectomy. These are all operations to clear out necrotic and infected tissue. One of the main reconstructive operations is myringoplasty — repair of the tympanic membrane: for this operation a small piece of fascia is often used (Fig. 13.20). The other operations are tympanoplasty and ossiculoplasty in which the ossicular chain is restructured using a variety of techniques and prostheses (Fig. 13.20). The nursing care is much the same for all procedures differing only in a few details. The surgeon will make his wishes known.

Preoperative care
The patient will be admitted a few days before the operation so that a full range of audio-metric tests can be performed. Sometimes these tests are done on an outpatient basis. Either way they are essential for pre- and post-operative comparison.

The patient requires all the normal preoperation care given before major surgery. In addition hair is shampooed using a medicated shampoo and the head is shaved on the affected side (Fig. 13.21). The scalp and post-auricular sulcus must be cleaned with an antiseptic solution. Care must be taken to keep any of the solution from running into the ear. The hair is kept in place using hair fixative and the area covered using a head bandage. (Fig. 13.21).

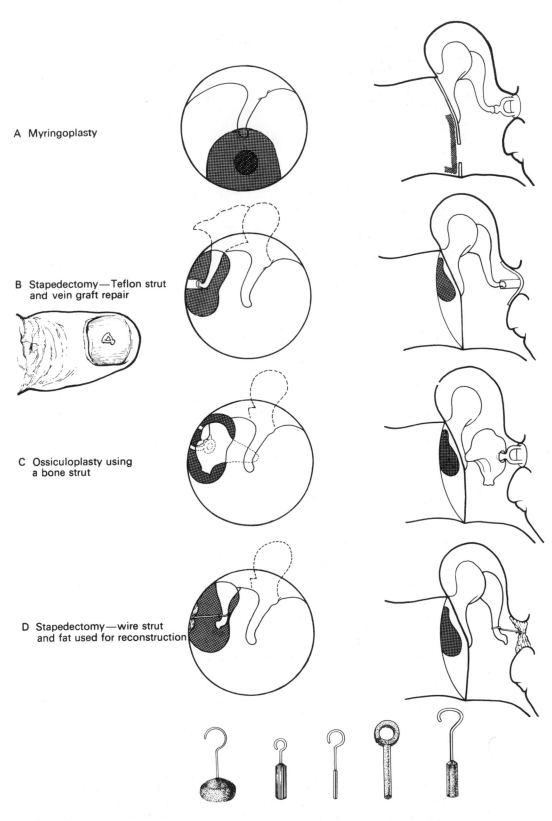

A Myringoplasty

B Stapedectomy—Teflon strut
   and vein graft repair

C Ossiculoplasty using
   a bone strut

D Stapedectomy—wire strut
   and fat used for reconstruction

Figure 13.20
Four examples of microscopic
surgery of the middle ear
Bottom row—A selection of
prostheses developed for
reconstructing the ossicular chain

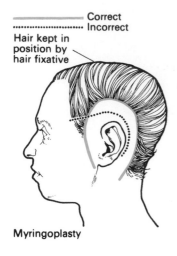

Correct
Incorrect
Hair kept in
position by
hair fixative

Myringoplasty

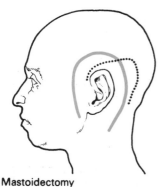

Mastoidectomy

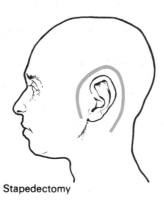

Stapedectomy

Figure 13.21
Skin preparation before ear surgery

Postoperative care
In the immediate postoperative period the patient is usually nursed flat. Despite this he may experience nausea and vomiting due to disturbance of the labyrinth.

Nursing observations are of particular importance:

The patient's temperature, pulse, respirations and blood pressure are recorded half hourly.

Signs of increasing intracranial pressure (see Ch. 3) must be reported immediately.

The patient must be observed for signs of facial palsy, denoted by asymmetry of the face. This is because the muscles on the affected side are unable to counteract effectively the pull of muscles on the unaffected side.

The patient should be asked to 'show his teeth' and any paresis (weakness) of the facial muscles is usually obvious. Should this complication develop the bandage is loosened and the surgeon and operating theatre staff are informed. To counteract the vertigo and the dizziness which many patients experience the patient is sat up gradually using one additional pillow at a time. If the dizziness persists a pillow is removed for a time. Occasionally a labyrinthine sedative may be required.

Ménière's disease

Ménière's disease is a very distressing condition caused by a disturbance in the labyrinth. Excess fluid accumulates in the membranous labyrinth causing distension. This results in malfunction of the nerves of balance and hearing. There are three main symptoms of which the patient complains:

1. Increasing deafness.
2. Tinnitus.
3. Repeated attacks of vertigo.

The diagnosis is made on the basis of the history, audiometry, caloric tests and X-rays of the petrous bone. More specialized X-rays, for instance computerized axial tomography (p. 95), may be required if tumours of, or in the region of, the acoustic nerve are suspected.

Treatment and nursing care
Medical treatment is tried first, consisting of dietary modification such as reduced salt intake and labyrinthine sedatives. If medical treatment fails, a small number of patients require surgery. Upwards of a dozen different operations have been devised. Some of these operations are quite radical: the patient's hearing is sacrificed on the affected side to relieve the terrible distress of tinnitus and vertigo. Other operations, such as endolymphatic shunt, have been devised to divert excess endolymph into the subarachnoid space. The pre- and postoperative care is essentially the same as for other major ear surgery.

THE THROAT

The lowest part of the pharynx and larynx comprises the throat.

Anatomy and physiology

The larynx is composed of several cartilages (Fig. 13.22) which give it a rigid structure to prevent it from collapsing easily. The opening into the larynx is closed during swallowing by a flap of elastic cartilage tissue called the epiglottis. Stretched across the inside of the larynx are the vocal cords. The vocal cords are attached to the movable arytenoid cartilages of the larynx. A complex arrangement of muscles is attached to the arytenoids and other cartilages and these muscles 'open' and 'close' the vocal cords. As air passing from the lungs is forced over the tensed vocal cords, sound is produced. The different pitches of sound depend on the degree to which the cords are stretched and the flattening or thickening of the cord edge. Speech, which is a learned activity, is controlled by an area in the left frontal lobe called Broca's area. The nerve supply to the

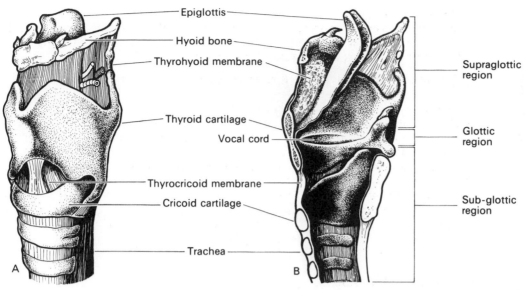

Figure 13.22
The larynx A. Front view B. Saggital section

larynx and vocal cords is via the recurrent laryngeal nerves which arise from the vagus nerves in the thorax, and branches of the superior laryngeal nerve.

Tumours of the throat

Benign tumours of the throat such as papillomata and fibromata are uncommon but can be troublesome when they do occur. In a child they may easily obstruct the free passage of air and on occasion may necessitate a tracheostomy. There is always a danger of damage to the vocal cords when such tumours are removed.

Various polyps (Fig. 13.23C) nodules and cysts also arise mainly on the vocal cords and may require surgical intervention.

The nursing care is the same as that given to any patient requiring surgery. Great care must be taken postoperatively on recovery from anaesthesia to ensure that the patient can swallow properly. The surgeon will advise the nursing staff on this and may well forbid food and fluid for several hours following the operation. Histopathology of the tissue removed is necessary so that the patient can be reassured that the growth was benign.

Carcinoma of the larynx

Carcinoma of the larynx makes up about 2 per cent of reported cases of malignant disease. The condition is more common in males than females. It has been suggested that the undesirable habit of smoking is a predisposing factor. There are also racial differences in the incidence of laryngeal carcinoma. The prognosis of the condition varies according to the site of the primary tumour. This is because of the anatomical arrangement of the larynx, its blood supply and in particular its lymphatic drainage. Spread is by local invasion of the growth and via the lymphatics to the neck and mediastinum; blood-borne metastases are uncommon.

Clinical features
These depend on the site of the tumour (Fig. 13.23). If the cords are not involved a vague discomfort in the throat, thickness of the voice, irritable cough, swollen lymph nodes in the neck and occasionally difficulty in breathing are the most common presenting features. If the cords are involved hoarseness is the main feature initially. Even in the very early stages, there is some alteration in the voice no matter how small the lesion. Hoarseness persisting for more than 14 days should always be investigated.

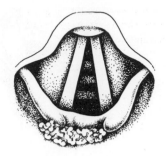

A. Supraglottic tumour

B. Glottic tumour

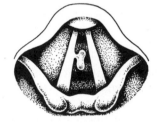

C. Polyp on cord

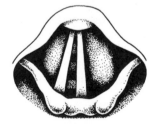

D. Paralysis

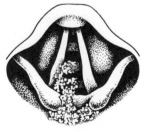

E. Subglottic tumour —
extensive spread

Figure 13.23
Lesions of the larynx

Diagnosis
This is not always easy, as several conditions can present with similar clinical pictures. These conditions include chronic laryngitis, syphilis and tuberculosis. The diagnosis is made on the basis of a careful history, direct laryngoscopy and tissue biopsy for histological examination. X-ray examination of the chest and neck are also carried out, the former to exclude bronchial carcinoma which may be causing pressure on the recurrent laryngeal nerves.

Treatment and nursing care

Once the diagnosis is established there are two main forms of treatment — surgery and irradiation.

For tumours in supra- and subglottic regions of the larynx the usual treatment consists of a combination of irradiation and surgery. Many patients do not seek treatment early enough because of the vagueness of the symptoms. Patients with supra- and subglottic tumours undergo a course of irradiation followed by surgical removal of the tumour. Localized glottic tumours respond very well to radiation exposure, with a high cure rate. The voice returns to more or less normal.

Preoperative care

The surgery required is extensive; for this reason the patient must be as fit as possible before the operation. As with all major surgery the management of the patient is very much a team effort involving surgeons, radiologists, physiotherapists, speech therapists and nurses as well as the resources of many other departments within the hospital. The patient is admitted a few days before the operation. This enables the team to get to know him and to prepare him to manage without a larynx, with all that this entails. The speech therapist instructs the patient in oesophageal speech; even quite elderly patients show a remarkable ability to master this form of communication. The physiotherapist instructs the patient in breathing exercises as the patient will have a permanent tracheostomy following removal of his larynx and chest infections must be avoided.

The doctors and nursing staff are responsible for carrying out all the normal preoperative care. A positive, optimistic approach by all members of the team will do much to instil confidence in the patient and his relatives. An opportunity to meet a former patient who has had a successful laryngectomy will do much to instill confidence. Most patients accept the situation philosophically, having already undergone irradiation therapy, an exhausting experience in itself. The anaesthetist will also visit the patient as the nature of the surgery presents him with several problems in providing adequate ventilation of the lungs during operation.

The general preoperative care is the same as for all major surgery. Some surgeons may request that a nasogastric tube be passed before the patient goes to theatre; other surgeons pass the tube during some stage of the operation.

Postoperative care

On return from theatre the patient should be under constant surveillance; for this reason and to protect him against infection he will be nursed in an intensive care area or in a side room in the ward. Once back in the ward the patient will be nursed in the upright position well supported by pillows, as soon as it is safe to do so. He will have a tracheostomy tube in position; usually this will be a plain plastic or rubber tube (Fig. 13.24). Some surgeons

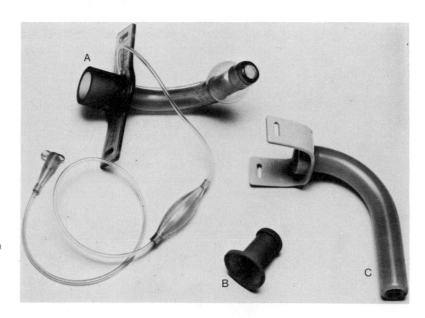

Figure 13.24
Tracheostomy tubes A. Single cuffed tracheostomy tube—balloon (cuff-inflated) B. Medasil silicone stoma button C. Plain plastic tracheostomy tube

prefer to use cuffed tubes to prevent blood and other secretions from flowing down the trachea into the lungs (Ch. 6). Pressure from the cuff on the walls of the trachea quickly causes a troublesome necrosis (a pressure sore), which can erode through to the oesophagus causing a tracheo-oesophageal fistula. For this reason a regime for regular release of the cuff must be established. The other alternative is a two-cuffed tracheostomy tube, only one cuff needing to be inflated at a time. Most surgeons will fit the patient with a silver tube later in the postoperative period (Fig. 13.25).

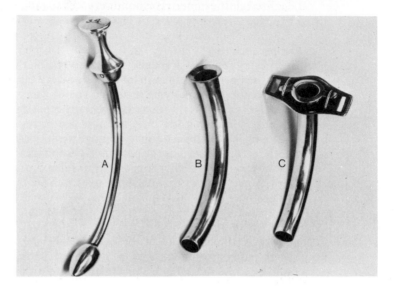

Figure 13.25
Silver tracheostomy tubes
A. Obturator
B. Inner tube
C. Outer tube

The tracheostomy tube will require very frequent cleaning using suction every 15 or 30 minutes. (Ch. 6). Strict asepsis must be observed. As the normal humidification of incoming air by the nasal passages is absent, some form of humidification will be required. This may be achieved by instilling 5 mls of sterile normal saline into the trachea before and after suction. Special attachments for giving oxygen via a tracheostomy tube are available.

The wound should be inspected for any sign of haemorrhage and the dressing changed using a strictly aseptic technique. If a vacuum drain is in place, it must be maintained to prevent the accumulation of blood and serum within the wound area, which could give rise to pressure resulting in respiratory distress. A tray with spare tubes and all necessary equipment should be available to change or replace the tube if the need arises.

The patient's intravenous infusion will be maintained as prescribed. The stomach contents are aspirated hourly via the nasogastric tube to prevent regurgitation during the initial period. Frequent and careful oral toilet is essential to prevent infection from developing in the mouth. Prescribed analgesics are given as required to control pain. The usual postoperative observations and blood pressure should be recorded half hourly.

Depending on how well the patient progresses—and every patient behaves differently — the intravenous fluids may be discontinued the first or second postoperative day. The patients fluid and nutritional needs are given via a nasogastric tube. This method of feeding is maintained up to the tenth post operation day. This allows the wounds to heal properly and lessens the risk of infection.

Before oral feeding is recommended it must be ascertained that there are no fistulae communicating with the respiratory system. This is common in patients who have undergone radiotherapy treatment, and it tends to delay healing. The existence of fistulae can be established by, for example, running a few drops of an aqueous solution of gentian violet on to the patient's tongue and asking him to swallow. The tracheostomy and wound are then observed to see if any gentian solution appears. If no solution appears, normal feeding is gradually introduced. The patient may be allowed up to sit in a chair by the second or third post operation day and may even manage a short walk. Early ambulation is desirable. The physiotherapist and speech therapist will attend to fulfil their respective roles and the patient should be ready for discharge by the end of the second week or even earlier.

Unfortunately, not all patients respond to treatment either because they have been slow to seek medical aid or because of the position and nature of their tumour. In a few instances the tumour erodes through the skin, becomes infected and causes an offensive odour. Many patients remain in this unpleasant state for quite a long time causing great distress to their families. Necrosis of the skin and fistulae are common features in patients who have undergone irradiation. There are often difficulties in swallowing and breathing and palliative surgery may be necessary. Pain is not a common feature. Many of these patients die of uncontrollable haemorrhage. During this terminal illness drugs to relieve any pain and allay anxiety will be necessary.

The many successful treatments make the management of these patients a rewarding exercise especially when one sees the patient months and then years later, having mastered oesophageal speech and leading an almost normal life. Swimming is impossible, but otherwise the patient can indulge in almost anything he fancies which is within his physical and mental capacity.

SUGGESTED ASSIGNMENTS

Projects

1. What services and facilities are available for the deaf and hard of hearing in the community in which you live and nationally?

2. From your knowledge of speech production and from listening to people communicating orally, list the qualities of speech. From this list predict which qualities you think will be absent in the patient who has had a laryngectomy and has learned oesophageal speech.

If possible interview a patient who has had a laryngectomy or listen to a tape recording of a patient using oesophageal speech and see if your predictions are valid.

Discussion topics

1. Should the government pass laws compelling people to wear ear defenders to prevent deafness or is this an individual responsibility?

2. Loss of hearing is a worse handicap than loss of vision.

FURTHER READING

Casey T, Walker H 1976 The special senses. Penguin Library of Nursing Series. Churchill Livingstone, Edinburgh

Hudson G C 1972 Handbook of tracheostomy care. Portex Ltd, Hythe, Kent

Marshall S, Oxlade Z 1975 Ear nose and throat nursing, 5th edn. Bailliere Tindall, London

Miles-Foxen E H 1978 Lecture notes on diseases of the ear nose and throat, 4th edn. Blackwell Scientific, Oxford

Pracey R, Seigler J, Stell P M, Rogers J 1977 Ear nose and throat surgery and nursing. Hodder & Stoughton, Sevenoaks

Rotter K 1972 The ear nose and throat for nurses, 3rd edn. Faber, London

Saunders, Havener, Keith, Havener 1979 Nursing care in eye ear nose and throat disorders, 4th edn. Mosby, St. Louis

14. *The Skin*

This chapter deals with some ways in which skin damage occurs. It also gives an introduction to the principles of nursing care and treatment of some common skin disorders. The reader seeking more specialized knowledge will find an increasing number of excellent textbooks becoming available.

STRUCTURE AND FUNCTION OF THE SKIN

Figure 14.1 shows clearly the component parts of the skin and its appendages. The outer layer, the **epidermis**, has a **basal cell layer**. These cells are constantly dividing and moving towards the surface. Here they become *keratinized* and are constantly being removed by friction and washing. Other cells, called **melanocytes**, are in the basal cell layer. These produce a pigment, **melanin**, which gives the skin its colouring; it is increased by the action of sunlight.

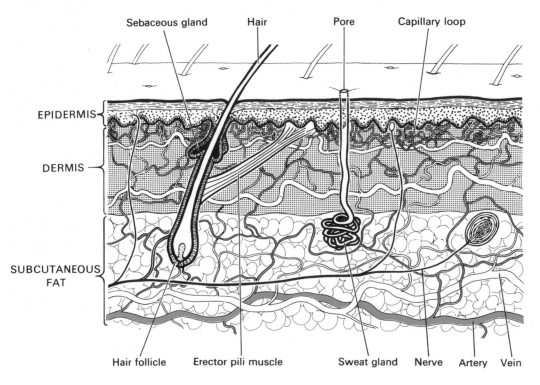

Figure 14.1
The skin

Hair follicles are invaginations of epidermis into the second layer of skin, the **dermis**. **Sebaceous glands** open into the hair follicles and secrete **sebum**, which helps to keep the skin soft and pliable. Also in the dermis are **sweat glands** — coiled tubes which open on the surface through ducts. Sweat glands provide an important way for the body to lose excess water and keep itself cool.

The dermis is also a supporting tissue for blood vessels, lymphatic vessels and special sensory nerve endings. At the junction of dermis and epidermis, undulations can be seen; these are called **papillae** and help to prevent the separation of the two layers. The dermis has a rich blood supply with many capillary networks extending into the papillae. As well as promoting rapid healing of injuries the extensive blood supply permits the body both to lose heat when necessary by dilating skin blood vessels and to conserve it by constricting them (Figs. 14.2 and 14.3).

Skin manufactures **vitamin D** as the result of the action of sunlight upon it (Fig. 14.4). At one time, when low living standards and inadequate, low-vitamin diets were common, children living in smoky towns often had rickets as a result of being deprived of sunlight.

Another important function of skin is **protection**, not only against micro-organisms but also against other harmful agents such as acids and alkalis (Fig. 14.5). Occasionally, however, a hair follicle becomes infected producing a boil.

Skin is also **waterproof** (Fig. 14.6). Not only does it prevent the body from losing all its water; it also prevents it from becoming water-logged in the rain or in the bath. Some water is lost in a controlled way by sweating, but uncontrolled loss, as might occur in severe burns, is very serious and can lead to death.

Special nerve endings in the skin also keep the brain informed about the environment. Different sensations, such as heat, cold, touch, pressure and pain, are caused by nerve endings being stimulated, the stimuli then being transmitted to the brain.

The changing skin

Everyone admires the soft, smooth skin of babies, yet softness means tenderness, so special care must be taken of the skin of infants. It should be remembered that the surface area of a baby's skin, in relation to its weight, is much greater than that of an adult so proportionately more heat is lost. Because the heat-regulating mechanism in infants takes time to develop, heat loss can be dangerous. Environmental temperatures for babies must therefore be adequate and constant, and exposure avoided (Ch. 17).

As years go by, changes occur in the skin. Often the first remarkable change is during the period of adolescence when acne may be a problem (Fig. 14.7). Not only is it unsightly but it occurs at a time when young people are at their most sensitive. Acne usually clears up by the mid-twenties, but in the meantime, sympathetic treatment is essential. The cause of acne is believed to be related to the increase in sex hormones which occurs at this time of life. Sometimes eating chocolate makes it worse; if so this, and also fatty foods, should be avoided. Washing the skin with soap and water should be encouraged, and patients should be warned about picking at the spots as this habit may result in scarring. Various forms of treatment are used. Some are preparations which cause peeling of the epidermis, such as *salicylic acid* and sulphur. Ultraviolet light will have the same effect. In severe cases, long courses of *tetracyclines* may help.

During the menopause further skin changes may occur. This, too, is a period of endocrine change often accompanied by emotional upsets. Thinning of the hair may be noticed, as well as the appearance of facial hair. Weight gain increases the possibility of intertrigo (inflammation occurring in folds of skin). *Pruritus*, especially around the external female genital organs, may also begin to be troublesome.

The effects of ageing on the skin are probably in part due to changes in the dermis, the supporting part of the skin. Contrasted with that of a baby, aged skin is wrinkled and loose. Often it is very thin and almost transparent. Patches of brown pigmentation occur. Dietary deficiencies leading to symptoms of pellagra or scurvy may be the result of poverty or apathy (Ch. 4). In old age, there may be nail thickening and distortion as well as skin changes. This problem is best dealt with by a chiropodist.

KEEPING SKIN HEALTHY
Washing

Skin becomes covered with sweat, sebum, dust and dead epithelial cells. Decomposition of sweat by bacteria gives rise to unpleasant odours, particularly in the axillae and groins. Daily washing with soap and water is required and many people find deodorants helpful. (By and large, expensive brands of deodorant tend to be no better than cheaper ones.) Special attention must be paid to folds of skin — between toes, and in the groin, scrotum and anal regions. This is particularly true of the helpless patient

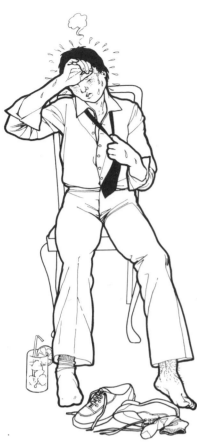

Figure 14.2
Losing heat

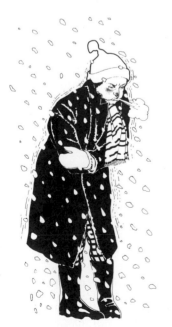

Figure 14.3
Conserving heat

being nursed in bed for whom the old maxim 'as far down as possible and as far up as possible' is not good enough. 'Possible' must also be washed thoroughly. Occasionally a person's skin may react to certain soaps and deodorants, and these must then be avoided.

Nutrition

No special diet is required to keep skin healthy, only one containing the necessary nutrients. Protein deficiency, seen in underdeveloped countries, causes kwashiorkor, one feature of which is skin ulcers. Vitamin C deficiency causes scurvy, while pellagra, the result of nicotinic acid deficiency, has among its features skin disorder. Of these three, the only one likely to be seen in developed countries is scurvy, which may occur among the elderly (Ch. 20).

Clothing

Although warmth is important, clothing should be comfortably loose. Undue tightness causes chafing and damages the skin. Nylon and other synthetic materials are not very absorbent and are therefore not suitable for wearing next to the skin. They also tend to keep the body too hot in summer and too cool in winter. Tight-fitting shoes and elevated heels can cause untold damage to feet, the least of which will be corns. Socks should be changed daily, more frequently if the feet sweat profusely. Metal hooks and fasteners, especially if nickel-plated, cause skin reactions in some people.

Cosmetics

Although cosmetics are useful for covering blemishes and often enhance the appearance, it is nonetheless true that most women have no idea what they are putting on their skins. Many ingredients go into cosmetics, and occasionally some people will find that their skin reacts to certain varieties. These they must avoid.

BREACHES IN THE SKIN

Skin normally remains intact unless damaged in some way. A common form of injury is burning. An inadequate blood supply due to impaired arterial circulation will also lead to skin death; so too will inadequate venous drainage such as occurs with varicose veins. A common result of skin damage is an ulcer. This is defined as a circumscribed lesion in which loss of skin and possibly subcutaneous tissue has occurred.

Pressure Sores

Patients who are confined to bed for long periods and who have a limited degree of movement are liable to suffer damage to skin and possibly also to underlying tissue. Pressure sores, or decubitus ulcers, are mainly the result of prolonged pressure being exerted on the skin at various points. This localized pressure diminishes the blood supply to the skin, which becomes devitalized and susceptible to damage by even the most trivial injury. Often a reddening of the skin appears first, then a break in its integrity. Unless vigorous measures are taken, an ulcer, which is often infected, develops. A distinction is sometimes made between this and the death of deeper tissue, which can extend to bone; but in both cases pressure is the principal cause.

Figure 14.8 shows the parts of the body most likely to be affected by prolonged pressure. These are parts where tissue is compressed between bone and the surface on which the person is lying. The surface can vary in hardness. Operating tables tend to be fairly hard in spite of cushioning; so too do stretchers in ambulances. A long period spent on such surfaces can begin the process that results in the development of sores. Softer surfaces that change to fit the body contours will achieve a more even and wider distribution of body weight and are consequently less likely to be damaging.

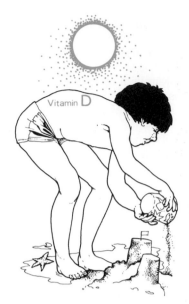

Figure 14.4
Skin makes vitamin D

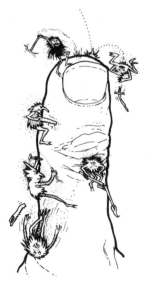

Figure 14.5
Skin protects

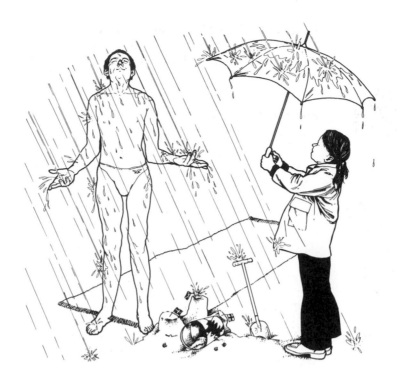

Figure 14.6
Skin is waterproof

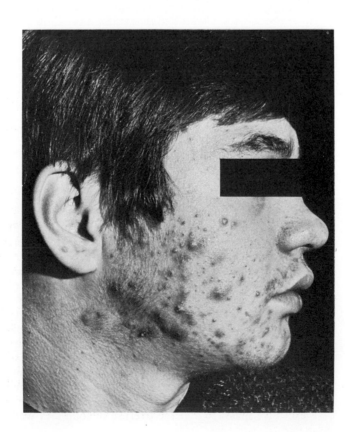

Figure 14.7
Acne vulgaris (Courtesy of Mr
McIntyre, Department of Medical
Photography, Victoria Hospital,
Kirkcaldy)

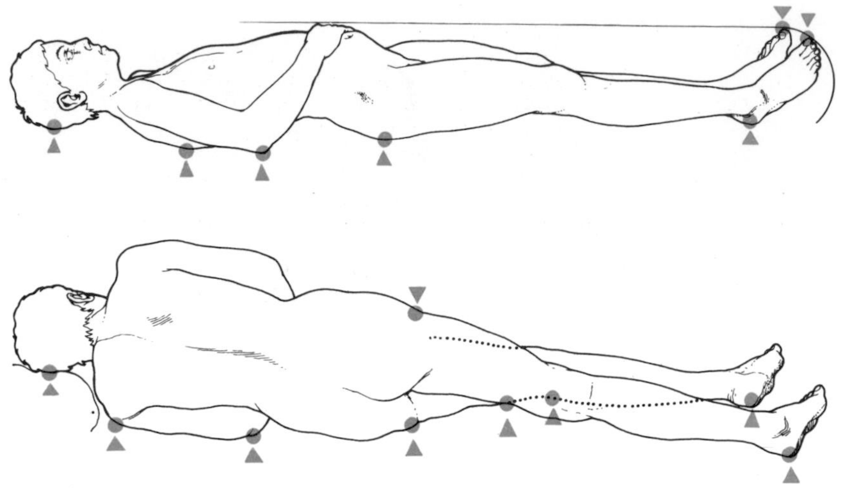

Figure 14.8
Pressure areas

Causes

Although pressure is the main cause of pressure sores, there are several other contributory factors. These can be divided into two groups; those relating to the condition of the patient himself, and those relating to his environment — his bed, and so on.

Causes relating to the patient

Malnutrition, especially protein and vitamin C deficiency.

Other diseases — diabetes mellitus, anaemia, malignant disease, obesity, oedema of any origin.

Changes particular to old age — hypertension, lowered resistance to infection, impaired sensation, impaired consciousness.

Slipping down the bed because of lack of support.

Causes relating to the environment

Wrinkled or patched sheets.

Rubber mackintoshes on beds.

Draw sheets of rough texture.

Bread crumbs or other particles in the bed.

Soiled or wet sheets.

Friction caused by incorrect lifting.

Excessive skin massage.

Excessive use of soap on skin.

Bedpans.

Prevention

Prevention of pressure sores is a nursing priority. Provided preventive measures are begun before damage occurs, sores need not develop. The most important part of prevention is to recognize those patients who are prone to develop sores so that preventive measures of the appropriate intensity can be taken at the earliest possible moment. Research has provided an extremely useful method of measuring the degree to which any patient is at risk. The method, shown in Table 14.1, consists of assessing the patient on a scale from 1 to 4 on five different aspects of his condition. Those patients who score a total of 14 or less on these scales are considered to be at risk and require intensive measures to prevent pressure sores developing.

Traditional preventive methods of treating pressure areas include massage using soap and water, barrier creams and sometimes the application of surgical spirit to the skin. With the exception of gentle washing for hygiene and the use of barrier creams for incontinence, there is probably little or no value in any other of these measures. Indeed, excessive massage and the overuse of soap and water can be harmful.

Table 14.1

Assessment of a patient's risk of forming pressure sores (*From* Exton-Smith, A. N., Norton, D. & McLaren, R. (1962) *An Investigation of Geriatric Nursing Problems in Hospital.* Originally published by the National Corporation for the Care of Old People. Reprinted in 1975 by Churchill Livingstone, Edinburgh.)

Physical condition		Mental condition		Activity		Mobility		Incontinence	
Good	4	Alert	4	Ambulant	4	Full	4	Not incontinent	4
Fair	3	Apathetic	3	Walks with help	3	Slightly limited	3	Occasionally incontinent	3
Poor	2	Confused	2	Chair-bound	2	Very limited	2	Usually — urine	2
Bad	1	Stuporous	1	Bed-fast	1	Immobile	1	Doubly incontinent	1

Useful preventive measures include:

Regular changing of position (2 or 4 hourly).
Inspection of pressure areas at each change.
Keeping the skin clean and dry.
Avoiding friction and abrasion.
Changing linen when wet or soiled.
Using barrier creams for the incontinent.
Avoiding patched sheets.
Improving the patient's nutritional state.
Preventing sliding down the bed by use of a foot board, or slightly elevating the bed foot.
Lifting patients properly (Ch. 2).
Providing local protection for heels and elbows.

Where the patient's illness limits his ability to move or be moved, other aids may be necessary, for example:

Air rings.
Latex foam pads.
Sheepskins.
Pillow packs.
Ripple mattresses or water beds.

There is also a range of more sophisticated equipment, such as the Stryker frame, which is used in nursing spinal injuries (Ch. 3). Other devices include variations on the theme of the fluid-filled mattress. Which ever method is used, there is no substitute for the basic principles of prevention already mentioned, especially the early detection of 'at risk' patients.

Pressure sores should therefore never be regarded as inevitable. Though some will occur, early detection of skin damage and relief of pressure will prevent a superficial lesion becoming deep. Once established, every possible step must be taken to make sores heal as quickly as possible. Obviously further pressure must be avoided entirely. A diet rich in protein with sufficient carbohydrates and supplementary vitamins will aid tissue repair. Anaemia must be corrected, with blood transfusions if necessary.

Attention to the ulcer involves aseptic dressing technique, as would be practised for any wound. Infection is frequently a problem, so cleansing is necessary as well as the removal of dead tissue (sloughs). Packing the ulcer with gauze soaked in *Eusol* or Milton is valuable for cleansing and encourages healing by granulation from the base upwards. Swabs for bacteriological examination must be taken regularly to detect infection. Topical antibiotics in powder or aerosol form will help to control any infection.

Pressure sores heal more quickly if patients can be mobilized. This minimizes the effects of pressure and improves blood flow. Sores which are difficult to heal may eventually require plastic surgery.

Leg ulcers

Chronic leg ulcers are caused mostly by defective venous drainage from a limb. Adequate drainage depends on the pumping action of surrounding skeletal muscle and the presence of valves in the veins. It is significant that the only mammal to suffer from such ulcers is man, who is also the only one to have adopted the upright posture completely. Impairment of drainage often results from thrombophlebitis of deep leg veins (Ch. 7). Eventually valves become defective and blood becomes stagnant in the veins. Varicosities of superficial leg veins and chronic oedema of the lower part of the leg occur. Skin becomes undernourished and devitalized and may become eczematous. Sooner or later an ulcer forms, frequently precipitated by a trivial injury.

Other factors, such as pregnancy, obesity or intra-abdominal tumours, may also hinder venous drainage and lead to ulceration. Ulcers may also result from insufficiency of arterial blood supply. Arteriosclerosis of large arteries in the lower limb cuts down blood flow and, if severe enough, leads to gangrene. Small areas of skin gangrene will develop into ulcers on the legs and feet. Infection of ulcers frequently complicates the situation and hinders healing.

Management

The management of varicose ulcers is aimed mainly at relieving the local oedema and improving venous drainage. If drainage is improved, oedema will subside and healing will begin (Fig. 14.9).

Reduction of weight

Since obesity is often a causative factor of ulcers, weight may have to be lost and the loss maintained.

Exercise

Treatment of varicose ulcers in bed is rarely necessary. Walking should be encouraged and, when standing, calf muscles should be kept contracting and relaxing. When resting, keeping the legs above the level of the trunk promotes venous drainage.

Local treatment

Most methods of treating venous ulcers involve the use of compression bandages and may include local massage. First the ulcer crater is cleaned thoroughly with a solution such as Eusol or Milton. The skin around the edges may then be massaged, gradually working away from the ulcer. Strips of an impregnated bandage such as Uraband, Quinaband or Ichthaband are used to pack the crater. The same bandage is used to bandage the leg up to the knee. An adhesive bandage such as Lestreflex, with lengthways stretch only, is used as a compression bandage applied from the foot up to the knee.

A week is allowed to elapse before the next treatment. After healing, support is still needed. *Tubigrip* is an alternative to elasticated stockings, which may be difficult for patients to put on properly. Recurrence of the ulcers means that varicose veins must be treated.

If the ulcers are due to impaired arterial supply, treatment is often doomed to failure and amputation may be necessary. Some ulcers will heal, but only with difficulty. It is important to screen such patients for diabetes mellitus (Ch. 11). Patients with impaired arterial circulation must be educated in the care of the *ischaemic* limb in order to avoid injury. Cleanliness is essential, with daily washing in warm water and careful drying. The skin between the toes should receive particular attention. Woollen socks are less harmful than nylon but should be free from darns. Well-fitting footwear is necessary, and in cold weather fur-lined boots, though expensive, are valuable. Extra care is needed with corns and toe-nails; these should be left to the skills of a chiropodist.

BURNS

A burn is an injury to tissues which results from the application of heat (moist or dry), electricity, chemicals (acids or alkalis), radiation or friction. Burns may be either superficial or deep. A superficial burn is one in which only the epidermis has been

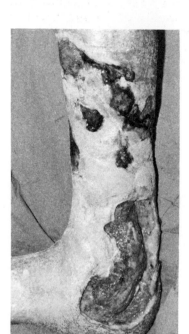

Figure 14.9
Leg ulcer in early stages of healing

injured; this may peel off, leaving the basal cell layer, but it will heal without scarring. A deep burn involves complete skin destruction and possibly the destruction of deeper tissues as well.

Once skin has been destroyed two of its most important functions are lost — the prevention of loss of fluid from the body and protection against infection. Obviously, the more skin that is destroyed the greater will be the effects of losing these two functions. Thus in estimating the seriousness of a burn, the area of skin lost is a very useful guide. It is also useful initially as an indication of how much fluid has been lost and which must, therefore, be replaced quickly. Calculation of the area burned is easily and quickly carried out using the percentages given in Wallace's 'rule of nine' (see also Fig. 14.10):

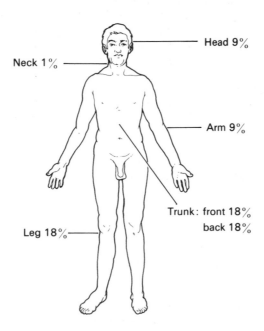

Figure 14.10
Wallace's 'rule of nine'

The depth of a burn will determine how it heals. When only epidermis is destroyed, regeneration will occur from epidermal cells left in sweat glands and sebaceous glands, as well as any remaining basal cell layer. However, if the dermis is also destroyed, regeneration cannot take place. A small amount of epithelium will grow inwards from the margin of the burns, but most healing will be by granulation followed by scar formation. The only way of minimizing this is by skin grafting.

Table 14.2
Percentage of body area of various parts.

Area of body	Per cent of body area
Surface of head	9
Surface of each upper limb	9
Surface of front of trunk	18
Surface of back of trunk	18
Surface of each lower limb	18
Surface of neck	1

Prevention of burns
There are many cases of burning each year and a great number are preventable. Most occur in the home and could be prevented by the exercise of a little common sense. The

vulnerable groups are children between the ages of 1 and 15 years and the elderly. The following are among the most obvious preventive measures:

Young children should never be left alone in the house.
All fires should have approved guards.
Flexes of electrical appliances should be out of the reach of children.
Matches or lighters should never be left out.
Saucepan handles should be turned away from the front of cookers (which should preferably be fitted with guard rails).
Gas cookers are safer if placed away from draughts.
All electrical equipment and flexes should be properly maintained.
Inadequate lighting should be corrected.
When not in use, electrical appliances should be switched off and unplugged, especially at night and on leaving the house.
Care must be taken not to overload power points with too many appliances.
Containers of hot water should not be left unattended nor put on table-cloths, which may be pulled on by a child.
Flame-resistant clothing and nightwear is advisable for children.
Hot water bottles should be protected with a suitable cover.

First aid for burns
The first step is to remove the cause of the burns or extinguish the flames. This can be accomplished by wrapping the part or person in a rug or blanket to exclude air (providing the rug is not made of synthetic material). The first step in dealing with electrical burns is to switch off the current and, if necessary, stop any machinery. Burning clothing must be removed, though not if charred and adherent to the body.

Burned patients are severely shocked. Initially this is neurogenic shock due to pain, but it quickly becomes *oligaemic* as a result of fluid loss and reduction in the volume of circulating blood. Casualties should therefore rest, preferably lying down. Superficial burns should be immersed in cold water or held under cold running water. This cools the part and reduces pain. Also important in minimizing shock is reassurance. Oral fluids may be given, though only small quantities at a time are advisable in case of vomiting. Cold drinks are best.

Scalds will necessitate the removal of soaked clothing. All that is necessary is for the burned area to be covered with clean, dry material, such as part of a clean sheet or a pillow-case. No other substance should be applied.

With chemical burns, as much of the chemical as possible should be washed off with cold running water. A bath or shower may be necessary if large areas are affected.

Finally, there must be no delay in getting the victim to hospital. It must be borne in mind that even a burn of a small area can cause considerable shock, so the patient should be seen in a hospital casualty department.

Hospital care
Shock
In hospital, the primary objective of treatment is to lessen shock, which may be life-threatening. Burns of 10 per cent or more in children and 15 per cent or more in adults can produce shock severe enough to kill. Before treatment begins, a quick assessment of the patient is necessary, though it should not delay treatment. Records of temperature, pulse, respiration rates and blood pressure are essential and should be taken at 15-minute intervals, A blood sample is taken in order to carry out a haemoglobin estimation and *haematocrit*. Fluid replacement begins with an intravenous infusion. A self-retaining catheter is inserted into the bladder and measurement of urinary output is carried out hourly, as well as a record of all fluid intake. The extent of the surface area burned is also considered when deciding on the amount of fluid which should be replaced. Most fluid is lost in the first few hours, so replacement is greatest at that time. Less fluid can be given after the first 24 hours. Nasal, throat and rectal swabs are taken from the patient because of the risk of autoinfection. Pain is severe, so analgesics are given. Regular and frequent observations of the patient's vital signs and a fluid balance record are continued until his condition improves.

Fluids

As was noted before replacement of fluids is a matter of urgency. Since plasma has been lost, plasma is the most suitable replacement. This will maintain osmotic pressure within capillaries and prevent leakage of water into the tissues, a process which would decrease the circulating blood volume and increase shock. *Dextran* solution (high molecular weight), sometimes referred to as a 'plasma expander', has a similar effect. The oral intake of fluids should be encouraged unless vomiting occurs. In the early stages, restriction to 30 or 60 ml of fluid per hour by mouth will help prevent vomiting.

Infection

Prevention of infection is second only in importance to controlling shock. When the patient's condition permits, the burn is cleaned carefully under general anaesthesia. All dead tissue and foreign material are removed. Blisters are snipped with sterile scissors. As well as the risk of septicaemia, infection delays healing and may cause unsatisfactory results. Important among preventive principles are:

Routine nasal swabs from all staff.
Exclusion and treatment of nasal carriers of pathogens.
Exclusion of all staff with respiratory infections and septic skin lesions.
The use of barrier nursing techniques.
The use of sterile bed linen if the exposure method of treating the burn is used.

It should also go without saying that a high standard of environmental hygiene is imperative.

Local treatment

After the initial treatment of a burn, two possible methods of management are available.

Exposure

This allows cooling and drying of the burned surface. Bacterial growth is inhibited by drying and a protective *eschar* forms. In time this will separate and infection beneath it is likely. Surgical excision of the eschar is carried out before this can happen, followed by skin grafting. The advantage of the exposure method is that the risk of infection is minimized and a clean wound suitable for skin grafting is provided. Patients are also generally more comfortable. Total barrier nursing is essential, in a room where the air is filtered and a temperature of 25° or 26°C can be maintained. Sterile bed linen is also necessary.

Occlusion

The other method, using occlusive dressings, has many disadvantages. The most serious of these is that dressings quickly become saturated with exudate from the burn and are an admirable medium for bacterial growth. The dressing next to the burn must be of *Sofra-tulle* or similar material to prevent sticking. It must be covered with layers of sterile absorbent material in a thick pad. The dressing must extend 8 or 10 cm beyond the edges of the burn and be held in place with a crepe bandage. Infection is difficult to prevent, and the patient is frequently uncomfortable.

Skin grafting

Destruction of the skin means that its regeneration is impossible. Unless a skin covering is provided, infection is inevitable and scar tissue will form. A covering for the raw area is provided by split-skin grafts taken from elsewhere on the body and placed on the surface in sheets. The donor area will regenerate its own epithelium from that left in hair follicles and sweat glands; the process takes 2 to 3 weeks. It may be difficult to find sufficient skin to cover a large area, so the grafts may be cut into pieces about the size of postage stamps and laid about 1 cm apart. The gaps then close by growth of epithelium from the edges of the grafts.

To provide immediate covering in very extensive burns where the situation is urgent, a *homograft* may be used. This will be rejected in time but can be life-saving. Early grafting of eyelids and fingers is important to prevent further damage to the eyes and finger tendons, respectively.

Routine skin grafting is usually carried out about 3 weeks after the injury. During this time, dead tissue will have been removed, infections controlled and the patient's nutritional state improved. Care of the grafted area mainly means preventing displacement of the grafts. Unless infection occurs, it will be left covered for about a week. It is then dressed under general anaesthesia, when sutures are removed, collections of blood, serum or pus evacuated and grafts which have not taken removed.

When healing is complete, gentle massage of the graft with lanolin stretches it and keeps it pliable. Grafts over joints may require splinting at night and exercises during the day to preserve the greatest possible range of movements. The donor area is protected by a dressing of Sofra-tulle and left undisturbed for about 2 weeks. When healing is complete the dressing automatically separates from the skin.

Nutrition

Burned patients require a diet rich in protein and high in kilojoules. Daily protein intake should be as high as 150 g, and 16 000 or more kJ should be supplied, depending on the patient's weight. Extra vitamins, especially vitamin C, are also necessary. Correction of anaemia may necessitate the administration of oral iron.

In the early stages, the situation is likely to be complicated by the fact that the patient is severely ill and unlikely to be able to take a normal diet. Nasogastric feeding may then become necessary.

Nursing the burned patient

All the above points require considerable expertise and technical skill. It must also be remembered that basic care, such as washing and treatment of pressure areas, is necessary and will demand considerable patience. Even apparently simple matters such as making the patient comfortable in bed require imagination and ingenuity. Inconceivable difficulties can arise for the patient even when using the bedpan or feeding himself.

The aspect of nursing burned patients most likely to tax the nurse's skill to the utmost is that of maintaining the morale of the patient. It is stating the obvious to say that kindness, sympathy and patience are essential qualities; however, firmness and the ability to encourage self-help rather than dependence are also necessary. Above all, the nurse must remember that the eventual objective is to rehabilitate the patient, returning him to as near normal a life as possible.

NURSING CARE OF PATIENTS WITH SKIN DISORDERS

Rashes, spots and blisters on the skin can be so readily seen that patients are extremely conscious of them, and also very sensitive to the reactions of others to their appearance.

Patients with severe skin disorders will therefore benefit from being nursed in a dermatology unit. Here they will see other patients with similar conditions making progress, and be cared for by nursing and medical staff with expert knowledge. In these units the emotional needs of patients are taken into account, and, as they are not usually incapacitated, they can mix together on a social basis.

Many patients with diseases of the skin do not need to be admitted to hospital, but can be treated as outpatients and care for their skins at home with the help of the family. Regular attendance at clinics provides the psychological support and practical advice necessary. Admission to hospital only occurs as the result of an acute exacerbation of the disease.

The following principles of care will help the nurse to understand the problems encountered by patients and their families, and be able to help them both at home and while in hospital.

Alleviation of itching

Itching is a common experience and can be exhausting and frustrating for the patient. It is first of all essential to observe when itching occurs and to attempt to discover the reason for it. The problem may be more severe at night for example or be aggravated by a particular food or drug. Rest is as important for an inflamed skin as for any other inflamed organ of the body. While it may seem unnecessary to the patient, he should rest in bed initially for a short period to reduce any external stimuli. Mild sedation is sometimes prescribed to help achieve this rest.

The environment should not be too hot, with adequate ventilation, light bed clothes and loose cotton nightwear rather than nylon or wool. Foods that may produce flushing of the skin such as hot, strong tea or coffee, spices or alcohol should be avoided.

The danger of causing secondary infection by scratching must be explained to the patient. Sometimes it is necessary, with a very young child, to apply splints or cotton gloves to prevent the skin being damaged in this way.

If lotions or creams are to be used they should be applied directly after the patient has had a warm bath (33.5–35.5°C) and his skin has been gently dried.

An over anxious patient will be more prone to scratching and if the nurse can help him to identify and deal with his problems he will become more relaxed, and in turn the intensity of itching will be reduced.

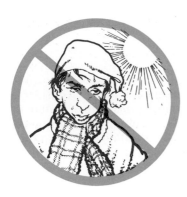

Figure 14.11
Avoid overheating

Maintenance of body fluid
When a large amount of fluid is lost due to formation of *bullae* or in the form of exudate then there must be adequate replacement of fluid by mouth. The patient will also require a diet high in protein to replenish losses.

Emotional adjustment
The nurse can be an active agent in promoting and helping her patient to achieve a state of mind and an attitude towards his skin condition which not only will hasten recovery, but may minimize recurrences of it. She can develop a relationship with her patient which is characterized by his confidence in her, and in which he becomes an equal partner in his care. She must know the effects of skin disease, both conscious and unconscious, on her patient's emotional state. She must also be able to relate these to the severity of the disorder and to the patient's behaviour. Only in this way can the nurse maintain an approach to her patient which is supportive, positive and objective yet sympathetic. The nurse's own behaviour is of paramount importance. She must overcome the natural revulsion that occurs on seeing some forms of skin disease for the first few times, and on no account allow any expression or implication of revulsion or distaste to occur.

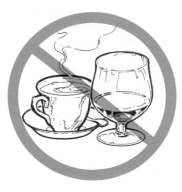

Figure 14.12
Avoid foods causing flushing

Positive steps can be taken to establish communication by taking the patient's hand to examine his fingers or nails. Some of the simple creams can be applied directly by hand if they do not contain steroid preparations. The nurse can also encourage relatives to take part in applying treatment and therefore getting used to touching the patient's skin.

Taking time to sit and talk to her patient also implies that the nurse is not reluctant to spend time in his company.

Apart from the disorders mentioned on page 462 few conditions are infectious or contagious. Patients and relatives need to be aware of this and patients should be encouraged to mix freely together to chat or watch television once they are no longer confined to bed.

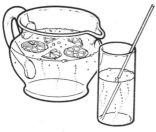

Figure 14.13
Adequate fluid intake

Avoidance of further skin damage
When the patient is bathed it is important to remove moisture from the skin gently by patting dry with a soft towel rather than rubbing a towel briskly on a tender skin. Simple Soap or Emulsifying Ointment B.P. are both suitable cleansers for use in the bath.

No form of 'self medication' should be used by the patient, for example proprietary antiseptics, which if added to the bath water may cause further damage to the inflamed skin. Aperients containing phenolphthalein should also be avoided because it may cause a drug eruption.

Topical treatment should be applied to lesions only, not the surrounding healthy skin.

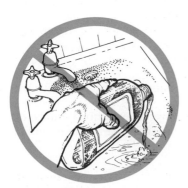

Figure 14.14
Avoid 'self-medication'

Efficient application of medication
The nurse must follow the instructions of prescriptions carefully when applying topical medication. If a patient is to apply medication at home it is usual to give him written instructions which he can read and refer to at leisure. It is important to ensure that he

fully understands these and this is a further opportunity to involve relatives and help them to understand how best they can assist the patient.

Rehabilitation

When an acute exacerbation of a skin disorder has settled, the patient should return to work wherever possible. Occasionally it may be necessary for him to consider a different occupation if it is established that work conditions or some form of irritant or allergen related to his work caused the exacerbation. In cases of this sort, substances known to irritate the skin must be avoided. Sometimes identification of the irritating agent can be confirmed by the use of *patch tests*. (Fig. 14.15).

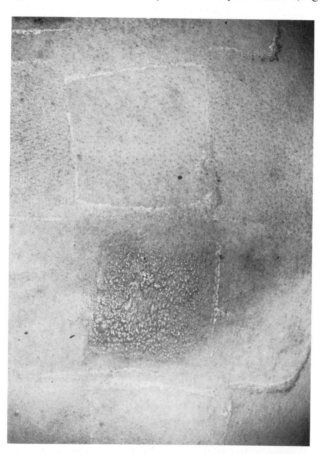

Figure 14.15
Patch test—positive. (Courtesy of Department of Medical Illustration, North Staffordshire Hospital Centre)

Where the skin of the hands is involved, then it is advisable that they are protected when carrying out wet work by wearing rubber gloves lined with cotton ones.

Special cover creams are available which will help to disguise scars or marks on the skin. This is particularly important if the skin of the face is involved. Young adolescents with acne for example need a great deal of help and encouragement to maintain a normal life style.

Topical skin treatments

These are varied as no one treatment is beneficial to all patients or beneficial for the same patient when a skin disorder is at different stages.

Baths, paints, lotions, creams, ointments or pastes may be prescribed singly or sometimes for use in conjunction with each other. It is important to use the treatment in the prescribed form.

Baths
A bath for the patient before application of dressings will help to remove any exudate or crusts that have formed on the skin. Dilute potassium permanganate solution may be prescribed for addition to the bath to reduce the risk of secondary infection developing, and other medicated baths may also be prescribed.

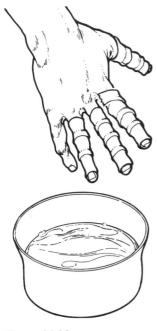

Figure 14.16
Wet dressings
  1. Soak strips of linen in solution
  2. Apply strips to overlap each other
  3. Cover with tubular gauze bandage

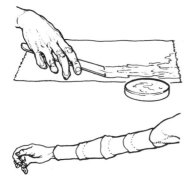

Figure 14.17
Ointment spread dressings
  1. Prepare the spread
  2. Apply the strips of linen, each piece overlapping the previous strip by two-thirds
  3. Secure with tubular gauze or elasticated net

Paints
These may be applied directly to the area required using cotton wool or a small soft brush.

Lotions
Lotions are cooling to the skin and will frequently help to relieve itching. Simple lotions e.g., Calamine Lotion, B.P. may be dabbed on the skin as frequently as the patient desires. Some lotions may be applied in the form of wet dressings (Fig. 14.16) of cotton or linen soaked in the solution. If this method is used then the dressings must be constantly kept in a wet state by adding further lotion or renewing them daily or twice daily. The patient's bed may need to be protected by use of a polythene sheet during treatment.

Creams
These also have a cooling effect on the skin as the water content evaporates and they may need to be reapplied liberally three to four times daily. If dressings are used they should be of cotton or linen as gauze allows the cream to seep through the mesh and is therefore ineffective.

Ointments
Ointments are greasier and may be rubbed in gently and covered with tubular gauze. An ointment may also be spread thinly onto a piece of linen, torn into strips and applied to the area, each strip overlapping the previous one (Fig. 14.17). These are renewed daily and if large areas are to be covered then ideally the patient will wear a pair of old cotton pyjamas in place of the linen strips.

Pastes
Pastes are much thicker and may be applied either using a wooden spatula or a gloved hand. The area is then covered with the tubular gauze.

Paste impregnated bandages are also available which may be left in place for one to three weeks. Pastes will not wash off the skin but can be removed gently using swabs soaked in olive or arachis oil.

Steroid preparations
When these are prescribed they must be used sparingly and with care and on the relevant lesions only, the nurse being sure she does not get them on her own skin. Steroids may also be prescribed in a diluted form.

Occasionally, polythene occlusive dressings are prescribed to enhance the effect of these preparations (Fig. 14.18). The area to be treated is smeared with the prescribed cream and covered with a piece of polythene. The air is excluded from beneath and the edges sealed with adhesive tape. This dressing is left in place for 12, 24 or 48 hours. This method of treatment tends to be reserved for particularly stubborn lesions because of the possible complications, which include increased absorption of steroids, development of infection in the area covered, atrophy of the skin, and development of striae in the area treated.

SOME COMMON SKIN DISORDERS

It has been said, and often quoted that the skin can be affected by anything under the sun, including the sun. Practically any substance which comes into contact with the skin may cause a reaction in some individual. Particularly potent in this respect are chemicals, more of which are being manufactured daily, and used with increasing frequency both in the home and in industry.

Eczema

Eczema and dermatitis are interchangeable terms describing a process taking place in the skin. The epidermis develops small areas of oedema called primary vesicles. Serous fluid escapes when these vesicles are damaged. As the condition becomes more chronic

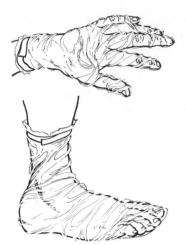

Figure 14.18
Polythene occlusive dressings
1. Apply cream to skin
2. Cover with polythene
3. Smooth to exclude air
4. Seal edge with adhesive tape

Figure 14.19
Contact eczema from rubber in bra
(Courtesy of Department of Medical
Illustration, North Staffordshire
Hospital Centre)

Figure 14.20
Atopic eczema (Courtesy of
Department of Medical Illustration,
North Staffordshire Hospital Centre)

the epidermis becomes thickened, especially if the patient rubs or scratches the area continually. Painful cracks may also appear.

Classification of eczema is difficult because there are so many types, with characteristics of more than one type sometimes appearing in the same patient. The eczema may follow repeated contact with substances such as chemicals or plants causing an allergic or hypersensitive reaction. This is known as contact eczema (Fig. 14.19). Some nurses develop it following handling of penicillin solutions or wearing rubber gloves.

When the reaction has settled down then *patch tests* help in identifying the substance, which can then be avoided. Some substances, known as primary irritants, will produce an eczematous reaction on any person's skin if left in contact for a sufficient length of time. These may be caustic substances such as strong chemical solvents or weaker ones such as detergents.

In endogenous or constitutional eczema the classification tends to be related to the pattern and distribution of the lesions on the body surface (see Table 14.3). One of the commonest types is atopic eczema (Fig. 14.20) which appears in babies a few weeks after

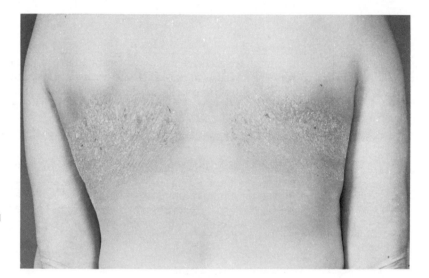

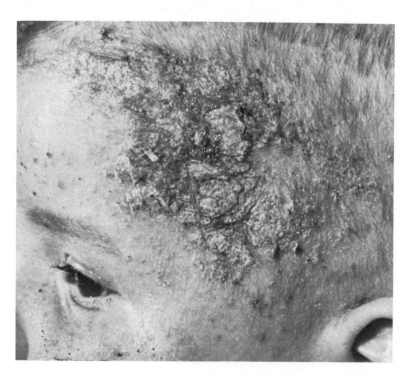

birth. As the child grows the flexures become involved and itching may be intense. There is frequently an associated hay fever or asthma in the patient and a family history of similar disorders.

Table 14.3
Some types of endogenous eczema

Type	Age group	Area of body involved
Atopic	Usually appears at approximately three months Toddlers, young children May persist into adult life	Face, scalp, arms, legs Flexures
Seborrhoeic	Infants Adults	Scalp, forehead, napkin area Face
Nummular or discoid	Young and middle aged	Limbs
Pompholyx	Young adults	Palms and soles
Varicose/stasis	Elderly, poor circulation	Lower leg

Treatment

Treatment of eczema is elimination of any aggravating factor if possible, rest if the eczema is widespread and application of prescribed medication according to the state of the skin. Wet dressings or paints are applied when the skin is very inflamed, and creams, ointments or pastes when the skin is dry and scaly.

Psoriasis

In normal skin the cells of the epidermis move upwards from the basal layer in approximately 25 to 28 days. In psoriasis this process is speeded up creating areas of skin with a rapid turnover of cells which present as raised red plaques covered by silvery scales. The extent of the lesions may vary from one or two small areas, which present very little problem, to widespread plaques causing major disability. Fingernails,

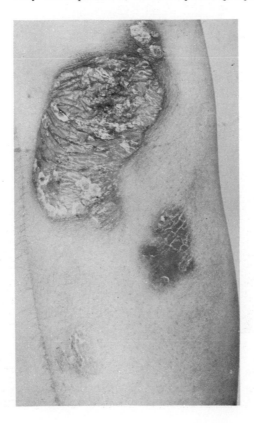

Figure 14.21
Chronic psoriasis, elbow (Courtesy of Department of Medical Illustration, North Staffordshire Hospital Centre)

toenails and the scalp may also be involved. Scalp treatment is particularly difficult because of the hair.

Treatment

This is aimed at remission of the disorder as there is no permanent cure. Individual patients may benefit from different treatments. Topical steroids are only occasionally used because quite often there is a rebound occurrence of the lesions when treatment is stopped.

Tar preparations and dithranol may be used for patients admitted to hospital when psoriasis is particularly disabling. At the present time photochemotherapy (PUVA) is being used in some areas of Britain with success. This involves patients taking a psoralen preparation by mouth or having it applied topically, followed by exposure to long wave ultraviolet light (UVA) for a short time at regular intervals. The possible long term effects of this treatment are still being evaluated.

Patients with widespread psoriasis may become very depressed but they can gain both psychological and practical help and support by joining the recently formed Psoriasis Association in Britain.

Basal cell carcinoma

This is a malignant local tumour which arises from the basal cell layer of the epidermis but rarely metastasises. It is often known as a rodent ulcer which in its commonest form begins as a small *papule* spreading outwards leaving a central ulcer that fails to heal. The edges are raised and pearly. Basal cell carcinoma usually occurs on the face and is a condition mainly of the middle-aged or elderly. It affects, particularly, fair skinned people who have spent a great deal of time in sunshine. It is a very common condition in Australia: in Britain it tends to occur in people who have spent most of their working lives out of doors or who have had some form of arsenic therapy many years before.

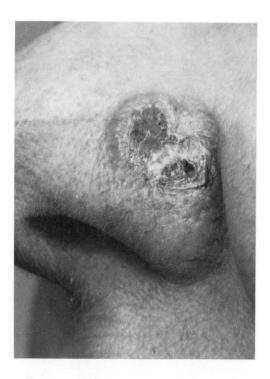

Figure 14.22
Basal cell carcinoma, nose
(Courtesy of Department of Medical
Illustration, North Staffordshire
Hospital Centre)

Treatment

Following biopsy to confirm diagnosis, radiotherapy or surgical excision are the main treatments of choice and patients will normally be treated on an out-patient basis.

Squamous cell carcinoma

Squamous cell carcinoma also arises in the epidermis but is more likely to metastasize. The tumour begins as a small *nodule* which grows to become oval or circular. It may develop into an ulcer with rolled edges. This cancer may arise on the face, lips or back of the hand. These are areas exposed to sunlight but they could have been exposed to chronic trauma or carcinogens such as oil or tar.

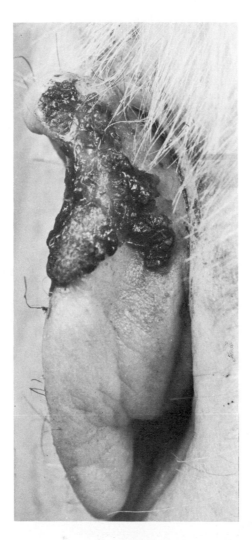

Figure 14.23
Squamous cell carcinoma, ear
(Courtesy of Department of Medical
Illustration, North Staffordshire
Hospital Centre)

Treatment
Following diagnosis by biopsy, treatment is either surgical excision or radiotherapy or both and if treatment is carried out early then prognosis is good.

Drug reactions

Almost any drug given systemically is capable of causing a skin reaction. Some people taking penicillin may develop *urticaria* or a widespread *erythema*, whereas sulphonamides may produce a bullous eruption. Not all drug reactions are allergic. Individuals may have an intolerance to some drugs due to impaired function of the liver or kidney. In this instance the drug cannot be excreted. It builds up to a toxic level and a skin reaction may occur. The drug may have been taken for some time before the reaction occurs. It is important to remember that patients may not even class medications as drugs if they are very familiar with them, for example aspirin.

Treatment

Once the suspected drug has been discontinued, treatment is largely symptomatic. This is a condition in which the nurse who adheres to the previously mentioned principles of skin care can really feel rewarded at seeing the speedy recovery of her patient.

The patient must be made aware of the name of the suspected drug so that he can avoid taking it in the future. Information on drug reactions should always be recorded clearly in the patient's case notes.

INFECTIONS OF THE SKIN
Impetigo

The common causative micro-organism is the staphylococcus, although frequently the streptococcus is also present. Impetigo is usually the result of autoinfection, staphylococci carried in the nose being transferred to the skin by the hands and inoculated by scratching. The scratching may be caused by itching rashes, scabies or lice. Children are especially liable to damage the skin in this way. In men, impetigo may be spread over the face by shaving. Vesicles form, followed by crusting; removal of crusts may actually impede the healing going on beneath. The condition is more unsightly than dangerous (Fig. 14.24) except in babies, in whom it can be fatal. Usually an antibiotic ointment such as Aureomycin clears the condition quickly; widespread lesions may respond to antiseptic baths or may require systemic antibiotic therapy.

Spread of infection to others must be prevented by keeping face flannels and towels separate. Bed linen must not be used by anyone else, and hair-brushes and combs should be used only by the infected person.

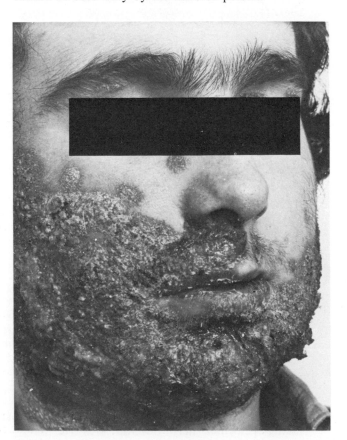

Figure 14.24
Impetigo (Courtesy of Mr McIntyre, Department of Medical Photography, Victoria Hospital, Kirkcaldy)

Boils

These are common infections of hair follicles. More common in seborrhoeic people, they may occur singly or in groups and may recur. Because susceptibility to infection is a complication of diabetes mellitus, people who have outbreaks of boils should be screened for this disease by having their urine tested. Eventually a boil will come to a point, rupture and discharge its contents. This will be followed by healing. Interference with boils should be kept to a minimum. Boils on the face are potentially serious, as septic material may find its way into the bloodstream if they are squeezed and this infection may spread to the brain. The only local treatment necessary is cleansing with antiseptic and application of a protective dressing. Locally applied antibiotic creams may help. Nasal swabs may be taken to identify micro-organisms carried in the patient's anterior nares and to enable specific treatment to be applied.

Spread of infection is especially likely when the boil is discharging. Therefore, frequent change of dry, sterile dressings is important. Carbuncles are similar to boils except that a large area of *necrosis* occurs; they point at a number of places and discharge through multiple *sinuses*. Patients are usually ill, have a pyrexia and should rest in bed. Systemic antibiotic therapy is usually needed.

Erysipelas

The same micro-organism which causes scarlet fever, the haemolytic streptococcus, also causes erysipelas. It usually enters through a break in the skin. At the onset, patients are usually quite ill and pyrexial. The skin around the point of entry becomes inflamed and swollen and there is direct spread of infection to adjacent skin. The face is the commonest site of infection with the organism entering through a small crack in the nostril. The condition responds well to penicillin, administered orally or intramuscularly.

Warts

These are very common virus infections of the skin. They occur often among school children, probably because of the opportunity to spread via towels, swimming pools and gymnasium floors. Most children lose their warts within a few years. Warts on the soles of the feet are known as verrucae or plantar warts. They are painful because of the pressure on them. Warts may be treated in a variety of ways, including the application of carbon dioxide snow, silver nitrate or podophyllin combined with salicylic acid in jelly form. Diathermy can also be used. Verrucae are usually treated with carbon dioxide snow or removed surgically.

Herpes simplex

A cold sore on the lip is a common example of herpes simplex. It is believed that, once acquired, the virus lies dormant, erupting only from time to time and often in association with the common cold, influenza or pnuemonia. The lesion clears up in about 10 days. There is no specific treatment, though an antibiotic cream will prevent secondary bacterial infection.

Herpes zoster

Commonly known as shingles, this painful rash is caused by the virus of chickenpox. The patient is usually adult and not uncommonly elderly when both the rash and the pain, which may persist long after the skin lesion has cleared, cause considerable distress. The virus attacks a posterior root ganglion of the spinal cord and travels along a sensory nerve fibre to reach the nerve endings. A vesicular rash outlines the path of the affected nerve. Treatment consists of analgesics for the very severe pain which occurs. Isolation from as many people as possible prevents spread, especially to children. If, as occasionally happens, the trigeminal nerve is involved, vesicles occur on the face and may cause corneal ulceration on the affected side (Ch. 12).

Fungus infections

The commonest fungus infections of the skin are ringworm and athlete's foot (tinea pedis). Ringworm usually affects the scalp but may affect other parts of the body as well. Recently there has been a decline in scalp ringworm, which is mainly caused by a variety of fungus acquired from cattle. Griseofulvin, an antifungal antibiotic, is effective in treating ringworm but involves a long process of treatment.

Athlete's foot is almost impossible to eradicate completely. Griseofulvin will allay the symptoms but the infection invariably reappears. It may be impossible to decide if it is a relapse or a reinfection, for instance, by other members of the household. Various local applications, each containing a fungicide in a cream base, are available. Castellani's paint helps, as does *Whitfield's ointment*, but neither is used much now.

SKIN INFESTATIONS

Scabies and lice are two of the most common infestations of the skin.

Scabies

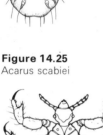

Figure 14.25
Acarus scabiei

Scabies is caused by a mite, the acarus scabiei (Fig. 14.25), and is acquired by direct contact with another person. Several weeks elapse before the main characteristic — itching — commences. Meanwhile the female mite burrows her way into the skin and lays her eggs. These hatch into mites. The burrows can be seen as dark lines about $1\frac{1}{2}$ cm long, usually between fingers, on wrists and in flexures. Scratching causes excoriation and may lead to secondary bacterial infection. Spread to others can occur as a result of prolonged, intimate contact, and nurses and doctors are at risk from infested patients.

Treatment is effective if carried out properly and if it includes all members of the family. First a bath is taken and the whole body thoroughly washed. Then an emulsion of benzyl benzoate must be applied over the whole body surface, from the neck down to the toes. The entire skin must be covered. When this has dried, the patient may dress in clean clothing. Each time the patient's hands are washed the emulsion must be reapplied to them. After 24 hours, a bath may be taken again. Usually one treatment is adequate, though a second may be given if necessary. Quellada is sometimes prescribed as it is effective after only 12 hours.

Lice

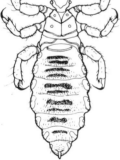

Figure 14.26
Pediculus capitis

Three types of lice infest the human body, **head lice** (pediculus capitis) (Fig. 14.26), **body lice** (pediculus corporis) and **pubic lice** (pediculus pubis). Head lice are the most common and, in spite of generally good standards of hygiene, are still prevalent among many children. Spread occurs easily in schools, so that lice may be found on children whose standard of hygiene at home is high. Head lice live on human blood and lay eggs (nits) which adhere to the hair with a cement-like substance. DDT preparations, never effective for nits, have become less harmful to lice also. However, malathion, in the form of Prioderm lotion, kills both lice and nits.

Table 14.4
Examples of common drugs prescribed topically in skin disorders

Drug	Brand name	Preparation	Condition
Betamethasone valerate	Betnovate	Lotion, cream, ointment	Eczema
Benzyl benzoate	Ascabial	Paint	Scabies, lice
Crude coal tar		In Lassar's paste	Psoriasis
Dithranol	Dithrocream	Cream	Chronic psoriasis
Gamma benzen hexachloride	Quellada	Paint	Scabies, lice
Hydrocortisone acetate	Hydrocortone	Cream, ointment	Eczema
Resorcinal sulphur	Eskamel	Cream	Acne
Zinc paste and icthammol	Icthopaste	Impregnated bandage	Eczema
Potassium permanganate solution		Wet dressings, baths	Eczema

Body lice lay their eggs in the seams of clothing, and an effective way of dealing with them is by dusting with DDT powder. A bath, followed by dressing in clean clothing should result in freedom from infestation.

Although it can be very demanding, nursing patients with skin disease can be greatly rewarding and enjoyable. It is one of the branches of nursing where the nurse is frequently involved in the long-term support of a patient and often his family as well.

SUGGESTED ASSIGNMENTS

1. Draw and label a diagram of the skin and the underlying structures. Show the position of the needle when an intramuscular injection has been given correctly.

2. How would you respond in the following situations?
    a. A friend has a 75-year-old grandmother being nursed at home following a 'stroke' and is worried about pressure sores developing.
    b. You are asked to talk to a group of teenagers at their school and to discuss the effect on the health of the skin of cosmetics and some types of occupation.

3. The skin, being on the outside of the body, is exposed to many harmful agents. It may also reflect internal disturbances, both physiological and psychological. Discuss the value of observing the skin of patients to the diagnosis and treatment of their illnesses.

4. A 17-year-old girl in your ward is recovering from extensive burns to her right arm and neck. Give an account of the emotional problems you might expect her to experience and of how you would help her to cope with these.

FURTHER READING

Huckbody E 1977 Nursing procedures for skin diseases. Churchill Livingstone, Edinburgh
Ingram J T 1970 Nursing care of the patient with skin disease. Heinemann, London
Laing J E, Harvey J 1972 Management and nursing of burns, 2nd edn. English Universities Press, London
Pegum J S, Baker H 1979 Dermatology, 3rd edn. Bailliere Tindall, London
Sneddon I B, Church R E 1976 Practical dermatology, 3rd edn. Arnold, London
Walker K A 1971 Pressure sores prevention and treatment. Butterworth, London
Wilkinson D S 1977 The nursing and management of skin diseases, 4th edn. Faber, London

15. Mental Handicap

This chapter is merely an outline of mental handicap. It is intended as an introduction for nurses who will be gaining experience in this field during training.

A student nurse's first experience in a unit for mentally handicapped people may be somewhat of a surprise, for a number of reasons. These units are run as homes, since most of the residents will spend the greater part of their lives in them. Mentally handicapped people are not to be expected to adapt to an existing ward routine; indeed they may be quite unable to do so. A primary objective of care is to meet their psychological needs, and their environment is arranged with this in mind.

It may also seem strange, to discover that the staff are far less concerned with diagnosis than with each person's abilities and potential for development. The arrangement of material in this chapter takes account of this difference in emphasis. The general approach to the management and care of mentally handicapped people appears first. A brief description of the causes, methods of diagnosis and the general features of individuals with mental deficits is given towards the end of the chapter.

CARE OF THE MENTALLY HANDICAPPED

At one time care consisted of providing a secure environment. It is realized now that many of these people have capacities for development; consequently opportunities and stimulation should be provided to enable and encourage them to attain their highest potential.

Philosophy

The mentally handicapped person is a human being with not only the right to life but the right to a quality of life in keeping with human dignity. Services for the mentally handicapped ideally should have the attainment of this right as their main objective. This presupposes the development of potential no matter how limited the final achievement may be.

The multidisciplinary approach to assessment

Assessment is carried out on a multidisciplinary basis. The mentally handicapped person's needs are assessed and individual programmes are tailored to meet these needs. Reassessment is an essential part of any programme to evaluate progress and for further planning.

Medical assessment is carried out by paediatricians, psychiatrists and orthopaedic and ENT surgeons. Clinical and educational psychologists have much to contribute in assessment, programme planning and remedial advice. Speech therapists, physiotherapists, occupational therapists, remedial gymnasts and teachers all have expertise which is invaluable in assessment. The social worker takes a full social history, which is necessary in identifying family problems. The nurse specially trained in mental handicap nursing is in a unique position in the assessment team, especially if the patient is in hospital. Nurses collectively are with the person 24 hours a day and are therefore able to observe behaviour patterns, frequency and types of epilepsy, communication problems, abilities in the activities of daily living and reactions to medication.

In recording behaviour, one of the most popular and useful charts available is the Gunzburg Progress Assessment Chart of Social Development. There are several types. Each type contains a useful chart of abilities related to self-help, communication, socialization and occupation and, properly used, these records show at a glance the areas in which the person has developed skills and where progress has yet to be made.

The multidisciplinary approach to management

Mental handicap is a 'life-sized' problem because in most cases there is no cure; therefore, the mentally handicapped person needs programmed management that extends from birth throughout his life. Mental handicap is a multifaceted problem: it occurs in childhood, but mentally handicapped children grow up; therefore services must provide for all age groups and for varying levels of intelligence.

Efficient management can only be achieved through a multidisciplinary approach where each 'specialist' uses his skills to develop the individual's potential to the fullest. Services should be the responsibility of a multidisciplinary team serving an area. The family with a mentally handicapped child is a family with stress: for the parents there is the strain of knowing that the problem will remain throughout their child's life, and for the other children a handicapped brother or sister can cause various problems. The family needs to be in touch from the very beginning with some person or group who can not only give support but also offer concrete, practical advice about programmed management all along the line. Ideally, services should provide early identification of the handicap, assessment of the potential development, a planned schedule from childhood through to adulthood and genetic counselling. The pivot of such services would be residential accommodation on either a long- or a short-term basis.

The physical environment

The ward, home unit or group home should be as home-like as possible, with colours, textures and ornamentation used skilfully to provide sensory stimulation; but there should also be a more subdued, restful area where patients can relax and be quiet on occasion. This is important for all age groups. Where rooms are set aside for specific learning activities, however, it is more practical to have the minimum of distracting stimuli so that the person with the patient does not have to compete for his attention. Necessary materials can be brought in for the session. In this way the environment can be manipulated to promote learning.

Adequate ventilation, heating and lighting are also very important. In some instances extractor fans may be necessary to allow the air in a room to be changed quickly. Lighting can be used effectively in adding to the overall home-like effect. Surfaces should be easily cleaned. Facilities for bathing and toilet training should be adequate both functionally and in providing privacy. In children's units play equipment of a suitable type should be provided as well as the space to store it.

Experiments have shown that ideally patients should be cared for in small groups in a family-like situation. The environment must also be safe as the mentally handicapped are very accident prone due to physical clumsiness and their inability to judge distances. They are also unable to recognize a potentially harmful situation.

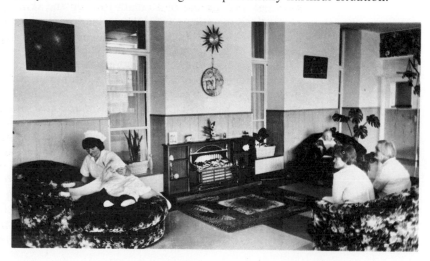

Figure 15.1
Restful area where patients can relax

Nursing care

Nursing care means doing for patients what they are unable to do for themselves. However, nursing the mentally handicapped also includes teaching patients to do these things for themselves. It involves providing for the physical, psychological and social well-being of the patient. There are two main areas of nursing activity. One is to ensure that the person's basic needs are met; the other is to see that the patient uses and develops, as fully as possible, whatever abilities he possesses. Considerable importance is attached to the surroundings in which these activities take place and much thought is expended to make the milieu as normal as possible.

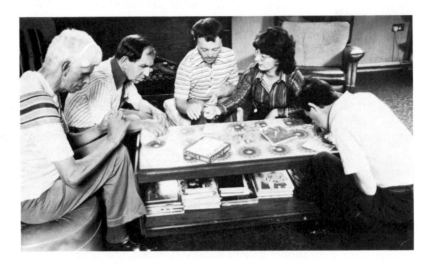

Figure 15.2
A small group of patients enjoying a game of bingo

The concept of normalization, which was first developed in the Scandinavian countries, is that the mentally handicapped individual should be allowed to develop in as natural a setting as possible and be given access to facilities, pleasures and comforts enjoyed by ordinary people.

The aim of a nursing care programme for the mentally handicapped is to develop potential in such a way that the person is capable of returning to the community or, if this is not possible, of living a useful and contributory life in a sheltered environment. In very high dependency patients where the above aims are unrealistic, the objective is to improve the quality of life in any way possible; for example a patient who is mobile, if only in a wheel-chair, has more opportunities than a patient confined to bed.

Nursing care of a high quality is the first step in socialization. Good basic cleanliness does much to dispel the all too familiar image of hospitals for the mentally handicapped. Careful attention to grooming can camouflage defects, and the individual consequently becomes more socially acceptable. Attention must be paid to skin care. Daily bathing is essential and the use of a cream to keep the skin soft and supple is recommended, particularly in patients with Down's syndrome; older patients can be taught to attend to their own skin care. Oral and dental care is of particular importance for all patients; it becomes of even greater moment when certain anticonvulsants are being given. Phenytoin, for instance, causes gingivitis.

Care should be taken of the eyelids with emphasis on the prevention of *blepharitis*. The nose should be kept clean and, where possible, children should be trained to do this for themselves. A persistent discharge from the nose or ear should be investigated since it could mean the patient has pushed a foreign body into one of these orifices (Ch. 13), which might not be obvious on initial examination. Nails should be kept short and clean. Clothing is very important and should be attractive, well-fitting, individual and durable, with colours and materials properly matched.

A well-balanced diet is important and foods likely to cause diarrhoea, particularly in the high dependency patient, should be avoided. On the other hand, the inclusion of roughage can help prevent constipation. Adequate fluid intake must be maintained because patients are often unable to indicate thirst. Special diets are necessary in certain conditions such as phenylketonuria (Ch. 4). In the management of bladder and bowel the objective is, if possible, to train the patient to control these functions. Where this is impossible, nursing ingenuity is taxed in caring for the incontinent patient and, at the same time, maintaining a fresh, well-ventilated environment.

Special nursing care is necessary in the management of many conditions such as Sturge-Weber syndrome (p. 478–79), hydrocephalus (p. 479) and the biochemical disorders. It is also necessary in conditions which complicate mental handicap.

Complications of mental handicap requiring special care

Epilepsy

Epilepsy is a symptom of an underlying cerebral disorder. There are various types of epilepsy but the same principles of nursing management apply for all. It is important to ensure that blood levels of anticonvulsants are maintained and to observe the effects and side-effects of these drugs. Special care is necessary when anticonvulsants are being changed.

Cerebral palsy

This term refers to muscular disabilities resulting from either damage to or impaired development of the brain. The most important single cause is brain damage during birth. The special management of cerebral palsy includes the prevention of deformity, the management of appliances and the nursing care following orthopaedic surgery.

Hyperkinesis

The hyperkinetic syndrome describes a state of hyperactivity or violent motor unrest. It occurs in children, is associated with cerebral damage and is a condition requiring skilled management. The fostering of the nurse–patient relationship is all important in reducing the level of anxiety in the child. These children need periods of calm during the day when they can sit quietly with a nurse. Soothing background music is helpful. Constant observation is necessary to prevent accidents.

Treatment includes drug therapy and, in severe cases, brain surgery.

Disturbed sleep patterns

Disturbed sleep patterns call for ingenious nursing management. Patients are often unable to say if or why they are uncomfortable or that they are in pain. It is the nurse's responsibility to recognize and interpret the patient's behaviour; for instance screaming and head scratching may denote toothache. The development of observational skills is very important in caring for mentally handicapped people because of their difficulty in communicating normally.

Aggression

Aggressive behaviour can be very disruptive in a therapeutic environment. The nurse must first deal with the immediate situation and then find out the cause of the outburst. Management may need to be modified as a preventive measure.

Mental illness

Neuroses and psychoses (Ch. 16) may be superimposed on mental handicap and these conditions need special management.

Physical illness

Congenital heart defects, diseases of the respiratory system and skin conditions are fairly common among the mentally handicapped and require special nursing management. In some instances patients are returned to their parent hospital 48 hours after an operation and will need appropriate nursing care.

Promoting the development of abilities

Physical

Due to delay in maturation the mentally handicapped person's physical rate of growth is slowed down. Control of head movements, sitting and walking are delayed; muscle co-ordination is poor and patients with Down's syndrome have hypotonic (flabby) muscles.

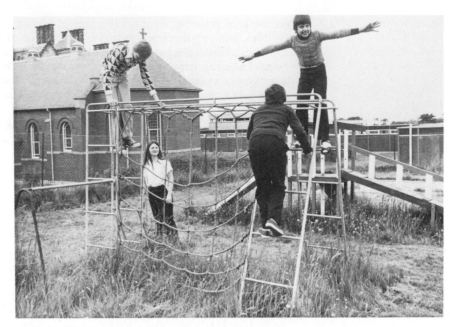

Figure 15.3 Opportunity for climbing and balancing in an adventure playground

When cerebral palsy is present there is an added problem of muscle spasm interfering not only with limb movement but also with swallowing and speech.

In some instances the development of muscle control and co-ordination is a preliminary to acquiring elementary self-help skills. The nurse, working in conjunction with the physiotherapist and remedial gymnast, can do much to aid physical development. Passive and active exercises and positioning to prevent or correct deformities can be programmed to meet individual needs. Muscle relaxation exercises using water play — if possible in a swimming pool — are beneficial. Movement to music can make exercises more fun. Allowing children scope and opportunity to walk, climb, balance, skip and sometimes ride ponies can also help. For children who have not learned to walk the use of standing and walking frames allows the experience of weight-bearing and balance and the development of *proprioception*.

Psychological
Psychological development can be considered in two areas — emotional and *cognitive*.

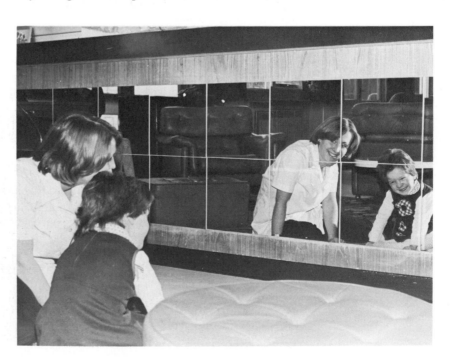

Figure 15.4
Using a floor level mirror to teach posture and body image

Emotional

An important aspect of nursing care is to provide an emotional climate which is warmly accepting, where the person is first of all an individual and only secondly a mentally handicapped individual. In this way a sense of security, which is necessary before any learning can take place, is developed. A positive approach where praise rather than blame is used can be strongly motivating.

Consistency in approach is important because inconsistency causes confusion in the mentally handicapped person who has difficulty in adapting to change. When environmental changes have to be made, the patient should be well prepared for them by simple explanations. Such measures can do much to prevent the emotional outbursts that are caused by frustration when the patient is unable to cope with differing demands.

Expectations of achievement should be realistic: patients can feel hopeless and give up trying if they sense staff disappointment, and low dependency patients can be surprisingly perceptive. Nurses and other team members should be able to establish

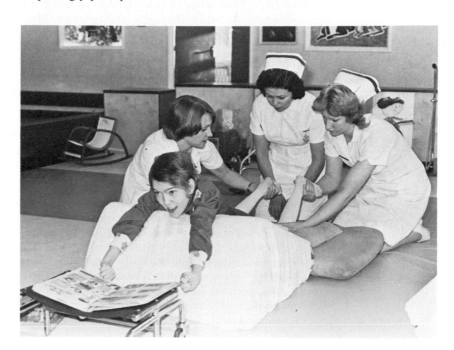

Figure 15.5
Positioning to correct deformity

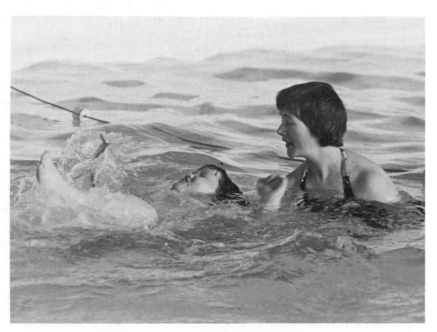

Figure 15.6
Water, a necessary therapeutic tool

rapport with the patients as this is essential in meeting and assessing emotional and other needs. Parents or parent substitutes should if possible be kept in close contact with children. The nurse's role is that of a therapist and not a parent substitute. However, when a child has no parents the nurse should ensure that he does not suffer emotional deprivation while in the nurse's care.

Cognitive

A knowledge of cognitive development is necessary in understanding the mentally handicapped person's difficulty in learning. The mentally handicapped person receives information through the senses, but he has difficulty in interpreting and giving a meaning to these sensations. The nurse in constant contact with mentally handicapped children should ensure that all the various aspects of a situation are clearly seen, felt and heard so that *perception* is made easier. Meaningful perception also depends on past experiences; therefore, the nurse should give the children as wide a variety of experiences as possible so that the introduction of new stimuli can be more easily assimilated.

Because a child's language ability helps him to correlate his memory of past experiences and his understanding of new ones, it is important to extend his vocabulary. He should be encouraged to use words in ordinary conversation. Signs or other forms of communication should not be accepted if a patient is capable of verbalizing, but when there is no verbal ability it is important that the nurse talks to these patients and develops a communication link on non-verbal levels. Since these children have a short *attention* span, simple sentences should be used in giving instructions; the child's name should be called first to attract his attention; and where possible the nurse should sit or kneel in front of the child on his physical level. If such methods are not used, verbal instructions may be lost in the background noises surrounding the child. The nurse, speech therapist, psychologist and teacher work closely together in developing language ability.

Social

It is generally accepted that almost all human behaviour is learned including basic skills such as walking, eating, washing, dressing and control of elimination. These skills are generally recognized as the activities of daily living. In normal children this learning takes place informally at home. In mentally handicapped children, however, these skills will not be acquired automatically but will need to be taught, that is informal learning is unlikely. Nursing care, therefore, must include the assessment of stages of readiness for training, provide base line data and record and report accurately observations on behaviour, both orally and in writing. Nurses must be able to programme and facilitate the learning of these basic skills.

THERAPEUTIC TECHNIQUES
An outline of skill training

Some basic principles can be applied in teaching either simple or (later) more complicated tasks:

1. The target behaviour should be defined and an assessment made of the individual's readiness for the particular type of response.

2. The task should be analysed, that is the skill to be taught should be closely examined and broken down into simple steps.

3. Each step should be taught using the same sequential pattern at each performance.

4. As each step is being taught, simple verbal instructions should be given together with a demonstration, making sure the child can see clearly and follow what is being done. It may be necessary to sit or stand beside the child to avoid confusion between right and left.

5. Corrections should be made where necessary, but at first slow, clumsy attempts should be accepted until the child becomes more adept. Encouragement should be given when the child shows even the slightest approximation of the desired result.

6. The child should be allowed to practice the skill until it is overlearned, that is until it becomes habitual.

7. Later, observation will be necessary to ensure that the skill is maintained.

8. Mirrors can be used in teaching skills such as hair care and dressing.

9. Distractions should be removed while trying to gain the child's attention.

Behaviour modification

Behaviour modification is the application of learning theory to the changing of human behaviour. It is based on the stimulus–response (S–R) theory. The principle involved is that if a behaviour is reinforced or rewarded it will be repeated.

Reinforcements

Reinforcements can be positive (pleasant) or negative (unpleasant); it is usually better to use positive reinforcements. Before deciding on reinforcements an assessment must be made as to what will be rewarding to the person. For children incentives such as sweets, social praise or social approval can be used. In some instances tokens are given which can be exchanged later for money or other suitable rewards.

The reinforcer should be given as soon as the desired behaviour has occurred. Care must be taken not to reinforce undesirable behaviour that may occur at the same time. It is also very important to be invariably consistent in the use of reinforcements. Initially one cannot expect a perfect response, but when the child's response approximates desired behaviour he is rewarded; this is called shaping. In this way the behaviour required is gradually 'shaped' or built up. A negative reinforcement is used when correcting undesirable behaviour and could take the form of suitable punishment such as ignoring attention seeking when it occurs.

Behaviour modification is becoming more widely used in the care of the mentally handicapped. Nurses are involved in these programmes and need to understand the underlying psychological principles. In conjunction with psychologists they help to devise and supervise these programmes.

Play therapy

Children learn through play; therefore nurses with the help of psychologists should devise and carry out play programmes suitable for individual children to help develop imagination, language, body image and sensory and motor abilities. It must be understood that play will not occur spontaneously in mentally handicapped children but must be developed by adults who guide but do not intrude. A box of clothes for dressing up, a full-length mirror, a play house, dolls that can be dressed and undressed are among useful, easily obtained equipment.

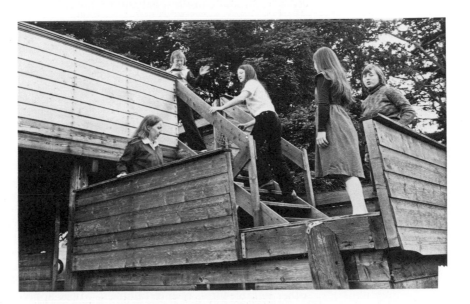

Figure 15.7
Most children enjoy playing in a tree house

An adventure playground planned with imagination and insight into children's developmental needs can be an asset. Most children love a tree house where they can really let their imagination run riot. Safety precautions must, however, be implemented.

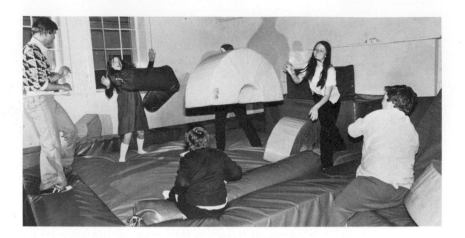

Figure 15.8
Fun and games in a safe
environment

The use of 'self' as a therapeutic tool

'Imitation is the sincerest form of flattery'
Mentally handicapped persons also learn by identification and imitation; the nurse, therefore, can use her own personality as a therapeutic tool in teaching sociotherapeutic skills either to individuals or to groups. In this way the nurse can help the patient to establish meaningful relationships, behave in a socially acceptable way in a group situation and communicate his needs and opinions to others. Depending on the strength of the nurse–patient relationship the nurse is in a position to use social approval as a reinforcer and to counsel and guide patients. For teenagers and older mentally handicapped persons group therapy can provide a useful learning situation.

Socialization

For both children and adults more sophisticated social training should take place as far as possible outside the hospital, using community resources. When the hospital has a holiday home at its disposal there is a tremendous opportunity for social orientation. Resourceful staff can allow patients to shop, plan menus and organise leisure activities in much the same way as do normal people. However, much teaching must go on at hospital level before this kind of adaptation can occur. For adult patients training in self-help and self-care form the basis for socialization. Ideally children should be so trained that when they reach adulthood they will have achieved at least marginal independence, provided they have the initial potential.

Education and training

Since the mentally handicapped are late developers it is only reasonable that education should be nearly continuous. Further education in areas such as cookery, housewifery, dressmaking, beauty culture, as well as academic subjects is invaluable for women. Various areas in the hospital can be used for occupational training. The laundry, kitchen and wards provide training opportunities which, if planned, supervised and evaluated, can provide patients with practice in various household and occupational skills.

Occupational and industrial therapy departments can provide both training for rehabilitation and work for long-stay patients. The ability to work and to receive financial remuneration for it satisfies an individual's ego. Acquiring self-confidence and social poise can be helped by recreational activities such as dancing, ice skating, clubs and other suitable forms of entertainment. Music appreciation, hand work and games can also be taught so that leisure time can be used constructively.

Sex education is important and for young adults individual and group counselling sessions are useful.

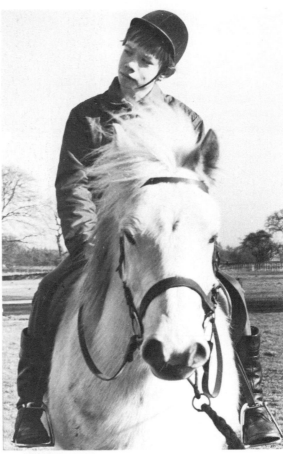

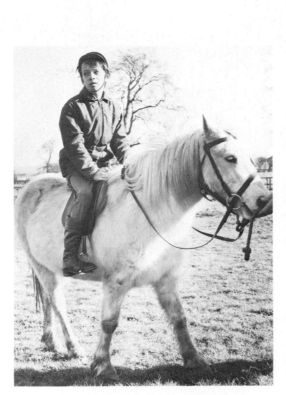

Figures 15.9 and 15.10
Riding

SUPPORT FOR THE FAMILY

The nurse trained in the field of mental handicap needs to be able to counsel, support and advise parents and others in aspects of caring and training. She should be able to identify stress in the family. Parents often have a guilt complex about their handicapped child especially if they are unable or unwilling to care for the child at home. Empathy alone is not enough, and the nurse must be able to support, guide and give practical help. It is possible for a ward sister to help to support a mother whose child has been discharged home, either by visiting or simply by being available at the other end of a telephone. In this way skills, knowledge and attitudes can effectively be imparted to parents and others.

The services available in Great Britain to patients living at home are noted in Chapter 18. Help may be offered by voluntary organizations too: the National Society for Mentally Handicapped Children gives help and advice whenever possible.

The emergence of the community nurse trained in mental handicap has been an added support for the family of a handicapped child living in the community. Her role is to assess the needs of the child in the home, devise programmes for the child's development and advise the parents about specific problems such as behavioural problems or physical problems. (Nurses can also use opportunities to educate the public in the understanding of mental handicap. Involvement in voluntary organizations gives an opportunity for education and support.)

CO-ORDINATION OF CARE

The nurse is in a position to co-ordinate the efforts of the other members of the therapeutic team. A patient's programme must be co-ordinated to gain the maximum effect from all the various specialist therapists. In some instances stimuli received from other therapists will need to be interpreted for the child. He will also need help and encouragement, as well as the opportunity, to practice new-found skills, and will need a

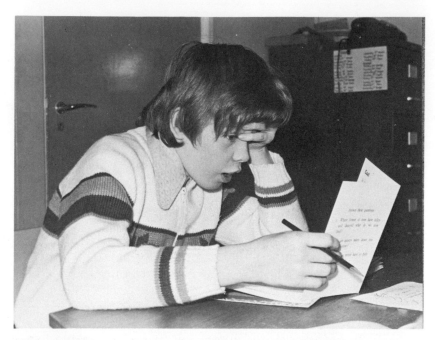

Figure 15.11
An individualized educational
programme meets the child's needs

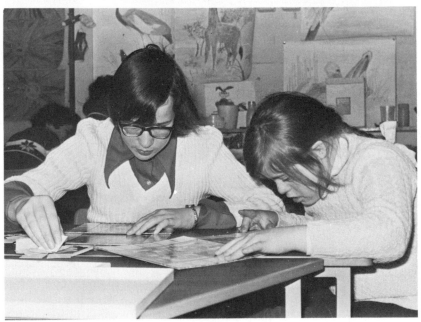

Figure 15.12
Interesting work will gain children's
attention

considerable amount of support and understanding when struggling with new learning experiences.

SOME CAUSES OF MENTAL HANDICAP

Genetic anomalies

This is a general term for a large group of conditions. There are two main subdivisions:

    1. Conditions associated with abnormalities of *chromosomes*, either the *autosomes* or the sex chromosomes.

    2. Disorders of metabolism. This range of maladies results from an inability to make normal use of a normal constituent of the diet.

Disturbances of development

Fetal development may be adversely affected during gestation (prenatally). *Perinatal* (around and during birth) and *neonatal* (within the first month of life) misfortunes may also result in mental handicap.

DIAGNOSIS

A history of the pregnancy and of the perinatal and postnatal periods is essential. Details of other pregnancies and of the mother's general health are taken. A physical examination including a full neurological examination is performed. Various diagnostic tests such as chromosome counts, haematological investigations, chromatography, X-rays and EEGs may be carried out. In the case of children a full developmental history should be taken.

GENERAL FEATURES OF MENTAL HANDICAP

A mentally handicapped person seems 'odd' because of appearance and behaviour.

Physical appearance

Many abnormal physical features can be present especially when mental handicap is as a result of genetic factors. (For an example, see below under Down's syndrome.)

Psychological features

Psychologically the mentally handicapped person cannot think or formulate ideas adequately; these defects together with a short attention span make learning difficult. Normal people appear to have a filtering mechanism whereby they can concentrate on one of several presenting stimuli. The mentally handicapped person is often unable to select the appropriate stimulus and therefore tries to pay attention to several at one time; he is consequently easily distracted.

Behavioural disorders

A mentally handicapped person may also suffer from behavioural disorders such as distractedness, hyperactivity, hyper-reactivity, perseveration, awkwardness, destructiveness and aggression. Motor performance habits such as head banging, rocking and other stereotyped mannerisms may be present.

Social immaturity

As learning is slow in all areas, social maturity is delayed or non-existent. For the normal person much social learning is acquired informally in the family situation and later among peer groups. The mother, once she begins to say 'no' to her child, is interpreting society's standards for him and he consequently learns what is acceptable and unacceptable in the society. For the mentally handicapped child this kind of learning is a very slow process. He lives very much in the 'here and now' and is unable to carry over learning from past experiences and to foresee the results of his actions, thereby impairing the acquisition of social maturity.

Associated conditions

Associated conditions such as epilepsy, cerebral palsy, congenital heart defects, susceptibility to chest infections and visual and hearing defects may also be present.

Emotional disturbances resulting from socially inadequate or culturally defective homes or from disturbances in the mother – child relationship may also occur.

THREE EXAMPLES OF COMMON CLINICAL PROBLEMS

The following disorders are among the commonest conditions associated with mental handicap.

Down's syndrome

People with Down's syndrome have many obvious physical characteristics in common. The thick, everted lips, large, fissured tongue, eyelids with an *epicanthic fold* and flattened bridge of nose give the typical 'mongoloid' features. The short stature, clumsy gait due to poor muscle co-ordination, awkwardness of hand movements and undersized stature complete the picture. Hands and feet show *dermatoglyphic* peculiarities. These characteristics are so noticeable that a preliminary diagnosis will probably be made soon after birth.

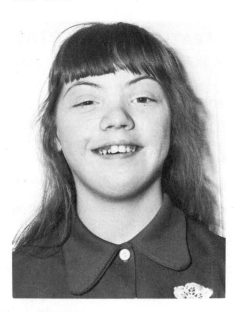

Figure 15.13
Down's syndrome

Nursing care

Many physical defects are associated with the syndrome, notably heart malformations (Ch. 7), susceptibility to mouth and gum infections and, most marked of all, predeliction to respiratory disease. About half the children born with Down's syndrome die of bronchopneumonia (Ch. 6) in the early years of life. The physical manifestations of disease require the same care and treatment as that accorded to any other child.

The degree of mental retardation varies considerably. Some children are severely handicapped, others may become self-supporting, especially if employment can be offered in a sheltered workshop.

It is generally accepted that children with Down's syndrome need intensive mental and physical stimulation during the first year of life. Marked improvement in development has been claimed when this form of therapy has been used.

The happy and affectionate dispositions of these children evoke correspondingly warm and tender responses from their families and from other people who become responsible for their care.

Sturge–Weber syndrome

Sturge–Weber syndrome is a condition of obscure aetiology associated with mental handicap. The essential pathology is angiomatosis of the skin and the leptomeninges. The facial haemangioma is usually confined to half the face in a pattern similar to that of the branches of the trigeminal nerve. It may, however, be bilateral and present on other parts of the body. The areas of meningeal thickening with venous angiomatosis are

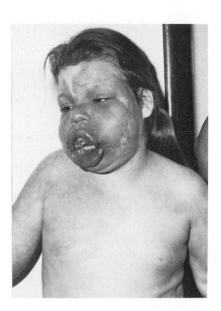

Figure 15.14
Sturge—Weber syndrome

usually found over the occipital lobe and on the same side as the facial naevus. Most patients have focal motor seizures. They may also have spastic hemiplegia.

Nursing care

Special nursing care involves care of the eyes and the mouth. Following epileptic seizures observations are very important as intracranial bleeding may occur. The same precautions are necessary if the child should fall and have even a slight head injury.

Hydrocephalus

In hydrocephalus there is an increased accumulation of cerebrospinal fluid within the ventricles of the brain. (Ch. 3.) There are many possible underlying causes, some of which may be treated surgically. The resulting pressure causes the bones of the skull to separate, the skull circumference to increase, the ventricles to become distended and the brain substance to be compressed.

Nursing care

If the head is grossly enlarged these children are unable to move from their cots. Therefore, imagination is necessary to improve the quality of life they can enjoy; in particular, they like to be able to see people and their surroundings and their posture in bed should permit this. The weight of the head causes great pressure on the scalp and pressure sores can occur; careful positioning with the use of soft pillows can prevent them.

When lifting the child from the cot the head must be supported before moving the child's body. It must be remembered that a hydrocephalic child has the same need for love and cuddling as a normal child and this need not be neglected provided the nurse acquires skill in handling the child.

GROWTH POINTS

There is need for much more research in the field of mental handicap particularly in the area of behavioural management. Community care needs to be extended far beyond that available at present. There should be more support for the mentally handicapped and their families, more training centres for children and adults in the community and more sheltered workshops. Finally it is important to realize that mental handicap is a multifaceted problem for which no one discipline has all the answers. There is need for efficient co-operation and participation on the nurse's part as a member of a therapeutic team.

SUGGESTED ASSIGNMENTS

Project

1. Think about a patient with Down's syndrome you are helping or have helped to nurse in hospital. Could she have been looked after in her own home? What help would the family have needed? Was it available? What would the advantages and disadvantages have been for your patient and her family?

2. Select one or two patients who for some reason have been prevented from carrying out their usual occupation for a period of time. Study carefully the effect this has had upon the behaviour of each individual and the reactions of his family and other patients.

Discussion topics

1. How has the experience you gained during your time in a unit for the mentally handicapped helped you to improve nursing care in other clinical areas?

2. Mental handicap is commonly regarded as causing a range of disadvantages. Consider ways in which mentally handicapped persons make a positive contribution to our society.

FURTHER READING

Crome L, Stern J 1972 Pathology of mental retardation, 2nd edn. Churchill Livingstone, Edinburgh
Finnie N R 1968 Handling the young cerebral palsied child at home, 2nd edn. Heinemann, London
Gunzburg H C 1973 Social competence and mental handicap, 2nd edn. Bailliere Tindall, London
Kirman B, Bicknell J 1975 Mental handicap. Churchill Livingstone, Edinburgh
Marais E, Marais M 1976 Lives worth living. Souvenier Press Educational and Academic Ltd, London

16. Mental Disorder

To be sick in body evokes sympathy; to be sick in mind incurs laughter, disgust and ridicule, bringing shame to the individual and his family. In the early nineteenth century such sentiments resulted in the building of huge, self-contained asylums, places of refuge for the mentally disturbed. The asylums were built on the out-skirts of towns, surrounded by high walls and camouflaged by trees. Their inaccessibility discouraged frequent visits and, once committed there, the inmates soon became the forgotten people.

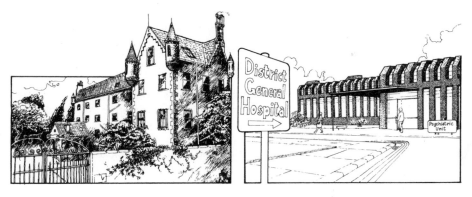

Figure 16.1
Changing face of psychiatric treatment Left: Asylum 1950 Right: Psychiatric department 1980

Remnants of the stigma attached to mental illness linger on, but fortunately more people are recognizing that treatment in the early stages of mental disease can make life more worthwhile for the patient and his family. Instead of hiding the sick relative from prying eyes, they are bringing him forward for treatment.

This change in attitude is reflected in the change in psychiatric hospitals from places of custodial care to places providing a therapeutic environment around which the whole range of psychiatric services can revolve.

Much active treatment is done in out-patient departments, particularly for people suffering from the 'stress' diseases of modern living. With the help of new treatment methods, including drug therapy, more and more people are managing to cope with their illnesses at home, perhaps requiring only short periods in hospital.

Long-term psychiatric hospital patients are mainly psychotics who have lived most of their adult lives in hospital and now have nowhere to go. Many of these have been rehabilitated — or could be if sufficient places were available — to live in half-way houses, which provide a form of community living away from the hospital environment but not completely out of its control. This move towards community psychiatry has been aided considerably by organizations which, among other services, provide essential transport for patients to out-patient clinics, day hospitals and recreational activities. They give care and support where it is desperately required.

Mental disease can be just as debilitating as physical disease and can cause even more disruption to the life of the patient and his family. The psychiatric services try to improve and maintain not only the patient's mental health but also that of the family unit.

The WHO has prepared a classification of mental disorders (Table 16.1), and the nursing care of patients with the commonest of these conditions is outlined in this chapter. The nurse should realize, however, that it is very difficult to categorize psychiatric illnesses because a patient's symptoms do not always fit neatly into pigeon-holes.

The **neuroses** are a group of mental disorders, without any demonstrable organic basis, in which the patient may have considerable insight and unimpaired reality testing; that is, he usually does not confuse his morbid, subjective experiences and fantasies with external reality. Behaviour may be greatly affected, although usually remaining within socially acceptable limits; personality is, however, not disorganized. The principal manifestations include excessive anxiety, hysterical symptoms, phobias, obsessional and compulsive symptoms and depression.

Table 16.1
Mental disorders (Based on WHO international classification)

Neuroses	Psychoses	Dementia
Reactive depression	Endogenous depression	Presenile
Anxiety states	Involutional depression	Senile
Obsessive compulsive states	Manic depressive psychoses	Arteriosclerotic
Phobias	Organic psychoses	
Hysteria	Schizophrenias	
Anorexia nervosa	Paranoid states	
	Alcoholism	
	Drug addiction	
	Personality disorders	

The term **psychoses** encompasses those conditions in which impairment of mental functions has developed to a degree that interferes grossly with insight and the ability to meet some of the ordinary demands of life or to make adequate contact with reality.

Mental disorder can also be described in relation to normal behaviour. Normal behaviour can be defined as socially acceptable behaviour in a given culture. Any exaggeration of or deviation from this concept of mental health can be described as mental illness.

Many people are unable to cope with the stresses of everyday living and express their difficulties through an extravagant response that is termed a neurotic illness. Neurosis is based on learnt behaviour and does not involve the whole of the personality; it is a reaction to stressful circumstances in a personality predisposed to such a reaction by previous learning.

Most neurotic patients are able to distinguish between reality and the symptoms of their individual illness, for instance the compulsive hand-washer can admit that what he is doing is absurd but cannot stop doing it. Insight is generally present in neurotic illness, but it can be absent, notably in hysteria, where the patient has no insight at all into his illness.

Psychotics are generally regarded in lay terms as being mad. For them reality becomes so distorted as to be out of the range of normal experience. Their behaviour is bizarre, and in the more severe cases they are unable to distinguish between reality and the disorders of perception which are a feature of the illness. This lack of insight is sometimes considered diagnostic of psychosis, but this is not completely accurate, since many schizophrenics and depressives in the early stages of their illness are aware that they are ill.

Aetiology

Mental illness results from stress within the social environment aggravated by personality traits and heredity factors. It is commonly thought that the inherited factors consist not only of a genetic element but also of a pattern of behaviour learnt from example.

Other factors related to the causation of mental illness are:

Local damage to the brain, such as tumours, head injuries, viral infections and deterioration accompanying arteriosclerosis.

Certain physical illnesses, in particular pernicious anaemia and myxoedema which cause depression, and thyrotoxicosis which causes an anxiety state.

Chemical factors, in particular alcohol, drugs and poisons. A great deal of research is being done in the field of biochemistry in an attempt to isolate causative factors of mental illness.

Clinical features

The clinical features of mental illness are manifestations of disordered function of mood, behaviour, perception, thought and memory. The most commonly seen features are the following:

Anxiety

Anxiety expresses a distressed mind. It is the commonest of the unpleasant human emotions and is fear of an unknown situation. It arises from a basic insecurity and is accompanied by lack of concentration, insomnia and physiological disturbances such as sweaty palms, dryness of the mouth, indigestion, frequency of micturition, diarrhoea, palpitations and headaches.

Agitation

Agitation is associated with anxiety. The distress is expressed in constant motion which may take a variety of forms, often drumming of the fingers, movements of the lips and groaning sounds. The individual gives the impression of being constantly 'on edge', twittering, anxiously moving about, never able to rest.

Depression

Depression is a state of deep sadness, dejection and despondency. It is accompanied by lethargy and the slowing down of body functions, resulting in dry skin and hair, anorexia, constipation, tiredness, insomnia, lack of energy and loss of libido. Emotions are flattened and the individual, who appears dull and uninteresting, is usually unable to explain or justify such apparent misery. Suicide attempts are always a possibility.

Elation

Elation is an elevation of mood which may be inappropriate to the individual's present circumstances.

Obsession

An obsession is a fixed thought or idea which persists in the patient's mind although he is aware that it is often illogical and out of keeping with his beliefs.

Compulsion

A compulsion is an act which the patient feels compelled to carry out regardless of how painful or illogical it seems. A common example is washing hands after touching anything other than the patient's own body.

Phobia

A phobia is an abnormal fear of a particular object or situation. It may be based on early learning — for instance a fear of dogs or a fear of crowds — or it may result from an early, forgotten, unhappy experience.

Insomnia

Insomnia or sleeplessness is a very common complaint of the mentally ill. Irregularities may include:

Difficulty in getting to sleep.
Waking early.
Sleeping during the daytime but being unable to sleep at night.
Nightmares.

Anorexia

Poor appetite is a feature of depression, chronic alcoholism and drug addiction. Delusions and hallucinations may cause a patient to refuse food.

Delusions

A delusion is a false belief which has no rational basis and which is out of keeping with the individual's educational and cultural background.

Illusions

An illusion is a misinterpretation of an external stimulus, for instance a bush in the dark interpreted as being someone skulking.

Hallucinations

An hallucination is a false perception dependent upon one of the senses: hearing, smell, taste, touch, sight. In this instance there is no external stimulus present: the patient may smell the scent of flowers when neither flowers nor perfume is present.

Thought disturbance

Thought disturbance takes a variety of forms and is observed in the patient's talk:

Neologisms: coining new words.
Thought blocking: sudden gaps in the thought process.
Flight of ideas: a constant stream of different ideas with little connection between them.

The patient may also be seen to exhibit a strong emotional reaction to particular topics.

Memory disturbance

A patient showing signs of memory disturbance may simply appear to be easily distracted and lacking in concentration. His memory may be good for events long past but poor for recent events. There may be gaps in his memory to which he admits, or he may confabulate, that is fill in the gaps with imagined events. There may be clouding of consciousness, confusion and disorientation shown by the patient being unsure of his identity and unable to estimate rationally time and place. He may also have complete loss of memory (amnesia).

It is essential for the nurse to have some understanding of the normal psychology of the human maturation process so that she can appreciate where the patient deviates from the normal. It is also useful for the nurse to be aware of the recognized psychological defence mechanisms.

Psychological defence mechanisms

Rationalization is a means of self-deception by which facts are distorted to produce satisfactory and socially acceptable reasons for bad conduct.

Sublimation is the direction of socially unacceptable or forbidden tendencies into more acceptable channels. For example, sport can be an outlet for unconventional sexual and aggressive desires.

Projection is the attribution of one's own unacceptable feelings and attitudes to someone else or to the environment.

Repression is an unconscious symbolic expression of an unconscious impulse which is incompatible with one's ideals.

Regression means reversion to earlier stages of individual and social development, reacting and behaving accordingly.

The nurse may also find it useful to know some of the terminology associated with the various schools of analytical psychology led by figures such as Sigmund Freud, Carl Jung, Alfred Adler and Melanie Klein (see Further Reading, p. 504).

Investigations

The investigations required to diagnose psychiatric illness are carried out concurrently with initial treatment, which may be in an out-patient clinic or may follow admission to hospital, whichever is more suited to the needs of the patient and his family. An attempt is made to assess the patient's personality and environment, which may provide indications as to how the symptoms have occurred.

This detective work usually involves a number of professional staff. The doctor compiles a history of the patient's physical and mental illness. He wants to know if there is a family tendency towards a particular disease or a common behavioural pattern passed on from one generation to the next. Assessment of the patient's present physical and mental state is necessary. Psychologists' reports on the patient's intelligence, abilities, aptitudes and personality traits are submitted. The psychiatric social worker is asked to compile a report on the patient's home background and work situation. It may be possible for the psychiatric social worker or community nurse to meet the patient in his own environment and to observe the family's interaction. The general practitioner's help is sought to confirm the social and medical history of the patient and his family. The psychiatrist interviews relatives. These discussions often give a totally different perspective to statements made by the patient.

If the patient is admitted to hospital during this period, the nurse's role may be most crucial. Nursing staff are with the patient 24 hours a day observing all his daily activities. In many centres the nurse may also participate with the patient in occupational and recreational therapy. As a result nursing staff have continuous exposure to the patient during all his activities and, provided their method of reporting is efficient, all relevant observations can be communicated to the whole team, particularly those observations which might indicate a change in the patient's behaviour pattern.

Any significant encounter between the patient and a staff member, a relative, a friend, a workmate or another patient should be reported to the therapeutic team for consideration.

A physical illness may cause psychological disturbances, and the possibility of such a disorder will be taken into account when considering the differential diagnosis. For this reason a thorough physical examination is performed on all psychiatric patients and any indications of somatic disorder are followed up, for example pernicious anaemia mimicking depression or thyrotoxicosis resembling an anxiety state.

Assessment

Once the patient's case history is compiled a possible diagnosis can be reached and the treatment deemed suitable for the individual decided on. This decision is arrived at in ways which vary, depending on the administration and philosophy of the hospital or unit.

Hierarchical structures
The decision-making process depends on the structure of the particular unit or hospital. In a hierarchical structure a junior doctor examines the patient and compiles his history. He then confers with his senior colleagues regarding the diagnosis and possible treatment, which he then prescribes. Treatment is administered by the appropriate member of staff.

Therapeutic community
Most psychiatric units pay at least lip service to the concept of the therapeutic community, which is described as a multidisciplinary approach to patient care. In this community all members of staff, from the consultant to the ward maid, have a role to play in creating an environment conducive to treatment and all must have an opportunity to present their views.

Case presentation
About 1 week after admission the junior doctor presents his case history of the patient to the psychiatric team, which includes doctors, nurses, psychologists, social workers, occupational, industrial and recreational therapists and learners from all these professional groups. Most of the team know the patient by this time and are able to contribute to the discussion concerning his treatment, which should be based on an agreed, consistent approach known and understood by all staff.

Review session
A similar group meeting is held at regular intervals to review each patient's progress and to assess the effect of treatment. Also, consideration is given to new developments

and decisions are made concerning, for instance, a patient's fitness to go home for weekends prior to discharge.

Treatment methods

Group psychotherapy

Within a therapeutic community treatment invariably includes participation in group psychotherapy. When treating neuroses these sessions should be analytical in character, making the patient dissect his problems and recognize the part his own behaviour plays in their occurrence. Psychotic patients benefit from supportive psychotherapy, which provides reassurance, encourages and supports 'good' and positive behaviour and gently points out 'bad' or negative behaviour. (This is in contrast to analytical psychotherapy, in which patients themselves are pressurized to interpret their own behaviour.) Supportive psychotherapy should be honest and realistic so that the patient is helped to live as full a life as possible.

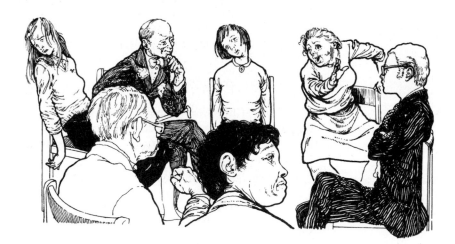

Figure 16.2
Verbal and non-verbal communication during group psychotherapy

In addition to staff, other patients act as therapeutic agents in group psychotherapy. Indeed, patients are often more persistent in pressurizing one of their members than are staff.

Such a group should be directed by a staff member recognized as leader, who encourages group members to comment and analyse throughout the meeting. The leader or another staff member who participated in the group is encouraged either to write a summary of the meeting or to give an oral report to the rest of the team.

A staff meeting usually follows each group meeting to pick out relevant points relating to the progress of individual patients and to provide material for discussion of the interaction and feeling in the unit at that particular time. These sessions can be used as teaching sessions for the learners.

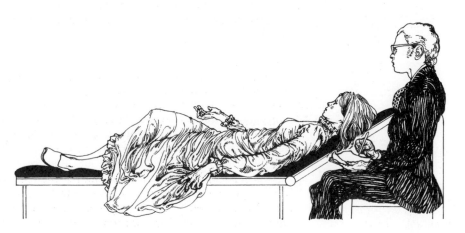

Figure 16.3
Individual psychotherapy

Figure 16.4
Family therapy

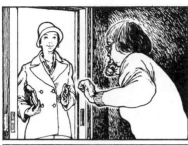

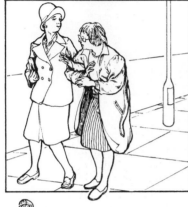

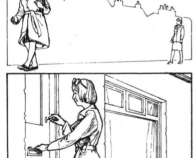

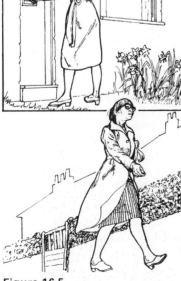

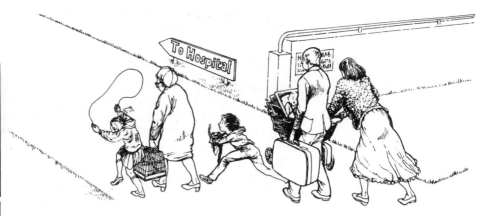

The nurse observer may write in the nursing notes of the patient's record a summary of the part individual patients played in the group meeting.

Didactic or individual psychotherapy

This is psychotherapy on a one-to-one basis. Many psychiatrists consider this the only true psychotherapy. It is a very time-consuming method and only a few patients can be treated in a given period, whereas in the same amount of time a psychiatrist can treat many patients using the group method.

Family or marital therapy

The marriage partner or other family members may be included in the talking session between the patient and the therapist, particularly if it is considered that these people have been involved in causing or aggravating the patient's illness or can help in any way to resolve it.

In some units, such as the Cassel Hospital in England, entire families are admitted to hospital for treatment.

Behaviour therapy

Behaviour therapy is based on learning theories and is a deconditioning or desensitization process by which the patient is retrained to cope with a situation which has previously illogically distressed him. This may take the form, for instance, of a fear of leaving home that causes the patient to become a prisoner within his own house. In behaviour therapy a therapist must work for a period of time almost exclusively with one patient, exposing the patient to ever increasing doses of the fear-provoking situation. For example, in the case of the patient who will not leave home, at first the therapist accompanies him on short excursions from the home. Then, once he can cope with going out with an individual he trusts, the next step is for the patient to go out alone but with the therapist not far away. Ultimately the patient will be able to leave home knowing that the therapist is not in the vicinity.

Nurses have been found to be very good at this type of work, possibly because they are used to spending long periods of time with patients as part of everyday living in hospitals.

Abreaction

Abreaction can be used in the treatment of hysteria and in other conditions where it is thought that the patient may be sublimating. This can be a long drawn-out procedure and requires careful explanation to the patient.

An intravenous injection of sodium thiopentone or sodium amylobarbitone induces the patient to relax sufficiently to speak without inhibition. It is hoped he will reveal long-forgotten incidents from his childhood that may be relevant to his present condition.

This is usually in a one-to-one situation between the patient and the psychiatrist. The nurse may only be required to assist with the administration of the drug. She may be excluded completely from the proceedings or allowed to remain as an observer or chaperone. During a long session the nurse may be expected to relieve the therapist,

Figure 16.5
Behaviour therapy successfully used in the treatment of agoraphobia

particularly during the early stages when the patient is allowed to talk freely about whatever comes into his mind. In such a case the nurse must be given guidance by the therapist as to what tactics to employ if the patient requires direction.

Aversion therapy

Aversion therapy is rarely used nowadays, some therapists find it useful in treating alcoholism and sexual deviations. The object is to guide the patient's stimulus in a healthier direction by giving him an aversion to what was formerly a pleasurable activity. This is achieved either by drug-induced distressful vomiting or by subjecting the patient to electric shocks when practising the asocial behaviour. Psychological support is required if this treatment is to be effective.

During this procedure the nurse may have to monitor the patient's physical condition regularly in case the side-effects of the treatments are too harsh.

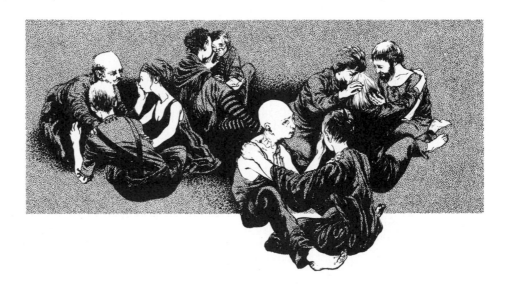

Figure 16.6
Encounter group

Encounter groups

Many patients suffering from neurotic illnesses are extremely inhibited. Some psychiatrists and psychologists, particularly in the United States, advocate the use of encounter groups to encourage people to express their feelings through physical contact with each other. Encounter groups have not been used to any great extent in the U.K. where most psychiatry is provided by the National Health Service, possibly because the sexual overtones inherent in this treatment method could be at variance with what is commonly regarded as professional etiquette.

Cultural differences are noticeable when people meet in a group. For instance British people tend to stand farther away from those they are talking to than do people from Eastern countries. At a party it can be amusing to watch an Englishman backing away from a persistently advancing Arab. Each is trying to maintain what he considers to be the correct social distance from the other. So, in spite of valiant efforts by both to observe the proprieties the unfortunate consequence of the encounter is embarrassment and disharmony. We in Britain also tend to reserve touching for our intimates whereas touching is part of conversation in some parts of the world. In areas where there are multi-racial societies such as in many large hospitals an encounter group can be a valuable teaching tool in promoting understanding and awareness of cultural differences.

Electroconvulsive therapy (electroplexy)

This procedure, known simply as ECT, is effective in the treatment of endogenous depression and early schizophrenia.

The patient is prepared as for a general anaesthetic. Electrodes are applied to the temples and an epileptic-type fit is induced, controlled by a short-acting anaesthetic, sodium thiopentone, and a muscle relaxant such as suxamethonium chloride.

The inital care is the same as for an unconscious patient. Once he has regained consciousness following the anaesthetic the patient is allowed to sleep for a few hours and then is encouraged to get up, dress and participate in the usual ward activities. If the procedure has been performed on an out-patient basis he will then be allowed home, accompanied by a friend or relative.

Temporary confusion and memory loss often follow this procedure, which is otherwise painless. A course of eight treatments of electroconvulsive therapy is usually prescribed.

Drug therapy

Drug therapy does not cure mental disorders, but most psychiatric symptoms can be relieved by the judicious use of drugs.

The main groups of drugs used in the treatment of the anxiety states and depression are the antidepressants (Table 16.2) and the mild tranquillizers (Table 16.3). The major tranquillizers (Table 16.4) are used in the treatment of confusional and delusional states and hallucinations.

The tricyclics are effective antidepressants which take 10 to 14 days to act. The monoamine oxidase inhibitors (MAOI) are not generally effective antidepressants, but some patients respond well to them. If taken in conjunction with tyramine-containing foods such as cheese, yoghurt, alcohol, broad beans, meat extracts (Bovril) and yeast extracts (Marmite), a severe hypertensive reaction can result. A similar reaction is caused if the MAOI group of drugs are taken at the same time or within 2 weeks of completing a course of tricyclics.

Table 16.2
Antidepressant drugs

Tricyclics	Monoamine oxidase inhibitors (MAOI)
imipramine (Tofranil)	phenelzine (Nardil)
trimipramine (Surmontil)	tranylcypromine (Parnate)
amitriptyline (Tryptizol)	

Table 16.3
Mild tranquillizing drugs

Benzodiazepines	Barbiturates
chlordiazepoxide (Librium)	phenobarbitone
diazepam (Valium)	amylobarbitone

Table 16.4
Major tranquillizing drugs

Phenothiazines	Butyrophenomes
chlorpromazine (Largactil)	haloperidol (Serenace)
thioridazine (Melleril)	trifluperidol (Triperidol)
trifluoperazine (Stelazine)	
promazine (Sparine)	
fluphenzine enanthate (Moditen enanthate)	
fluophenazine decanoate (Modecate)	

The benzodiazepines are very effective in the treatment of anxiety states, particularly if the patient is agitated. They are much safer to use than the barbiturates, small doses of which are effective in relieving anxiety. The barbiturates produce drug dependence and tend to make elderly patients confused.

The phenothiazines first came into use in 1951. They are effective particularly in schizophrenia, but are palliative only and the symptoms reappear if the drug is discontinued. Moditen and Modecate are long-acting drugs administered intramuscularly at intervals of 2 to 4 weeks; therefore they are particularly useful to the chronically ill patient living in the community. There are many side-effects to these drugs, notably pseudoparkinsonism, which is treated with antiparkinsonism drugs, for instance orphenadrine (Disipal). Jaundice, skin rashes and photosensitivity are other side-effects.

The butyrophenomes are newer drugs which are effective in treating schizophrenia and particularly in controlling mania. If prescribed in a low dosage, anxiety can be alleviated. The important side-effects of these drugs are also extrapyramidal symptoms, which include rigidity, shuffling gait, lack of facial expression, coarse tremor of the hands and head at rest, excessive salivation, rocking of the body backwards and forwards and posturing.

Most patients suffering from mental disorders are victims of insomnia and hypnotic drugs are usually prescribed to induce sleep.

THE LAW AND MENTAL DISORDER

The law related to mental disorder is designed to protect the patient, his property, his family, the people looking after him and the public.

The existing Mental Health Act 1959 (1960 Scotland) revolutionized people's attitudes to mental illness by making admission and discharge to a mental hospital as informal as admission and discharge to a general hospital.

Within the Act provision has been made to detain compulsorily patients who require treatment but do not recognize that they are a danger to themselves or others. The Mental Health (Amendment) Act 1975 was passed to strengthen the Mental Health Act 1959 to enable potentially dangerous patients to be detained in institutions. This Act does not extend to Scotland or Northern Ireland.

Application for detention can be made by the person's nearest relative or by a social worker and must be supported by medical evidence. Whenever possible this advice is obtained from two doctors, the patient's general practitioner and one appointed by the local authority for the purpose.

At any time, if his condition warrants it, the patient can be discharged or can be accorded informal status. Under these sections of the Act the patient can be discharged by a doctor, or on written application from his nearest relative, or by the Mental Health Tribunal (Table 16.5).

Under Section 136 of the Act the police have the power to take a person to a place of safety, which may be a mental hospital if they consider it most appropriate, for a period of up to 72 hours (7 days in Scotland and Northern Ireland) until appropriate arrangements can be made to take care of the person.

Various health agencies issue leaflets setting out the rights of patients detained in hospital, which should be given to the patient and his relatives. The doctor should explain to the patient the conditions of detention and how he may appeal against detention.

In some cases the criminal courts seek medical advice regarding the mental state of a person accused of an offence. If the court concurs that the person concerned would benefit more from psychiatric treatment than from a prison sentence, a hospital order is issued under Section 60 of the Act.

A patient committed under a hospital order must stay in hospital for 1 year. A hospital order may be renewed for another year and subsequently for 2 years, then reviewed every 2 years. The patient can be discharged by a doctor or by the Mental Health Review Tribunal.

If the person is detained under a hospital order for the safety of the public then he should be placed under a restriction order (Section 65 of the Act). By this order he may not be discharged for a fixed period of time, from anything over 1 year. The Home Secretary alone has the power to discharge this patient.

If a detained patient absconds from hospital, the police, social worker and the patient's nearest relative are informed. If the patient is able to maintain himself outside hospital without being traced for a certain period (28 days to 6 months, depending on his age and type of mental disorder) he is considered discharged.

The Mental Health Act is a comprehensive coverage of all aspects of the law that could possibly affect the patient. One aspect which may concern nurses in hospital is the section dealing with correspondence.

The doctor can censor letters and stop letters from being posted if they are obscene or if the individual to whom they are being sent requests that they should not be posted. The doctor has no authority to open a letter or prevent its being posted if it is addressed to any of the following:

The Prime Minister.
The Department of Health and Social Security.
A Member of Parliament.
The Mental Health Review Tribunal.
The Court of Protection.
The patient's solicitor.

Table 16.5
Summary of detention powers of Mental Health Act 1959 (Amendment Act 1975)

Section of the Act	Maximum period detained	Application for admission supported by	If still ill but unwilling to undergo treatment
25	28 days (21 days in Northern Ireland)	Two doctors (one doctor in Northern Ireland)	Detained under Section 26
26	1 year	Two doctors (one doctor in Northern Ireland)	Detained for 2 years and case reviewed every 2 years
29 (Emergency powers)	72 hours (7 days in Scotland and Northern Ireland)	One doctor	Detained under Section 25

State mental hospitals are provided for the care of the criminally insane. The Secretary of State is responsible for admission and discharge, and provision is made for transfer both to and from the area hospitals. There is one in Scotland at Carstairs and three in England and Wales: Broadmoor in Berkshire, Rampton in Nottinghamshire, Moss Side in Liverpool.

MENTAL DISORDERS

Depression

Depression is one of the most common conditions encountered in psychiatric hospitals. In lay terms it is a mood, but in psychiatric terms it is a syndrome with a number of variations:

Reactive (exogenous) depression.
Manic-depressive psychosis.
Endogenous depression.
Obsessional depression.
Involutional depression.
Puerperal depression.

Reactive depression is regarded as a neurotic condition. The other variations have psychotic features.

Reactive depression. This is described as exogenous because there are precipitating stressful factors outside the individual's personality that provide an understandable psychological cause for the behavioural response. Examples of precipitating factors are circumstances such as bereavement and loss of status. The reaction is, however, exaggerated.

Such a reaction usually occurs in individuals who are hypersensitive, anxious and resentful and who have difficulty coping with stressful situations. It could be said that reactive depression occurs in people with a predisposed personality who are subjected to adversities.

Most people have experienced the mood of depression and can therefore understand the patient's feelings, but they will have difficulty in appreciating the distorted response of the syndrome.

Reactive depression can be distinguished from other types by its accepted clinical picture: there is a recognized cause for the deep unhappiness experienced by the individual, who is usually anxious and resentful, blaming others for his illness; he will have great difficulty in getting to sleep, but if diurnal variation is present he will feel better in the morning, becoming more depressed as the day wears on.

Endogenous depression, manic-depressive psychosis. In contrast, endogenous depression usually occurs in the absence of any apparent environmental stress. There is usually a heredity factor and there may be a history of recurrent attacks of mania. The condition is known as manic-depressive psychosis.

It is a severe depression marked by strong delusions of guilt, unworthiness, hypochondriasis and persecution. Sometimes hallucinations are present. The patient usually gets to sleep easily enough but experiences early morning waking. The risk of suicide is considerable.

Spontaneous recovery will eventually occur.

Obsessional depression. This is a mild depression commonly occurring for the first time in middle-aged obsessional personalities with no family history of the disease. In women, it is often associated with the menopause.

Involutional depression. Rarer, but seen in the same type of people, is a severe depression labelled involutional depression. The features of this condition are intense agitation and delusions of guilt, persecution, and hypochondriasis (usually concerning the bowels). Sometimes nihilistic delusions are present, when the patient insists that everyone including himself is dead. No attempt should be made to reason with the patient regarding his delusions.

Puerperal depression. During the first few days of the puerperium (Ch. 10), because of the rapid changes taking place in the woman's endocrine balance, many women are slightly depressed and emotionally labile. This should not be confused with the severe depression called puerperal psychosis, which may occur early in the puerperium.

The main features of this illness are suicidal tendencies and a strong compulsion to kill the child. Admission to hospital is essential to prevent harm to the baby and to avoid suicide attempts. The other children in the family are usually safe.

Whenever possible, the baby is admitted with the mother, so that she can continue to look after it with the help of the nursing staff.

Complete recovery usually occurs within a month but relapse is common.

General features of depressive illness

All depressed patients suffer from a sad, despairing mood characterized by a feeling of hopelessness which lasts for weeks, months or even 2 or more years. Misery and dejection are apparent in the facial expression, stance and the way the clothes are worn. The patient looks weary, tired and lethargic and is unable to react with a normal show of emotion to events around him. He finds life dull, unexciting and worthless. He is unable to concentrate and experiences memory impairment and loss of libido.

This flattening effect on the spirit also affects his physical health. He complains of anorexia, loss of weight and constipation.

Some individuals become so retarded that they sit silent and immobile, while others become so tense and anxious that they become agitated.

In spite of their underlying depression some patients are able to put on a smiling, chatty, but usually brittle, front to conceal their inner despair. These patients are suicide risks because they have the inclination and the initiative to be able to commit suicide successfully.

Treatment and nursing care

Many patients can be treated effectively by the general practitioner with antidepressant drugs. In addition to drug therapy some patients may require sessions with the

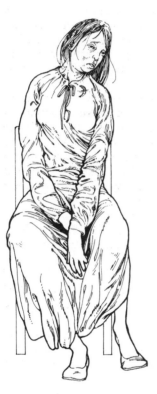

Figure 16.7
Depression

psychiatrist on an out-patient or day-patient basis, during which they can discuss their feelings and relationships.

Hospital admission is desirable for the severely depressed individual who cannot be safely managed at home, possibly because of the high degree of agitation he displays or because he constitutes a potential suicide risk.

Antidepressant drugs form the basis of treatment. Hypnotics are invariably prescribed to counteract insomnia, and agitated patients require mild tranquillizers to control their restlessness and distress. Endogenous depression responds well to electroconvulsive therapy but it is rarely used in the treatment of reactive depression unless agitation is a feature of the illness, in which case it can be useful.

Didactic and group psychotherapy can be usefully employed in assisting depressed patients to analyse their distress and pinpoint problem areas. Social problems can often be identified and, if possible, corrected, with the patient being helped to reach a new freedom of discussion with family members.

Occupational and recreational therapy provides some mental stimulation for the patient, giving him the opportunity to mix with other people.

Depressed patients are apathetic and will deteriorate if allowed to sit alone in a dingy, unstimulating environment. Their mood may be lightened slightly if the ward is light, sunny and furnished attractively and comfortably. Homely touches such as fresh flowers and carefully tended houseplants help to provide a pleasant, caring atmosphere. The aim is to create an environment in which it is possible for patients to meet with understanding and to be assured that the staff are interested in them as individuals.

Apathetic patients have difficulty in making simple decisions. To help them the nurse must develop a positive approach, insisting gently but firmly that basic principles of hygiene and nutrition are observed and that the various therapies are attended. These patients should be encouraged to participate in ward activities but should never be forced to do so. They will take the line of least resistance and can be guided into a passive response provided someone takes the initiative for them. The nurse should encourage conversation, talk to them even when they do not respond, reinforce their accomplishments and try to boost their self-confidence.

Those who are filled with resentment, blaming anyone other than themselves for their illness, need to regain their trust in people. The nurse can best help these patients by being consistent and matter of fact in her approach. These patients are sometimes subject to panic attacks (see anxiety states, p. 499).

Every depressed patient can be regarded as a potential suicide risk and should therefore be observed carefully but unobtrusively day and night. The nurse must observe any change in the patient's appearance or behaviour and report any suicidal tendencies.

All personnel in the ward, including patients, should be made aware if a particular person has contemplated suicide and their co-operation should be sought in preventing future incidents. Discussion of the subject should be free but not laboured, especially in group situations. Nursing responsibilities are:

To ensure that the patient is not left alone.
To know if he has in his possession items with which he could injure himself.
To be prepared to challenge him about his intentions.
To ensure he swallows medication and does not secrete tablets until he has a sufficient number for an overdose.

Constant observation of this type of person is an extremely arduous duty, but negligence is dangerous. Most of these patients observe the staff more rigorously than the staff observe them particularly as their apathy lifts. At this time a patient may appear to be improving, but hopelessness and despair may remain and the patient is now able to plan coolly and calculatingly the strategy which will lead to his death.

Such constant observation may increase the patient's depression, therefore he must gradually be trusted to be on his own. This should be a deliberate policy agreed on by all staff.

A suicide attempt is often a cry for help.

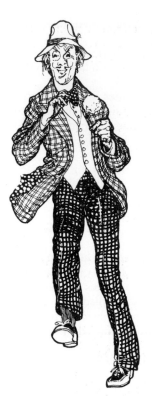

Figure 16.8
Hypomania

Manic states

In manic-depressive psychosis attacks of depression may alternate with the opposite mood state of mania. The first attack of mania is often precipitated by a crisis, and further attacks may occur at regular intervals or may accompany stressful situations.

Hypomania is a state of less severe excitement and overactivity than mania. All the symptoms of mania are present but they are less severe and the condition lasts longer than mania.

Clinical features of mania

Mania usually occurs in people who have a warm and friendly personality. With the illness these traits become exaggerated and the person becomes extremely elated and full of self-confidence, voicing complicated and ambitious plans which it would be impossible to fulfil.

They leap from one place to another with large, graceful movements, constantly moving and talking and dispersing largesse. They are unable to be still and cannot concentrate on any one task or topic of conversation. Their speech is sometimes difficult to understand because they talk rapidly and loudly using puns and rhymes and displaying 'flight of ideas'. They become hypersensitive to noise and space, feeling hemmed in, particularly indoors. They often feel that their skin is easily irritated even by clothing, hence they may strip their clothes off.

These patients often become undernourished and dehydrated because they do not take time to eat and drink and are so very easily distracted. The mouth and tongue can become dry and furred due to dehydration and from talking so much. The excessive amount of energy expended by these patients is not balanced by adequate nutrition and rest, and the result may be complete exhaustion. They become irritable and aggressive if stopped from doing what they want.

Initially their behaviour is infectious, but ultimately it becomes irritating to others and they become unpopular.

Treatment and nursing care

The aim of treatment is to provide the patient with rest and nourishment and to protect him from injury. Sedation is essential; haloperidol has been found to be extremely effective in controlling mania. The phenothiazine group of drugs are also useful in tranquillizing manic patients, and electroconvulsive therapy sometimes dampens their elation.

If the patient is very disturbed he may have to be nursed in isolation. In any event the nurse should try to provide a tranquil atmosphere. She can do this by being particularly quiet, slow and deliberate in her movements and speech; by the use of subdued lights; and by nursing the patient in dull, monotonous surroundings with an absence of noise.

The nurse must use initiative in coaxing the patient to eat. Snacks, sandwiches and high protein drinks should be encouraged throughout the day.

Occupational and recreational activities are an outlet for energy, however manic patients should be given jobs which are quickly done, do not require much concentration and do not excite, stimulate or frustrate the patient. Active activity should not be encouraged. A quiet walk out of doors in open space and fresh air is ideal for these patients.

The nurse can utilize the patient's distractedness to avoid injury or further disruption when the patient becomes aggressive, for example she can walk him up and down, chatting pleasantly to him all the time, drawing his attention away from the irritation. She should avoid struggling with the patient either physically or verbally.

Other patients must be protected from his overexuberance. This may mean that the manic patient requires a special nurse with whom he can build up a relationship and who will keep him away from other patients and from situations liable to excite him.

Clinical features of hypomania

Like a manic patient a hypomanic is extroverted, happy and elated, with lots of drive and energy and a very colourful appearance. He appears interested in everything and everybody and takes on the job of spokesman, leader or organizer of the patient group.

Other patients are at first amused by him and willing to follow his lead. Gradually, however, they become irritated because he is unable to carry out ideas. Eventually they become hostile towards him, seeing him as an interfering individual who tries to ingratiate himself with newcomers. This condition tends to become chronic and the patient may be in hospital for years because he cannot be tolerated in the community outside hospital.

Treatment and nursing care

Treatment is with sedation and tranquillizers. The nurse must protect the patient from other patients, whose tolerance levels may be low, and from overdoing things and exhausting himself. Unlike manic patients hypomanics are often plump because they tend to be greedy; therefore they may need reducing diets.

Schizophrenia

The schizophrenias are a group of illnesses of a psychotic nature characterized by a splitting off of the personality from the refinements of thinking and feeling.

About 45 per cent of mental hospital beds are occupied by schizophrenics. The incidence in the general population is about 0·85 per cent.

The main features of schizophrenia are disturbances of emotion, thought, perception and volition, resulting in abnormal and sometimes bizarre behaviour in which the patient is divorced from reality and living in a fantasy world.

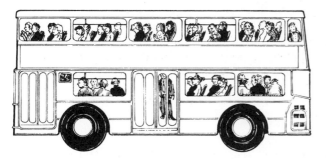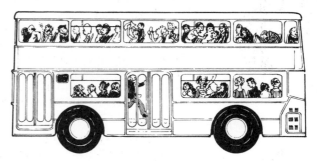

Figure 16.9
Incidence of schizophrenia—at least one of these people is a schizophrenic

Types of schizophrenia

The classical categorization of schizophrenia into four types — simple, hebephrenic, catatonic and paranoid — will be followed here. However, it should be pointed out that this classification is not perfect: there is considerable overlap between the four groups and patients will not fall neatly into one or the other.

Simple schizophrenia first appears in young people and has an insidious onset. A previously intelligent and apparently stable person becomes increasingly solitary and more and more detached from reality. He appears preoccupied, incapable of an emotional response and unable to communicate his thoughts to others. Ultimately he may withdraw completely from society, ceasing to go to work or school, remaining in his room and neglecting his appearance and physical needs until finally he requires hospital care. He may manage to maintain sufficient interest in his health and appearance to live in the community, but he is usually alone and friendless, living at a low economic level and working at unskilled work well below his original capacity.

Hebephrenic schizophrenia also first occurs in young people and is usually acute. The illness generally starts with a period of withdrawal followed by a short phase of wild excitement. The patient will display *incongruity of affect*, flattening of emotion, thought blocking, neologisms (p. 484), *ideas of reference*, strange delusions and hallucinations (p. 484), mainly of an auditory or tactile nature. He usually recovers enough to resume normal life, but relapses are common and flattening of emotion may persist. The personality never quite reverts to its premorbid state and each attack leaves the patient less well than before.

Catatonic schizophrenia is commoner in females and occurs for the first time in young adulthood. Periods of stupor and excitement alternate. Mutism is often a feature, possibly in obedience to hallucinations. The patient may repeat what has just been said to her. She displays resistiveness and negativism and may adopt strange postures and mannerisms. She develops 'waxy flexibility' in that her limbs can be moved into incongruous positions and the pose maintained. During stupor the patient appears to be unaware of what is going on, but afterwards she can relate events quite accurately.

Paranoid schizophrenia first occurs in late life. It is characterized by suspiciousness, delusions and hallucinations of a persecutory nature. The delusions are often plausible and the patient tries to fit his hallucinations into his delusional ideas. The patient behaves as if his delusions were true.

General features of schizophrenia

The cause of schizophrenia is unknown. There is an obvious heredity factor which is thought to be due to a recessive gene.

Commonly the schizophrenic is a day-dreaming, shy, introverted person. Some psychiatrists and psychologists think there is a prepsychotic personality which develops psychotically due to a disturbed family environment that does not allow the individual to mature normally. This fits in with a feature of schizophrenia: the patient seems to retreat from the stresses of reality into the seeming security of a fantasy world.

Certain drugs can produce schizophrenic-type reactions in normal people, for example lysergic acid (LSD), mescaline and amphetamine addiction. This indicates that there is a possible biochemical change in schizophrenia.

SCHIZOPHRENIA

Cause Unknown

Types

Simple
Hebephrenic
Catatonic
Paranoid

Common features

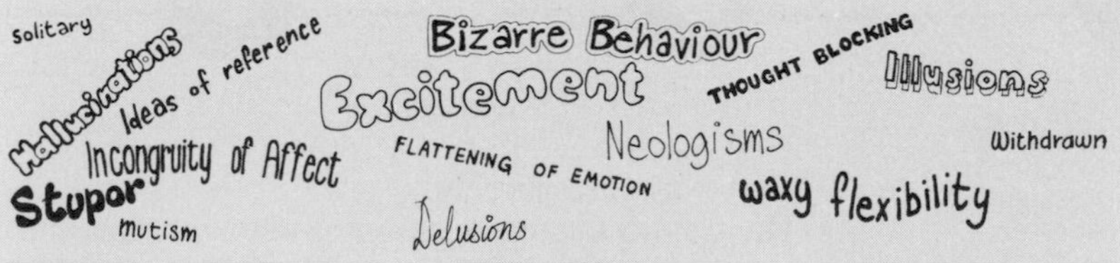

Treatment

Phenothiazines
Community support
Compassion

Figure 16.10
Schizophrenia

Treatment and nursing care

Treatment is palliative to control the symptoms. The major tranquillizers, particularly the phenothiazines, form the basis of treatment. The particular drug of this group that best controls an individual patient's florid and bizarre symptoms is found by trial and error. It is essential that the patient continues drug therapy as long as prescribed; in some cases this will be for life. These drugs have some unpleasant side-effects so that the patient is often reluctant to take them, consequently suffering a relapse. The introduction of the long-acting phenothiazines has helped to solve this problem. Many schizophrenics can now be maintained in the community, attending a Modecate clinic regularly or being visited in their homes by the community nurse who administers their drugs and monitors their effects and the reciprocal influences of patient and environment.

Electroconvulsive therapy is sometimes used, and *leucotomy* may be performed as a final resort. The aim is to reduce the symptoms so that it will be possible to rehabilitate the patient socially.

These patients are emotionally isolated and withdrawn from reality. It is often necessary to retrain them to cope with basic hygiene and nutrition. Group therapy on an occupational, recreational and supportive level helps to socialize an asocial patient by ensuring that he spends some time in the company of other people, participating, albeit passively, in activities.

The nurse can help a schizophrenic person to establish and maintain relationships with other people by first establishing a relationship with him. Much perseverance is needed to find a point of contact and to assist the patient to tolerate and later to participate in normal social interchanges. He learns by example to form and sustain interpersonal relationships, and he may need repeated stimulation and prolonged support from a perceptive nurse before he is able to live comfortably with other people.

Care must be taken to ensure that the patient is given suitable work. At first, repetitive, boring and simple jobs may be necessary, but more complex work providing stimulation and some responsibility should be included gradually.

Some patients are able to work out their disturbance through poetry, painting or music. These dimensions may act as a catalyst, opening the flood gates and allowing him to express some emotion.

Difficult behaviour of a violent, obstructive or destructive nature is usually based on fear and is possibly due to the patient's hallucinations and delusions. The nurse should not take such behaviour as a personal affront and should help the other patients and relatives to react helpfully.

If the patient has a secure family environment to go back to, day hospital facilities may be ideal for him. Others may be able to find accommodation and community life in half-way houses or after care hostels.

The prognosis is better for those whose first attack occurred later in life and for those with a stable family background. Most schizophrenics in the long-term need at least the help of the community psychiatric service and benefit from attachment to voluntary organizations that provide them with some form of social life.

Paranoia

Paranoid states have similar features to paranoid schizophrenia except that, apart from the delusions of persecution, the personality is usually normal. Also, the age group affected is usually older.

Paranoid reactions are a feature of most mental illnesses.

Organic psychoses

In the organic psychoses an organic condition is responsible for disturbed cerebral function causing the psychotic symptoms of confusion, memory impairment, disorientation and hallucinations.

ORGANIC PSYCHOSIS	
Causes	
Systemic	*Cerebral*
Infection	Infection
Metabolic disturbance	Tumour
Endocrine disorder	Degeneration
Deficiency disease	Trauma
Drug/alcohol intoxication	Epilepsy
Prominent feature	
CONFUSION	
Treatment	
Correct cause	

Figure 16.11
Organic psychosis

The origin of the cause may be infection, metabolic or endocrine disorder, deficiency diseases or drug intoxication. Cerebral disease including infection, tumours, epilepsy, trauma and degeneration are particularly important.

The nurse in the general hospital will be familiar with delirium and confusional states. In these instances the cause — say, dehydration — is found and treated and the condition is reversed. Sedation provides the patient with rest. Isolation, preferably in a cubicle, provides privacy until the acute stage is over. The presence of relatives and friends at his bedside will help to reorientate the patient. This is one occasion when nurses should try to impress their own identities on the patient so that he can easily recognize individual nurses and not be further disorientated by exposure to numerous faceless creatures in uniform.

Senile dementia

In the mental hospital the nurse will meet many cases of senile dementia, which is a disease of brain cell degeneration.

There tend to be more females than males with this condition and the onset is about 70 years of age. Some conditions with similar effects are known as the presenile dementias, and in these the onset may be as early as 55 years.

The normal changes of old age become steadily more marked. Early signs may be deterioration of memory and social behaviour. Memory for recent events fails but for remote events remains intact. Some physiological disorders, for instance dehydration, may cause symptoms which mimic senile dementia, but these symptoms disappear when the condition is reversed.

The features of the illness are a blunting of emotion, displaying petulant, irritable and childish behaviour. Apathy and depression accompanied by delusions of guilt may also feature. The patient shows obvious intellectual defects, for instance, difficulty in following an argument, perseveration, train of thought easily lost, becoming muddled even with the simplest tasks and mislaying articles.

Eventually talk becomes a mere babble of words and the patient is completely disorientated and unable to comprehend the simplest tasks or instructions. Delusions may be present.

Such people often have a sleep disturbance, turning day into night, and are often found pottering around the house or wandering in the streets during the night. Eating habits become depraved and urinary and faecal incontinence the norm.

When this stage is reached people require hospitalization and need to be separated from the elderly with sound mind, in the interest of the latter. They require intensive, constant care with many precautions for their safety. If at all possible they should be nursed out of bed because they will deteriorate more quickly both physically and mentally if confined to bed.

The patient should be encouraged to do things for himself for as long as possible and should take simple exercise and participate in occupational therapy. If not able to be ambulant the patient should be washed, dressed in daytime clothes and sat comfortably in an armchair with a group of other patients. Care should be taken over the patient's appearance. Many hospitals employ a beautician and hairdresser for this purpose.

These patients are like babies. They can sense approval even though they do not understand what you are saying. The words are unimportant as long as the tone is gentle, kind and approving.

Diet should be light, nutritious and soft. Care should be taken in feeding to ensure that sufficient quantities of food and drink have been consumed by the patient.

There is a possibility that incontinence of urine may be psychological, resulting from regression into babyhood. If the patient has been allowed to lie in bed, warm and understimulated, regression to babyhood occurs when excreta was voided automatically without the voluntary control of the patient. This can be treated by stimulating the patient, getting him up and dressed, giving him simple occupational therapy and providing toilet training. In conjunction with this, habit training can be introduced in washing, dressing, feeding and toileting. This can be done in small groups with the same activity being practised at the same time each day for each patient and the same series of actions performed on each occasion. This may help to give back to the patient some independence and can help to arrest deterioration.

The nurse should ensure that the patient's bowels are emptied. Use of a commode or toilet is preferable so that he is in the natural position for defaecation. He should also be warm and comfortable. An impacted faecal mass is often a complication and may be masked by apparent diarrhoea. This may be a cause for restlessness and should always be investigated and treated. Often the patient is uncomfortable or in pain. If no cause can be found sedation may be prescribed.

With adequate nursing care and attention deterioration can be arrested and a certain amount of rehabilitation achieved. The greater the amount of activity and interest which can be provided the better the patient will retain his failing faculties.

Anxiety states

The anxiety states are common neurotic reactions which may be treated on an outpatient basis, although many people require treatment in hospital.

Anxiety is a normal, understandable reaction to a threat. Once this stress has been removed the symptoms of anxiety usually abate. Anxiety is a feature of depression, schizophrenia, mild brain damage and some physical diseases, such as thyrotoxicosis, but it can also be a neurotic condition in its own right.

Stress affects individuals differently but always in the areas in which they are already vulnerable. A situation which may seem trivial to one will be overwhelming to another. In an anxiety state the reaction is severe and prolonged and is usually precipitated by difficulties experienced by the individual in coping with a disturbing change in his occupational, social or domestic milieu.

Clinical features

Anxiety is fear, usually of the unknown, which gives rise to recognized physical symptoms affecting all the body systems. These include palpitations, tremors of the hands and feet, profuse sweating, frequency of micturition, diarrhoea, dryness of the mouth, indigestion and unpleasant sensations in the epigastrium, such as 'butterflies in the stomach'. Tension symptoms are frontal headache, mild aching of the muscles and fatigue.

Many anxious people overbreathe and therefore lose excessive quantities of carbon dioxide, which causes alkalosis and tetany.

Anxious people are more responsive to incoming stimuli and the resultant increased distractedness causes the psychological features associated with the condition, namely memory problems, lack of concentration, muddled feeling and fear that they are going mad.

The level of anxiety will fluctuate according to the amount of stress present. Colds and urinary tract infections can make the condition worse. Fear breeds fear and anxiety is habit-forming. An individual can learn to react to stress in a particular way.

An acute exacerbation is described as a 'panic attack' and may occur for little or no obvious reason. The features of a panic attack are palpitations, gasping respiration, unpleasant epigastric sensations, intense fear and a sense of impending death or doom.

Reassurance and sedation form the basis of treatment for such an attack.

Treatment and nursing care

The aim of treatment of an anxiety state is to help the patient recognize and cope with the problem areas of his life. He must be guided into developing insight into his condition.

Many of these patients dwell on the physical symptoms to the exclusion of all else. To help him understand the true nature of his illness these symptoms must be fully investigated and, as each cause is eliminated, it is hoped that he will be nearer recognizing that the symptoms will only improve once he resolves his difficulties.

Symptomatic relief for the physical symptoms must be administered. Tranquillizers will be prescribed to help control the anxiety, and hypnotics if there is a sleep disturbance.

The patient must be helped to analyse his problems and this is best done in group, family or marital psychotherapy. Abreaction may help him to uncover the unconscious root of his difficulties. Supportive psychotherapy will encourage the patient to look at his reactions in relation to stress. Occupational and recreational therapy ensures that he is forming relationships with other patients; he can be helped to tolerate stress by being placed in increasingly stressful situations, always provided he has been successful in managing the previous test.

Co-operation from relatives should be sought and the patient should be seen coping with the stressful environment before being finally discharged from care.

The nurse must be sympathetic but firm with this patient to help him face reality.

Other manifestations of anxiety

Anxiety sometimes takes the form of a **phobia** which is an abnormal fear of a particular situation, such as going into crowds. The best treatment for this is behaviour therapy.

Obsessive, compulsive states are another form of anxiety in which the patient is obsessed with a disturbing thought or is compelled to perform repeatedly an act according to a ritual. The previous personality of many of these patients was that of a neat, tidy, punctilious individual who loves order for its own sake. There is often an overlay of depression.

Treatment is with the mild tranquillizers and antidepressants if appropriate. Supportive psychotherapy may be useful.

Hysteria is a way of resolving an anxiety conflict by the production of socially acceptable physical and mental symptoms. It is a common device with the primary aim of modifying the environment to suit the individual; frequently there are secondary advantages, such as gaining much attention. The individual is at least partially unaware of what he is doing.

Treatment is by tranquillizers, abreaction, sedation and analytical psychotherapy.

Anorexia nervosa

Anorexia nervosa is classified by the World Health Organisation as a form of neurosis, characterised by starvation and its hormonal consequences. The age of onset is usually between 11 and 35 years. Normally those affected are of above average intelligence and belong to social groups 1 and 2.

There are two recognised types:

Primary anorexia nervosa which is a disturbance in body image concept characterised by the wish for 'thinness' achieved by a refusal to eat. This type commonly occurs in adolescents, mainly girls.

Secondary anorexia nervosa is a ploy of individuals, of both sexes and any age but again mainly women, to manipulate others by losing weight. Every case is different and atypical cases from both these groups are common.

The clinical features are a direct result of starvation. These patients refuse to eat, are emaciated and have serious depression of all vital functions. They present with facial pallor, cyanosis of the extremities, dry skin and head hair, downy growth on face and body, and amenorrhoea in the females. Characteristically they are restless, full of energy and guile.

The aim of treatment is to restore the patient to normal body weight and correct the underlying psychopathological disorder. This is best achieved by bed rest in hospital until the body weight is within normal limits. This allows rapport to develop between the psychiatric team and the patient as well as separating the patient from the family and friends emotionally involved in his/her illness. Treatment is continued in the psychiatric outpatient department.

Alcoholism

Alcoholics cannot control their drinking, which may be continuous or in bouts. Ultimately their physical and mental health is damaged. It is a social disease that disrupts the family and society. Many alcoholics have an underlying depression or anxiety state. By the time the patient comes for treatment it is not always obvious whether the home environment caused the addiction or results from it.

Aversion therapy and group psychotherapy have been used to treat this condition. Neither form of treatment has been very successful in the long term. In response to a government working party some special units were set up in the U.K. specifically for the treatment of alcoholism. Patients had to demonstrate that they were strongly motivated towards cure before being admitted to such a unit. These of course are expensive to run and it is difficult to measure their success rate.

Generally clinical treatment is mainly by sedation and the administration of vitamins to help counteract the withdrawal effects of alcohol. This is known as 'the drying out process' and mainly occurs in the surgical wards of general hospitals following admission from the Accident and Emergency Department.

If further treatment is considered necessary, the patient may be referred to a psychiatrist. His task is to treat any underlying psychiatric conditions although at this stage it is often difficult to gauge which came first — the psychiatric condition or the alcoholism. Other forms of help are given within the social setting, particularly from organizations such as Alcoholics Anonymous. Because all the members of Alcoholics Anonymous have been alcoholics themselves they are uniquely able to provide the support and discipline the wavering alcoholic needs.

Alcoholism is now recognized as a social problem affecting people in all walks of life and more help and understanding is being given to the alcoholic at work and in society than ever before.

Moderation in the use of alcohol is advocated and real attempts are being made to make people aware of the unfortunate results of alcoholic abuse while they still have time to change their drink pattern.

Drug dependence

Drug dependence arises from repeated administrations of a drug on a periodic or continuous basis. The clinical features vary according to the drug or drugs involved. Barbiturates, cannabis, amphetamines, morphine, cocaine or LSD (lysergic acid diethylemide) are all examples of preparations which may be misused, either alone or in combination.

People likely to become drug addicts vary from the middle-aged housewife attempting to slim or with an insomnia problem, who becomes addicted to amphetamines or barbiturates, respectively, to the adolescent out for kicks taking LSD or cannabis.

Basically society is at fault. Drugs are readily available and money can be made from selling them. Taking them adds initial excitement to someone's life.

Increased doses are needed to provide the required effect, and unpleasant psychological and physical symptoms occur when the drug is withdrawn.

Co-operation is necessary for treatment. Hospitalization is best so that the drug can be 'tapered' off slowly. In some cases replacement therapy is given in the form of a synthetic drug, methadone (Physeptone).

The patient's nutritional state is improved and tranquillizers and antidepressants are prescribed if appropriate.

Long-term treatment requires some sort of social support and psychotherapy. Many fall into their old ways. For some death results.

Personality disorders

A psychopathic disorder, according to the Mental Health Act 1959, refers to a persistent disorder or disability of mind resulting in abnormally aggressive or seriously irresponsible conduct by a patient; it is considered to require medical treatment.

These patients are usually devoid of guilt or shame for their actions, are emotionally labile and do not appear to be able to form lasting friendships or respond to social training. They are often in trouble with the law and many are housed in the state mental hospitals.

The aim of treatment is to try to redirect their energies into more socially acceptable channels.

People who practice sexual deviations are also considered to have personality disorders. It is thought that they have regressed or not matured psychologically in their sexual development.

Tranquillizers, psychotherapy and abreaction can all be useful. Aversion therapy is employed to control a perversion such as fetishism.

NURSING IN A MENTAL HOSPITAL

A mental hospital provides a sheltered environment permitting the normal functions of sleeping, eating, work and recreation. In such an environment the patient can be trained — or can relearn — how to cope with everyday living. To meet this function most wards in mental hospitals provide separate sleeping and living accommodation similar to that of the average home.

Patients lead ordered lives: up and dressed for breakfast, off to work, treatment sessions or industrial or occupational therapy by 9 a.m., a break for coffee, more work or therapy before a break for lunch followed by a similar regime in the afternoon. Recreational activities may be confined to evenings or may also be encouraged in the afternoons.

Many patients need to be coaxed to adhere strictly to such an ordered life. Due to their illness many are lethargic and apathetic and much of the nurse's time can be spent in rousing enthusiasm for the various activities. As part of treatment and rehabilitation programmes the nurse participates with patients in all their daily activities therefore she can be found doing domestic work or some routine job in industrial or occupational therapy or perhaps dancing or playing games. By the example of her interactions with people the nurse teaches patients how to relate to others in simple situations, as well as by the part she plays in the various psychotherapeutic treatments. The nurse works, plays, talks and listens to the patient, becoming a confidante and mentor; she helps to develop the patient's potential to live as normal a life as possible by tolerating his eccentricities and by raising his expectations of his own behaviour.

The nurse also participates in discussions on the patient's progress with other members of the therapeutic team. To do this she must be able to report accurately and succinctly significant conversations held with the patient. Similarly, she must observe and report accurately the behaviour of the patient when he is alone and thinks himself unobserved and also his interactions with other patients, visitors and staff.

Many nurses entering mental hospitals for the first time are afraid that they will meet violence and strange behaviour with which they will not be able to cope. Actually, violence in the mental hospital is comparatively rare. Seeming violence is often impulsive behaviour that arises in response to hallucinations. Most patients are so well controlled by drug therapy that outbursts are uncommon, and in most cases a trained nurse is usually able to anticipate such behaviour and distract the patient successfully. Special arrangements are made for the criminally insane.

Nurses and new patients, very quickly become accustomed to the eccentric behaviour displayed by some patients, particularly the rituals of obsessive patients, and once this behaviour is understood it is soon tolerated and accepted as part of a person's individuality.

Boredom is the main complaint of new nurses working in the field of mental health. Many find it hard to get involved in patient activities, and the quiet, even tenure of life in the mental hospital seems to contrast sharply with the rat race of the world outside the hospital walls. Great enjoyment, job satisfaction and personal development is experienced by the nurse who is able to involve herself in her patients' affairs while retaining a measure of objectivity and who does not allow her professional life to encroach on her personal life.

Mental nursing

All nurses must be able to give basic nursing care so that their patients will be clean, warm, and well nourished. They also require some technical knowledge and skills to be able to administer prescribed treatments. They must also develop the ability to deal with people tactfully and with kindness and understanding so that patients and their relatives will be reassured and trusting relationships formed.

To meet the physical and psychological needs of patients basic skills must be learnt, modified and adapted. For example, while working in a surgical ward the nurse learns how to dress and care for a wound. When working in a medical ward the nurse may meet a patient with a wound. The skills learnt in the surgical area are utilized so that the wound is given the same expert care it would have received if the patient had been nursed in a surgical ward.

Similarly when working with patients with mental illness the nurse has the opportunity to develop her capacity to form professional relationships with patients and staff. The knowledge and expertise which develops out of this experience should be utilized when nursing patients outwith the psychiatric hospital whether it be in the community, the obstetric department, the general medical or surgical wards or areas providing special care.

The psychological care of sick people and their relatives ranks in importance with the physical care required by patients. The nurse prepares herself to provide the physical needs of patients by studying human biology. Knowledge of the normal allows the nurse to understand the requirements necessary to correct any deviation from the normal.

Since nurses deal with people of all ages and circumstances in order to meet the psychological requirements of patients the nurse studies the psychology of: childhood, learning, the maturation process, ageing, bereavement, fear, and guilt. In particular the nurse should develop an understanding of the mental defence mechanisms. This will help her to appreciate the behaviour not only of patients and their relatives but also her own behaviour and that of her colleagues and superiors. Therefore, knowledge of the accepted normal behaviour in a given situation allows the nurse to cope with individual reactions.

This particular skill is one which the nurse will develop and use in her domestic and social life as well as in the work situation. Some may have a natural talent in this direction but all can learn the mechanisms of behaviour and use this knowledge to modify their own behaviour and develop some understanding of the behaviour of others. In her working life it is a skill the nurse will utilize daily wherever she is working and from the first day in the clinical area. She will also learn by observing and following the example set by more experienced nurses.

A period of experience in the psychiatric field gives the nurse the opportunity to consolidate the learning related to this skill. In the group setting she can study and experiment with her own behaviour and observe the behaviour of other members of staff and patients. Psychiatric patients are usually reasonably fit physically, therefore it is possible for both them and the staff caring for them to concentrate on their mental symptoms which usually demonstrate either some deviation from the normal or some exaggeration of the normal. In the environment of the psychiatric hospital the nurse is able to spend time listening to patients and observing their behaviour. Much of what is learnt from this experience can be utilized wherever the nurse is working. For example, anxiety manifests itself in similar ways regardless of whether the cause is real as in childbirth, preoperatively, or as in relatives watching a loved one die, or, with no apparent cause, as in agitated depression. Therefore by learning the responses of psychiatric patients to anxiety the nurse develops an awareness of how everyone reacts to anxiety. She can now work out how to combat or modify these reactions according to individual needs.

If a nurse is to be truly compassionate and at the same time able to offer practical help to patients and their relatives with their emotional needs, it is essential that she develops her skills so that she is able to meet the psychological needs of people as well as the physical needs.

SUGGESTED ASSIGNMENTS

Project
Find out to what extent the following are involved in the social rehabilitation of psychiatric patients in your area:

Halfway houses.
Day centres.
The local community.

Discussion topics
1. Is attempted suicide 'a cry for help'?

2. What do you understand by the term 'blurring of roles' in the context of the therapeutic community?

3. From your own observation does the community psychiatric nurse play a viable role in supporting the mentally ill patient outside the hospital?

4. Alcoholism is the commonest form of addiction in some countries, including Great Britain, and has profound social and psychological effects on the individual and his or her family. How can this problem be tackled nationally?

FURTHER READING

Brown J A C 1969 Freud and the post Freudians. Penguin, Harmondsworth

Burkhalter P K 1975 Nursing care of the alcoholic and drug abuse. McGraw Hill, New York

Dally P 1979 Anorexia nervosa. Heinemman, London

Department of Health and Social Security 1976 Review of the Mental Health Act 1959. A consultative document. HMSO, London

Drew L R H, Moon J R, Buchanan F H 1974 Alcoholism a handbook. Heinemann, London

Fleming A C, Paterson H F 1969 Mental disorder and the law. Churchill Livingstone, Edinburgh

Fowlie H C, Stokes R F 1972 Psychiatry in comprehensive nursing. Collins, Glasgow

Kneish C R, Ames S A 1974 Mental health concepts in medical surgical nursing. A handbook. Mosby, St. Louis

Kramer J F, Cameron D C (eds) 1975 A manual on drug dependence. WHO, Geneva

Longhorn E 1975 Psychiatric care and conditions. HM & M Publishers, Aylesbury

Maddison D, Day P, Leabeater B 1976 Psychiatric nursing, 4th edn. Churchill Livingstone, Edinburgh

Mental Health Act 1959 HMSO, London

Mental Health (Amendment) Act 1975 HMSO, London

Mental Health (Scotland) Act 1960 HMSO, London

Mental Health (Northern Ireland) Act 1961 HMSO, London

Pitt B 1974 Psychogeriatrics. Churchill Livingstone, Edinburgh

Saxton D F, Hyland P A 1975 Planning and implementing nursing intervention. Mosby, St. Louis

Silverstone T, Turner P 1974 Drug treatment in psychiatry. Routledge & Kegan Paul, London

Thompson S, Kahn J H 1970 The group process as a helping technique. Pergamon, Oxford

Tredgold R F, Wolff H H 1975 UCH notes on psychiatry, 2nd edn. Duckworth, London

WHO 1974 Glossary of mental disorders and a guide to their classification. WHO, Geneva

Section B

Individuals in Hospital and Community

17. The Newborn

The birth of a baby is a family event in every culture, race and creed that is generally accompanied by joy and celebration. This precious, new life must be nurtured, protected and watched over with meticulous care.

Present-day obstetric and paediatric practice and improved nutrition and housing have contributed greatly to the reduction of *neonatal mortality* rates so that babies begin life with a much greater chance of survival. During the antenatal period the expectant mother and father attend classes to prepare them for labour, delivery and parenthood. The expectant father is encouraged to remain with his wife during delivery and thus the unique experience of parenthood is shared from the moment of the baby's birth.

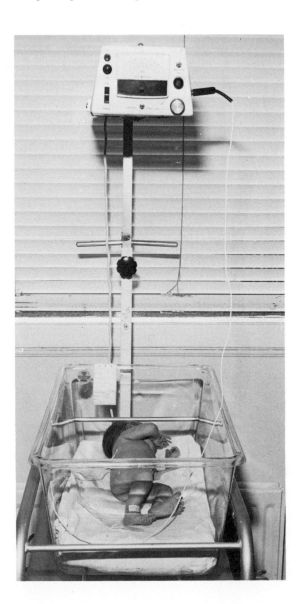

Figure 17.1
Baby warmer showing thermo-couple in position

PREPARATION FOR DELIVERY

Warmth is essential. The baby will emerge from the uterus as it were from a warm bath — very wet — and so the skin cools rapidly. The delivery room temperature should never be below 25°C and if possible is best kept at 30°C. A cot is prepared with warm blankets, and a specially designed 'baby warmer' is available which provides heat directly over the baby's cot with servo temperature control (Fig. 17.1). The thermo-couple is attached to the baby's skin and the baby's temperature is recorded on a dial on the baby warmer.

A sterile delivery pack must be at hand and resuscitation equipment must be ready for immediate use (Fig. 17.2).

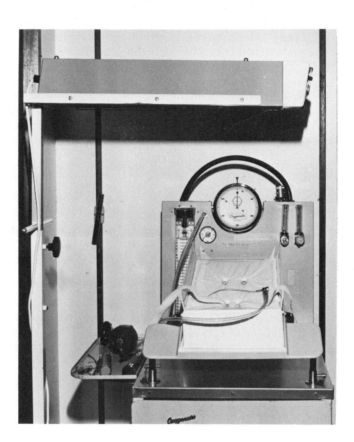

Figure 17.2
Resuscitaire with equipment

DELIVERY

When the baby's head is born the midwife quickly feels for the umbilical cord which may be round the baby's neck. The cord is only clamped and cut if it is tight and likely to cause strangulation of the baby during birth. The midwife then wipes the baby's eyelids to remove secretions from the birth canal which might contain pathogenic organisms. With the next contraction, the head rotates and the shoulders are born, followed quickly by the trunk and limbs.

IMMEDIATE CARE AT BIRTH
Airway

It is imperative that mucus extraction is carried out at once to prevent inhalation of mucus and secretions which could seriously endanger the baby's life. When the baby is completely born the head is tilted down for a few moments to allow drainage of mucus from the trachea and pharynx. Aspiration is carried out by the midwife using a mucus extractor (Fig. 17.3). A healthy baby cries immediately.

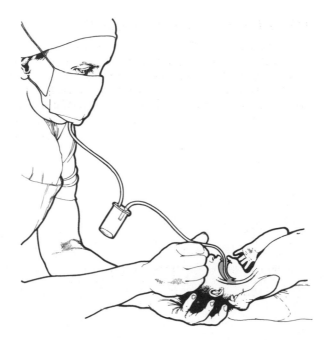

Figure 17.3
Mucus extractor in use showing
catheter in nasopharynx

Assessment at birth

The baby's general condition is rapidly assessed and care is taken to record the exact time of birth and onset of regular respirations. If the baby's condition gives any cause for anxiety the midwife immediately begins resuscitative measures and sends urgently for the paediatric team.

Apgar score

This is a method of estimating, in numerical terms, the heart beat, respiratory rate, colour, muscle tone and response to stimuli of a newly born baby (Table 17.1). It gives an assessment of the total condition and allows comparison of one baby with another. The method was first described by Dr Virginia Apgar.

Sex

The sex is determined and medical aid sought if the genitalia are such that the sex of the infant is in doubt.

Preliminary examination

The baby is quickly examined for any obvious abnormality, but detailed examination is left until later.

Table 17.1
Apgar score sheet

Name	Date		Age	(Min.)
	0	1	2	Score
Heart rate	Absent	Below 100	Over 100	
Respiratory effort	Absent	Slow, irregular	Good, crying	
Muscle tone	Limp	Some flexion of extremities	Active movement	
Response to catheter	No response	Grimace	Cough or sneeze	
Colour	Blue pale	Body pink Extremities blue	Completely pink	

The cord

Following cessation of pulsation the cord is clamped with Spencer Wells artery forceps 5 cm from the umbilicus. The second clamp is applied 6 cm from the umbilicus and the cord is divided between the two forceps. The baby is placed in a sterile towel and dried carefully. This towel is then discarded and the baby is wrapped in a fresh sterile towel and placed in the warmed cot until the delivery of the placenta is completed. The cord is finally occluded. There are several different methods in current use for accomplishing this:

1. The application of sterile cord clamps which may be removed in 48 hours or left until the cord drops off (Fig. 17.4).

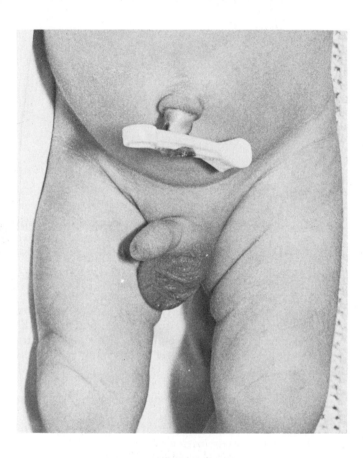

Figure 17.4
Cord clamp occluding umbilical vessels

2. Ligation. Ligatures must be strong and made of material such as nylon tape which will not cut through the cord; otherwise it will cause immediate and profuse haemorrhage. As the substance of the cord (called *Wharton's Jelly*) shrinks, the ligatures may become loose and may need to be reapplied (Fig. 17.5). Cord haemorrhage is a real danger and can have very serious consequences for the baby; therefore frequent examination of the cord must be made during the first 24 to 30 hours. No dressing is applied but the cord may be treated with an antiseptic preparation in surgical spirit.

Identification of the baby

This is an important duty of the midwife. Identification is carried out in the presence of the mother and possibly also the father; ideally it should be checked by them. Various methods are available. One of the most common is a transparent bracelet into which a card is inserted with the baby's particulars recorded on it. The bracelet is placed on the baby's ankle and secured by a special press stud (Fig. 17.6). It can only be removed by cutting it off. On admission to the nursery a second bracelet can be applied to the other ankle as an added safeguard.

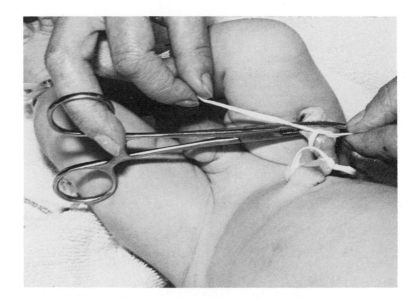

Figure 17.5
Application of cord ligatures

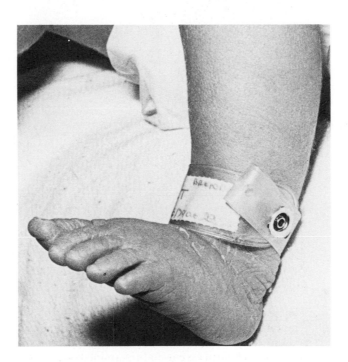

Figure 17.6
Identification bracelet in position

The mother

Care of the mother during and after the third stage of labour is described in Chapter 10. It is essential to allow time for the mother to fondle her baby, examine him in minute detail, and put him to the breast if she so wishes. This skin contact, one with the other, is known as 'bonding' and forms the first vital link in the relationship of the mother and her baby. All her thoughts are centred around the baby's safety and physical needs and the mothering and protective instinct is very strong at that time. It is desirable to avoid separation of the mother and her newly born baby and in purpose-built maternity hospitals provision is made to have the baby beside the mother so that she may watch over him and feed him when he demands it. (Fig 17.7). However, rest during the day and sleep during the night are essential for the mother so separate accommodation must be provided to enable the baby to be removed if necessary.

SUBSEQUENT CARE OF THE NORMAL BABY

The baby is left to rest for 1 to 2 hours in his cot in the nursery. Special care must be taken to ensure that the baby's body heat is maintained and that the cord is examined frequently for bleeding. The rectal temperature should be 37°C; the room temperature should be 30°C.

Detailed examination

This is undertaken by the midwife and the paediatrician. Measurements of length, head circumference and weight must be very carefully checked and recorded as an error can cause great anxiety and distress to the parents.

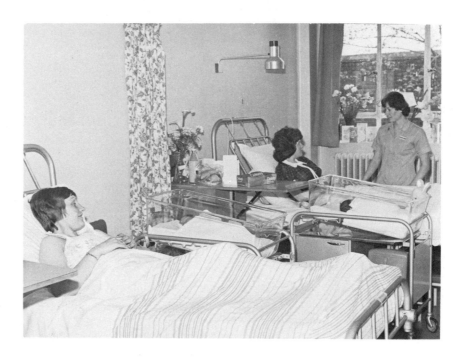

Figure 17.7
Rooming in

General inspection, noting the size, cry, colour, limb movements, respiratory rate and chest movement and general reaction to touch, noise and light, is carried out before noting the following particular anatomical details.

The head
This is inspected generally and any swellings such as *caput succedaneum*, which may be present from birth, or *cephalhaematoma*, which may develop later, are noted.

The **mouth** must be carefully examined with a good light for cleft palate. A cleft lip is obvious but a posterior cleft in the palate could be missed unless looked for specifically.

An excessive amount of mucus may indicate an abnormality of the alimentary tract and must always be reported immediately.

The limbs
The limbs should move freely. All babies are examined for congenital dislocation of the hips (Fig. 17.8).

The **hand** must be opened out gently to examine the fingers. Occasionally there is an extra digit attached to the little finger (Fig. 17.9). When inspecting the feet the toes are also carefully examined for the same reason. The presence of club foot (*talipes*) (Fig. 17. 10) would also be noted.

The back
The back is inspected for *spina bifida* (Fig. 17.11). This condition is described in Chapter 3.

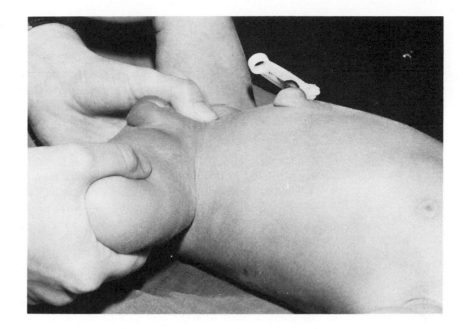

Figure 17.8
Examination for congenital dislocation of the hips (Courtesy of Keay and Morgan—Craig's care of the newly born infant. Churchill Livingstone, Edinburgh)

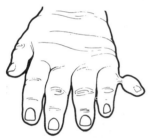

Figure 17.9
Extra digit

The external genitalia
These are examined carefully. In a male child the urethra may not extend to the end of the penis but open on to the under surface. This condition is known as hypospadias. If the urethra opens on to the upper surface of the penis the condition is known as epispadias (Ch. 9). Surgery may be required in childhood to correct either condition.

The anus
Occasionally the anus may be covered with a thin, anal membrane giving rise to an imperforate anus. It can be corrected by incision of the membrane. There may, however, be atresia of the anal canal and if so a colostomy (Ch. 5) will be necessary to relieve the obstruction.

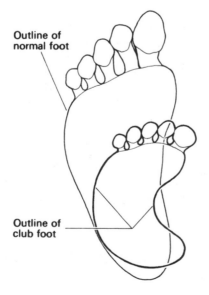

Outline of normal foot

Outline of club foot

Figure 17.10
Bilateral club foot (Talipes)

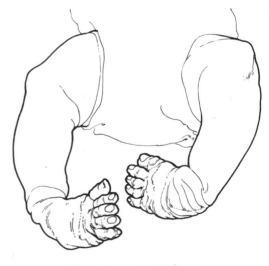

Bilateral club foot (Talipes)

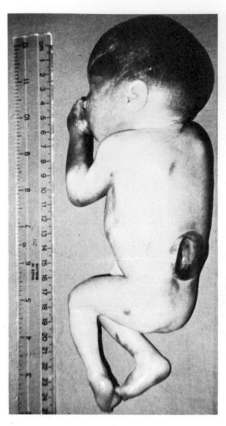

Initial cleansing

Immersion of the baby in a bath is undesirable because it may cause severe chilling and because the newborn baby's skin is very susceptible to infection.

Cleansing may be carried out in the baby's cot using sterile cotton wool swabs moistened in sterile water or in a diluted solution of an antiseptic detergent such as Phisohex. The Phisohex solution should be wiped off the skin with sterile water. The prolonged use of Phisohex can be dangerous but the advantages of short-term use outweigh the risk of staphylococcal infection of the skin. Special attention must be paid to the skin folds in the neck, axillae and groins.

The cord should be treated with an antiseptic such as 0·5 per cent Hibitane in 70 per cent surgical spirit and if necessary ligatures may have to be reapplied.

The baby's temperature should always be checked at the end of the procedure. The baby is then dressed in light, simple clothing allowing free movement without constriction.

Feeding

The rate of growth of the baby should continue at much the same rate as it did in the uterus before birth. In order to achieve this and to keep the infant healthy, he must be fed sufficiently often with the correct amount and type of food.

Breast feeding

Breast feeding for the newborn is ideal from both a nutritional and an emotional point of view and every encouragement should be given to the mother to attempt it, even if only for a short period. Antenatal classes will have helped to educate her and she will have had the opportunity to discuss breast feeding at the antenatal clinic and during parentcraft teaching. In preparation for breast feeding advice will have been given regarding a good fitting brassiere and gentle, daily massage of the nipples with a lanoline-based cream preparation.

The baby is usually offered his first feed within a few hours of birth. The early feeds must be fully supervised. Patience and tact are required as this is an unfamiliar experience for the new mother who may become despondent if the baby does not suck readily. Sufficient time must be taken to ensure that she is comfortable and holding the baby correctly (Fig 17.12). If possible, demand feeding should be encouraged since the baby will feed well when he is hungry.

Colostrum is present in the breasts from the 16th week of pregnancy. It has a higher protein content and a smaller amount of sugar and fat than milk and is easily digested. It also contains immunoglobulins (Ch. 1). During the first 2 or 3 days the colostrum increases in amount and gradually alters in composition and by the fourth day milk is being produced. At this stage the breasts may be tense and feel uncomfortable. Warm bathing will stimulate the flow of milk through the lactiferous ducts to the nipple and will relieve the tension. A good supporting brassiere should be worn.

Early breast feeds should be of short duration to avoid damage to the nipple. Care must be taken to ensure that the baby draws the nipple back to the soft palate so that the gums exert pressure on the areola, **not** on the nipple itself.

Before and after feeds the breasts and nipples must be carefully inspected, washed and dried. If there is pain associated with feeding, the affected breast is rested, the milk gently expressed by hand and a soothing ointment applied. The mother quickly gains confidence in her ability to feed her baby so long as she has maximum support and reassurance in the early days.

Artificial feeding

If breast feeding is not possible there are many baby milk preparations available.

Prepared feeds

During the last few years a number of firms have produced prepared and sterilized feeds in sealed bottles for use in hospital (Fig. 17.13). A separate sterile disposable teat unit is supplied. This system is costly to use but no milk kitchen or staff is required and there is no risk of the feeds becoming contaminated during preparation. Prepared feeds are

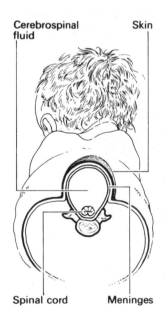

Cerebrospinal fluid   Skin

Spinal cord   Meninges

Figure 17.11
Spina bifida
(Courtesy of Dr J. B. Scrimgeour, Consultant Obstetrician and Gynaecologist, Western General Hospital, Edinburgh)

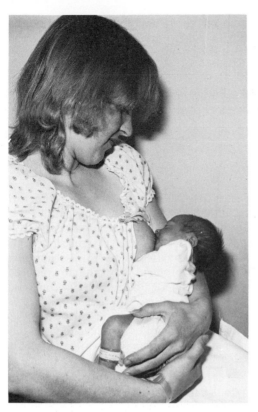

Figure 17.12
Breast feeding

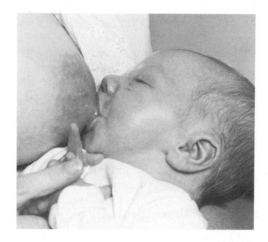

coming into production for use at home also, but at the moment they are too expensive for the average household.

Dried milk
Dried milk is used widely. It is reconstituted by adding 30 ml boiled water to one level scoop of powder. It may be necessary to add sugar as recommended on the packet if this

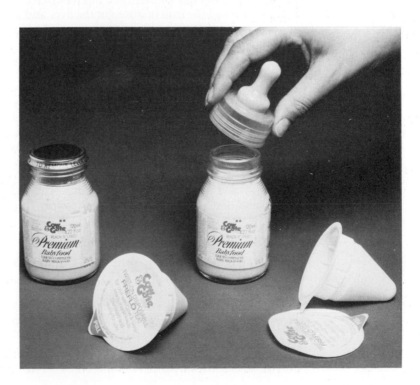

Figure 17.13
Prepared feed and teat unit

has not already been done by the manufacturer. The recommended volume of feed the baby requires should only be used as a guideline; his activity and maturity should also be considered. In 7 to 10 days the baby should be taking 150 ml per kg of body weight divided into five feeds. For example, a baby of 3·5 kg will take 100 ml per feed and five feeds per 24 hours.

It is essential to teach the mother the importance of sterilizing bottles, teats and equipment, how to prepare feeds and the dangers to the baby of faulty technique.

Daily observations and care

A healthy, thriving baby has a clear, pink skin, moves freely, cries lustily, feeds eagerly and has good muscle tone.

During intrauterine life some antibodies pass across the placenta from the mother to the baby. Most mothers have antibodies to common virus diseases such as measles and chickenpox, so most newborn babies have a degree of passive immunity to these diseases, which may last for about 3 months (Ch. 1). Babies are, however, very susceptible to bacterial infection and must be protected by good nursing technique and scrupulous cleanliness of the nursery and equipment. Individual equipment for each baby reduces the possibility of cross-infection. Handling of the baby by friends and relatives must be discouraged.

Accurate recording of all observations is of prime importance in caring for the newborn, and it should be remembered that the paediatrician has to depend upon the nurse to carry out this duty and to rely on her judgments. Some observations are best carried out when feeding the baby or changing him. These include:

Respirations
Any change in respiratory pattern during feeding or crying, particularly if accompanied by a change in colour, is noteworthy and could indicate, for example, respiratory infection or a congenital heart lesion.

Colour
Undue pallor or blueness are always serious signs and should be reported immediately.

Physiological jaundice
The newborn baby has an excessive number of red blood cells. The surplus RBCs are broken down and the iron is stored in the liver and spleen; as the newborn baby's liver cannot cope immediately with conjugating all the bilirubin produced, it accumulates in the bloodstream staining the skin yellow.

This type of jaundice appears around the third day of life and often causes drowsiness and disinclination to feed. The doctor may wish to estimate the serum bilirubin level. In a mature baby the jaundice clears up by the sixth or seventh day and the baby suffers no ill effects. It can however be dangerous to low birth weight babies.

Jaundice occurring during the first 24 hours of life is always of serious significance and jaundice occurring later than the normal physiological type can also be ominous. Thus the time of onset of jaundice must be recognized promptly and recorded correctly.

Vomitus
Records should show when the vomiting occurred in relation to feeding and the character of the vomitus. It may be due simply to poor feeding technique or it may indicate a serious complication.

Urine
Urine is often voided during birth; if so this must be noted as it may not be passed again for 24 hours.

Stools
Meconium is usually passed within the first 24 hours of birth; over the next few days the stools alter to a greenish-brown colour known as the 'changing' stool. After 3 or 4 days the breast fed baby's stools become yellow and soft in consistency and are passed three to four times per day. The artificially fed baby has more formed stools which are greyish

in colour and have an offensive odour. The total number of stools must be carefully recorded over a 24-hour period.

Care of the buttocks

The buttocks require thorough cleansing and drying each time the napkin is changed. Zinc and castor oil cream may be applied as a prophylactic measure to the perianal region to prevent soreness. If sore buttocks do occur the cause must be carefully investigated. The soreness may be due to:

1. Faulty washing and rinsing of the napkin. Modern detergents are not suitable for washing napkins and a change in laundering method may produce immediate improvement.

2. Unsuitable feeding. Frequent stools are a source of irritation to the skin. This condition can be caused by too much sugar in the feed or by the feed being prepared incorrectly.

3. Infection. Gastroenteritis also causes frequent loose stools. This is a most dangerous condition in a newborn baby — it results in rapid dehydration and collapse. Speedy diagnosis is vital to the baby's life and any suspicious case must be isolated immediately since the disease readily becomes epidemic. Treatment is directed at removing the cause and restoring fluid and electrolyte balance. Antibiotic therapy is essential. In a severe case the buttocks can be exposed in a warm environment to promote healing. Various soothing creams can be used.

General care of the skin and mucous membranes

From birth until the fourth or fifth day the baby is usually 'top and tailed' in his cot. The technique has already been described for initial cleansing. Special note must be taken of the following points during the procedure:

Eyes

There should be no discharge from a newborn baby's eyes. Tears are not formed during crying in the early weeks and any discharge must be treated as infection.

Mouth

Inspection of buccal mucosa and tongue for thrush infection must be carried out. This condition is most commonly seen in the mouth of an artificially fed baby and seldom in a breast fed baby. It is caused by the *Candida albicans* and is contagious. It can be spread round a nursery by the nurses' hands and equipment. The baby does not feed well and, on examination of the mouth and tongue, there are greyish-white spots which look like milk curd but on gentle examination cannot be removed. Should thrush infection arise the nursery techniques must be carefully investigated, paying special attention to the preparation of feeds and the handling of bottles and teats. The baby will be isolated or barrier nursed with all his equipment including feeding utensils. The doctor may order a course of nystatin oral drops 100 000 units 3 or 4 times daily for 4 to 7 days. Thrush responds quickly to treatment. Early recognition is essential because it can spread very quickly.

Skin flexures

The skin flexures are cleansed, dried and inspected for infection.

Cord

The cord stump and surrounding tissues must be examined for signs of infection and treated at least twice daily with Hibitane in spirit.

Skin

Bathing of the baby is usually permitted by the fifth or sixth day of life. A demonstration is given to the mother who should then be allowed to bath her own baby with guidance from the midwife at least twice before she goes home.

Temperature

The temperature must be taken and recorded at least once daily using a special low reading rectal thermometer (scale down to 25 °C).

Weight

This may be recorded daily, but care must be taken to ensure that the mother does not become obsessed with the baby's weight pattern. For the first 2 to 3 days the weight falls mainly due to the passage of urine and meconium and because of a small fluid intake. By the fourth to fifth day it should begin to rise again and a mature and healthy baby will regain his birth weight in 7 to 10 days.

Identification

Identification bands should be checked daily.

The baby should be beside his mother as much as possible and the mother should be encouraged to care for her baby under sympathetic supervision.

SPECIAL CARE OF LOW BIRTH WEIGHT BABIES

If a baby at birth weighs 2500 g or less he is classified as being of **low birth weight**.
This may be because:
1. He has been born too soon—**preterm**.
2. He has not grown normally before birth—**light-for-dates**.

The preterm baby

In Chapter 10 the method of working out the EDD (expected date of delivery) was described. A baby is considered to be at term if delivered between 37 and 41 weeks. If he is born early, that is before 37 weeks' *gestation*, he is known as a preterm baby. The chances of survival are reduced as the gestational period becomes shorter, especially if it is less than 34 weeks. Most maternity hospitals or units have a special care nursery designed to provide the best possible conditions for nursing low birth weight babies under the direction of a consultant paediatrician.

A high standard of nursing care must be maintained with careful attention to detail, and it is crucial that the paediatrician is provided with accurate records. Continuous observation of these babies is essential and in many instances intensive nursing care is required. The survival of special care babies depends on a team effort involving medical and nursing staff.

Modern incubators with an infant servocontrol give a continuous record of the baby's body temperature as well as controlling the incubator temperature to maintain the baby's temperature at a preset level (Fig. 17.14). The baby is nursed naked which

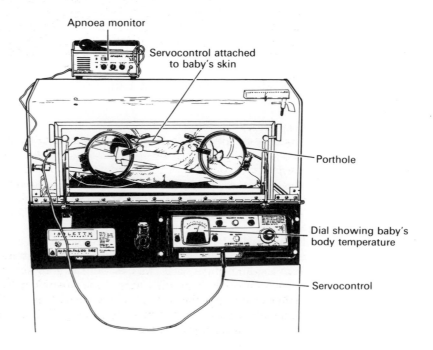

Apnoea monitor

Servocontrol attached to baby's skin

Porthole

Dial showing baby's body temperature

Servocontrol

Figure 17.14
Incubator showing apnoea monitor with alarm, which sounds if the baby stops breathing

makes observation much easier; in particular the colour and respiratory pattern can be readily noted. Oxygen administration must be carefully monitored and regulated and the humidity controlled.

Feeding

Feeding can be started soon after birth. Human milk is most easily digested but is not always available and it may be necessary to use an artificial milk preparation. Preterm babies have poor sucking and swallowing reflexes and may need to be fed with expressed breast milk via a nasogastric catheter which can be left *in situ* (Fig. 17.15). Abdominal distension causing respiratory embarrassment following a feed can occur, and therefore the volume of each feed must be carefully worked out according to the baby's weight and capacity. There may also be problems with the digestion of the feed.

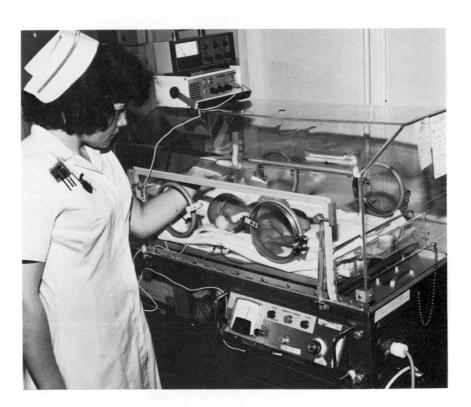

Figure 17.15
Tube feeding showing use of incubator porthole

Daily care

Minimal handling with as little disturbance to the baby as possible is essential. The detail of daily care has been already described for the normal baby. All procedures should be carried out prior to feeding, working through the incubator portholes (Fig. 17.15). Weighing may be carried out using a special scale designed for use inside the incubator. The weight usually falls and levels out during the first 7 to 10 days and then slowly rises and the birth weight may be regained in 2 or 3 weeks.

The mother

Because the baby must be nursed in a special care nursery some separation from the mother is inevitable. It is vital to the infant–mother relationship that every effort be made to involve the mother as much as possible in the care of her baby. It is now the policy of most paediatricians to allow the mother into the nursery and to encourage her to handle her baby under supervision (Fig. 17.16), even if it only involves holding her baby's hand for a short time.

Complications

Some common complications that are liable to occur in preterm babies include:

Respiratory Distress Syndrome (RDS)

This condition is characterized by cyanosis — rapid respirations with marked indrawing of the ribs and the sternum accompanied by apnoeic attacks which may gradually become more prolonged and severe. This condition manifests itself soon after birth and requires intensive nursing care. High concentration oxygen therapy or the infant ventilator may be required combined with intravenous administration of electrolytes, particularly sodium bicarbonate, via the umbilical vessels. Feeds may be given by continuous drip method via the nasogastric catheter. Many babies do recover but there are a number who die, particularly those of low gestational age.

Oxygen concentration levels must be estimated frequently using a special oxygen analyser. Prolonged administration of a high concentration of oxygen may cause damage to the blood vessels of the retina of the eye causing irreversible blindness. Oxygen should be reduced as soon as the baby's condition shows improvement and discontinued altogether as soon as possible.

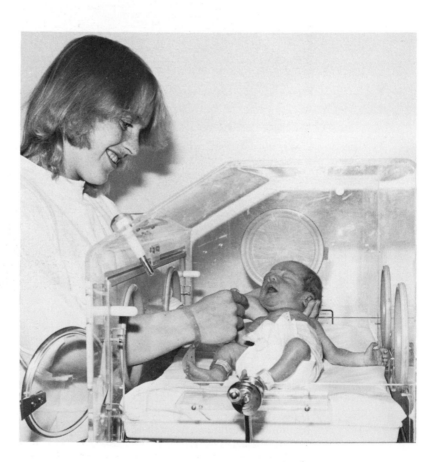

Figure 17.16
Mother making physical contact with her baby

Jaundice

Physiological jaundice, which often occurs in the normal full-term baby, tends to be more severe in the preterm baby due to immaturity of the liver. The jaundice becomes more intense as the serum bilirubin level rises steadily in the circulating blood. If untreated the baby may suffer permanent brain damage or even die. The serum bilirubin level in the blood is checked twice daily, sometimes even more frequently, and phototherapy may be given (Fig. 17.17).

Phototherapy is exposure of the baby (naked) to fluorescent light which is a source of blue light. Care must be taken to expose the baby for the prescribed number of hours, maintain the body temperature and shield the eyes with a light pad of protective material. The bilirubin is altered by the blue light and as it is excreted the level slowly falls.

In severe cases it may be necessary to carry out a replacement blood transfusion and thus reduce the circulating bilirubin level.

Infection

Infection used to be one of the commonest causes of death in low birth weight babies. Modern paediatric practice using improved techniques combined with antibiotic therapy has cut down the mortality rate. All precautions must be taken to ensure that the nurseries, furnishings and equipment including incubators are kept scrupulously clean. All staff must be free from infection, and visitors other than than the parents must be excluded from inside the nursery area. Frequent screening by the bacteriologist of the nursery environment, equipment and staff helps to control infection.

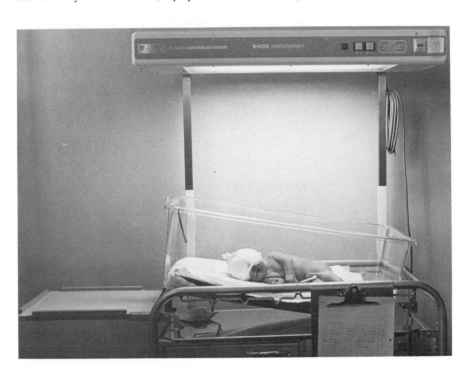

Figure 17.17
Phototherapy

Follow-up

After the baby's initial problems of survival he may be slower to reach the milestones of development (Ch. 18) than a mature baby of the same age. His progress is carefully monitored by the paediatrician since there is a considerable risk of cerebral palsy and mental retardation.

The light-for-dates baby

Babies who fall into this category are those who have been subjected to inadequate nourishment *in utero* due to poor placental function, for example in *pre-eclampsia*. Labour is usually induced early when there is evidence of poor fetal growth because intrauterine death might occur. The baby's weight is less than anticipated for the gestational age.

Nursing care

The light-for-dates baby also requires expert care, which is provided in the special care baby unit.

Feeding

Feeding by nasogastric catheter is not usually necessary since the light-for-dates baby can swallow and suck satisfactorily.

Complications

Complications which are likely to occur in a baby which is light-for-dates are the following:

Hypoglycaemia

This condition is liable to occur in the first 48 hours and serious brain damage may occur following convulsions. It may be precipitated by lack of oxygen and chilling. **Prevention** is essential. Resuscitation at birth must be prompt and in a warm environment. Early feeding will also prevent the development of hypoglycaemia. Screening may be carried out with Dextrostix and blood specimens examined for glucose every 4 hours during the danger peroiod.

Hypothermia

The light-for-dates baby is lacking in subcutaneous fat and loses heat very quickly. It is an essential part of nursing care to maintain the body temperature and it may be necessary to nurse the baby in an incubator.

Infection

The light-for-dates baby is also at risk, as is the preterm baby.

Follow-up

Follow-up care is carried out by the paediatrician. The outlook for the light-for-dates baby has greatly improved with modern care but he may remain small throughout his life.

MOTHERCRAFT TEACHING

Mothercraft classes in the postnatal period are of great importance (Fig. 17.18). They are more meaningful than those in the antenatal period as the baby is now born and imminent discharge home with the potential problems this involves is almost upon the new mother. Topics covered in these classes may include:

Preparation of feeds.
Role of the district midwife and health visitor.
Prevention of home accidents.
Demonstration of modern baby 'aids'.
Introduction to family planning with leaflets and location of clinics so that the mother can discuss this important matter with her husband.

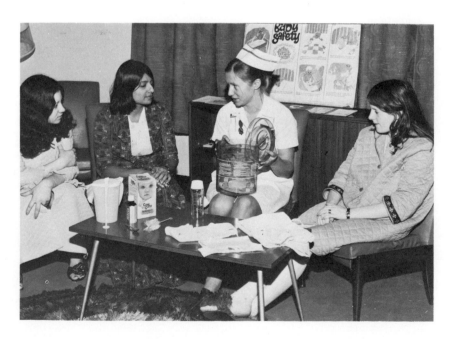

Figure 17.18
Mothercraft teaching

A close liaison between the hospital, district midwife, health visitor and general practitioner must be established so that when the mother and baby are discharged home all the relevant information is readily available. Nursing care of the mother and baby in the puerperium is different from general nursing. Patient dependency is minimal: the majority of the new mothers are not ill and are quickly ambulant. The role of the nurse is a supportive one — helping the mother to adapt herself to and accept the responsibilities of motherhood. A great deal of tact, patience and human understanding are essential.

FURTHER READING

Keay A J, Morgan D M (eds) 1978 Craig's care of the newly born infant, 6th edn. Churchill Livingstone, Edinburgh
Myles M F 1981 Textbook for midwives, 9th edn. Churchill Livingstone, Edinburgh
Scottish Health Education Group 1980 The book of the child. SHEG, Edinburgh
Vulliamy D G 1977 The newborn child, 4th edn. Churchill Livingstone, Edinburgh

18. Children

This chapter gives an introduction to the special needs of children and outlines the services in the community and in hospital which are designed to meet those needs.

The nurse must remember that children are not small adults; their tolerance of illness and response to treatments cannot be assumed to be in proportion to their size. Indeed their reactions are often markedly different and may bear no relationship to those of adults. In general, children respond quickly and dramatically both to illness and to treatment. Early signs of adverse reactions must be noted and reported with the minimum of delay because a small child's condition can deteriorate so rapidly. For this reason the paediatric nurse must be forever vigilant. A junior nurse should remember that it is better to raise a false alarm than run the risk of irreversible worsening of a young patient's condition through hesitation because of uncertainty.

It is essential to have an understanding of the growth and development of the healthy child so that any deviation from the normal which the sick child may show can be easily and quickly recognized.

GROWTH AND DEVELOPMENT OF THE NORMAL CHILD

Growth refers to an increase in size, development to the processes whereby a child matures physically, mentally, emotionally and socially. The normal rate of growth is not constant throughout the growing years; it is most rapid in the first 2 years of life and during adolescence. Each child has his own pace of development although most children follow the same sequence. The pace is determined by both the child's innate potential and his environment; the physical care and mental stimulation he receives are important influencing factors.

Development depends on the maturation of the nervous system. No amount of teaching will enable a baby to perform a skill before the necessary areas of the nervous system are mature. The direction of development is cephalocaudal, that is from the head downwards through the trunk to the lower limbs. The infant can grasp with his hands before he can co-ordinate with his lower limbs, and he can hold his head up before he can sit. A child learns to sit before he can walk, and the age at which he learns to walk varies considerably from one child to the other.

There is progression from general responses to the more specific. The baby demonstrates his emotions by activity of his arms and legs, increased respirations and by becoming pink with excitement, whereas an older child shows his emotions by facial expression only.

Formulae have been devised from studies carried out on infants and children which provide average standards for growth and development; these are known as milestones or norms.

Stages of growth and development

During the first few months of life activity is instinctive, for example sucking, swallowing, grasping and eliminating. A baby develops an awareness of his surroundings, of being loved and adequately nourished and of security through the care given by his mother. He sleeps most of the time, wakening only for feeds, and he will cry in response to hunger or discomfort. Later crying may indicate fear, anger or frustration.

At 3 months old he sleeps less, recognizes and enjoys his mother's company, smiles and is interested in quiet play. He listens to music and his eyes will follow a moving object which he will attempt to grasp. At 5 months he chuckles and makes babbling sounds, can sit with support for a short time, discovers his fingers and toes and plays by himself briefly, enjoying repetitive play. Also around this time, he can recognize familiar faces and show his pleasure. He may show fear when approached by the unfamiliar.

At 6 months he can determine sound direction and turn his head towards it. He develops a need to bite and, by this time, primary teeth begin to appear, the central lower incisors being the first. At 7 months he can sit unsupported and propel himself in any direction using his arms and hands.

At 9 months he tries to feed himself and can grasp small objects using finger and thumb, often protesting when the object is taken away from him. By now he can raise himself on hands and knees in an attempt to pull himself upright. He speaks in monosyllables and can imitate a variety of sounds. If thumb sucking develops this may signify hunger, distress, tiredness or insecurity.

The toddler is dependent on his mother and a familiar routine. He becomes insecure if the pattern of his daily life is altered. He strives towards independence by attempting to dress and feed himself; these attempts are initially untidy and messy, but with patience and encouragement the child will eventually succeed. At this stage the child is full of curiosity and activity; he sleeps well and requires a nap during the day.

Voluntary control of bowel and bladder begins at the age of $1\frac{1}{2}$ to 2 years. There is extreme urgency initially, but this decreases as he grows older so that by the age of $2\frac{1}{2}$ to 3 years, he attains sphincter control and may demand privacy for toilet purposes.

He lives entirely in the present and time is associated with a familiar routine. He has no concept of sharing. He requires play materials of differing textures and shapes to stimulate co-ordination and learning capabilities. He plays happily on his own, alongside other children, without becoming involved in their play. If disturbed or restricted in his activities, he may display signs of frustration and anger. About this time, too, a child may notice and ask questions about sexual differences. Sibling rivalry may present problems to the 2 to 3 year old who may resent a new baby or the abilities of an older child. Vocabulary increases and he loves repeating simple nursery rhymes or listening to familiar stories.

Primary or deciduous dentition is complete by the third year. From the age of 6 years permanent teeth gradually replace the primary teeth.

Between the ages of 3 and 5, improved co-ordination and balance allow the child to run and climb confidently. He becomes socially aware and learns to share and play with other children. He particularly enjoys playing with sand and water, bricks, jigsaws, paint, construction toys and equipment, using imagination to act out domestic activities, pleasant and unpleasant. A greatly increased vocabulary and ability to articulate allow the child to construct simple sentences.

At this stage attendance at a nursery school or preschool group is invaluable; here the child will have the opportunity to increase his social experiences and will be provided with occupations that encourage concentration and learning.

From the age of 5, growth continues at a constant rate until the preadolescent state when there is a marked increase. This is known as the growth spurt. There is rapid growth of the limbs followed by growth of the trunk, and sex differences are demonstrated by the distribution of fat and muscle. These changes and the development of the secondary sex characteristics occur earlier in girls, although they are physically less strong than boys.

During the school years, emotions tend to fluctuate between feeling secure and feeling anxious. Sleep patterns may be disturbed and nightmares are common due to the fears caused by the demands of wider educational experiences. Competition is enjoyed but failure is not easily accepted. Learning continues rapidly, interests widen and the peer group becomes all important.

CARING FOR CHILDREN IN THE COMMUNITY

In the United Kingdom the responsibility for community care is shared by the Departments of Health, Education and Social Services. The facilities they offer are available to all children. The midwifery service takes care of the mother and baby until 10 to 14 days after delivery, whether a baby is born in hospital or at home (Ch. 17).

The preschool child

From this time the main adviser to the mother is the health visitor, unless illness occurs when the family doctor is consulted. The health visitor is concerned with the physical and mental health of the whole family; she has an important role in the prevention and early detection of health problems.

Her work includes visiting homes where there are preschool children. During these visits she advises mothers to attend the local child health centre or group practice 'well-baby' clinics. Such clinics are organized by the health visitors and provide advice on all aspects of mental, physical and social care as the need arises.

Routine medical examinations are carried out by the doctor at the first visit, and at 3, 6 and 12 months, then annually during the preschool years. Physical and developmental assessments are made at these times and the doctor will also be available if the mother or health visitor wishes the child to be seen between routine examinations. When the child is 9 months old, the health visitor carries out routine hearing tests. The clinic provides an immunization service. A sample immunization programme is shown in Table 18.1.

Table 18.1
Sample immunization programme

Year	Vaccine/Toxoid	Remarks
1st	(a) Triple antigen (diphtheria whooping cough, tetanus)	(a) At 3 to 6 months
	Poliomyelitis (Sabin)	
	(b) As above	(b) At about 8 months
	(c) As above	(c) At 10 to 12 months
2nd	Measles	May be given in third year to reduce the risk of reactions
5th	Diphtheria/tetanus Poliomyelitis	Booster dose
10th to 13th	BCG	Only if negative on tuberculin testing
11th to 13th	Rubella	Offered to all girls
15th to 19th	Poliomyelitis Tetanus	Usually at school-leaving age

Advice on health education, parentcraft and accident prevention is provided through group discussions, lectures and films. Any special problems such as those of the immigrant family can be dealt with or the family can be put in touch with additional services, if necessary. Welfare foods and vitamins are provided at reduced cost — for instance vitamin drops for the baby and vitamin tablets for nursing mothers. Free milk is available for children in special need. The centre becomes a meeting place where mothers can make friends and have discussions about their families.

Home visiting by the health visitor is continued at regular intervals. The main advantage of home visiting is to see the child in his own environment and thus assess more readily whether adequate care is being given. The health visitor checks that growth and development are proceeding normally. She advises on feeding, clothing, general hygiene and immunization and gives practical guidance on the prevention of home accidents. If she recognizes social or mental stress within the family she will advise and mobilize the relevant services. She maintains a record of progress for each child which is passed on to the school medical service when full time education begins.

Day nurseries for children from 6 weeks up to 5 years are available to families with temporary or long-term social problems. They are open 6 days each week from 8 a.m. to 6 p.m., are staffed by trained nursery nurses and are equipped to meet the needs of the different age groups.

Nursery schools are provided by the Education and Social Services Departments for children between the ages of 3 to 5 years. They may attend for a half day or a full day. Time is spent in constructive play and group activities organized by teachers assisted by nursery nurses. The objectives are to help children become happy, active members of a group, to gain experience with adults outside the family and to prepare them for the wider experience of infant school.

A registered child-minder may look after a small group of children in private premises if the facilities have been approved by the Social Services Department.

Private play groups with functions similar to those of nursery schools are supported by the **Preschool Play Groups Association**. Play groups financed by the Save the Children Fund are often sited in socially deprived areas where much of the work is carried out by voluntary help. These, too, must be approved by the Social Services Department.

The school child

In the U.K. it is the responsibility of the school medical service to continue the supervision of the child's health throughout his school years and to co-operate with the education service to help the handicapped child. The health team includes the school doctor, health visitor and/or school nurse. Medical examinations, including hearing tests, are carried out on all children on starting school and at intervals throughout the school years. This includes testing vision when the child is 7 years old. Dental inspection is carried out every 6 months. Reinforcing immunization programmes are continued and BCG vaccination is given to any child leaving school who has a negative response to a Mantoux test.

The school nurse or health visitor carries out regular examinations of the children to ensure that personal cleanliness is maintained. She looks in particular for lice infestation of hair, infections of scalp, skin rashes such as scabies and verrucae of the feet (Ch. 14). Appropriate treatment (which may include the whole family) is initiated as necessary.

The health team assists in promoting health education within the school curriculum and meets with parent–teacher groups. The topics discussed include personal hygiene, dental care, nutrition and eating habits, self-discipline related to the use of leisure hours, sex, smoking, alcohol and drugs.

A school meals service is available and children are provided with lunch at a nominal cost. In cases of need, lunches and extra meals are provided free of charge. Footwear and clothes can be provided when families have financial problems. Children not living within walking distance of school (2 miles for those under 8 years and 3 miles for older ones) are provided with transport to and from school. Representatives of road safety organizations and the police assist in school road safety programmes. To ensure the safety of children crossing busy roads, patrolmen are on duty to control traffic.

The handicapped child

Special care and education are provided by local education authorities for all physically handicapped and educable mentally handicapped children. Some of these services are assisted by voluntary organizations. Disabled children are examined at yearly intervals or more frequently as required. There is close liaison between the school health team, family doctor, parents and teacher to ensure adequate treatment and follow-up.

There are 10 categories of handicap:

Blind.
Partially blind.
Deaf.
Partially deaf.
Educationally subnormal.
Epileptic.
Maladjusted.
Physically handicapped.

Children with speech defects.
Delicate children.

Where possible, these children attend ordinary classes or they are placed in a special class within a normal school, thus enabling them to share in the general activities as far as possible. Others require special schools which may be either day or residential; those with multiple handicaps may be taught at home or in a hospital school. Ideally, all handicapped children should be educated in their home community and should interact with normal children, within the limits of their handicap.

Children whose mental subnormality renders them ineducable are cared for in occupational centres or in hospitals for the mentally subnormal where sociability and independence are encouraged (Ch. 15).

The deprived child

In Britain, the Children's and Young Person's Act of 1963 authorized local authorities to give assistance to deprived children in kind or in cash where necessary and also to work with voluntary organizations. It is an attempt to diminish the need to take children into care. Information about available voluntary and statutory social services can be obtained from the Citizens' Advice Bureau. Voluntary organizations such as Dr Barnardo's and the Woman's Royal Voluntary Service (WRVS) give advice and practical help to families in danger of breaking down. The WRVS helps the overworked mother and provides holiday homes for children.

The incidence of neglect and child abuse is increasing. Child abuse may be referred to as either 'the battered child syndrome' or 'non accidental injury'.

Child abuse takes many forms, from that of extreme physical battering to severe emotional and psychological deprivation. Any age group can be ill-treated though babies of less than six months old are especially vulnerable. One child in the family may be singled out for abuse.

In Great Britain approximately 3000–4000 children are deliberately injured each year, of these about 700 die; many suffer permanent injury, brain damage and neurological impairment.

The nature of battering is varied. Common forms include bruising from excessive pressure from fingers on face and trunk, burns from cigarettes or other sources of extreme heat, bite marks and swelling of the upper lip with tearing of the frenulum. Other forms are fractures of the long bones and ribs, head injury and retinal haemorrhages.

Child abuse is most common in families who are physically, financially, intellectually or emotionally deprived, and may occur in any social class. It often takes place when the parents are under stress. They are usually young and have themselves experienced battering in childhood.

The Royal Society for the Prevention of Cruelty to Children works closely with the social services, and the hospital and community health teams to identify and assess 'at risk' families. A multidisciplinary approach is needed to help the whole family and prevent further child abuse.

CARING FOR CHILDREN IN HOSPITAL

When caring for children it is essential to consider their emotional and physical needs. In order to do this account must be taken of each child's background — his family, his home and his environment. Parents are the most important people in the child's life especially when he is sick. They should be helped to feel comfortable in the ward environment and guided to help in the care of their child as much as possible.

Effects of admission to hospital

Separation from family caused by admission to hospital can readily lead to serious psychological trauma; this may be transient or lasting. Signs of psychological trauma in a child are persistent crying and refusal to be comforted, aggression, withdrawal, personality changes and regression in social behaviour such as bed wetting and thumb sucking.

In hospital a child's usual pattern of daily life is disturbed and he must accept a strange routine in unfamiliar surroundings. Nursing and medical care now take precedence and, of necessity, care has to be given by a variety of adults. His 'room' is no longer his own or shared with his family but shared with a number of other unknown children (Fig. 18.1). It is not, therefore, surprising that the majority of children suffer emotionally when admitted to hospital. How much a child suffers depends on his age, his personality and the degree of security previously experienced in his home environment. Predictably the preschool child is the most vulnerable because of his limited ability to communicate and to socialize.

Parents may also demonstrate anxiety when their child requires admission to hospital. They may have feelings of guilt, especially if the child has been involved in an illness or accident that could have been avoided. Loyalties may become divided because the demands of the sick child conflict with the needs of other family members, thus causing friction. Parental anxiety may be shown by the parents' failure to accept explanation or by complaints of a petty nature to other parents or junior staff. Parents require tactful handling, patience and consideration from all staff.

The adverse effects of hospitalization can be reduced, even in unsuitable buildings, but they are most readily minimized in purpose-built paediatric units.

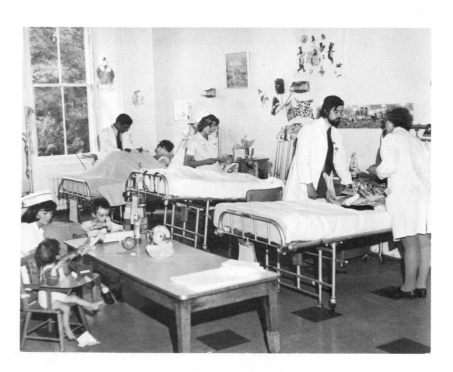

Figure 18.1
Sharing with other children

The paediatric unit

This may be one of several comprising a children's hospital or may be found within a general hospital. In a well-run unit the atmosphere will be kindly and welcoming because the doctors and nurses have a special regard for and understanding of children. The atmosphere is also created in part by the surroundings, which should be cheerful, warm, bright, colourful and safe.

Only in a specially designed unit can the sick child's needs be fully met. Here he can have emotional support, skilled medical and nursing care, opportunity for play and, if old enough, education.

Since emotional support is best given by the mother, accommodation should be available for her to live in the unit. This enables her to be admitted with her child, to help during the 'settling in' period and also to assist in giving care if she is able and willing (Fig. 18.2).

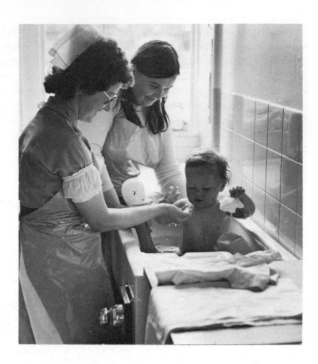

Figure 18.2
A mother helping to care for her child

Play helps the child to relax and allows safe working out of strong emotions such as fear and aggression. The play room should be of adequate size for the number of patients, contain a wide selection of toys and play materials suited to all age groups and be staffed by a play therapist. The play therapist will be able to assist in the rehabilitation of children with special needs. Furniture should be simple, attractive and of sizes suited to the age groups of its users.

Education for the school child is an on-going process and, whenever illness allows, it should be continued. The Department of Education requires that teaching be provided for children who are in hospital for more than 3 weeks (Fig. 18.3). Full-time teaching is an important part of the care of a child who is in hospital for a long time. Part-time teaching is generally sufficient in acute wards.

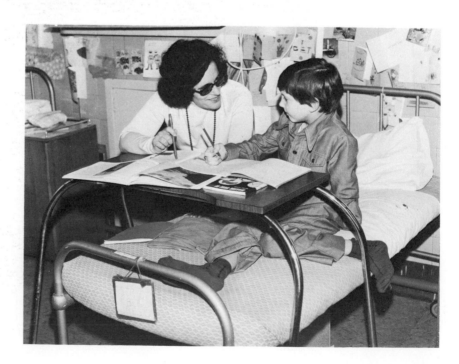

Figure 18.3
Teaching in hospital

Most paediatric units provide facilities for day care. This means that a child needing minor surgery or diagnostic tests who does not require elaborate preparation can be admitted in the morning and taken home again that evening.

General care of the child in hospital

Careful patient care planning is essential to ensure that the child has adequate periods of rest, occupation and play (Fig. 18.4). In this way exhaustion, boredom and frustration will be avoided. Thoughtful care can help to make the child's stay a pleasant experience.

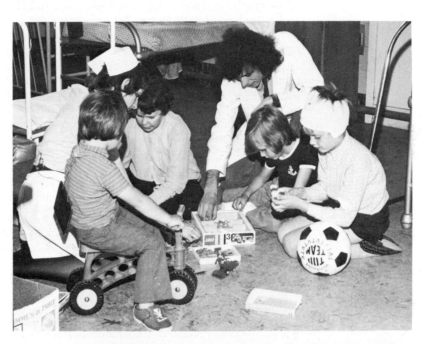

Figure 18.4
Play

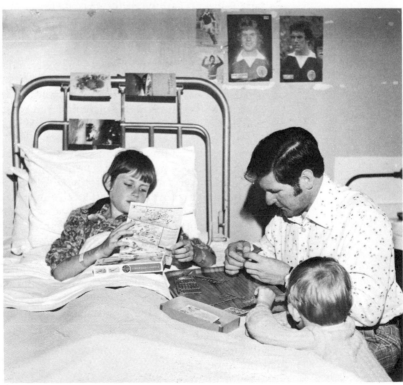

Figure 18.5
Visit from father

Ward routine should be geared to meet the needs of its occupants and not the other way round, as was so often the case in the past. Open or free visiting is essential in a paediatric unit. If it is not possible for the mother to live in, then she should be encouraged to arrange her home routine in order to be with her sick child as much as she can — especially at meals, play time and bed time when she would normally be closely involved with him. Sometimes the father is able to take a turn (Fig. 18.5), allowing his wife to be free to maintain contact with the home and the other children in the family. Alternatively, he may just look in on his way to or from work.

The child should have as much freedom as his illness permits; he will be happier and adjust more easily if he is allowed out of bed for meals and play. If he cannot be mobilized he should be dressed in his own clothes and nursed on top of his bed to give greater freedom of movement and maintain a more normal daily routine.

Meal times should be happy, relaxed occasions and free from rush. The food presented should be attractive and suitable for the different age groups of children. After attending to toilet needs and hand washing, children should be comfortably and safely seated at the table where they should be encouraged to remain until the meal is completed. Colourful nursery crockery and suitable sizes of cutlery should be provided and opportunity must be offered to each child to feed himself. He should be encouraged, not forced, to complete his meal. Children enjoy a little play and conversation at meal times. A doll, teddy or story can be used to persuade the reluctant child to finish his food.

Special aspects of care

Special elements of therapy and care merit more detailed consideration.

Admission

Children are admitted to hospital when medical treatment and nursing care cannot be carried out in the home. This may be because home conditions are inadequate, because the care required is highly technical or because special diagnostic tests are necessary. Admission to hospital is usually planned but it may result from an emergency.

Planned admission

This is arranged between the family doctor and the hospital consultant to whom the child has been referred. Visits to a hospital clinic will have preceded admission in most cases, and here full explanations of the reasons for admission, an indication of the date of admission and the approximate length of stay can be given. Good relationships develop at this stage if the information provided is clearly understood and the questions asked are fully answered.

The child and his parents should visit the paediatric unit where they will meet the sister. She will give guidance regarding the preparation for admission and make arrangements for the mother to live in with her child if she wishes.

At the time of admission, a welcoming and reassuring approach from the nursing staff will help to allay anxiety. One nurse should deal with the formalities of admission (Fig. 18.6) so that the child can identify with her. She should already know the child's name and the reason for his admission. She should encourage the mother to remain throughout the procedure, since this will calm the child and permit observation of the interaction between him and his mother. Observation should also be made of general health, nutrition and overall cleanliness. An identity bracelet should be made out and checked by the mother before being attached to the child's wrist. Enquiries as to his baptismal state should be made discreetly. If the child is not to be confined to bed, he should wear his own clothing, which must be adequately labelled and cared for. Discussion with the mother should include diet, for example the type of food the child likes and dislikes, and also his sleep pattern and toilet habits.

The following guidelines can be used by nursing staff to elicit information regarding a child during the admission procedure. The information can then be used as a basis for the development of a nursing care plan.

Name of child	Age	Birthday
Pet name	Baptismal status	
Name of brother(s)	Age	
Name of sister(s)	Age	

Does the child require help with
  dressing?
  bathing?
  combing hair?
  cleaning teeth?
Has the child been in hospital previously?
Does the child know why he is being admitted?
Does the child make friends easily?
Has the child a favourite comforter?
  e.g. dummy teat.
      piece of blanket.
      bye byes.
Has the child brought it to hospital?

Diet
  Is the child's appetite good?
  Is the child breast fed/bottle/spoon/cup.
    Breast feeding
      Regular times?
      Demand feeding?
    Bottle feeding
      Type of milk?
      Amount?
      Number of feeds?
  Feeds self alone.   Feeds self with help.
  What foods does the child like?
  What foods does the child dislike?
  What fluids does the child like?
  What fluids does the child dislike?
  Any food allergies?
  Any other food comments?

Toilet habits
  Is the child toilet trained
    bowel?
    bladder?
  Does the child wear a nappy
    all day?
    night only?
  Does the child use a potty?
  Does the child use a lavatory?
  What word(s) used for bowel movement?
  What word(s) used for micturition?
  Is the child taken to toilet at night?
    What time?

Sleep pattern
  Usual bed time?   Hours of sleep at night?
  Are naps taken?   What time?
  Does the child sleep alone?
  Does the child sleep in a bed?
  Does the child sleep in a cot?
  Any special bed time routine?
    e.g. Dolly's company?
        Teddy's company?
        Saying prayers?

Play/occupation
  Has the child a favourite toy?
  Has the child a favourite game?

Does the child play alone?
Does the child play with other children?
Does the child play with other adults?
Does the child watch TV regularly?
Does the child have special programmes?
Does the child have a pet?   Name.

School
Does the child attend nursery school?
Does the child attend primary school?
Name of the school.
List special interests
   Hobbies.
   Books.
   T.V.
   Radio programmes.

Any other comments.

A child from a secure, caring home who has been properly prepared for his stay in hospital will adjust more quickly to life in the ward. He is likely to have some impressions of hospital life learned from television, radio and story books. The National Association for the Welfare of Children in Hospital provides booklets, films and slides which are used as teaching aids when visiting schools and mothers' groups. The Association offers advice and practical assistance to mothers with children in hospital by providing baby-sitters and transport if necessary.

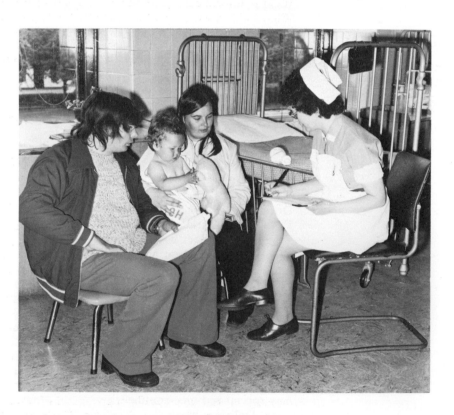

Figure 18.6
Admission to hospital

Emergency admission
An emergency admission presents difficulties because there is no time for preparation of either child or parents. After the clinical examination of the child, reassurance and explanation is of the utmost importance, particularly if the admission is the result of an accident or sudden illness. Child and parents should be separated as little as possible, for example only during the preparation for operation. In some instances, parents can

accompany their child to the anaesthetic room. There are very few situations where parents cannot remain with their child to the benefit of all.

Observation
A normal, healthy child looks bright, happy and interested, is rarely still during the day and sleeps soundly at night.

General observations
In illness the child becomes more dependent on mother. Changes in behaviour are, often, the earliest signs of disease process, e.g. lethargy, fretfulness, loss of appetite, restlessness.

Children adopt unusual postures when in pain and discomfort; for example a child with abdominal pain will lie curled up and flex his knees during bouts of colic and the child with severe cyanotic heart disease adopts a squatting position. Photophobia is demonstrated by turning the head away from the light or burying the head under the bed clothes.

The healthy infant may cry to be lifted up because he is wet, cold or too hot. Hunger is announced by strong, continuous crying accompanied by sucking of the fingers. Episodes of strong crying, accompanied by frowning and drawing up of the legs, may indicate flatulence or abdominal colic. The teething infant often cries with pain, gnaws anything that is hard and cool and has excess salivation and red patches on his cheeks. Head rolling or rubbing of the affected ear and loud crying often indicates earache. The cry of extreme pain and exhaustion tends to be feeble and moaning, and a sharp, shrill, piercing cry is associated with cerebral irritation.

The foregoing are generalizations and included solely for illustrative porposes. It cannot be overstressed that there is no substitute for nursing experience and that the art of observation can only be learned in the practical situation. The value and significance of nursing observations, particularly in relation to children, merit serious consideration . Of necessity doctors spend less time with their patients than do nurses and therefore rely heavily on nursing observations and records. What the nurse sees, hears, feels and smells in relation to her patient may be valuable pointers to his progress. The quick detection and reporting of a sudden change in a child's condition may be the first step in a life-saving measure.

It should go without saying that two of the nurse's most important responsibilities are to observe accurately and record or report faithfully.

Observation and recording of temperature, pulse, respiration and blood pressure
The relationship between temperature, pulse and respiration is important and the three are usually taken and recorded together. In most units this is done routinely twice each day and 4 hourly or more frequently in acute illness. There are two types of thermometers used to ensure the accurate measurement of body temperature:

1. *The standard clinical thermometer*, which is calibrated to record temperatures between 35°C and 45°C.

2. *The low registering thermometer* with a range of between 25° and 40°C.

The type of thermometer used is determined by the age of the child. The standard clinical thermometer is used for children aged 1 year and over and the low registering thermometer is used for all newborn, low birth weight and ill infants. The latter is used so that hypothermia can be recognized. The temperature regulating centre in the hypothalmus is not fully developed in the early years of life and infants are prone to extremes of body temperature if overheated or chilled. A low body temperature in an infant may indicate, for example, that infection is present whereas the older child with an infection will have a pyrexia. These variations are shown in Table 18.2.

The temperature will vary according to the site in which it is taken. The skin temperature, taken in the axilla or groin, is the lowest. The temperature in the mouth is about 0·6°C higher than that of the skin. The temperature in the rectum is about 0·6°C higher than that in the mouth. There is, therefore, a difference of 1°C between the skin temperature and that of the rectum.

To ensure that an accurate record of temperature is kept, the same site should be used each time. To avoid confusion and possible accident due to biting or breaking the thermometer, it is usual to take temperatures of children under 1 year per rectum and for children over 1 year in the axilla or groin unless otherwise instructed. Rectal surgery and enteritis are two examples of situations where taking temperatures per rectum would be contraindicated.

Table 18.2
Variation in body temperature

Body temperature	Range (degrees C)
Normal	36·3–37·2
Pyrexia	
Low	37·2–38·4
Moderate	38·4–39·5
High	39·5–40·6
Hyperpyrexia	Above 40·6
Hypothermia	Below 36·4

Table 18.3
Normal range of pulse and respiration

Age	Pulse rate per minute	Respiration rate per minute
Birth	150–130	60–30 irregular in rhythm and depth
3 months	130–110	50–30 regular
6 months	120	45–30
1 year	115	30–25
2 years	110–100	30–25
3–6 years	100–90	25
7–10 years	100–80	24–20
11–14 years	90–70	20

When using the rectum, the thermometer should be **held** in position for 1 minute. When using the axilla or groin, the area should first be dried with a towel and the thermometer held in position for 3 minutes. The pulse and respiration are usually in a 4:1 ratio. They vary with the age of the child, being rapid at birth and becoming slower as the child grows older (Table 18.3). They are also affected by physical and emotional activity, which increases the heart rate hence varying the pulse rate. To ensure an accurate record in the young child, pulse and respiration should be counted while the child is resting or sleeping and before he is disturbed to have his temperature taken.

Respiratory activity is assessed by placing the hand lightly on the child's chest. In the baby, observation of the movements of the abdomen will give a more accurate record because of the important role played by the diaphragm and abdominal muscles in respiration. A baby's respirations may be irregular in rate, rhythm and depth. However any irregularity occurring in the older child must be reported immediately.

The sites for locating the pulse are at the anterior lateral aspect of the wrist, over the temporal bone in front of the ear and, in an infant, at the anterior fontanelle. Rhythm and volume are also noted when counting.

The blood pressure is only taken when specifically requested. It is important to ensure that the correct size of cuff and stethoscope is used and that the child is resting and quiet.

Table 18.4
Variation in range of blood pressure

Age	Systolic	Diastolic
Birth	65–95	30–60
2–6 years	60–110	45–75
6–10 years	75–120	50–70

There are two methods of obtaining a reading by:

1. Auscultation. (See Chap. 7. p. 220)
2. Flush method. The cuff is placed on the wrist or ankle and a firm bandage is wrapped round the limb distal to the cuff. The cuff is then inflated to 20 mm^{Hg} and the bandage removed. The limb looks blanched and feels cold. The cuff is *deflated slowly* until the extremity flushes when the systolic pressure can be read using a stethoscope.

Pre- and postoperative care

Physical and psychological preparation is needed before surgery is undertaken. Some children, especially the older age group, have a fear of being put to sleep and having 'things done to them' so it is important that their preparation is carried out with thoughtfulness. An operation may be elective or emergency. Elective surgery gives time for preparation and ensures that the optimum level of health under the circumstances is achieved.

On admission the child is carefully observed for signs of infection which would contraindicate surgery. He is weighed and the routine records are maintained. A specimen of urine is collected for ward testing. Bowel preparation is not required unless the child is to have bowel surgery. A bath is given on the day of the operation. Attention should be paid to the cleanliness of hair, nails and skin folds such as the umbilicus, groins and axillae. A detailed medical history is obtained and a physical examination is carried out. The doctor obtains written consent for the operation from the parents.

The immediate preoperative care begins 4 hours before the operation when the older child is given a light meal and told that he must not eat or drink thereafter. An infant is given a half-strength milk feed. A 'nil orally' sign is then placed on the bed or cot. Prolonged periods without food are not tolerated well by children as the blood sugar falls rapidly. The child is encouraged to pass urine, bathed and dressed in an open-backed theatre gown then returned to a clean bed or cot. The hair is secured with a ribbon or cap. The mouth is checked for the presence of an orthodontic plate or loose teeth. Premedication is given as prescribed by the anaesthetist and the patient is encouraged to sleep and allowed to have his favourite toy beside him It is helpful if the nurse spends a little time talking quietly until he becomes drowsy. Case notes, X-rays and drug prescription records are collected and accompany the child when he is taken to the operating theatre. Careful checking is essential to ensure that the correct child and the correct notes are taken to the operating theatre; in particular, identity **must** be confirmed by looking at the arm band.

On return from the theatre, the child has an airway in position and he is placed in a semiprone position. His lower jaw is directed forward to ensure that the airway is adequately maintained. Consciousness is very quickly regained and the airway is usually ejected. He should be observed constantly until fully conscious. Colour, temperature, pulse and respiration are carefully noted and recorded and the wound dressing is inspected for signs of haemorrhage. Analgesia, ordered by the doctor, should be given if the child becomes restless and complains of pain.

The child's first request is usually for a drink; **small** sips can be given unless medical orders are to the contrary; then mouth care should be given to reduce the discomfort of a dry mouth. Hands and face are washed and he is put into his own nightwear and has his hair combed. He is allowed a pillow and encouraged to rest in a comfortable position. The older child can have easily digested food 6 to 8 hours after surgery if he wishes, especially if he is tolerating oral fluids well; normal diet is resumed the following day. The infant is given glucose fluids 3 to 4 hourly following surgery and his normal feeds are gradually reintroduced.

A child is usually anxious to regain his independence and early ambulation presents no difficulty. Parents are invited to be with their child as soon as possible after surgery and to assist where they can in giving care and reassurance.

Maintenance of fluid and electrolyte balance

In health the composition and concentration of body fluids are maintained within very narrow limits, and there is a delicate balance between them (Ch. 4). A child's body weight is composed of 80 per cent water compared with less than 70 per cent in the adult. In the infant the ratio of extracellular fluid to intracellular fluid is greater than in the older child and the adult. The infant also has a greater body surface area and higher basal metabolic

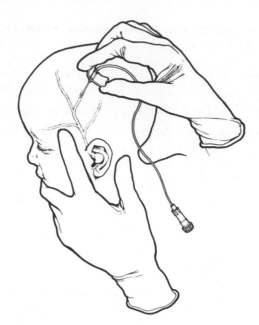

Figure 18.7
Scalp vein infusion using
butterfly needle

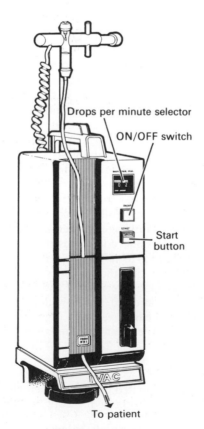

Drops per minute selector

ON/OFF switch

Start
button

Figure 18.8
IVAC pump

Figure 18.8

To patient

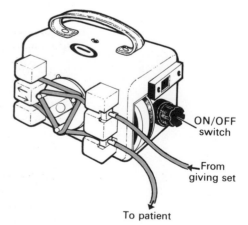

ON/OFF
switch

From
giving set

To patient

Figure 18.9

Figure 18.9
Holter pump

rate per unit of weight, the latter being approximately twice that of the adult. The loss of fluid through the skin, lungs, kidneys and alimentary tract is correspondingly greater. The kidneys of the infant are immature so they are less able to conserve and concentrate fluid. To maintain this balance within the body, the fluid requirement for the young child is 150 ml per kg of body weight over a 24-hour period. The fluid requirements decrease as age increases.

Fluid and electrolyte depletion occurs when there has been an inadequate intake or an excessive output of fluid, such as occurs in vomiting, diarrhoea or polyuria; the child is then said to be dehydrated.

The signs of dehydration are weight loss, sunken eyes which lack lustre, depressed fontanelle, loss of skin turgor, dry mouth, scanty urinary output, lethargy and poor muscle tone. Fluids can be given orally to correct dehydration provided the child is conscious and not vomiting. Other means of providing an adequate fluid and electrolyte intake are by intravenous or intraperitoneal infusion. The paediatrician will prescribe the type of infusion, the amount and nature of fluid and the rate at which the infusion is to be given (usually in millilitres per hour). He bases his decisions on the clinical signs of dehydration, the results of blood chemistry and the child's weight and needs in terms of fluids and electrolytes.

Common sites for intravenous infusion are the superficial temporal vein (Fig. 18.7), antecubital vein or long saphenous vein. The infusion must be carefully regulated to prevent overhydration and overloading of the circulatory system. To ensure the correct rate of flow the infusion must be checked at quarter to half hourly intervals. Various mechanical aids are available to help the nurse regulate the infusion accurately Examples are the IVAC pump (Fig. 18.8) and the Holter pump (Fig. 18.9). In the absence of these aids, the following formula may be used:

In the standard recipient set 15 drops equals approximately 1 ml;
$$\text{ml/hour} \times 15 = \text{number of drops per hour};$$

$$\text{therefore, ml/hour} \times \frac{15}{60} = \text{number of drops per minute}$$

$$\text{estimation of rate flow} = \frac{\text{ml/hour}}{4}$$

$$= \text{drops/minute}$$

The microdrip recipient set (Fig. 18.10) is calibrated at 60 drops/ml and enables the rate of flow to be more easily regulated; the number of millilitres per hour is equal to the number of drops per minute. The standard giving set (Fig. 18.11) is shown in comparison. It is important to remember that it is **dangerous** to administer intravenous fluids more rapidly than prescribed to the young infant because of the risk of overloading the circulation.

Accurate records of fluids administered and of the child's output are maintained to assist in the estimation of hydration. Other observations necessary are the rates of pulse and respiration. Any significant changes such as restlessness, dyspnoea, cyanosis or the development of oedema must be reported immediately. Should either of the latter occur the nurse should slow the infusion rate and seek medical advice forthwith.

The child should be kept comfortable and his position changed frquently to relieve pressure and prevent chest complications.

Administration of medicines

To ensure that medicines are safely and successfully administered, the nurse must approach the child in a calm, kindly manner. In some instances a great deal of patience and persuasion are needed although older children generally co-operate in taking medicine.

It is essential that the correct drug is given, in the prescribed amount, at the time specified. Careful calculation of the very small amounts of drugs prescribed for children is necessary (Table 18.5). Some drugs, such as phenobarbitone and digoxin, are prepared in doses suitable for children and in a palatable form such as elixirs or syrups, as well as in tablets or capsules.

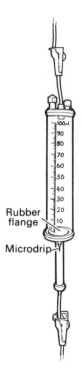

Rubber
flange

Microdrip

Figure 18.10
Microdrip infant recipient
set

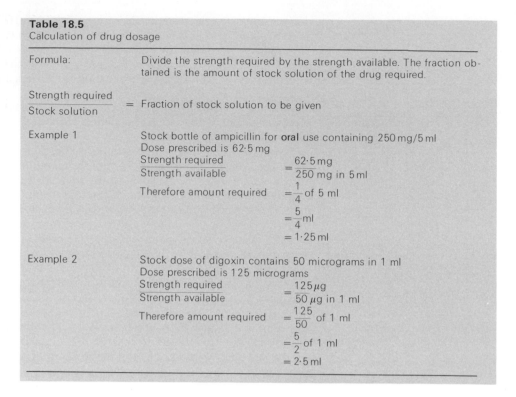

Table 18.5
Calculation of drug dosage

Formula:	Divide the strength required by the strength available. The fraction obtained is the amount of stock solution of the drug required.

$$\frac{\text{Strength required}}{\text{Stock solution}} = \text{Fraction of stock solution to be given}$$

Example 1
Stock bottle of ampicillin for **oral** use containing 250 mg/5 ml
Dose prescribed is 62·5 mg

$$\frac{\text{Strength required}}{\text{Strength available}} = \frac{62·5 \text{ mg}}{250 \text{ mg in } 5 \text{ ml}}$$

$$\text{Therefore amount required} = \frac{1}{4} \text{ of } 5 \text{ ml}$$

$$= \frac{5}{4} \text{ ml}$$

$$= 1·25 \text{ ml}$$

Example 2
Stock dose of digoxin contains 50 micrograms in 1 ml
Dose prescribed is 125 micrograms

$$\frac{\text{Strength required}}{\text{Strength available}} = \frac{125 \,\mu g}{50 \,\mu g \text{ in } 1 \text{ ml}}$$

$$\text{Therefore amount required} = \frac{125}{50} \text{ of } 1 \text{ ml}$$

$$= \frac{5}{2} \text{ of } 1 \text{ ml}$$

$$= 2·5 \text{ ml}$$

The child should be fully awakened and given a drink before his medicine is administered. The nurse must ensure that the drug has been swallowed. There are various ploys to aid this, such as crushing tablets and mixing them with drinks, jam or soft sweets, provided these are allowed. The nurse should talk and play with the young child to help him to accept his medicine. It may help to lift the child from his cot and nurse him and place small amounts at the back of the tongue with a spoon.

Young babies may need to be lightly restrained during drug administration and care must be taken to prevent inhalation of the medicine. This may occur if the drug is given too quickly and the baby splutters. Refusal to swallow, resulting in the loss of part or all of the medicine, must be reported and recorded.

Oxygen therapy
Oxygen is given when the child's condition necessitates concentrations of oxygen higher than the 21 per cent found in atmospheric air. Oxygen is supplied to the wards in metal cylinders (black with white top) or through pipes from a central oxygen supply.   Oxygen may be administered by using:

1. A disposable polythene mask, suitable for an older child (Ch. 6).
2. An oxygen tent, for a younger or very ill child.
3. An incubator, only suitable for a baby (Ch. 17).

Care of the child in an oxygen tent
Pressure tubing is used to attach the supply of oxygen to the tent, the rate of flow being controlled by a flow meter. Humidification and cooling, by diverting the oxygen supply through distilled water and a container of ice, is necessary to moisten the oxygen as it is very irritant to the epithelial lining of the respiratory tract. The relative humidity can be increased by using a humidifier (Fig. 18.12), atomizer or nebulizer.

When preparing the tent for use, it should be flushed with oxygen, 10 to 20 litres per minute for 20 minutes, and the oxygen content of the tent analysed. The doctor prescribes the concentration required and the flowmeter is adjusted accordingly. To ensure that the concentration is maintained, the rate of flow should be increased when it is necessary to open the tent. Analysis of the oxygen concentration is required 2 to 4 hourly and, if the child's condition does not show improvement, it may be necessary to increase the

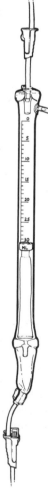

Figure 18.11
Standard infant recipient set

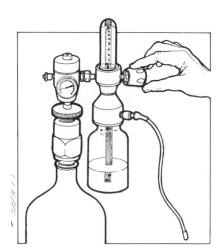

Figure 18.12
Humidifier and flowmeter

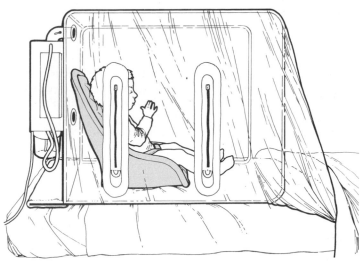

Figure 18.13
Child in baby sitter in oxygen tent

concentration. Care must be taken to ensure that the inlet and outlet of the tent is not obstructed.

In caring for the child, reassurance is given to help him to adjust to the confined space and it is often helpful if his mother remains with him. The child should be nursed in a comfortable position, supported by pillows. Toddlers and babies are more easily positioned by using a baby sitter (Fig. 18.13). Over exertion should be prevented and treatment arranged so that he can have adequate rest to increase the effect of therapy. If dyspnoea or cyanosis is present, all care should be carried out in the tent. The child's clothing and bed linen should be changed as often as necessary to prevent chilling by the dampness created by humidification. Fluids should be offered frequently to prevent dehydration. If respiratory distress inhibits the taking of fluids orally, a nasogastric tube may be passed.

When oxygen therapy is initiated, it is important to ensure that the child is observed closely — colour, temperature, pulse, respiration and general behaviour being noted and recorded to determine the child's response. It is also necessary to check the oxygen supply, flowmeter, oxygen concentration, fluid level in humidifier and temperature within the tent, which should be maintained at about 18 to 21°C. Ice is replenished as needed to aid cooling.

The nurse should know how to maintain the equipment to ensure adequate oxygen concentration. She should also be aware of the ignition hazard associated with the use of oxygen and prevent the use of friction toys which create sparks. Paper, grease and oils which are easily ignited must also be kept well away from the tent and the oxygen supply.

Discharge from hospital

'When can I go home?' is the thought uppermost in a child's mind. It does not always indicate that he is unhappy in hospital but rather that he would be happier at home.

Preparation for homegoing must be well planned, particularly if the child and mother have to continue care at home which may involve special diets, drugs or appliances. The special diets could include those peculiar to a child with diabetes mellitus, coeliac disease or with a colostomy or ileostomy. If drug therapy is to be continued, advice must be given on its correct dose, time of administration, storage and disposal of the drug once therapy is complete. Before leaving hospital, the mother and possibly the child should be competent in the use of any appliances such as calipers or colostomy bags. It is also important to ensure that the source of replacement, maintenance and repair of these items is known to the family.

The fact that the child may not readjust to family life immediately should be made clear to the mother so that she will understand the reasons for the child's regression in behaviour. Sleep may be disturbed and it is not uncommon for a child to have nightmares or to sleepwalk following a traumatic experience. On return home, the child may be demanding, perhaps resentful of having been 'left in that place' or unwilling to let his mother out of his sight. However, if the mother has been prepared for this behaviour she herself will avoid feelings of rejection and, with patient understanding, will help her child to readjust and feel secure.

The date and time of discharge should be decided as soon as possible so that transport, either provided by parents or in an ambulance, can be arranged. Any other services needed will be provided by the family doctor and the paediatric community nursing sister. The medical social worker may, if necessary, arrange for the child's education to be continued at home.

Very occasionally, parents decide for one reason or another to take their child home before treatment is completed. They should be encouraged to give a reason for their decision. During discussion with senior members of nursing and medical staff, they should be helped to understand the effects this may have on their child. The parents are asked to sign the relevant form indicating their acceptance of personal responsibility for this action. All possible guidance is given on continuing care. The family doctor is informed of the situation and any request for readmission to hospital is granted.

CARING FOR THE CHILD WITH A TERMINAL ILLNESS

Perception and sensitivity are needed when caring for the terminally ill child and in supporting his parents and relatives. Once diagnosis has been made and prognosis estimated by the doctor, he should talk to the parents in an attempt to help them understand and accept the situation. The ward sister should also be present during this interview so that she will be able to support the parents and answer their questions. The nursing staff must be aware of the need to provide a quiet room where parents can express their grief freely, overcome the initial shock and talk. Often a cup of tea and private discussion is of benefit to parents; the hospital chaplain or family minister may also be involved. The parents may find it helpful to know that staff are always available to talk to them at the time.

The child should be nursed in an area where he can watch the activities of other children. However, when his general condition becomes poor, it will be necessary to move him to a single room. It is essential, at this time, to avoid giving him a feeling of isolation.

It may be possible, in some instances, for the child to be nursed in his own home. This will of course depend on the child's condition, home circumstances, parents' ability and the availability of community care. Parents are assured that the family doctor, district nurse and health visitor will continue to support and assist with the practical aspects of care. Readmission to hospital can be arranged whenever necessary.

Whether the child is cared for in hospital or in the community, the nursing aims are to ensure that the child is kept clean and comfortable with adequate analgesia and sedation to ensure freedom from pain and restlessness. By involving the mother in the nursing care, some of her emotional needs and those of her child are partly satisfied. Parents should be encouraged to maintain their own health, particularly if there are other children in the family who will also need their care and attention.

As the child's condition deteriorates, the nursing staff can help to make the parents aware of the situation by asking if they wish to be informed of any changes, whatever the hour, and to be at the bedside during the final moments. In the absence of parents, a nurse who is familiar to the child should stay quietly by the bedside, talking to him if this is indicated. Parents who choose to stay with their child at this time may also appreciate the presence of a nurse.

After the death of their child, parents should be left at the bedside for a short time and then taken unobtrusively to a side room where they can share their grief and develop some composure before returning home. Any specific wishes regarding the child's belongings should be respected.

The need for support continues after the child's death and can be provided by both hospital and community care teams. Visits from or writing letters to those who have been involved in caring for the child are helpful to some parents while visiting the hospital and assisting in the care of other children is more beneficial to others. Great help may be provided by sympathetic friends and relatives who can give practical and psychological support.

PATIENT CARE STUDIES

The use of a variety of services and the involvement of the parents are illustrated in the following care studies.

Linda—age 7 months

History

Linda was admitted to hospital when she was 7 months old to be investigated for failure to thrive.

At birth she was 2·6 kg in weight having been born at 32 weeks' gestation. She was the third daughter of an unmarried mother who suffered from alcoholism. Although Linda was of low birth weight, her general progress was good and she was discharged home with her mother when she was 3 kg in weight. Her mother was advised to report to the baby clinic in 4 weeks' time so that Linda's progress could be assessed.

Her mother failed to report to the clinic on three occasions and a request for a progress report was made to the family doctor and the health visitor. The family doctor reported that Linda had been in the local hospital with a chest infection on two occasions but was now at home. The health visitor indicated that the home was poor and that Linda's mother showed a limited interest in her child. Linda was difficult to feed and appeared very thin and apathetic. Mother 'fortified' herself very frequently and generally was unable to give adequate care. Assistance had been sought from the Royal Scottish Society for the Prevention of Cruelty to Children (RSSPCC) and a social worker was assigned to work very closely with the family.

A fourth appointment was made, through the social worker, for Linda and her mother to attend the baby clinic. Transport and an escort were provided by the RSSPCC. Her mother was unable to give a complete progress report because of her inebriated state. Admission to hospital was arranged to observe Linda's dietary intake and general behaviour.

On admission she was a pale, pathetic, whimpering little girl of 5·8 kg in weight. She had an irritable cough, was fretful and difficult to comfort. Stools were loose and green.

Among possible reasons for her delay in development were malabsorption and the presence of infection; the appropriate investigations were made. Examination of stools proved negative and it was thought that the alteration in colour and consistency was due to underfeeding. An upper respiratory infection was diagnosed and the antibiotic therapy and physiotherapy were initiated, to which the infection responded well. Development was slightly below average and consistent with maternal deprivation.

Linda's appetite improved slowly, a weaning diet was started and she became very enthusiastic and excited when food appeared. Her general demeanour altered and she became a very attractive, lively and responsive child. Weight gain was slow but consistent.

Linda's mother did not visit her during her 5 week stay in hospital. Her father, however, demonstrated an interest, visited frequently and eventually encouraged her mother to take Linda home as he wished to help to support the family.

Summary

Linda is the third daughter of an unmarried 37-year-old woman in poor social circumstances who suffers from alcoholism. Her income is derived from social security benefit but she works as an office cleaner when able. Linda's father, not necessarily father to the other children, did not show interest or give support until Linda's admission to hospital. Since Linda's return home 6 months ago, the family have remained united but continue to need the support and advice of their social worker.

Peter—age 8 years

History

Peter was admitted to hospital from school complaining of severe abdominal pain, nausea and vomiting. The onset of pain was sudden although Peter had complained of two short episodes of vague abdominal pain a few days previously.

On admission, Peter was a well-nourished, healthy-looking child though rather pale. He appeared intelligent, bright-eyed but anxious. During examination, he was very co-operative and explained how the pain had been 'all over his tummy' and now was present only in his right side. Physical examination revealed guarding and tenderness in the right iliac fossa, and a diagnosis of acute appendicitis was made.

The diagnosis and operation necessary for the removal of the appendix was explained to Peter and to his parents who then gave permission for the operation to be performed.

Peter's mother remained with him until he was taken to the operating theatre 2 hours later. Meanwhile she was asked not to give him any further fluids. She also helped to prepare him for theatre by assisting with his bath and encouraging him to pass urine. An identification band was placed on his wrist. Following the preparation he rested quietly until the prescribed premedication was given.

The operation was performed for removal of the appendix and the wound was closed without drainage. The appendix was acutely inflamed.

Recovery from general anaesthesia was satisfactory and Peter was allowed small amounts of fluids later and a light diet was given the following day. Ambulation started on the first postoperative day and Peter was permitted to sit out of bed and take a short walk. His mother's visits were a great encouragement to him and he was soon moving around easily and playing with the other children.

As his progress was uneventful, he was eating and sleeping well and wound healing was normal, he was discharged home into the care of his parents, the paediatric district nurse and the family doctor. The sutures were removed on the sixth postoperative day as the wound was well healed.

He was visited by the family doctor 2 weeks later and discharged from medical and nursing care.

Summary

Peter developed acute appendicitis for which an operation was performed. Postoperative recovery was satisfactory. Home conditions were good: Peter had his own bedroom and his mother did not go out to work. His mother was advised to restrict his activities for 10 days to 2 weeks and to ensure that Peter had adequate rest and a nourishing diet. She was assisted in caring for her child by daily visits from the paediatric district nurse and supervision by the family doctor.

FURTHER READING

Bates S M 1979 Practical paediatric nursing, 2nd edn. Blackwell Scientific, Oxford
Dennison W M 1974 Surgery in infancy and childhood, 3rd edn. Churchill Livingstone, Edinburgh
Duncombe M, Weller B 1979 Paediatric nursing, 5th edn. Bailliere Tindall, London
Francis D E M 1979 Diets for sick children, 4th edn. Blackwell Scientific, Oxford
Harvey S, Tooke A H 1972 Play in hospital, Faber, London
Illingworth R S 1975 The development of the infant and young child normal and abnormal, 6th edn. Churchill Livingstone, Edinburgh
Latham H C, Heckel R V 1977 Pediatric nursing, 3rd edn. Mosby, St. Louis
Robertson J 1970 Young children in hospital, Tavistock, London
Wolff S 1973 Children under stress, Penguin, Harmondsworth

19. Adolescents and Adults

The aim of this chapter is to review briefly some of the many problems encountered when people between the years of childhood and old age become ill. The difficulties created for the patient, his relatives and the caring team will be explored. Although in most situations no clear-cut solution can be offered, it will help the nurse to have an appreciation of some of the factors involved.

Every individual is unique, and disablement brings problems which differ from one person to the other; nevertheless some generalizations may be made. Anticipation and understanding of some of the predictable difficulties may make it easier to find a solution for an individual patient.

Reactions to hospital

The patient's role in a general hospital is usually seen as a dependent one. This may be difficult for some patients to accept, particularly those whose social role has some status. The adolescent patient may respond to the influence of a male nurse or older woman, but friction may occur when those looking after him are young and female — people with whom he would normally expect to be on equal if not dominant terms.

The authority of nurses lies in the recognition of their level of competence by both colleagues and patients. This recognition may not now be as forthcoming, for a number of reasons — the reduced length of a patient's stay in hospital, the shorter working week and the shorter periods allocated for nurses in training. As a result conflicts may arise. Failure of the patient to accept a dependent role may be interpreted by some staff as a challenge, as undue independence, foolhardiness or sheer perversity. Such irreconcilable attitudes inevitably affect the standard of care given.

In the psychiatric field, similar problems may arise, but for opposite reasons. The patient may feel and exhibit the need to be dependent, whereas the staff, in their therapeutic capacity, may not think protective support is valuable in the long term for this patient.

ADOLESCENTS

The early teenage years (12 to 18) are characterized by the problems of adolescence. Changes in a teenager's physique, which may not occur at the same time for him as for his peers, and the identification and acceptance of the sexual role create difficulties under any circumstances. The strains of modern life — the number of one-parent families, for example — make identity development even more difficult. The struggle for independence, in both physical and emotional terms, often involves a reaction to parental and societal authority. The teenager must be given room to move so that he can establish himself as a unique and worthwhile person, and he needs a great deal of patience and understanding if the swings from child-like dependence to careless, aggressive independence are to be tolerated and supported.

This labile approach to life may create some of the troubles which bring an adolescent into the orbit of the health professions. His own social group may find him impossible and not react in the way he desires. His reaction to social pressures may lead to experiments with drugs, alcohol, sex and underage driving. All these areas involve health risks. Drug-taking and sexually transmitted diseases are on the increase in this age group and can have serious consequences.

Many young people nowadays drink alcohol regularly. It is difficult to estimate the age of a boy or girl partly because maturation occurs so early and partly because so many people in their 20s and 30s no longer appear old before their time. Increased incomes, with little to spend them on except pleasure, encourage the drinking habit, which in turn is responsible for much of the antisocial behaviour seen today and for many unwanted pregnancies.

Teenagers in hospital

Acute illnesses of short duration

An acute illness of short duration, such as appendicitis, may produce few difficulties. Indeed, the sufferer may enjoy a period of enhanced popularity as a result of his experience. But another short-stay situation, such as a therapeutic abortion, is not so easily managed. The attitude of the patient may be overtly brazen, or she may spend her time 'sleeping' to avoid the conversation and anticipated accusations of other patients and the staff. The situation may be further complicated by the presence of others in the ward who are desperately trying to preserve a pregnancy or who are undergoing investigations for infertility.

Nurses are not in a position to judge or moralize, although it is inevitable — and right — that they should have views on the subject of abortion. It is important to remember that an abortion for any reason is always physiologically stressful, and the emotional trauma is not discharged with the fetus. It is never a simple solution to the problem of an unwanted pregnancy and rarely does the patient feel only relief untinged with regret. It may be difficult for some nurses who have strong views on this subject to offer practical advice, but it is part of the nurse's role to ensure that a patient in any predicament resulting from an unwanted pregnancy does not leave the hospital without knowing where to turn for help. It may very well be the young, junior nurse who is the confidante, and she may have her own inner conflicts; but an appreciation of the traumatic nature of this event in her patient's life and the probability that the emotional crisis is yet to come may make her response more valuable.

Acute illnesses of long duration

By about 16 years of age, neuromuscular co-ordination is at its peak. Unfortunately, this is rarely accompanied by emotional maturity; a belief in personal immortality and the search for power often lead to many risky activities which may produce physical damage. This is especially true in relation to road accidents: the young driver may sometimes escape unhurt because of good reflexes but he may take unnecessary risks which involve others in injury.

Some of the injuries sustained, such as a fractured femur, may take a long time to heal and involve prolonged immobilization. As the general health of the patient is usually good, he gets bored and frustrated and may exhibit demanding behaviour which interferes with the care given to other patients who may be equally, or more, needy. The restriction of physical activity leaves time for teasing, which some nurses may find difficult to tolerate, and two or more of such patients may prove exhausting to ill or older patients in the same ward. It is part of the nurse's job to try to protect these patients from such horse-play and hilarity while at the same time recognizing the need for the young, basically fit patient to express himself.

If the injuries sustained are likely to involve permanent disability, such as paraplegia, a shortened or deformed limb, or even its loss (especially of an arm), it may be necessary to reconsider the future that was planned. The patient may have a circle of friends which depended for cohesion on a physical activity in which he can no longer participate. An older person may be capable of accepting a non-participatory role — for example becoming secretary of the football club instead of a player — but rarely do teenagers have the maturity to cope with such a major transition of role.

The future in terms of an occupation may also need to be reorganized. The individual who has a job in mind and whose schooling has been geared towards it, or who has begun or completed an apprenticeship for a particular trade, may have many difficulties accepting the need to start again. The physical adjustments often present a challenge which is met and overcome by a young person; however the need to go back to 'school' in any form, when he has just completed his formal education, may provoke strong feelings of resentment and aggression which, if expressed, are deemed antisocial and, if withheld, may ultimately require psychiatric help.

Should the injury cause mental damage, the patient will become dependent and, while he may prove a heavy nursing load, he may not cause many problems of management. His parents, however, and perhaps a wife or girl friend, may need great support. Not only are all their hopes for the patient shattered, but all their hopes for their own futures have to be adjusted to meet the new demands. Decisions will have to be made regarding long-term care and who will (or can) give it, and the opportunity to talk, learn, practice and adjust must be given; this is largely the nurse's responsibility.

Chronic illness

Chronic illness in children creates special problems when they reach the adolescent period. At a time when great emotional demands are made on the maturing individual, many of the chronic conditions become less stable and necessitate recurrent admission and adjustment of therapy involving, in consequence, periods of suffering.

At this stage, a paediatrician whose patient is expected to survive for many years often considers that care in a paediatric unit is inappropriate because the orientation of staff, the facilities and the time-table are more suited to small children. Frequently the child is suffering from a medical condition, for example diabetes mellitus, asthma or epilepsy; the change of physician and perhaps of hospital may create such insecurity that the management of the condition on an out-patient basis is impossible. Frequent admissions to a general medical ward, where the average age of patients may be well over 50 years at any one time, are equally unsuitable and the younger teenager gets a great deal of attention and protection which further delays the maturation process. Children with handicaps tend to be overprotected by their parents and to accept the attendant constraints for longer than normal: when the revolt comes it may be very dramatic.

Parents often fear that their offspring will never manage alone; they need to be helped to allow their child to plan a future as independent as that of his healthy peers. In some instances, however, the future may indeed be bleak; for example patients with cystic fibrosis may not survive beyond their teens. The parents may have known this since the time of diagnosis, and often the patient begins to realize, as adolescence passes, that he is not going to have the kind of future he had previously taken for granted. It then becomes a vital function of the nursing staff to provide support and to offer encouragement so that realistic goals are attained.

For many young people suffering from chronic disease, academic achievements, however meagre, are of paramount importance because of the reduced range of jobs which are suitable. Thus keeping them out of hospital and if possible in school and providing facilities for study when in hospital are important aspects of their management. Special units for young people are provided in some psychiatric hospitals but suitable provision in the general field is sadly lacking.

Psychiatric illnesses are becoming increasingly common among teenagers. As they may often come to light due to antisocial behaviour such as vandalism, the failure to attend school, or being beyond the control of parental influence, there may well be limited support from the family during therapy because they would see punitive measures as more appropriate. Some psychiatric establishments are setting up specialist Young People's Units, in which specially trained staff and suitable treatment approaches are available to meet the needs of these families.

ADULTS

The young adult

Physical fitness is usually at its peak in the third and fourth decades of life. Disorders, including those resulting from stress and degenerative processes, begin to make their appearance later. The most common problems in this age group result from accidents on the road or at work. In future, various legal measures may decrease the number of traffic accidents, and the provision of occupational health facilities and careful control of safety factors should reduced industrial injuries.

Effects of disability

Disablement, which may necessitate a complete change of life-style, requires the provision of facilities quite different from those provided for the elderly disabled — but frequently these are all that are available. The ability to undertake new learning successfully may not be seriously impaired in the under-40-year-old, but these factors, housing adjustments, transport facilities (or lack of them) restricted employment and entertainment opportunities all constrain the victim, who may have dependants and has learned to appreciate and enjoy his own independence. Fears about the future — the inability to provide for the family as planned, the inability to fulfil the marital or the parental role, the possibility that the patient may not see his children reach maturity — all prey on the patient's mind and, unless carefully thought through, may interfere with his adjustment to his adversities and result in failure to achieve even his reduced potential.

Social provisions

Provision for the young chronically sick or disabled person in the community is poor. Happily, an increasing number of public buildings are accessible by wheel-chair, but many are not. It is probably possible to go to the theatre or a concert in a wheel-chair, but only at the cost of stall seats for occupant and companions; this is an additional penalty for one whose income level suggests seats in the upper circle. For hygienic reasons, many hotels and restaurants refuse admission to guide dogs, and so reduce the social opportunities of the blind who are struggling to maintain an independent existence.

Transport

Transport for the disabled may be a problem; public transport may be unmanageable, and total dependence on friends and relatives for every outing is unacceptable in the long term. For some people, the use of a car with automatic gear change may suffice for a long period. The three-wheeled cars provided by the Department of Health and Social Security for disabled drivers may meet a need but have been criticized on grounds of instability. They are now to be withdrawn and replaced by a cash grant. The regular use of a taxi service is generally beyond a family's income.

Financial burdens

Special income supplements are available on application; in some cases tax relief (if the individual can earn at all) may be appropriate; in a few situations, when trauma was the cause and the victim was not at fault, he may be awarded costs against an insurance policy. None of these things will relieve the emotional stresses of the disabled, although they may meet some of the increased costs of fuel bills and food and make up for the person's reduced earning power. But unless rewards are immense (generally, judged prospectively, in terms of the victim's lost potential), fears for the future of his family must be an ever-present anxiety.

Reduced earning power, whether it be the result of an accident, slowly progressive disease or morbidity from an acute event such as a myocardial infarction, affects interpersonal relationships in a variety of ways. Marriages are put under strain, so great is the readjustment required of both partners to their new roles. The nature of the original relationship may now be seen for what it was and be found wanting. The woman who exchanged a protecting family for a dominating husband and finds herself in the breadwinning role may be quite unwilling or unable to adjust; the man whose needs were met by a mothering relationship and finds himself with a demanding but dependent wife may also be psychologically unable to cope. It should not be forgotten that many chronic invalids can be highly manipulative, particularly emotionally, and this can stretch the tolerance of all around. Many apparently stable relationships may break under these circumstances, leaving the patient without support, either domestic or personal. Admission to hospital — often a long-stay ward with a preponderance of very elderly patients — may be the only way of providing essential services. The needs of the geriatric patient and the facilities offered in long-stay wards are discussed in the next chapter; these facilities are, however, rarely suitable for the alert, young, but chronically sick patient who requires nursing care that is not available in the community.

The prime of life

During these years, the fulfilment of many ambitions, the achievement of potential and the confidence of being socially at ease are most likely to occur. The courage to allow oneself to be seen as an individual, without pretence, reduces the risks taken. The needs of a spouse and family responsibilities may provoke stress, but the resilience of a still-young physique and emotional tranquillity enable stress to be borne without undue trauma.

The effect of illness

Illness is less common in this age group although, when it does occur, its effect may be shattering to the entire family.

Financial difficulties may be related to inadequate insurance and loss of income as the result of the illness; subsequent reduced earning power may seriously affect not only the individual's ability to provide for the family, but also his own self-image as provider. The illness of a wife and mother places a very real burden on the family, and if her ability to resume her many roles is ever in doubt, the disruption to family life may be insupportable.

For many people in this age group, an illness may spell disaster because they are the sole supporters of young children; their hospitalization may involve the children being placed in foster homes or institutions, with all the long-term problems this involves.

Fear of these consequences may mean that a patient fails to seek expert advice early enough in the course of an illness. If the symptoms are bearable, a woman may suppress her fears and ignore the rational arguments put forward for early diagnosis. The fear of having her anxieties confirmed may delay her further. The need of a family for a steady income may make a man work too hard or cause him to ignore symptoms which, if diagnosed early, could enable curative measures to be taken.

The middle years

Although degenerative diseases may be apparent earlier, it is more often in the years between 40 and 55 that these conditions and the disorders resulting from stress become overt.

Threats to health

The workload at this time of life is high; positions of responsibility are held and stress is both self-imposed and externally applied to retain them. In technical and labouring jobs, the middle-aged worker becomes aware of tiring more easily and struggles to keep pace or do overtime in order to maintain and provide for a teenage family.

During these years obesity tends to increase and the stress factor increases the risk of myocardial infarction. The fear of losing a job to a younger, more able worker may produce hypertension, ulcers and depression. This is the most common age at which men commit suicide.

For women the reduced dependence on her by her children and her fading self-image which accompanies the loss of her reproductive function may provoke profound depression. If she has had a family, she now feels useless; if she hasn't, she feels life has passed her by. It is an age of increasing dependence on tranquillizer and antidepressant drugs and, more recently, of alcoholism in women. Unpleasant symptoms so often associated with the menopause may also complicate the situation.

Malignant conditions of the lungs and genital tract are more likely to appear at the beginning of this period and, towards the end, gastrointestinal tumours and the more severe effects of industrial lung diseases and cardiac failure may arise.

Chronic bronchitis and rheumatoid arthritis, causes of morbidity in a large part of the population of Great Britain in this age group, may result in recurring admissions to hospital. As people age, they may be at greater risk from loss of a job or enforced early retirement, for which they are ill-prepared, either emotionally, socially or functionally.

It is a feature of the aging process that multiple pathology becomes more common. Obesity, with its many complications, is the most common nutritional disease in the Western world; this time of life is possibly the last opportunity to tackle it with any chance of success. Once physical activity is reduced, as is usual with advancing years, it is extremely difficult, if not impossible, to lose weight unless there is underlying pathology.

The effect of illness

The early onset of chronic, disabling conditions creates a number of problems. The patient who has struggled long and hard to maintain an independent existence and who finally has to accept the inevitable may become deeply depressed and, suddenly, totally dependent. This return to childhood can be very frustrating to the health team professionals and to the friends and family of the patient, who may be straining to preserve the remaining abilities. Often strong feelings of anger against the patient may be felt at what appears to be deliberate waste of skills; this exasperation is replaced by guilt. A wave of protective care follows, further endorsing the dependency of the patient, setting up a vicious circle.

Alternatively, and more especially if the effects of the disability are not overt, a reversion to the irresponsibility of the teenage years may occur. This may result in unnecessary demonstrations of independence and disregard of instructions and advice. Such behaviour, which may meet the needs of the patient to prove he is still worthwhile, can create strong feelings of both fear and resentment in the rest of the family. Nurses, too, are not immune to these feelings — to have worked hard to preserve a life, only to see foolhardy behaviour destroy it, or threaten to destroy it, can be difficult to tolerate.

It is necessary to attempt to bring the needs of the patient into the open, to discuss his fears and to help him see that they are reasonable, even if his way of dealing with them is not. But the patient will need sound advice. Medical and nursing staff are, unfortunately, only too accustomed to using clichés like 'Take things easy for a while'. Just what does this statement mean? What is 'easy' to a steelworker may still be too hard for his heart or cerebral vessels. How long is 'a while' — a week, a month or a year? How does a patient progress along the path to finding his new potential? It is possible that much clearer guidelines and more careful discussion with the whole family might avoid some of the tragedies, either of recurring disaster or of chronic invalidism, the latter a refuge of the patient too frightened to get better.

Late middle years

Retirement, and its problems or joys, first looms ahead and later becomes a reality during this stage of life. For many, a shared lifetime is shattered and a lonely future is all that faces them. Reduced mobility and the loss of the more acute sensory perceptions may make life trying. For those who are blessed with good health, the reduced family responsibilities and increased freedom of retirement allow them to build an exhilarating new life and to plan for the time when they are less able. The joys of grandchildren, without the responsibility for their upbringing, may make these years very precious, a time when increasing infirmity may be faced with equilibrium.

SUMMARY

To adapt to illness of any sort requires a maturity that enables one to meet and cope with adversity. In the teenager, this may present unexpectedly, and when it does the natural resilience and learning abilities of youth may ride the storm. Older people have learned at least to appear to be able to cope. Only close observation, time and attention will elicit the signs of anxiety, fear, anger and resentment which must be discussed and resolved if any useful rehabilitation is to be achieved.

Grieving for a dead friend or relative is a natural process which should be allowed to take its course. In many situations where the trauma associated with disability was severe, the patient will usually grieve for his lost abilities, opportunities and aspirations; his family will also, and this process cannot be hurried without affecting the long-term adjustments for all concerned. Where chronic, progressive disease exists, the patient may indeed be grieving for his own death and, while perhaps resenting that he is not to live out his expected natural life span he may at the same time feel guilty at his level of dependence on relatives and friends.

For some, the clergy may be able to offer a great deal of support and practical help. For all, the role of the nurse is to listen: this is not a passive occupation but a demanding and exhausting one. It may be difficult because the patient may not be very approachable, but caring means attempting to meet the needs of the patient. It is usually easier to meet the physical needs, but the emotional claims, upon which the future well-being of the patient may depend more heavily, must not be avoided or ignored.

Nurses, too, are human beings. A high proportion of those giving care in hospital are still teenagers, coping with all the adjustments of this age group. At the same time they are acquiring the skills and taking the responsibility of an arduous professional role. In the community, whilst a slightly older age group is involved, the additional stress of being alone (though not unsupported by professional colleagues) and often coping with new relationships in personal life add their own pressures. The work itself is stressful at times and many of the less experienced nurses find it very difficult indeed to survive, let alone deal with the crises facing their patients. To learn objectivity without losing sympathy; to acquire a realistic approach without becoming hardened to the very real problems encountered; to be flexible but not inconsistent; to be wise beyond her years — what sort of human being can achieve these all the time?

Perhaps the most valuable lesson any nurse can learn is that no-one can be all things to all men, but what is generally appreciated, and patients can certainly expect, is that she should be willing to try, and to recognise individual limitations.

FURTHER READING

Altschul A 1975 Psychology for nurses, 4th edn. Bailliere Tindall, London
Anderson E R 1973 The role of the nurse. Royal College of Nursing, London
Franklin B L 1974 Patient anxiety on admission to hospital. Royal College of Nursing, London
Hayward J 1975 Information a prescription against pain. Royal College of Nursing, London
Roberts I 1975 Discharged from hospital. Royal College of Nursing, London
Stockwell F 1972 The unpopular patient. Royal College of Nursing, London
The seven ages of man 1964 Reprinted from New Society

20. The Elderly

This chapter deals with the commoner problems of the elderly sick and examines the role of the nurse as a member of the team that provides care for old people, living either in hospital or in the community.

Geriatric medicine is a branch of medicine concerned with clinical, social, preventive and remedial aspects of illness in the elderly. It has developed as a specialty concerned with old people with health problems and often with additional social difficulties. In geriatric care the emphasis is on supporting the patient to live with his disabilities, whatever they may be. Old age is not always attractive; the therapeutic benefits of treatment are often harder and slower to achieve, relapses are more common and the patient often returns from hospital to unfavourable conditions which militate against the efforts which have been made on his behalf.

Throughout his active life the elderly person has contributed to our society and to its improvement, and he may continue to do so, given suitable opportunities. However, he rarely reaps the benefit which his life work has gone to achieve. After retirement he often lives in a depressed state, financially and residentially. In many countries the proportion of people over 65 rises each year (Fig. 20.1). Many live alone, have no relatives near at hand and their neighbours are likely to be old themselves. Such people may not be 'geriatric patients' for they are not ill, but social services may enable them to find greater enjoyment and fulfilment in life. Health services both help to prevent illness and, when it does occur, provide for early diagnosis, treatment and care.

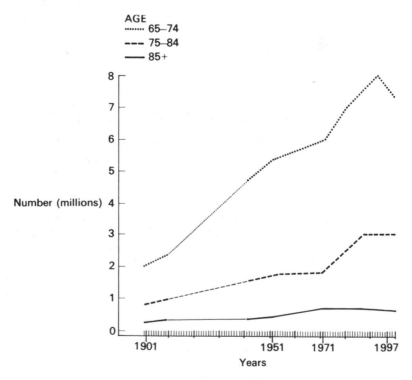

Figure 20.1
Population growth of the elderly in the United Kingdom

552

NORMAL AGING

The body's structure and functions undergo changes with the passage of time. These involve the following areas.

The musculoskeletal system

Height diminishes, muscles become smaller and the posture less erect.

The skin and hair

Skin becomes dry, loses elasticity and wrinkles appear. Hair grows grey as pigmentation disappears and it becomes more scanty, especially in men.

Respiratory system

The vital capacity is reduced as elasticity of lung tissue diminishes. The muscles, including those of the chest wall and diaphragm, become weaker.

Circulatory system

The heart has a smaller reserve of power and it has to work harder to achieve less. The blood vessels lose much of their elasticity.

Renal system

The excretory power of the kidneys reduces with age. The bladder capacity is also reduced.

Brain and mental faculties

Normally some brain cells die every day, but because there are millions of them the effect does not become obvious until old age. Mental faculties begin to diminish as one gets older. There is a decline in intelligence, although human experience compensates for this. Remote memory seems to be enhanced but recent memory is impaired: recall of events which took place many years ago is easy but remembering a shopping list becomes more and more difficult.

Interest in the world and in day-to-day living is reduced. Many factors may contribute to this diminished interest. A person who has difficulty in seeing and hearing may very quickly become withdrawn and apparently uninterested. As age progresses it becomes increasingly hard to adapt to new ideas or to a change in environment. Old people find it much easier to follow a set and well-established routine. This change in attitude may in part be a way of compensating for a failing memory.

Special senses

Eyesight begins to fail and reading glasses may no longer be adequate. Hearing becomes impaired with reduced high note reception; a hearing aid may help. The voice loses its timbre as the elasticity of the vocal cords decreases. The sense of smell is often lost.

ABNORMAL AGING AND DISEASES OF THE AGED

Diseases, deficiencies and depletions all result either in an identifiable illness or in some degree of ill-health. Old people tend to suffer from more than one disorder. The onset of mental disturbance may, for example, be precipitated by a physical illness. A deficiency disease may be a sequel to inadequate dentition, poor cooking facilities or difficulty in shopping. 'Multiple pathology' is a term frequently used in referring to disease in old age and pathological changes in this context may have environmental as well as medical causes. Disorders frequently affect the following systems.

Musculoskeletal system

    Rheumatoid arthritis.
    Osteoarthritis.
    Fractures.

Respiratory system

    Chronic bronchitis.
    Pneumonia.

Circulatory system
 Congestive cardiac failure.
 Degenerative arterial disease.
 Iron deficiency anaemia.

Endocrine system
 Diabetes mellitus.
 Hypothyroidism.

Nervous system
 Cerebral vascular accident.
 Confusion.
 Dementia.

These conditions are described in Section A of this book.

Memory lapses, confusion and dementia
Any one of us can become forgetful and slightly confused. A name, a date or a time may be forgotten for the moment. With advancing age **memory lapses** and subsequent confusion become more prolonged. The impaired short-term memory of the elderly can make them uncertain of time and place. **Confusion** occurs because of some disturbance happening outside the brain. Old people very easily become confused when their environment is suddenly changed, say, from home to hospital, from ward to ward and after there has been a change-over of staff. Chest infection and urinary tract infection can precipitate confusion. It is not permanent but is a transient difficulty which may perist for minutes, hours, days, weeks or months, depending on the patient's condition and what has caused it.
 Dementia is a permanent condition occurring, on the whole, in the elderly. Some brain cells are dying all the time in all individuals. However, in certain people the number of brain cells which have died are so numerous as to cause brain damage which results in severe mental failure. This is termed **senile dementia** (p. 498). **Atherosclerotic dementia** occurs when the vessels feeding the brain become diseased.
 The features of dementia are:
 Disorientation.
 Behaviour changes.
 Intellectual loss.
 Disturbance of normal personality.

HAZARDS OF OLD AGE

There are two well recognized dangers to bear in mind.

Accidents

The elderly are more prone to accidents than are those in the younger age groups. One reason is the mental and physical 'slowing down' that is inherent in the aging process.
 Falls are very common in old age both in the home and in hospital. Many falls are preventable but the nurse should realize that falls are a hazard of old age. Approximately a third of falls occur in the over eighty age group. Of accidental falls about one-third happen on stairs and another third are associated with slipping. As serious injury may result from falls, particularly fractures of the neck of femur, their prevention is important.

Causes of falls in old age
 1. Accidental falls.
 2. Vertigo:
  a. associated with central nervous system lesion.
  b. associated with cervical spondylosis and head back position.
 3. Trips.
 4. Postural hypotension.
 5. Drop attacks.
 6. Foot and leg abnormalities.

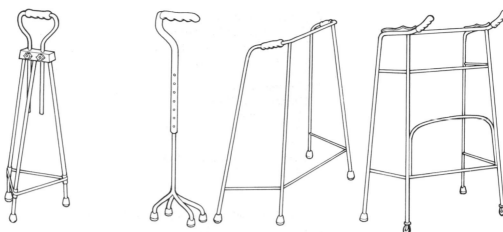

Figure 20.2
Zimmer aids, tripods, walking sticks

Nurses should endeavour to reach a compromise between imposing too many restrictions and exposing the patient to avoidable dangers.

When considering prevention of accidents to the elderly the effect of drugs must not be overlooked. Oversedation increases the likelihood of falls. The nurse should be aware that the response to drugs in the elderly is very often different from that in younger people. Barbiturates tend to be poorly tolerated and certain combinations of drugs may be positively harmful.

Ways of preventing accidents in home and hospital

Provide low level beds and good lighting.

Provide safe chairs, toilets, bathroom equipment, tables, crockery, electric, coal and gas fires.

Avoid loose-fitting carpets and overpolished floors.

Use cot sides (as infrequently as possible).

Provide aids such as Zimmer aids, tripods, walking sticks, raised toilet seats, non-slip bath mats and appropriate bath grips in bath, toilet and stairway, and help the patient to use them (Figs. 20.2–20.4).

Explain the need for, and if necessary provide, walking shoes, thereby discouraging the use of slippers, especially in the home.

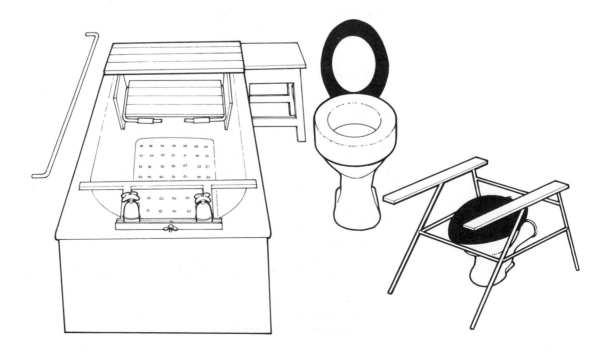

Figure 20.3
Bathroom aids

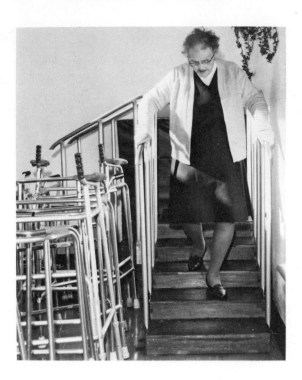

Figure 20.4
Walking aids (stairs)

Test sight and hearing and provide up-to-date glasses and hearing aids.

Teach the elderly the importance of adequate dietary intake and translate this into practical terms.

Wipe up floor spills immediately.

Provide chiropody services to minimize foot problems.

Ensure correct temperature of bath water.

Service equipment such as gas cookers regularly.

Hypothermia

This is another well-known hazard of the elderly in which the body temperature, especially the 'core' temperature, falls below 35°C. There is an increase in the incidence of old people dying of hypothermia especially in the winter months. It is a preventable condition. Provision of adequate heating, housing and warm clothing will minimize the risk.

Regulation of body heat is monitored by the hypothalamus through the autonomic nervous system. The efficiency of this mechanism can become impaired by age changes. The only way of establishing whether a person is in a state of hypothermia or not is to take the person's temprature with a low reading clinical thermometer rectally. There is no sign of shivering in elderly patients suffering from hypothermia. Pallor, bradycardia, shallow and slow respirations, a falling blood pressure, apathy, drowsiness and Cheyne-Stokes breathing are common signs. If the temperature falls below 32°C confusion progresses to coma.

Temperature above 35°C can be treated by insulating against further heat loss with blankets, recording hourly temperature, giving fluids, raising room temperature to a level (about 22°C) which will bring the patient's temperature up no faster than about 0.5°C every hour and if not rising fast enough increase room temperature to 28°C or 32°C. A patient whose temperature is down to 35°C or below will probably need treatment in an intensive care unit. Severe hypothermia requires more rapid re-warming to avoid irreversible tissue changes.

Some ways which help to prevent hypothermia are:

Ensuring adequate food intake and extra food intake in winter.

Encouraging as much activity as possible.

Ensuring effective roof insulation: double glazing, accessible power points for supplementary heating.
Using woollen mittens, bedsocks, long underwear and warm dry blankets.

The normal person of any age takes appropriate measures to combat the cold. The elderly person because of illness, confusion or poverty, may be unable to do this. Health visitors and district nurses are often the first to become aware of this situation and they try to educate and provide preventive measures for the elderly in their care.

CARING FOR THE ELDERLY
Community care

Approximately 90 per cent of elderly people live in the community, so it is here that most geriatric care is needed. Many families look after their old folk under very stressful conditions in their own homes. Of those at home one-third are cared for by relatives other than spouses. A wide variety of services are available both to the house-bound and to the mobile elderly (Figs. 20.5 and 20.6). The general practitioner is in the best position to assess the care required, to advise on and to mobilize these services.

Social and other services are provided in an attempt to keep the aged functioning in their own homes for as long as possible and also to help them maintain their independence.

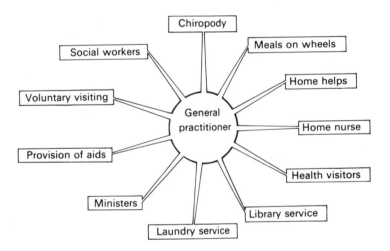

Figure 20.5
Services for the house-bound elderly

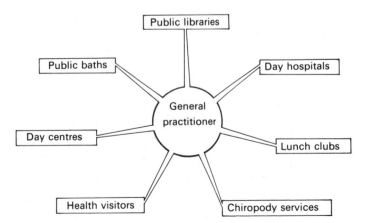

Figure 20.6
Services for the mobile elderly

Facilities available for the housebound elderly

Home helps

Home helps are provided by and are responsible to the Department of Social Services. Their job is to do the general housework, the washing, the shopping and now and again to cook a meal. They are not nurses so cannot undertake nursing care. A home help may visit the home as often as 5 days each week or as infrequently as once a week, depending on the particular situation. It should be noted that home helps do not normally work at weekends. The home help is a human contact for the house-bound elderly and so is not only a physical help but also, and perhaps more important, a psychological and social comfort.

District nurses

The home nurse is the trained community nurse. Her patients are in their own homes and the nursing care she provides is carried out in the home. It is the general practitioner who calls upon the home nursing service. The home nurse in turn is a vital 'feed-back' link to the doctor.

Health visitors

Health visitors are nurses who have undergone further training to equip them with knowledge of the preventive aspects of care in the community and the ability to assess an old person physically, psychologically and socially. As their title suggests health visitors are nurses who visit people in their own homes to advise on health (they can often discern difficulties before the patient or general practioner).

Social workers

Social workers are employed by the Department of Social Services to establish contact with the elderly and to supervise old people who appear to be failing to cope at home. They hope to detect social problems and to provide help to diminish or completely eradicate them. The social worker can advise on pensions, supplementary benefits, reduced rent schemes and other financial matters.

Meals on wheels

The Women's Royal Voluntary Service enables hot, nutritious meals to be provided. Food is prepared at a central kitchen and carried by voluntary helpers in vans or cars to the old person's home. The local authority may give financial aid. This service is not available at weekends.

Laundry service

In some areas the local authority provides valuable service, free, for incontinent patients at home. (Local voluntary day centres contribute this service to the house-bound elderly.)

Library services

Mobile library services are often provided either by the voluntary services or by the local authority. They supply a wide variety of publications in large print and Braille and also talking books for the blind.

Provision of equipment

Equipment for medical, nursing and social purposes can be supplied on loan by the local authorities, voluntary services and the British Red Cross. This equipment includes walking frames, bed cradles, mackintosh sheeting, incontinence pads, wheel-chairs, commodes, ramps and handrails.

Chiropody

This service can be provided in the patient's house, in a day centre or in a clinic by chiropodists employed either by the local authority or by the Red Cross. The services provided for the house-bound may also be made available for those who are more mobile.

Other facilities available for the mobile elderly

Day hospitals
These are described on page 560.

Day centres
Day centres differ from day hospitals in that they aim to provide social stimulation and supervision. They are usually run by voluntary organizations such as the Old People's Welfare Council. The facilities provided by day centres are numerous and include hot baths, hot nutritious food, chiropody and laundry service. Social activities include music, forming percussion bands, sewing classes, art classes, bus outings and holidays. Not only the ambulant elderly benefit from these centres; house-bound persons can be brought to the centre by the minibus attached to the clinic, or by car owner voluntary helpers.

Lunch clubs
These clubs provide meals suited to the needs of the elderly at a reasonable cost and also provide the lonely elderly with some social contact.

From these examples it can be seen that there are many ways of helping the elderly to remain contentedly and comfortably in the community.

Hospital care

An old person who requires hospital care may enter either a ward which receives patients of many age groups, often a general medical ward, or a department of geriatric medicine designed and run to meet the special needs of old people. The success of any department of geriatric medicine depends primarily on its ability to enable prompt admission of those who need it and to make considerate arrangements for the discharge of people no longer requiring the unit's care.

Assessment wards
These very active wards (and out-patient clinics) have facilities for a range of physical and psychological investigations, diagnosis and treatment. Decisions about continued treatment and care are based on the result of these investigations and on the patient's observed capabilities and deficits. The members of the team, each of whom makes her own contribution to the assessment of the patient, may include:

Consultant geriatrician.
Ward sister.
Physiotherapist.
Occupational therapist.
Social worker.
Health visitor.
Speech therapist.
Psychiatrist.

Each member also has her own, valuable part to play in caring for an old person. Nursing staff, collectively, are with a patient for most of the day and night and so are able to provide a considerable amount of information on his response to admission and treatment. Their 24-hour records depict, for instance, the patient's behaviour when awake, his sleep patttern, frequency of micturition and episodes of incontinence.

The ward sister has a special responsibility for co-ordinating the efforts of all members of the team and aiding communication between them. Relatives can supply information about the patients's abilities and difficulties and should be encouraged to maintain contact with and support for him. The condition which was the immediate reason for the patient's admission may or may not respond to treatment. His residual disabilities may or may not permit his discharge from hospital. A patient who is sensible, ambulant and continent will probably be allowed home if conditions there allow it.

A very important factor in making this decision is the amount of support available from people near him. It should not be forgotten that relatives may need a good deal of reassurance that they will neither be left without help and advice, nor expected to shoulder too great a burden of responsibility. Services available in the community should help meet these needs. A patient who cannot return home but does not require hospital care may be found a place in a private or local authority nursing home or in an old person's flatlet (sheltered housing). Severe difficulty in walking, intractable incontinence and behaviour disturbances usually result in plans for continuing care in hospital.

Continuing care wards

The term is self-descriptive. In many instances this care is given until the patient dies, but it should be remembered that many patients in continuing care wards regain independence sufficiently to be allowed home or to be transferred to a nursing home. The aim in continuing care wards is not to cure the patient — this is usually impossible — but to improve and maintain the quality of life the patient has left, that is to allow the person to live physically and psychologically within his own capabilities until he dies. Continuing care wards are the home of the patient. They have evolved because many elderly people, even with all the facilities available in the community, require, for their own safety, 24-hour care and supervision.

The main conditions which necessitate admission to a continuing care ward are confusion, dementia, urinary incontinence, faecal incontinence, impaired mobility and lack of responsible relatives or friends to give the 24-hour care necessary.

One of the disadvantages of continuing care wards is that they can quickly become drab, monotonous and unstimulating. Nurses should recognize that activity and interest are of paramount importance to the old people living in these wards. The social aspects of care are just as important as the physical and psychological ones. Simply listening and talking to the patient is the first step and this can gradually lead to something more fruitful. From conversation one can ascertain whether the patient can see or hear properly; the relevant aids can then be provided. Dental care and chiropody are other ways of helping to make patients more comfortable.

Some aids to stimulate social behaviour are:

Paints and large paint books.
Talking books.
Selected radio programmes.
Television.
Large print books.
Reading newspapers to patients.
Showing short films.
Providing large noticeboards for news items and football results and for patients' own use.
Holding church services.
Encouraging all visitors to visit and to take patients out on short visits.
Having a ward album for family photographs.
Celebrating birthdays
Decorating wards with pictures and plants and arranging flowers.

The ways of capturing interest are endless. Nurses must be aware that stimulation in continuing care wards is essential to maintain morale, diminish depression, reduce confusion and above all prevent isolation and introversion.

Day hospitals

Day hospitals are units attached to geriatric hospitals or general hospitals for investigation and daily supervision of the elderly. The idea originated from the psychiatric day hospitals. They provide care without actual hospital admission. They are bridges between in-patient care and a person's independent life at home.

Day hospitals help in several ways to preserve, maintain and develop physical and social competence in the elderly. They help to prevent hospital admissions by easing the load and responsibilities of the relatives, who may then be happier to continue to make their contribution to caring for their old folk. Treatment may be given which minimizes or resolves the need for hospital admission and, by providing regular follow-up, earlier discharge into the community may be arranged. They also help to maintain improvement and therefore reduce the incidence of hospital admission. They provide good hot meals, companionship and facilities for bathing, bowel control, chiropody and hairdressing — that is hospital facilities without sleeping accommodation.

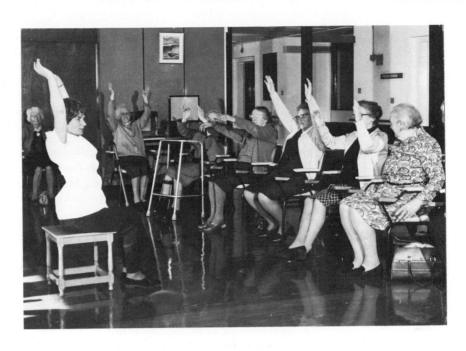

Figures 20.7 and 20.8
Day hospital

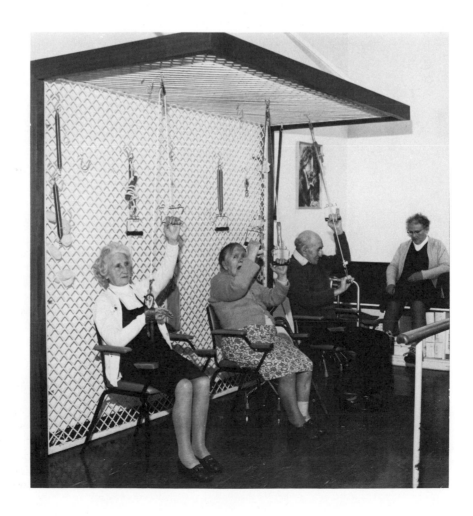

Day hospitals differ from day centres in that they are part of the National Health Service and provide medical and social care. They enable many elderly people who might have needed hospital care to remain in the community.

NURSING OLD PEOPLE

Old people in hospital are not found solely in departments of geriatric medicine. They are also admitted, for example, to medical, surgical and orthopaedic wards to have acute manifestations of diseases treated. In addition to this treatment they require nursing care appropriate to their special needs. These needs include the provision of an environment in which the patient is allowed, encouraged and stimulated to be as independent as his disabilities permit. It is not just administering basic nursing care, but often enlightened withdrawal of that care that is essential. It is not unfeeling to expect a patient to attempt to dress, eat and walk. It is unimaginative to do it all for him.

Nutrition

The elderly need to eat a diet which contains all the necessary constituents for maintenance of bodily functions, that is protein, fat, carbohydrate, vitamins, mineral salts and roughage in appropriate amounts. Many older people have a faulty dietary intake due perhaps to:

Bad teeth or ill-fitting dentures.
Difficulty in chewing.
Difficulty in swallowing.
Lack of money.
Reduced mobility and consequent difficulty in reaching shops.

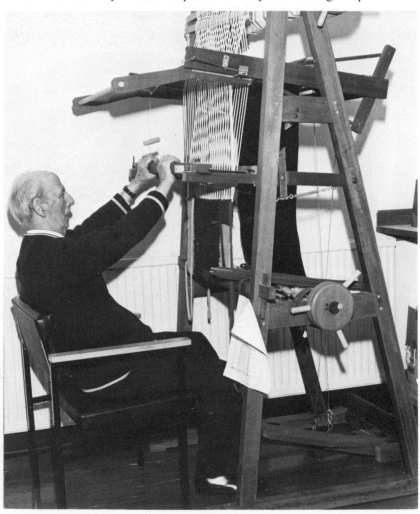

Figure 20.9
Day hospital

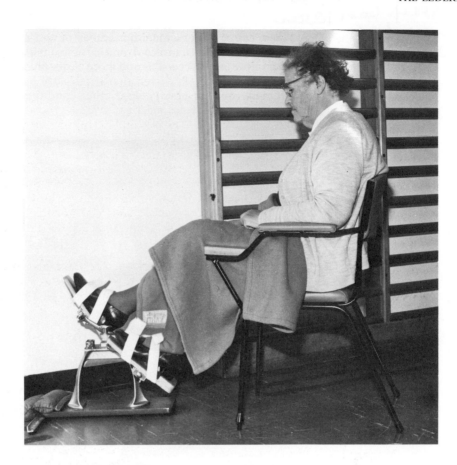

Figure 20.10
Day hospital

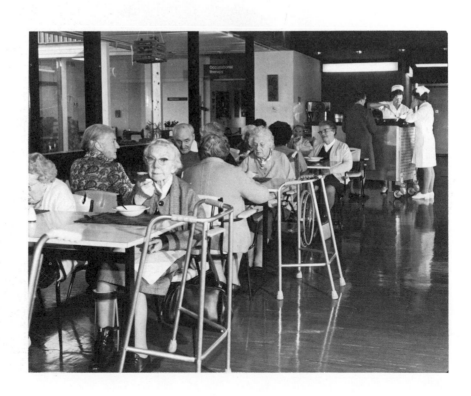

Figure 20.11
Meal time

*causes:- more common in women /men.
age 30-50
thyroid deficiency. can follow
partial removal of
thyroid gland.

For these reasons meat and fresh fruit may be avoided. They are too expensive and for some people too difficult to cook and eat. If protein foods are avoided in preference to cheaper, more easily accessible and more easily prepared and eaten carbohydrates, the diet is incomplete. It follows, too, that a high carbohydrate diet and diminished physical activity will result in obesity. Two other conditions associated with overweight are myxoedema and diabetes mellitus.

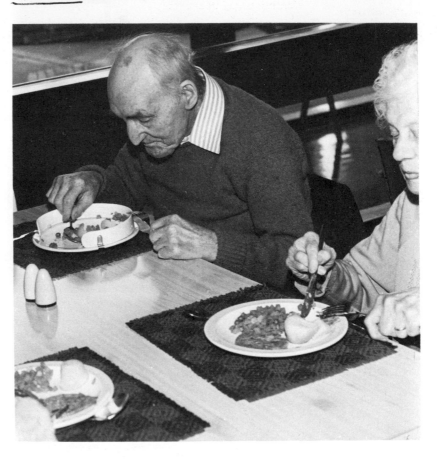

Figure 20.12
Plate guard

The nurse's observations should help in the discovery of where the main problem lies. She should notice whether the patient can chew food and if he has dentures which fit and are comfortable. If they are not comfortable either they will not be worn or they will make the mouth sore. Any discomfort or difficulty complained of or noticed involving chewing or swallowing should be reported. The patient's likes and dislikes and the amount of food eaten should also be noted. It may be that the patient needs to be re-educated; if he has been eating cakes and fry-ups for years it is very difficult to change these habits of a lifetime.

The person must be slowly and patiently re-educated about diet. Knowledge of the cheaper protein foods is a starting point. Adequate fluid intake is just as important as taking sufficient food. Making the most of meal times for persons of reduced activity is one of the more time consuming yet highly rewarding nursing responsibilities. How can a nurse ensure that her patients achieve as much independence as possible and consume a balanced diet?

She should ensure food is at the correct temperature.

The food should be attractively served in small minced or cut up portions.

Each course should be served separately.

She should know of and use appropriately the variety of aids available to allow the person to eat independently. These aids include non-slip table mats, plate guards, sporks, feeding cups and large napkins or bibs (Figs. 20.12 and 20.13A–D).

She should always encourage the patient to feed himself. In the beginning this may result in the patient managing only to drink soup out of a feeding cup or take two or three

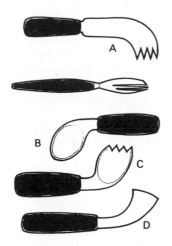

Figure 20.13
Special cutlery

spoonfuls of his main course unaided, but the fact that he is attempting and succeeding at all should be praised and the praise should inspire him to try harder.

Above all, the nurse **must give the patient time to do what he can.**

Special problems

Confusion and dementia

The nurse's attitude and approach to patients whose behaviour is abnormal is most important. She should show patience, perseverance and practical appreciation of the patient's difficulties. The aim is to help the patient regain touch with reality. The nurse can help him by constantly offering reminders as to the day, the time, the meal he is eating, the bath he is going to have, the visitors who come to see him and so on. Use of his proper name at all times to remind him of his identity is a practical and positive way to reduce confusion and dementia. If a patient suddenly becomes confused, the nurse from her observations may be able to ascertain and perhaps eliminate the cause. For example, faecal impaction is often a cause of temporary confusion.

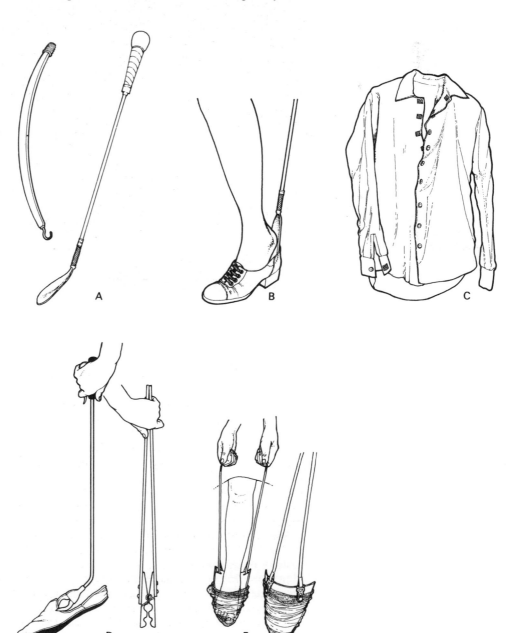

Figure 20.14A–E
Aids to dressing

Paralysis/stroke

Many patients in geriatric wards are suffering from some form of paralysis. The degree of paralysis depends on the cause and the area of the brain affected. A cerebrovascular accident (Ch.3) leaves the patient with some residual disability brought about by diminished blood supply to brain cells and absent or impaired function of peripheral nerves. Recovery from a stroke may be rapid and straightforward; more often it is frustratingly slow.

The nurse's responsibility in aiding the recovery of the stroke patient is great. If he is properly directed, the patient can be restored to modified independence; without it he may acquire mental as well as physical contractures, causing increasing disability, which will deny him the independence and activity which may have been well within his grasp. The patient who has had a stroke should attend the physiotherapy, occupational and diversional therapy departments. The treatment given in these departments must be continued in the ward. It is the nurse's responsibility to motivate the patient to do what he can for himself, even if he does so with difficulty. She can do this by:

Passive exercise of the paralysed limbs.
Assisting the patient to stand up independently.
Attempting to 'walk' the patient (Fig. 3.37, p. 107).
Assisting with bed-end exercise.
Encouraging the appropriate use of available aids (Fig. 20.14 A–E).
Using wheel-chairs only when absolutely necessary.
Assisting the patient to eat and drink with dignity.
Giving the patient time to do what he can for himself.

Aphasia/dysphasia

The term **aphasia** is used to describe varying degrees of language deficit. In the aphasic patient there is complete absence of coherent speech. In the **dysphasic** patient there is difficulty in speaking. Approximately one-third of stroke patients suffer from some form of dysphasia; this is the most common symptom found after a cerebrovascular accident. Aphasia is described as either receptive or expressive. **Receptive aphasia** is difficulty in understanding the spoken and written word, that is the in-going message is not received. In **expressive aphasia** the spoken word is understood but verbal communication to express wants is impaired or absent, that is the out-going message cannot be expressed. As with all aspects of stroke rehabilitation, treatment of dysphasia is a team effort. In this case the leader of the team is the **speech therapist**, but her work must be continued by other members. The nurse has a responsibility to aid the aphasic or dysphasic patient to communicate. She can do this by:

Speaking more slowly than usual and in full view of the patient.
Allowing the patient to observe lip movement and facial expression.
Helping the patient to identify himself by using his name at all times.
Introducing herself so that he learns to identify those around him.
Giving constant reassurance by explaining all events which concern him.
Keeping the patient informed, for instance about the day, date and 'highlights' (everyday things with which he is normally familiar, such as happenings in relation to time of day or time of year).
Making use of all channels of communication—hearing, touch, vision.
Providing aids to assist him to communicate (Fig. 20.15).

The first step towards recovery may indeed be the ability of the nurse to make eye contact with the patient. This may be his only means of communication. The nurse's attitude should verbally and behaviourally always portray respect, realism and hope. Aphasia makes the patient dependent on the nurse; this dependence should never be abused.

Urinary incontinence

Many old people have malfunctioning bladders but they manage to cope without becoming incontinent by arranging their environment to fit in with their limited bladder function. They do this by keeping a commode at the side of the bed, avoiding long bus journeys and regularly emptying the bladder. Older people may find their own solutions to avoiding incontinence, but if a situation arises to interfere with their routine

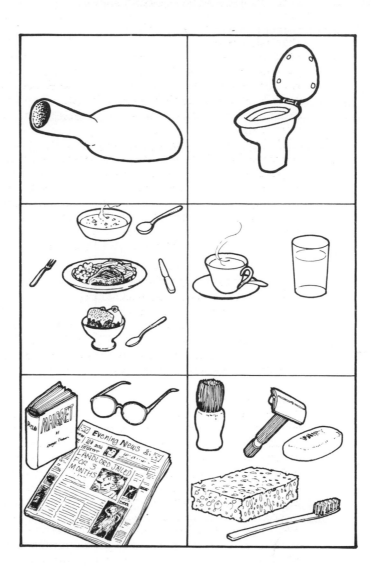

Figure 20.15
Communication card

incontinence may occur. Nursing responsibility in temporary and established incontinence varies. In temporary incontinence, caused perhaps by urinary tract infections, the emphasis is on curing the cause; in established incontinence, often associated with disorders of the central nervous system, the emphasis is on encouraging the person physically and psychologically to be as independent as his incontinence will allow.

Urinary incontinence is dealt with more fully in Chapter 9.

Nursing care
The most important care the nurse can give is to take the patient to the toilet as often as necessary. An 'incontinence chart' (Fig. 20.16) is a great help. It can show quite clearly how often and when a person will benefit from toileting. It may be that a person needs to be toileted 2-hourly or 4-hourly or perhaps 4-hourly during the night. When this is done the nurse should note whether the patient is wet or dry, then over a period of a week a chart will show the whole time scale of incontinence, for instance whether the patient is incontinent only at night, all day long or perhaps only at 6 a.m.

It is just as important to chart the incidence of incontinence as it is to chart the incidence of sugar in the urine. It is often thought that if the fluid intake is decreased the patient will not be incontinent. This is not so; many incontinent patients become dehydrated and need an increased fluid intake. However, it does not make sense to give a patient a large amount of fluid before going to bed.

Obviously the more mobile a patient is the more likely it is that he will reach the toilet; therefore it follows that if the nurse encourages mobility she is at the same time

HOSPITAL .... UNIT No.

INCONTINENCE CHART

NAME

DATE OF BIRTH

DIAGNOSIS

DATE		DAY 08.00 10.00	10.00 12.00	12.00 14.00	14.00 16.00	16.00 18.00	18.00 20.00	NIGHT 20.00 22.00	22.00 24.00	24.00 02.00	02.00 04.00	04.00 06.00	06.00 08.00	REMARKS
	U													
	F													
	U													
	F													
	U													
	F													
	U													
	F													
	U													
	F													
	U													
	F													
	U													
	F													

DATE		DAY 08.00 10.00	10.00 12.00	12.00 14.00	14.00 16.00	16.00 18.00	18.00 20.00	NIGHT 20.00 22.00	22.00 24.00	24.00 02.00	02.00 04.00	04.00 06.00	06.00 08.00	REMARKS
	U													
	F													
	U													
	F													
	U													
	F													
	U													
	F													
	U													
	F													
	U													
	F													
	U													
	F													

IF INCONTINENT, OF URINE, AND/OR FAECES, CROSS HATCH SQUARE, U OR F
AT THE TIME OF THE EVENT

NORMAL URINATION OR BOWEL ACTION MAY BE MARKED BY A DIAGONAL
STROKE IN THE APPROPRIATE SQUARE

Figure 20.16
Incontinence chart

diminishing the risk of incontinence. Another way the nurse can help is to provide toilet facilities as soon as the patient asks for them. Delay in giving a commode or urinal encourages incontinence. One is well aware of the patient who constantly asks for a bedpan or urinal. Every time a nurse appears a urinal is needed. This state of affairs occurs because, when the patient genuinely requires the toilet, no nurse is available, so to compensate for this he asks as soon as a nurse appears. In fact, he tries to gear his toilet requirements to the availability of the nurse. People do not enjoy being incontinent, but on occasions apathy, rejection and depression set in and the patient gives up trying. Avoiding this situation is an explicit nursing responsibility.

Catheterization and care of in-dwelling catheters
Catheterization is not invariably carried out on all incontinent patients but only after all else has failed. The decision to insert a permanent catheter is made after all aspects of the patient's condition have been considered. It is inserted for the psychological and physical comfort of the patient, not to reduce the work load of the nurses or to help the laundry service. One of the hazards of an in-dwelling catheter is infection. Often this is accepted as 'one of those things'. The nurse can minimize the risks associated with catheters in the following ways:

Encouraging the patient to drink at least 1·5 litres of fluid in 24 hours.
Ensuring the catheter is not kinked and is draining freely into a uribag or closed drainage system.
Taking aseptic precautions when changing the bag.
Keeping the urethral orifice scrupulously clean. Daily or twice daily toilet is usual.
Nursing observations for patients who have in-dwelling catheters include:

Measuring and recording fluid intake and output.
Noting the appearance and smell of the urine.
Taking and recording the temperature and pulse twice daily.
The catheter will be changed and specimens of urine sent for microbiological examination regularly, according to the routine of the ward or unit.

Faecal impaction and incontinence
Faecal impaction occurs when a mass of faecal matter is lodged within the lumen of the large bowel. The mobility of the gastrointestinal tract slows down in old people which makes the movement of the waste matter sluggish. Normally a person becomes aware that the rectum is full and its contents are expelled at an appropriate time. In faecal impaction this does not happen. The slower onward movement of the intestinal content allows more time for water to be reabsorbed and the residue becomes abnormally solid. Eventually the constipated faeces, which cannot be expelled unaided, accumulate in the rectum. This state may be accompanied by leakage of fluid faecal material, which seeps around the impacted mass and through the anus, an occurrence sometimes called **spurious diarrhoea**. It is possible to distinguish it from true diarrhoea by reference to the patient's general condition and the invariably fluid faecal discharge. The faecal mass will be felt on rectal examination.

Additional indications which would make the nurse suspect faecal impaction are lower abdominal pain and a distended abdomen. Once impaction has occurred it can take as long as 3 weeks to clear the bowel completely. The first step will be to empty the rectum digitally. Mild oral aperients may be prescribed to soften the faeces to facilitate easier passage.

Regular per rectum examination is imperative. If there are faeces in the rectum the appropriate suppositories or enemata are used, but there is no point in injecting an enema into an already empty rectum. The treatment of faecal impaction involves a great deal of nursing care and patient discomfort. On the whole it is something that can be avoided. It is on the nurse that this responsibility lies.

Care of the dying

When a patient is dying the aim of all those looking after him is to promote his physical and mental comfort and to provide support and help for his relatives. Death may occur suddenly, but more often the warning signs gradually increase and the patient's condition slowly deteriorates until the functions of vital organs cease.

It is difficult to instruct a nurse on the art of caring for the dying as dying and death are unique experiences. One can demonstrate a caring attitude but how can one aid a nurse to be prepared for such an event? She is confronted with this without prior experience. Each nurse, patient or relative is a different individual, therefore it follows that each dying experience is different. How the nurse approaches this experience will depend on her own personality, knowledge and understanding.

One can offer guidelines such as allowing the patient to express feelings but it is only in the actual experiencing of it that the nurse learns when to listen, when to talk and when to act. It is only with experience she learns to 'hear' the cues the patient or relative give. An example of a cue are words like: 'I have had a good life nurse'.

Rapport between the dying patient, relative and nurse cannot be established quickly. Some relationships will develop more quickly than others but most two-way meaningful and mutual communication takes a certain length of time. In a busy ward this is difficult to achieve but one must be aware that 'successful' care of the dying has more chance of achievement if all who are involved in this care show willingness and readiness to participate in this experience.

The physical comfort of the dying person often takes priority over the psychological needs. To 'do' is easier than being prepared to listen. When one 'listens', one has to be ready to acknowledge the patient's feelings and the effect those feelings have on one's own. Nurses often realise this and to protect their vulnerability withdraw or even ignore that these feelings exist.

The first experience of death for any nurse is usually a traumatic experience. One does not know what to expect. There is a fearfulness of this unknown experience. To help to diminish this trauma the nurse should not be expected to participate in the care of the dead patient (whether she has nursed the patient or not) but rather observe the body then depart to express feelings verbally or emotionally. At her next experience of death she should watch the dressing of the dead person and ideally only participate in the last offices at subsequent deaths.

The junior nurse is often in the ambivalent position of being the one the patient confides in, yet is in no position to give positive answers to questions such as 'am I going to die'. Beware of curtailing a chance of finding out what a patient's feelings are by resorting to the standard 'I will have to ask sister', but rather allow the person to speak.

When confronted with questions of death or dying the nurse should answer honestly. If she is asked 'am I going to die?', she can honestly answer 'I do not know. Do you feel you are going to die?'. The patient may reply 'yes' to this question and the nurse can now allow the patient to express his feelings and thoughts. She could then offer to get a sister or a doctor or a minister to speak to him if he wishes. The patient may or may not want this but whatever he wants and whatever his feelings are can be reported to senior staff and perhaps discussed at report time and then further discussions with the relatives could follow.

A certain amount of pretence is tolerable when caring for the dying but too much encourages the patient to pretend and deny his true feelings and diminishes opportunities for expression of real anxieties from the patient and his relatives. One wants to strive, for a compromise between compassionate 'honesty' and blunt truth.

Drugs, such as narcotics, may be prescribed if the patient is likely to suffer severe pain. Any prescribed drug will be given as frequently as the patient needs it; possible addiction will no longer be a consideration and the comfort of the patient will be of paramount importance. Often simple measures, such as alteration of his position and change of bed linen, relieve distress and help to prevent the additional pain which would accompany pressure sores. Mouth breathing occurs frequently in terminal illness and the mouth and lips should be treated as often as necessary. Attentions of this sort, which may seem of little practical significance, make a very important contribution to the patient's care, mainly because they enable the nurse to demonstrate care, sympathy and respect for the patient and understanding of his difficulties.

The psychological care the dying person receives contributes as much as, if not more than, the physical care. It falls to the nurse to allay fears and anxieties. She should listen, look and touch. The dying person should not be left to die alone and the presence of his relatives should be encouraged. Once it is known that the patient's condition is deteriorating they are informed. The doctor or ward sister talks to them and they are allowed to visit or stay with the patient at any time. Having a relative close by is a great comfort to the patient but a severe strain for his relatives. Often relatives feel frustrated because there seems to be so little they can do; allowing and encouraging them to visit gives them a chance to perform little acts of kindness. It is a sad time for them; they should be allowed to express their grief and worries and be given every consideration. They, almost as much as the patient, need the nurse's reassurance and support.

The spiritual aspects must always be considered when caring for the dying. Faith is a powerful factor in the make-up of man. Nurses should recognize this and accept that a dying patient may find solace and contentment in the words and ritual of his religion, whatever his particular faith may be. The relevant minister, priest or rabbi will be informed if the patient and his relatives wish it. In the Roman Catholic Church the last rites must be given before death. Consultation between patient, relatives and the respective minister regarding ritual after death is desirable; for example an orthodox Jew must not be touched after death by a gentile without permission from a rabbi. If possible, instructions about wedding rings and personal valuables should be known before the person dies.

Another feature of death that the nurse should be aware of is the effect it has on the other patients. A death in a ward cannot be kept a secret. The nurse should calmly and quietly go about caring for the rest of the patients and, if asked, should tell the truth, simply.

Once the patient has died the caring emphasis moves from the patient to his relatives. Sister's duty room or a sitting room can provide a place in which to comfort them and give them some privacy. The nurse then informs the doctor, who comes to certify the death. If the death occurs during the day the relatives can collect the death certificate prior to leaving. If the patient dies during the night the relatives are asked to come back in the morning. A death should be registered within 3 days. The relatives are advised to take the death certificate and any relevant insurance policies to the registrar of births, deaths and marriages as soon as possible. Once the death has been registered the appropriate funeral arrangements can proceed. Once the patient has been certified dead the last offices are carried out. This should be done quietly and with respect. The last offices are the last services of the nurse to her patient.

Guidelines to aid nurses when caring for the dying and their relatives

Understand that the nurse does not fail when the patient dies but rather succeeds if her patient dies physically and psychologically painfree and without excessive anxiety.

Try not to interrupt when a patient or relative starts to talk about dying or death with cliche expressions like 'Come, come, don't talk like that'.

Spend as much time as you can with the dying person yet remember the needs of other patients.

Be accessible to relatives and allow them to express concern and emotion. Give them as much information as you can. Be patient with relatives who require constant reassurance.

Accept anger, anxiety and frustration in the patient and his relatives. Anger may be directed at you but not with you.

Accept that your own feelings of sadness and helplessness are natural and human.

Do not be afraid to show emotion through words and actions.

TEAM APPROACH TO CARE

The following two case histories help to illustrate the contribution of various health and social services to the care of the elderly.

Mrs B — age 78 years

History
Mrs B was fit and independent up to the day of her admission to hospital. She was able to do her own shopping, cooking and housework until 2 months ago when she fell to the

ground and was unable to rise. She was observed to develop some twisting of her face, and her left arm and left leg were partially paralysed. While in hospital there was a substantial return of power in the left leg and at the end of 2 months of intensive rehabilitation she was able to walk with the help of a Zimmer aid and was even able to manage stairs slowly. Although incontinent of urine for a week or two after admission, bladder control was regained and at the end of 2 months she was fully continent and able to help dress herself and to walk to the toilet without assistance. In spite of her good functional recovery she tended to tire readily, and when this happened her walking deteriorated somewhat and she was in danger of falling.

Mrs B lived alone and her flat was four flights up with an outside lavatory and no bath. With better housing and one caring relative she would have been fit for home discharge, but because she became weary quickly and because of the poor quality and situation of her house, she was transferred to a local authority home.

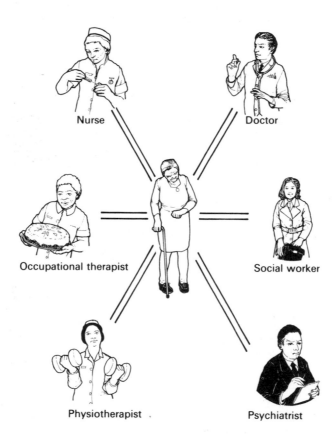

Figure 20.17
The multidisciplinary team: caring for the elderly in hospital

Summary

This patient suffered a left-sided stroke, made an excellent recovery but tended to tire rather easily and had no supportive relative in the home. She was, however, continent, ambulant with the help of a Zimmer aid and sensible, so that she was eminently suitable for a residential home or sheltered housing.

It is probably worth stating that many patients are considered suitable for a residential home who are not as independent as Mrs B; some help with walking and occasional incontinence may not debar a patient from such provision. Serious urinary incontinence and behavioural problems absolutely exclude a patient from being considered for special accommodation provided by a local authority.

Mrs C—age 85 years

History

Before admission to hospital Mrs C was able to go out for short walks and do some of her own shopping. She had a home help twice a week who was able to do some of the shopping and most of the housework. The new trainee assistant general practioner decided to take Mrs C's blood pressure and found the diastolic reading to be 105 mmHg. Treatment with a hypotensive agent was started and following this she developed postural hypotension, which led to a fall and a fractured neck of the femur. She was admitted to hospital for surgery; after 3 months of intensive rehabilitation she was able to walk with a Zimmer aid and was continent and sensible.

Mrs C lived in a comfortable ground floor flat with her elderly, though fit husband. The flat was adequately heated and had a bath and an indoor toilet. Although Mrs C was able to walk with a Zimmer aid she needed help with washing and dressing and was not able to bath herself. It was also felt that, although she had improved dramatically while in hospital, if rehabilitation ceased her walking would probably deteriorate and she would become chair-fast.

Arrangements were made for a home help to attend 3 days a week to help with the shopping, cooking and housework although her husband was able to contribute to these activities.

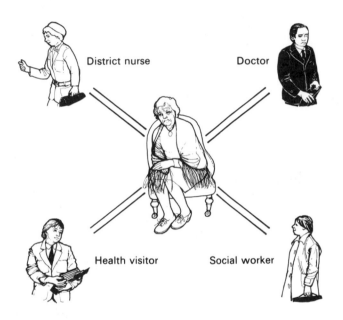

Figure 20.18
The multidisciplinary team: caring for the elderly at home

The district nurse was asked to visit once weekly to help bath Mrs C. It was arranged that she should attend the day hospital twice weekly for continuing physiotherapy and occupational therapy.

The unit health visitor arranged to visit Mrs C at first once fortnightly and then once every 6 weeks ro review the circumstances and report back to the consultant geriatrician and the general practioner. If the situation started to deteriorate and the husband was unable to cope then the health visitor would be able to warn the general practioner and the geriatrician at a fairly early stage. Preventive action could be taken and if necessary Mrs C could be readmitted to hospital for a short period.

Summary
This patient was given a hypotensive agent and (as a result) fell and fractured her leg. In spite of some residual disability and because of the quality of her accommodation and the presence of a willing and relatively fit though elderly spouse, she was able to return home with appropriate domiciliary support.

In the final analysis continence and the ability to transfer safely from bed to commode and then back to bed are essential prerequisites for home discharge if no able and caring relative lives with the patient. If the patient is continent and is able to go to the toilet herself then even a badly disabled patient can be supported at home by means of domiciliary help and day hospital attendance.

FURTHER READING

Agate J N 1979 Geriatrics for nurses and social workers, 2nd edn. Heinemann, London

Anderson W F 1976 Practical management of the elderly, 3rd edn. Blackwell Scientific, Oxford

Brocklehurst J C (ed) 1978 Textbook of geriatric medicine and gerontology, 2nd edn. Churchill Livingstone, Edinburgh

Brocklehurst J C, Hanley T 1976 Geriatric medicine for students. Churchill Livingstone, Edinburgh

Carver V, Liddiard P 1978 An ageing population. Hodder and Stoughton in association with the Open University Press

Hyams D 1972 The care of the aged. Priory Press, London

Norton D 1970 By accident or design. A study of equipment development in relation to basic nursing problems, Churchill Livingstone, Edinburgh

Norton D, McLaren R, Exton-Smith A N 1975 An investigation of geriatric nursing problems in hospital. Churchill Livingstone, Edinburgh

Glossary

(Abbreviations: F = French; L = Latin; G = Greek)

Abduction (L *abducere* to draw away, separate) Movement of a limb away from the midline of the body.

Adduction (L. *adducere* to bring towards) Movement of a limb towards the midline of the body.

Adynamic ileus (paralytic ileus, ileus paralyticus) Ileus resulting from inhibition of bowel motility which may be produced by numerous causes, most frequently by peritonitis.

Aetiology (G *aitia* cause, *logos* discourse) The study of the causes of disease.

After pains Spasmodic painful uterine contractions occurring during the first 48 hours following delivery, most commonly seen in multiparous women. They may be caused by clots in the uterus.

Allergen (G *genein* to produce) A substance capable of producing a specific hypersensitivity in an individual, for example drugs, pollens, eggs.

Allergy (G *allos* other, *ergein* to work) Hypersensitivity to some foreign substance, often certain foods or pollens. These substances, allergens, are usually of a protein nature and can include eggs, strawberries, oranges, pork, cauliflower, fish, dust from feathers or from the hair of horses, cats or dogs.

Alopecia (G *alopex* fox) Baldness. It often occurs in sharply defined patches in disease.

Alpha fetoprotein (AFP) A protein of fetal origin found in liquor amnii (amniotic fluid). In a normal pregnancy there is a small amount which diminishes as the pregnancy develops. In some abnormal conditions of the fetus such as myelomeningocele the level is considerably raised. Maternity units offer a screening test around the sixteenth week of pregnancy.

Amaurosis (G *amauroein* to darken) Complete loss of vision especially that in which there is no evidence of a pathological condition of the eye.

Amaurotic Pertaining to one afflicted with amaurosis. A family idiocy. Term for a group of related familial diseases, marked by dementia, impaired vision and lipid defect.

Amblyopia (G *amblys* dull, *ops* eye) Dimness of vision or loss of sight.

Amnion (G the fetal membrane) The innermost membrane of the fetal sac in which is contained the liquor amnii or amniotic fluid. This fluid acts as a shock absorber to the fetus and allows free movement.

Amyloid disease (G *amylon* starch) A condition in which tissue, especially liver and kidneys, degenerates and becomes waxy in appearance due to deposition of fibrous tissue.

Ankylosis (G *agkylos* crooked) Condition in which a joint is stiffened either by fibrous tissue (fibrous ankylosis) or by bony fusion (bony ankylosis).

Anomaly (G *anomalia* irregularity) 1. Anything contrary to general rule. 2. Any organ or structure which is abnormal with reference to form, structure or position; a malformation.

Anoxia (G *an*, oxygen) A state of deficiency of oxygen in the tissues.

Apnoea (G *a* without, *pnein* to breathe) Temporary cessation of breathing.

Arthrodesis (G *arthron* a joint, *desis* binding together) Fixation of a joint by destruction of the articular surfaces, followed by bony fusion of the bones involved.

Arthrogryphosis (G *arthron* a joint, *gryphosis* a curve) Flexure of a joint — a congenital deformity.

Arthroplasty (G *arthron* a joint, *plassein* to form) The formation or production of a movable joint by surgery.

Ataxia (G *ataxia* lack of order or arrangement) Lack of co-ordination of voluntary movements.

Atelectasis (G *ateles* incomplete, *ektasis* a stretching) A condition in which a lung (or lungs) is incompletely expanded.

Athetosis (G *athetos* not fixed) Useless, purposeless, disordered movements.

Atrophy (G *a* without, *trophe* nourishment) Lack of growth and wasting of an organ or limb.

Attention (L *attendere* to stretch) Power to focus on some phase of consciousness including some aspect of the world of reality.

Autosomes (G *autos* self, *soma* body) Any of the paired chromosomes other than the sex chromosomes (X and Y). In man there are 22 pairs.

Avulsion (L *avulsus* torn away) Forcible separation of two parts

Blepharitis G *blepharon* eyelid, *-itis* inflammation) Inflammation of the eyelid, particularly chronic inflammation of the lid margins, causing crust formation and eventually trichiasis. Attention to hygiene, improvement of general health and local applications are of help. It is akin to dandruff of the scalp.

Bougie (F candle) A solid, cylindrical-shaped instrument used for insertion into a natural orifice such as the urethra, oesophagus or rectum, usually for the purpose of dilatation.

Braxton Hicks contractions Painless uterine contractions felt on abdominal palpation from the 16th week of pregnancy.

Breech presentation The term used to describe the fetus lying with its buttocks in the lower part of the uterus. The baby is born with the buttocks coming first, as opposed to the more common vertex presentation (95 per cent of all deliveries), when the baby is born head first. (*See* Vertex).

Bronchography (G *brogchos* windpipe, *graphein* to record) An examination by X-ray of the bronchi following the introduction of a radio-opaque dye.

Bronchoscopy (G *brogchos* windpipe, *skopein* to watch) An examination of the inside of the bronchi using a bronchoscope.

Bulla (L bubble) Large blister.

Calcaneus (L *calx* the heel bone) In a calcaneus deformity the heel bone becomes abnormally prominent due to acute dorsiflexion of the foot at the ankle joint.

Caput succedaneum (L head) A localized area of oedema which forms under the baby's scalp caused by vascula congestion from pressure of the cervix during birth. It subsides in 24 to 48 hours without treatment.

Carcinogen (carcinoma, G *genein* to produce) Any substance which causes living tissue to become carcinomatous.

Carcinoma (G *karkinos* crab, *-oma* tumour) A malignant tumour which tends to spread, destroying normal tissue as it progresses.

Carina (L *carina* keel) The area at which the trachea bifurcates.

Cavus (L *cavum* cavity, hollow) Longitudinal arch of the foot which is abnormally high.

Cephalhaematoma (G *kephale* head, *haima* blood, *-oma* tumour) A firm, circumscribed swelling on the skull due to an effusion of blood under the periosteum. It most often occurs when there has been a very short labour and rapid delivery and is caused by friction between the baby's skull and the mother's pelvis. No treatment is required but, as it usually persists for six to eight weeks, the mother requires considerable reassurance.

Chondromalacia (G *chondros* cartilage, *malakia* softness) Erosion of artecular cartilage.

Chorion (G a skin) The outer protective and nutritive membrane covering the fetal sac.

Chromatography	Chemical analysis by which a mixture of substances is separated by fractional extraction or absorption on a porous solid (column of aluminium oxide or filter paper) by means of flowing solvents.
Chromosomes	(G *chroma* colour, *soma* body) Microscopic rod-shaped bodies which develop from the nuclear material of a cell and are especially conspicuous during mitosis; they stain deeply with basic dyes. Chromosomes contain the genes or hereditary determiners. The number of chromosomes is constant for each species, being 46 in man (23 pairs in all somatic cells).
Clinical examination	(G *kline* bed) A physical examination.
Cognitive	(L *cognoscere* to know) A general term covering all the various modes of knowing, perceiving, remembering, imagining, conceiving, judging, reasoning.
Commensal	(L *cum* combined with, *mensa* table) An organism which lives on or within another but which does no harm to the host. Commensals are normally found on various mucous surfaces of the body.
Concept	(L *concipere* to take in) An idea.
Constipation	(L *constipatio* to crowd together) Infrequent or difficult evacuation of faeces; it results from the non-passage of motions for a longer period than is normal for that individual.
Coxa	(L) The hip joint.
Craniotomy	(L *cranium* G *kranion* skull + *tome* cut). Any operation on the skull.
Cubitus	(L *cubitus* to lie down) When reclining on couches during meals, the Romans leaned on their elbows. Hence the present connotation = the elbow, as in cubitus valgus deformity.
Cyto	(G *kytos*, vessel, hollow) Describes relationship to a cell.
Cytology	(G *logos* science) The science of the structure and function of cells.
Dacryocystitis	(G *dakryon* tear, *-itis* inflammation) Inflammation of the lacrimal drainage system, usually an acute painful suppurative inflammation which requires treatment with systemic antibiotics. It tends to occur in the very old and the very young.
Dermatoglyphics	(G *derma* skin, *glyphe* a carving) Study of surface markings of the skin especially those of the hands and feet.
Dextran	A plasma substitute for transfusion purposes which contains complex carbohydrate molecules. Its effect is to exert osmotic pressure, attracting water, thus preventing loss of water from capillaries in shock. Various forms are available, including the low molecular weight Lomodex and Rheomacrodex. Dextran 150 has a higher molecular weight.
Diarrhoea	(G *dia* through, *rhein* to flow) Abnormal (for the individual concerned) frequency and liquidity of faeces. Also described as looseness of the bowels.
DNA	Deoxyribonucleic acid, which is found in the cell nucleus.
Doptone	An ultrasonic device used to monitor the fetal heart. It may also be used to detect pregnancy at an early stage.
Dorsiflex	To flex the ankle or wrist towards the dorsum of the foot or hand.
Dysarthria	(*Dys* + G *arthrun* to utter distinctly + *ia*) Imperfect articulation of words due to disturbance of muscular control resulting from damage to the nervous system.
Dyscrasia	(G *dys* bad, imperfect, *krasis* mixture) An abnormal state of the body.
Dysfunction	(G *dys* bad etc., L *functio* performance) Absence of completely normal function.
Dysplasia	(G *dys* bad etc., *plasis* forming, shaping) Abnormality of formation or development.
Dystrophy	(G *dys* bad etc., *trophic* nourishment) Abnormal nourishment, therefore imperfect growth.
Eclampsia	(G *ek* centr, *lampein* to flash) An advanced stage of serious pre-eclampsia, characterized by convulsions; the mother's life, as well as the fetus's, is at great

risk. Because of the prompt diagnosis and treatment of pre-eclampsia, eclampsia is now rarely seen. (*See* Pre-eclampsia).

Ectropion (G *ek* centre, *trepein* to turn) Eversion or rolling out of the eyelid. It can result from scarring of the lids or, in the senile form, from loss of muscle tone.

Emphysema (G *en* into, *physema* a blowing) A condition in which the alveoli of the lungs are permanently dilated due to bronchial obstruction.

Encephalopathy (encephalon, G *pathos* disease) Any dysfunction of the brain.

Entonox Inhalation analgesia consisting of oxygen 50 per cent and nitrous oxide 50 per cent. The Central Midwives Boards of the U.K. permit the midwife to administer it during the late first stage of labour and during the second stage of labour to relieve pain.

Entropion (G *en* into, *tropos* a turning) conversion or turning in of the lid margins. It is usually caused by contraction of scar tissue.

Enucleation (L *e* out + *nucleus* kernel) To shell out whole. The removal of an organ or tumour from its covering. Used in connection with the eye it means removal of the eyeball after the optic nerve and the extrinsic muscles of the eye have been severed.

Epicanthic fold (G *epi* upon, *kanthos* lip of a vessel) A fold of skin extending from the root of the nose to the median end of the eyebrow, covering the inner canthus and caruncle. It is a characteristic of the Mongolian race.

Episiotomy (G *episeion* pudenda, *teinein* to cut) An incision made into the perineum under local anaesthesia to allow more room for the delivery of the baby's head and to prevent damage to the pelvic floor and soft tissues.

Equinus (L *equinus* of the horse) In an equinus deformity the forepart of the foot is plantar flexed in the manner of a horse's hoof.

Ergometrine Drug used to control haemorrhage following the birth of the baby. Given by i.m. injection or i.v. injection — dose 0.5 mg.

Erythema (G redness) A rash which appears as a superficial reddening of the skin.

Eschar (G *eschara* scab) A slough, resulting, from death of tissue due to gangrene or burning.

Eusol A form of antiseptic containing hypochlorous acid and boric. The name is made up from the initial letters of Edinburgh University Solution of Lime.

Evisceration L *e* out + *viscus* the inside of the body) Used in connection with the eye it means removal of the contents of the eyeball leaving the sclera intact.

Exostosis (L *ex* out of, G *osteon* bone, *osis* a condition of) A condition in which there is a bony outgrowth.

External version Turning the fetus in the uterus from a breech to a vertex presentation. The manoeuvre is carried out by the obstetrician.

Fetal development 1. The term **embryo** is used up to the 12th week of pregnancy.
2. The term **fetus** is used from the 12th week of pregnancy to birth.
3. After birth, the fetus is known as the **baby**.

Forewaters The liquor amnii contained in the membranous sac lying in front of the presenting part; it may rupture spontaneously prior to the onset of labour or during labour. (For artificial rupture of membranes, *see* Induction of labour.)

Fructose (L *fructus* fruit) Laevulose. Fruit sugar.

Galactosaemia (G *gala* milk, *haima* blood) The presence of galactose (see below) in the blood.

Galactose (G *gala* milk). $C_6H_{12}O_6$ A monosaccharide or simple hexose sugar. Galactose is an isomer of glucose and is formed along with glucose in the hydrolysis of lactose. Galactose is readily absorbed in the digestive tract; in the liver it is converted into glycogen.

Gene (G *genein* to produce) The basic unit of heredity. Each gene occupies a certain place on a chromosome.

Genetics	The science that accounts for natural differences and resemblances among organisms related by descent. The study of heredity and its variations.
Gestation	(L *gestare* to bear) Period of intrauterine fetal development from conception to birth.
Glyconeogenesis	(Glyco + G *neos* new + *gennan* to produce) The formation of carbohydrates from molecules which are not themselves carbohydrates as amino acids, fatty acids or related molecules.
Guthrie test	A means of screening used between the fifth and tenth day of life to detect phenylketonuria and other metabolic disorders. Capillary blood is collected from a heel-prick on to specially prepared blotting paper and allowed to dry before being sent to the laboratory.
Haematocrit	(G *haima* blood, *krinein* to separate) Packed cell volume. When blood is centrifuged and prevented from clotting, it separates into layers. The bottom layer is red cells, which account for 45 per cent of the total volume of blood. In any condition where fluid has been lost from the circulation, as in burns, this figure will be increased.
Hepatolenticular	(G *hepar* liver, L *lens* lentil) Related to the liver and the lenticular nucleus. Hepatolenticular degeneration (Wilson's disease). Progressive lenticular degeneration in cirrhosis of the liver.
Histamine	(G *histos* tissue) A substance found in body tissues. The concentration varies in different organs. In man tissue histamine may be released in response to trauma, antigens, trypsin and bile salts.
Homograft	A portion of tissue removed from a donor to be applied to a recipient of the same species; such a graft survives for a very short period except in the case of cornea, artery, bone, cartilage and perhaps endocrine tissue.
Hordeolum	(L *hodeum* barley) A stye; inflammation of one or more glands of Zeis (sebaceous glands of the eyelids). Application of heat helps to speed discharge of pus.
Hydramnios	(G *hydor* water, *amnion* the fetal membrane) Excessive accumulation of amniotic fluid.
Hyperostosis	(G *hyper* above + G *osteon* bone + *osis*) Hypertrophy (overgrowth) of bone; exostosis.
Hypo-	Prefix, from the Greek preposition *hypo*, meaning under, deficient, beneath.
Hypochromic	(G *hypo* deficient, *chroma* colour) A term applied to red blood cells which contain less haemoglobin than normal. It is usually associated with microcytosis and is characteristic of iron deficiency anaemia.
Hypopyon	(G *hypo* deficient, *pyon* pus) Pus in the anterior chamber of the eye. It may occur as the result of a severely infected corneal ulcer.
Ideas of reference	A symptom of psychological illness. The patient believes that even the most casual remark and action of others refer in some special way to him. The most obvious example is the paranoid or suspicious individual who is convinced that every time he leaves a room everyone present begins to talk about him.
Ileus	(L; G *eileos* from *eilein* to roll up) obstruction of the intestines.
Incongruity of affect	Display of inappropriate emotion in response to a situation, for instance, to giggle when told of a tragic happening.
Induction of labour	This procedure is usually undertaken in the interests of the other and the fetus. ARM (artificial rupture of the membranes) is carried out and the uterus may be stimulated to contract by administering i.v. Syntocinon, which is a synthetic form of oxytocin.
Intelligence	(L *intelligentia* perception) The capacity to comprehend relationships. The ability to think. The ability to solve problems and to adjust to new situations.
Intelligence quotient	The measure of intelligence obtained by dividing the individual's mental age (according to the Binet scale) by his chronological age and multiplying the result by 100.

International unit (iu)	A given quantity of a substance having a recognized effect. The active principals of many nutritional compounds have now been discovered, and specific weight equivalents are generally used when discussing intake of these compounds.
Ischaemia	(G *ischo* to restrain, hold back, *haima* blood) Inadequate or deficient blood supply to some part of the body.
Keratin	(G *keras* horn) A protein substance found in the horny layer of the epidermis (keratinize: to make or become horny).
Kernicterus	(G Kern kernel, icterus = jaundice) A form of icterus neonatorum occurring in infants in which nuclear masses of the brain and spinal cord undergo pathological changes accompanied by deposition of bile pigments within them.
Ketoacidosis	Acidosis accompanied by the accumulation of ketone bodies (ketosis) in the body tissues and fluids as in diabetic acidosis.
Ketosis	A condition characterized by an abnormally elevated concentration of ketone bodies in the body tissues and fluids. It arises when there is insufficient carbohydrate in the diet and increased amounts of fat are used for energy as in starvation or severe vomiting (it can be accompanied by a metabolic alkalosis).
Kyphosis	(G *kyphos* hunch-backed) Forward concave curvature of the spine.
Lanugo	(L down) Fine downy covering of hair on the skin of the premature baby.
Leucotomy	(G *leukos* white, *temnein* to cut) A surgical operation in which the association fibres running from the frontal lobes of the brain to the thalamus are severed. It is performed to alleviate debilitating mental distress when other methods of treatment have failed. The operation can be performed using a variety of techniques. Inevitably personality changes occur ranging from happy-go-lucky attitudes to apathy, emotional blunting and a vegetable-like existence.
Lochia	(G *lochos* childbirth) The name given to the discharge from the uterus following the birth of the baby until the end of the puerperium. (Lochia is pleural, e.g. 'the lochia *are* heavy'.)
Lordosis	(G *lordos* bent with a frontal convex curve) Spinal curvature which is convex anteriorly, e.g. exaggerated lumbar curve.
Low grade intelligence	An intelligence quotient below 25.
Macrocytic anaemia	(G *makros* large, *kytos* cell) This refers to red blood cells of a greater diameter than normal and is found in some types of anaemia, notably pernicious anaemia.
MB tube	Mousseau Barbin tube. A type of plastic catheter with an expanded upper end used to maintain patency of the oesophageal passage in patients with carcinoma of the oesophagus. It can be passed into the oesophagus but requires open operation on the stomach in order to secure it.
Meconium	The first stool passed by the newborn baby. Meconium is dark-green in colour and is present in the intestine from the 16th week of pregnancy.
Mediastinoscopy	(L *mediastinus* midway, G *skopein* to watch) Examination under direct vision of an area on both sides of the carina.
Megaloblastic anaemia	(G *megas* large, *blastos* germ) A type of anaemia in which the red blood cells are of larger diameter than normal and possess an abnormal nuclear structure. It is typical of pernicious anaemia.
Meibomian cyst	A very common condition of distension of a meibomian gland with secretion due to obstruction of its duct. It appears as a small tumour of the eyelid and generally requires excision (performed in the out-patient department).
Meta	(G among, between, besides, etc.) Using as a prefix, meta implies a change of order, position, kind, shape, etc.
Metastases	(G *stasis* a standing) Transfer of disease from its primary site to distant parts of the body via the circulatory or lymphatic system or by direct invasion.
Metatarsalgia	(L *tarsalis* of the tarsal bones, G *algos* pain) Pain in the part of the foot beyond the tarsal bones, i.e. the metatarsus.

Microcytic anaemia	(G *mikros* small, *kytos* cell) This refers to red blood cells of a smaller diameter than normal such as those found in iron deficiency anaemia.
Motor neurones (upper)	Axons which extend from cells in the motor cortex of the cerebrum, down the pyramidal tracts and end at a synapse in the anterior horns of the spinal cord.
Motor neurones (lower)	Axons which originate in the anterior horns of the spinal cord, pass out in the anterior nerve root to form part of a mixed nerve and are distributed to voluntary muscle fibres.
Moulding	The shaping of the baby's head that occurs as it adjusts to the size and shape of the birth canal.
Movements (active)	Movements of joints which are performed by the patient's own muscles. They may be made with gravity eliminated, e.g. in the hydrotherapy pool, against gravity or against resistance, e.g. weight lifting.
Movements (assisted)	A combination of active and passive movements.
Movements (passive)	Movements of a patient's joints made by a nurse or physiotherapist with no assistance from the patient.
Multigravida	(G *multus* many, *gravidus* pregnant) A pregnant woman who has had two or more pregnancies.
Myelitis	(G *mylos* marrow, *-itis* inflammation) Inflammation of the spinal cord. (The spinal cord used to be regarded as the marrow of the spinal column.)
Myeloma	(G *myelos* marrow, *oma* a tumour) A locally malignant tumour. Cells are the type normally found in bone marrow.
Myositis	(G *mys* muscle, *-itis* inflammation) Inflammation of voluntary muscle. In myositis ossificans, bony deposits are laid down within the muscle.
Necrosis	(G *nekros* dead, *-osis* condition) The death of a limited amount of tissue, e.g. a group of cells.
Neonate	(G *neos* new, L *natus* born) A newly born child.
Neonatal mortality	Infant deaths occurring in the first four weeks following birth.
Neonatal period	The period of time from birth until the end of the first four weeks of life.
Neuroglioma	(G *neuron* a sinew; later, 2nd century, a nerve; *glia* glue, *-oma* a tumour) A tumour of the special connective tissue of the nervous system.
Neuroma	A tumour involving a nerve.
Nodule	(L *nodulus* little knot) Raised discrete lesion on the skin, deeper and firmer than a papule.
Nystagmus	Involuntary rapid movement of the eyeballs from side to side, up and down or in a rotary manner from the original point of fixation. There are various causes including lesions of the eye, ear and brain.
Oligaemia	(G *oligos* little, *haima* blood) A diminished amount of blood in circulation.
Ophthalmia neonatorum	(G *ophthalmos* eye) Any purulent discharge from a baby's eyes occurring within three weeks of birth. It is a notifiable condition. Micro-organisms causing the condition are the staphylococcus, streptococcus, pneumococcus and still occasionally the gonococcus.
Osteochondritis	(G *osteon* bone, *chondros* cartilage, *-itis* inflammation) An inflammatory condition affecting bone and cartilage. Commonly affects the epiphyses, and the clinical picture is one of degeneration, followed by regeneration, e.g. Perthes' disease.
Osteomyelitis	(G *osteon* bone, *myelos* marrow, *-itis* inflammation) Pyogenic infection of bone and marrow. In 80 per cent of cases the causal organism is *Staphylococcus aureus*.
Palliative	(L *palliare* to cloak) Serving to alleviate symptoms or suffering.
Panophthalmitis	(G *pan* all, *ophthalmos* eye, *-itis* inflammation) A purulent infection of the whole eye. There is a danger of meningitis or cerebral abscess from spread of infection back via the optic nerve or ophthalmic veins to the brain. (The ophthalmic veins empty into the cavernous sinuses.)

Papule	(L *papula*) Discrete lesion raised above the skin surface.
Patch tests	Potential sensitisers are applied to the skin of the patient's back and covered for 24 hours. If positive, a patch of eczema develops at the site 48 to 72 hours later.
Perception	(L *percipere* to perceive) Process of being aware of objects.
Perinatal period	(G *peri* around, L *natus* birth) The period of time from birth until the end of the first week of life. Infant mortality is highest during this period. (Stillbirths are recorded as occurring in the perinatal period.)
Periphery	(G *periphereia* a circumference) The outermost boundary or limit.
Perseveration	(L *perseverare* to persist) Continued repetition of a meaningless word or phrase, or repetition of answers which are not related to successive questions asked.
Pes	(L *pes, pedes* a foot, feet) As in pes cavus—*see* Cavus.
Phthisis bulbi	(G a wasting away) Degeneration, atrophy and shrinkage of the whole eye, following a severe progressive inflammation.
Physiotherapy	(G *physis* nature, *therapeia* treatment) The use of physical measures to correct deformities and restore function after disease or injury.
Plantar/palmar flex	(L *planta* sole of foot, L *palma* palm) Flexion of ankle/wrist towards the sole of foot/palm of hand.
Podophyllin	A caustic chemical used to destroy unwanted tissue.
Post-partum haemorrhage	Bleeding during the third stage of labour or within 24 hours following the expulsion of the placenta. It is a very serious complication of delivery and the mother's life can be in danger.
Pre-eclampsia	A condition peculiar to pregnancy which can adversely affect the survival of the fetus because it causes a reduction in the blood flow to the uterus and the placenta. The three main features of the disease are rise in blood pressure, oedema and proteinuria. Early diagnosis and treatment are essential and the patient may be admitted to hospital with only one of the above signs.
Primigravida	(L *primus* first, *gravidus* pregnant) A woman who is pregnant for the first time.
Proprioception	(L *proprius* one's own, *capere* to take) The awareness of posture, movement and changes in equilibrium, and the knowledge of position, weight and resistance of objects in relation to the body.
Pruritus	(L *prurire* to itch) Severe itching irritation of the skin.
Prosthesis	(G addition) An artificial part which is attached to the patient.
Pseudarthrosis	(G *seudes* false, *arthron* joint) A false joint formed between the fragments of a fractured bone which have failed to unite.
Quickening	The feeling of fetal movements by the expectant mother. Movements are first felt at about 16 weeks in a multigravid woman and at about 18 to 20 weeks in a primigravid woman.
Retinoblastoma	(L *rete* net, G *blastos* germ, *-oma* tumour) A rare malignant tumour of the eye which occurs in young children (0 to 3 years). It commences in the retina and can spread forwards to involve the rest of the eye and/or back along the optic nerve to the brain.
Retinopathy	(L *rete* net, G *pathos* disease) Any abnormality of the retina, with formation of exudates and haemorrhages. It is associated with general diseases such as diabetes mellitus, atherosclerosis and hypertension. The behaviour depends on the cause.
Retrolental fibroplasia	(L *retro* backward, *lens* a lentil; L *fibra* fibre, G *plassein* to form) A condition, mainly of premature babies, resulting from hyperoxygenation. There is growth of embryonic tissue, causing the formation of new vessels in the vitreous, which in turn causes retinal detachment. The end result is total blindness. The condition is rarely seen now, because oxygen concentration in incubators is kept below 40 per cent.
Rheumatoid factors	Antigamma globulin antibodies found in the sera of most patients with rheumatoid arthritis and in some patients with other chronic diseases and chronic infections.

Rigor	An attack of intense shivering. The internal temperature rises rapidly and may either remain elevated or fall rapidly as profuse sweating occurs.
RNA	Ribonucleic acid, which is found in the cell cytoplasm and nucleolus.
Salicylic acid	A caustic chemical used to destroy unwanted tissue.
Sarcoma	(G *sarx* flesh, *-oma* a tumour) A highly malignant neoplasm affecting bone tissues.
Satiety	(L *satis* sufficient + *-ety* state or condition of) sufficiency or satisfaction as full gratification of appetite or thirst.
Sinus	(L curve, hollow) An unhealed passage leading from an internal lesion to the surface of the body.
Sofra-tulle	Tulle gras impregnated with Soframycin (framycetin).
Spasticity	(G *spastikos* drawing in) In a state of spasm. The movements of a spastic person show imperfect voluntary control. The muscles relax slowly under continued steady pressure but jerk back when pressure is removed. Tendon reflexes are exaggerated.
Spondylitis	(G *spondylos* a vertebra, *-itis* inflammation) Arthritis of the vertebral column.
Spondylosis	(G *spondylos* a vertebra, *-osis* a condition) Literally an abnormal state or condition of the spine, non-infective in origin, but with some ankylosis.
Stillbirth	The birth of a dead child.
Stimulus	(L *stimulare* to incite) Any agent or factor able to influence directly living protoplasm, as one capable of causing muscular contraction or secretion of a gland, or of initiating an impulse in a nerve.
Symblepharon	(G *syn* together, *blepharon* eyelid) Adhesions between the conjunctiva lining the lids and the conjunctiva of the eyeball and the cornea. It is generally the result of burns of the eye, e.g. lime burns.
Syntometrine	Syntocinon 5 units and ergometrine 0·5 mg combined, given to control haemorrhage during the third stage of labour.
Talipes	(L *talus* ankle) Congenital deformity called, in lay terms, 'club foot'. The deformity is not at the ankle proper, but at the tarsal joints.
Tendovaginitis	(L *tendo* tendon, *vagina* sheath, G *-itis* inflammation) A mild, chronic, non-bacterial inflammation of a tendon sheath prevents free movement of the tendon.
Tenosynovitis	(G *tenon* tendon, *syn* together, L *ovum* egg, G *-itis* inflammation) Inflammation of the epithelial lining of a tendon sheath. There is pain on moving the affected tendons. The cause may be mechanical (overuse) or bacterial (acute or chronic) infection. Commonest site is the flexor tendons of the forearm and hand.
Tetracycline	A broad spectrum antibiotic.
Thoracoscopy	(L *thorax* chest, *skopein* to view) Examination of the pleura under direct vision.
Thoracotomy	(L *thorax* chest, G *tremnein* to cut) The operation of opening the chest.
Tomography	(G *tome* section, *graphein* to record) The X-ray of layers of body tissues at any required depth.
Trachoma	(G roughness) A very severe form of conjunctivitis, resulting in many complications. It is associated with hot, sandy conditions, inadequate water purification, flies, poor sanitation and poor living conditions.
Transillumination of sinuses	Inspection of the interior of a cavity by using a light strong enough to pass through its walls. The nasal sinuses can be inspected by placing a lighted torch in the patient's mouth.
Trichiasis	(G *thrix* hair) Turning in of the eyelashes, causing them to scratch against the cornea with the risk of corneal abrasion and ulceration.
Tubigrip	A proprietary name for a form of elasticated leg support.
Ultrasonography	A diagnostic technique using vibrations of the same nature as audible sound waves but of greater frequency. It does not carry the hazards of exposure to X-rays and has therefore largely replaced X-rays in specialities such as obstetrics.

Urticaria (L *urtica* stinging nettle + *ia*) Vascular reaction of the skin in which there is transient appearance of smooth slightly elevated patches (wheals). These are redder or paler than the surrounding skin and are often attended by severe itching.

Valgus (L wandering) Divergence of part of the body away from the midline. In coxa valga the angle between the neck of the femur and the shaft is increased. In hallux vulgas the great toe is angulated towards the other toes, i.e. away from the midline of the body.

Varus (L facing) Angulation towards the midline of the body. In coxa vara the angle between the shaft and the neck of the femur is decreased. Talipes varus is inversion of the foot.

Venous sinuses Dilated channels for venous blood found within the cranium. They anastomose with each other and run between the layers of dura mater.

Vernix caseosa (L cheese-like varnish) The greasy substance composed of sebum and shed epithelial cells which covers the skin of the baby at birth. It retains the heat and is protective.

Vertex (L summit) The area of the fetal head which presents in 95 per cent of all babies born head first.

Vesicle (L *vesicula* small bladder) A small blister.

Wharton's jelly The soft, pulpy, embryonic connective tissue forming the basis of the umbilical cord. The umbilical vessels lie within. (Name derived from Thomas Wharton, English physician and anatomist, 1614–1673.)

Whitfield's ointment A treatment for skin diseases containing 3 per cent salicylic acid and 6 per cent benzoic acid in petroleum jelly base.

Wilson's disease A rare disease of degeneration of the corpus striatum and cirrhosis of the liver, characterized by tremulous distortion of the muscles, dysarthria, dysphagia and emotionalism. It is thought to be the result of abnormal copper metabolism.

Index